CLINICAL HANDBOOK
OF PSYCHOLOGICAL DISORDERS
IN CHILDREN AND ADOLESCENTS

Also Available

Treating Tourette Syndrome and Tic Disorders:
A Guide for Practitioners
Edited by Douglas W. Woods,
John C. Piacentini, and John T. Walkup

Clinical Handbook of Psychological Disorders in Children and Adolescents

A Step-by-Step Treatment Manual

edited by
Christopher A. Flessner
John C. Piacentini

THE GUILFORD PRESS
New York   London

Copyright © 2017 The Guilford Press
A Division of Guilford Publications, Inc.
370 Seventh Avenue, Suite 1200, New York, NY 10001
www.guilford.com

Printed in the United States of America

This book is printed on acid-free paper.

Last digit is print number: 9 8 7 6 5 4 3 2 1

The authors have checked with sources believed to be reliable in their efforts to provide information
that is complete and generally in accord with the standards of practice that are accepted at the time
of publication. However, in view of the possibility of human error or changes in behavioral, mental
health, or medical sciences, neither the authors, nor the editors and publisher, nor any other party
who has been involved in the preparation or publication of this work warrants that the information
contained herein is in every respect accurate or complete, and they are not responsible for any errors
or omissions or the results obtained from the use of such information. Readers are encouraged to
confirm the information contained in this book with other sources.

Library of Congress Cataloging-in-Publication Data

Names: Flessner, Christopher A., editor. | Piacentini, John, editor.
Title: Clinical handbook of psychological disorders in children and
    adolescents : a step-by-step treatment manual / edited by Christopher A.
    Flessner, John C. Piacentini.
Description: New York : The Guilford Press, [2017] | Includes bibliographical
    references and index.
Identifiers: LCCN 2016049825 | ISBN 9781462530885 (hardcover : alk. paper)
Subjects: | MESH: Mental Disorders | Child | Adolescent
Classification: LCC RJ503 | NLM WS 350 | DDC 616.8900835—dc23
LC record available at *https://lccn.loc.gov/2016049825*

To Dave and Yvonne, the best parents
(and Packer fans) a son could ask for
—C. A. F.

To my family and to the children and families
with whom I've worked over the years
—J. C. P.

About the Editors

Christopher A. Flessner, PhD, is Associate Professor in the Department of Psychological Sciences at Kent State University and a clinical child psychologist with KidsLink Neurobehavioral Center. He has been Director of the Pediatric Anxiety Research Clinic at Kent State since 2011. Dr. Flessner's research focuses on biological and psychosocial risk factors that may be linked to the development of childhood anxiety and related problems—such as obsessive–compulsive disorder, trichotillomania, and tic disorders—and how a better understanding of risk factors might be used to improve existing therapeutic interventions.

John C. Piacentini, PhD, ABPP, is Professor of Psychiatry and Biobehavioral Sciences in the David Geffen School of Medicine at the University of California, Los Angeles (UCLA). He is Director of the Center for Child Anxiety Resilience Education and Support and of the Childhood OCD, Anxiety, and Tic Disorders Program at the UCLA Semel Institute for Neuroscience and Human Behavior. Dr. Piacentini is Chair of the Behavioral Sciences Consortium of the Tourette Association of America, a Founding Fellow of the Academy of Cognitive Therapy, a Fellow and past president of the Society for Clinical Child and Adolescent Psychology of the American Psychological Association, and a Fellow of the Association for Psychological Science. His research focuses on the etiology, assessment, and treatment of obsessive–compulsive, tic, anxiety, and body-focused, repetitive behavior disorders in children and adolescents.

Contributors

Jennifer R. Alexander, MS, Department of Psychology, Texas A&M University, College Station, Texas

Amy Altszuler, MS, Center for Children and Families and Department of Psychology, Florida International University, Miami, Florida

Tony Attwood, PhD, private practice, Brisbane, Queensland, Australia

Caroline Boxmeyer, PhD, Department of Psychiatry and Behavioral Medicine, University of Alabama, Tuscaloosa, Alabama

Elle Brennan, MA, Department of Psychological Sciences, Kent State University, Kent, Ohio

Mark Burton, BA, Department of Psychological Sciences, Case Western Reserve University, Cleveland, Ohio

Simon P. Byrne, BPsych, Centre for Emotional Health and Department of Psychology, Macquarie University, Sydney, New South Wales, Australia

Tammy Chung, PhD, Department of Psychology, University of Pittsburgh, Pittsburgh, Pennsylvania

Stephanie Davis, PhD, Department of Psychiatry and Human Behavior, Alpert Medical School, Brown University, Providence, Rhode Island

Maria DiFonte, MA, Center for Anxiety and Related Disorders and Department of Psychology, Boston University, Boston, Massachusetts

Casey Dillon, MA, Department of Psychology, University of Alabama, Tuscaloosa, Alabama

Jill Ehrenreich-May, PhD, Department of Psychology, University of Miami, Coral Gables, Florida

Dawn M. Eichen, PhD, Department of Pediatrics, University of California, San Diego, La Jolla, California

Christianne Esposito-Smythers, PhD, Department of Psychology, George Mason University, Fairfax, Virginia

Lara J. Farrell, PhD, School of Applied Psychology and Menzies Health Institute Queensland, Griffith University, Southport, Queensland, Australia

Norah C. Feeny, PhD, Department of Psychological Sciences, Case Western Reserve University, Cleveland, Ohio

Christopher A. Flessner, PhD, Department of Psychological Sciences, Kent State University, Kent, Ohio

Elizabeth Frazier, PhD, Bradley/Hasbro Research Center, Brown University, Providence, Rhode Island

Rachel D. Freed, PhD, Department of Psychiatry, Icahn School of Medicine at Mount Sinai, New York, New York

Jennifer Freeman, PhD, Department of Psychiatry and Human Behavior, Alpert Medical School, Brown University, Providence, Rhode Island

Tracey Garcia, PhD, Department of Psychology, Florida International University, Miami, Florida

Allison G. Harvey, PhD, Department of Psychology, University of California, Berkeley, Berkeley, California

Tyler A. Hassenfeldt, MS, Department of Psychology, Virginia Polytechnic Institute and State University, Blacksburg, Virginia

David C. Houghton, MS, Department of Psychology, Texas A&M University, College Station, Texas

Anna M. Karam, MA, Department of Psychological and Brain Sciences, Washington University at St. Louis, St. Louis, Missouri

Francesca Kassing, MA, Department of Psychology, University of Alabama, Tuscaloosa, Alabama

Stephanie M. Keller, PhD, Department of Psychological Sciences, Case Western Reserve University, Cleveland, Ohio; Bradley/Hasbro Research Center, Brown University, Providence, Rhode Island

Sarah M. Kennedy, MS, Department of Psychology, University of Miami, Coral Gables, Florida

Ashley Korn, MA, Center for Anxiety and Related Disorders and Department of Psychological and Brain Sciences, Boston University, Boston, Massachusetts

Richard Liu, PhD, Department of Psychiatry and Human Behavior, Alpert Medical School, Brown University, Providence, Rhode Island

John E. Lochman, PhD, ABPP, Department of Psychology, University of Alabama, Tuscaloosa, Alabama

Fiona Macphee, BA, Center for Children and Families and Department of Psychology, Florida International University, Miami, Florida

Katharina Manassis, MD, FRCP(C), Department of Psychiatry, University of Toronto, Toronto, Ontario, Canada

Jamie A. Mash, MS, Department of Psychology, University of Miami, Coral Gables, Florida

Brittany Merrill, MS, Center for Children and Families and Department of Psychology, Florida International University, Miami, Florida

Anne Morrow, MS, Center for Children and Families and Department of Psychology, Florida International University, Miami, Florida

Yolanda E. Murphy, MA, Department of Psychological Sciences, Kent State University, Kent, Ohio

Ella L. Oar, PhD, School of Applied Psychology and Menzies Health Institute Queensland, Griffith University, Southport, Queensland, Australia; Centre for Emotional Health and Department of Psychology, Macquarie University, Sydney, New South Wales, Australia

Thomas H. Ollendick, PhD, Child Study Center and Department of Psychology, Virginia Polytechnic Institute and State University, Blacksburg, Virginia

William E. Pelham, Jr., PhD, Center for Children and Families and Department of Psychology, Florida International University, Miami, Florida; Department of Psychology, University at Buffalo, The State University of New York, Buffalo, New York

Tara S. Peris, PhD, Department of Psychiatry and Biobehavioral Sciences, David Geffen School of Medicine, and Semel Institute for Neuroscience and Human Behavior, University of California, Los Angeles, Los Angeles, California

John C. Piacentini, PhD, ABPP, Department of Psychiatry and Biobehavioral Sciences, David Geffen School of Medicine, and Semel Institute for Neuroscience and Human Behavior, University of California, Los Angeles, Los Angeles, California

Donna B. Pincus, PhD, Center for Anxiety and Related Disorders and Department of Psychological and Brain Sciences, Boston University, Boston, Massachusetts

Cameron Powe, MA, Department of Psychology, University of Alabama, Tuscaloosa, Alabama

Nicole Powell, PhD, Department of Psychology, University of Alabama, Tuscaloosa, Alabama

Angela Scarpa, PhD, Department of Psychology, Virginia Polytechnic Institute and State University, Blacksburg, Virginia

Nicole K. Schatz, PhD, Center for Children and Families and Department of Psychology, Florida International University, Miami, Florida

Benjamin N. Schneider, MD, Department of Psychiatry and Biobehavioral Sciences, David Geffen School of Medicine, and Semel Institute for Neuroscience and Human Behavior, University of California, Los Angeles, Los Angeles, California

Anthony Spirito, PhD, Department of Psychiatry and Human Behavior, Alpert Medical School, Brown University, Providence, Rhode Island

Elyse Stewart, BA, Department of Psychology, Binghamton University, The State University of New York, Binghamton, New York

Saneya H. Tawfik, PhD, Department of Psychology, University of Miami, Coral Gables, Florida

Eric F. Wagner, PhD, FIU-Banyan Research Institute on Dissemination, Grants, and Evaluation, Florida International University, Miami, Florida

Sally M. Weinstein, PhD, Department of Psychiatry, University of Illinois at Chicago, Chicago, Illinois

Amy E. West, PhD, Department of Psychiatry, University of Illinois at Chicago, Chicago, Illinois

Denise E. Wilfley, PhD, Department of Psychiatry, Washington University School of Medicine in St. Louis, St. Louis, Missouri

Ken Winters, PhD, Department of Psychiatry, University of Minnesota, Minneapolis, Minnesota

Jennifer Wolff, PhD, Department of Psychology, Brown Medical School and Rhode Island Hospital, Providence, Rhode Island

Douglas W. Woods, PhD, Department of Psychology, Marquette University, Milwaukee, Wisconsin

Preface

Our inspiration for this volume came from David H. Barlow's influential edited volume *Clinical Handbook of Psychological Disorders: A Step-by-Step Treatment Manual*, now in its fifth edition. Barlow's volume was one of the first to show how to base effective clinical practice on reliable research evidence. As a young student, I (C. A. F.) was exposed to Barlow's book in my first cognitive-behavioral therapy course, and it provided me with working knowledge on how to translate research into practice. When I began to work with real clients, and my need for immediate help became increasingly urgent, this volume became my go-to resource. As a guide to understanding and treating psychological disorders in adults, showcasing evidence-based psychotherapy models, and offering a step-by-step guide for treatment implementation, the book became the premier sourcebook not just for me, but for many trainees and therapists.

What has been lacking in the child and adolescent world is just such a book: an easily accessible, one-stop resource for understanding the evidence base for clinical treatment and for explaining how to implement it in a step-by-step fashion. The initial impetus for this book arose after I was charged with preparing a syllabus for a child psychotherapy course at Kent State, where I was then an assistant professor. I had assigned seminal articles for students on the evidence base for therapeutic interventions but couldn't find a complementary book that provided the practical information needed to implement evidence-based treatments for children and their families. What I really wanted was a text that incorporated knowledge about the disorder, offered clear explanations of available evidence-based treatments, and provided a rubric for how to go about conducting sessions with children and their parents.

In our collaboration, John and I sought to design a book that would offer just what I had been looking to provide to my students: a volume that included a review of the evidence-based treatments available for a range of different child and adolescent disorders, and a session-by-session treatment plan that would be effective for each disorder. Although working with children and adolescents and their families can be one of the most rewarding experiences of any clinician's professional life, the clinical work often presents what may seem like insurmountable difficulties. We hope this volume will help you, the reader, meet the challenges that this work gives rise to and provide you with effective, evidence-based interventions to help any client who comes to your clinic or office get back on a healthy developmental trajectory.

Our goal from day one was to recruit an outstanding group of authors with expertise across myriad psychiatric disorders afflicting children and their families. We are both grateful for the time and effort these authors have put forth. Without hesitation or exception, we can say that they have exceeded even our grandest expectations and we cannot thank them enough. We are greatly appreciative to the expert publishing team at The Guilford Press, most notably Carolyn Graham, who worked with us on nearly every phase of the production process, and Kitty Moore, Executive Editor. Kitty has been a constant and enthusiastically contagious champion of this project—never wavering in her support of this book and what we were trying to accomplish. She contributed significantly to conceptualizing, improving, and refining the book's primary aims and message, and we look forward to the possibility of working with her again on a second edition! We greatly enjoyed working with each other and look forward to additional opportunities for collaboration on other projects.

CHRISTOPHER A. FLESSNER
JOHN C. PIACENTINI

Contents

PART I

AN EVIDENCE-BASED APPROACH TO WORKING WITH YOUTH

CHAPTER 1

Introduction:
Aims and Scope of This Book

Christopher A. Flessner and John C. Piacentini

Therapists are increasingly called on to provide evidence-based treatments to the children and families with whom they work—and rightly so, since to ignore what the research tells us means not offering our clients the most effective treatments. Unfortunately, and in spite of this, there are few places to find one volume that translates evidence-based research into clear guidelines to provide appropriate assessments and interventions in real-time clinical work.

Few of us have the time to become experts in the evidence-based treatment of each of the myriad of presenting problems we encounter daily in our professional lives. Moreover, integrating knowledge about the etiology and phenomenology of evidence-based treatments for these problems and their effective implementation is daunting for even the most seasoned therapist. This book represents an efficient and multifaceted resource that covers the broad range of child and adolescent disorders within a single volume, thus mitigating the need for multiple texts or resources that might otherwise be required by busy practitioners.

More specifically, our rationale for writing this volume is twofold. First, the constantly evolving science-based changes to our understanding and pathophysiology of psychiatric disorders and problems in childhood and adolescence require an updated, concise, and clinician-friendly overview of those disorders most commonly encountered in clinical practice. Second, clinical child and adolescent psychologists and other evidence-based practitioners need an easily accessible, comprehensive, and succinct review of not only the evidence-based treatment literature for a given disorder or problem but also the corresponding literature on evidence-based tools for diagnosis and monitoring treatment progress. Importantly, the chapters in this volume not only guide readers through the details required to evaluate and conduct interventions for both common and less familiar disorders but also provide an important resource and opportunity for even seasoned therapists to brush up on their assessment and treatment skills. As an example, formal sleep disorder diagnoses are relatively rare in children and adolescents, yet many treatment-seeking youth report sleep-related problems. Harvey (Chapter 18, this volume) describes an easily accessible, evidence-based psychosocial intervention for sleep problems in youth and identifies appropriate measures to administer during the course of treatment. This chapter may prove indispensable to both new and experienced therapists who have less familiarity with clinical approaches to this common problem.

This book presents relevant clinical information in a concise, accessible, and comprehensive manner. Most chapters are organized to provide (1) a careful overview of the clinical phenomenology and etiology of the topic disorder or presenting problem; (2) a critical review of extant evidence-based assessment and treatment protocols for the disorder, including evidence related to posited mediators/moderators of treatment efficacy; and (3) a step-by-step description of how one might go about implementing each evidence-based treatment. We believe this volume will be valuable as both a textbook for use in training tomorrow's therapists and as a portable reference for more experienced therapists in need of immediate guidance. Our goal is to offer a unified text in the child therapy literature able to convey "what to use" and "how to use it" across the full range of more common to less common presenting problems.

A FOCUS ON EVIDENCE-BASED ASSESSMENT AND TREATMENT

The central focus of this book is to provide readers with immediate access to the background and information necessary to effectively help the children and families with whom they work. We deemed a comprehensive and succinct review of both the literature supporting the evidence-based assessment and treatment of these disorders to be imperative. In general, the term "evidence-based" is simple enough to understand. Understanding more explicitly what it means and the background behind the establishment of this "evidence base" is somewhat more confusing. For example, in speaking with their child's pediatrician over the years, parents may quickly discover that multiple derivatives of penicillin exist (e.g., amoxicillin, amoxicillin and clavulanate potassium), all of which demonstrate evidence in support of their use for the child's infection. How that evidence was determined, the strength of those claims, and which is best for that child's particular situation may be less clear. The same can be true for readers seeking to evaluate assessment instruments and treatment options for their patients. Our aim in this book is to make this evaluative process more straightforward.

This book's approach to defining evidence-based treatments is a familiar one. The most recent Division 12 (American Psychological Association) Task Force criteria (Chambless & Hollon, 1998; Southam-Gerow & Prinstein, 2014) have been used to classify interventions for a variety of child mental health disorders as *well established, probably efficacious,* or *possibly efficacious,* based on the strength of their underlying evidence base (see Brennan, Murphy, & Flessner, Chapter 2, this volume, for a detailed description of these criteria). As readers of this text are likely aware, the classification of an intervention on such a basis is not without its limitations or detractors, including perhaps most notably questions about the clinical generalizability of the treatment studies on which these classifications are based (Chambless & Ollendick, 2001). This system, or others like it, has provided the backdrop against which recent generations of clinical psychologists and other therapists have been trained, and which the majority of clinical researchers use to evaluate the efficacy of therapeutic interventions. These guidelines provide a common language for professional communication regarding the relative merits of various interventions for specific clients and clinical presentations. It is for these reasons that we have asked each of the contributing authors of this book to use the most recent Division 12 Task Force criteria (Southam-Gerow & Prinstein, 2014; see Brennan, Murphy, & Flessner, Chapter 2, this volume) in their reviews of the extant literature for the clinical problem area about which they write.

The focus of this book is psychosocial interventions, yet each chapter also includes an overview of available evidence-based pharmacological treatments in order to provide a more complete treatment overview of the disorder in question, since many youth presenting for psychotherapy are currently receiving psychotropic medication or have past histories with this treatment modality. We also note that combining medication and psychotherapy has been shown to result in better outcomes than either therapy alone for some disorders, including anxiety (Walkup et al., 2008), attention-deficit/hyperactivity disorder (MTA Cooperative Group, 1999), and major depressive disorder (Glass, 2005), among others. This is not to say that youth presenting for treatment with these disorders should automatically be referred for medication as a first-line intervention, but rather that medication may be an option for some patients, depending on presenting characteristics or should a course of quality, evidence-based psychotherapy not achieve the desired gains.

In this same vein, we have also asked each of our teams of contributing authors to review available mediators and moderators, when applicable, of treatment efficacy for the evidence-based treatments described within each chapter. For some disorders, this review is necessarily briefer (e.g., tic disorders and trichotillomania; see Houghton, Alexander, & Woods, Chapter 15, this volume) due to the lack of substantial research within this area, while the discussion for other disorders (e.g., anxiety disorders; see Kennedy, Mash, Tawfik, & Ehrenreich-May, Chapter 6, this volume) is more extensive. Given our goal to provide the best possible care, we need the ability to provide families with the most up-to-date information regarding *all* available and evidence-based interventions, and the specific populations for whom these interventions work best.

Formal criteria for delineating the evidence-based assessment of childhood psychological disorders do not enjoy the same level of detail as found for evidence-based treatments. As such, this book allows experts in the diagnosis, assessment, and treatment of various forms of child psychopathology to develop their own conceptual framework for the evidence-based assessment of a particular problem (e.g., obsessive–compulsive disorder, substance use) in practice. While this approach may lack uniformity across disorders, we can rely on the knowledge provided by well-informed therapists about integrating psychometrically sound diagnostic instruments and self-/parent-report measures to conceptualize a child's case and inform treatment planning. Each chapter provides an overview of important differential diagnoses to consider as well. Evidence-based assessment does not stop after the first or second meeting with a child and his or her family. It is an ongoing process. As such, each chapter provides guidance as to the appropriate tools for use in the ongoing assessment of relevant symptoms during the therapeutic process, thus allowing the reader to identify recalcitrant symptoms and "course-correct" along the way as needed.

A STEP-BY-STEP TREATMENT MANUAL

How can a therapist with strong training in evidence-based treatments yet limited training in a particular disorder implement these treatments equally well for the myriad presenting children and families with whom they may work? How can a clinical psychologist in training gain a fundamental understanding of various evidence-based treatments and, at the same time, gain insight into how each session is to be set up, what topic to cover in each session, and how to broach difficult topics with their patients? This book seeks to answer these questions in a manner that is unique within the child therapy literature by detailing evidence-based treatment approaches for over 15 of the most commonly occurring presenting problems in treatment-seeking children and adolescents. Developing the skills and expertise necessary to become an effective therapist and practitioner of these interventions is a long and arduous process, requiring nearly a decade of time, commitment, and training. Few therapists emerge from this process with the knowledge, skills, and expertise necessary to help all children and families equally well. A by-product of the approach taken in the vast majority of clinical psychology training programs is to develop future therapists that demonstrate core competencies (e.g., science, application, systems) in the field of clinical psychology. Often, these students obtain some degree of expertise within a subdomain of the broader field (i.e., anxiety, mood, obsessive–compulsive spectrum). Although we wish that it could, this book is not designed to eliminate the need for this long journey, nor is it designed to make everyone who reads this text an expert in each topic. Sorry! What this book does provide, however, is a detailed blueprint, in a session-by-session format, necessary for trainees and seasoned therapists alike to provide cutting edge, high-quality evidence-based treatment to children and families presenting with problems or concerns in which the trainee/therapist may be less familiar.

ORGANIZATION OF THE CHAPTERS

We begin each chapter within this book with a succinct macro-level overview of the disorder in question, followed by a description of treatments meeting criteria as well established and probably or possibly efficacious according to the most recent guidelines of Division 12 of the American Psychological Association (Southam-Gerow & Prinstein, 2014). In addition, this review provides information on newer psychosocial interventions that, while currently lacking substantial empirical support, show promise (e.g., attention bias training, cognitive remediation). Finally, each evidence-based treatment review closes with available evidence regarding predictors of treatment response, as well as a brief overview of evidence-based pharmacological interventions for the disorder in question. With this overview in hand, the reader is well positioned to make informed choices regarding the treatment of choice for his or her patient and how best to make use of this intervention in practice. What follows is a step-by-step approach to implementing the chosen evidence-based treatment. This is the real meat of the chapter. Initially, a thoughtful and careful description of the core components of each session is provided. An overview and description of key treatment components (e.g., cognitive strategies, relaxation, exposures) are offered alongside important items to consider in administration of these components and tips for maximizing the success of each skill or tool provided. When appropriate, evidence-based recommendations regarding the use of key measures, tools, and/or recording sheets are provided. A scripted transcript of the treatment provides the reader a session-by-session understanding of how the protocol might actually look in practice. Throughout this elaborated description of the treatment protocol, authors have also provided sample dialogue that provides a context for explaining core components of the intervention and offers insight on how to broach sometimes tricky facets of sessions. For example, authors provide dialogues relating to how exposure tasks might be explained (e.g., see Kennedy et al., Chapter 6, this volume), why reward programs are different from bribing (e.g., see Stewart & Freeman, Chapter 17, this volume), and how to explain to parents their part in a child's behavior (e.g., see Peris & Schneider, Chapter 10, this volume). It is our hope that, by the end of each chapter, readers are left with a greater degree of confidence in understanding and tackling a perhaps unfamiliar clinical problem or simply brushing up on existing skills. The authors contributing to this book are expert clinicians and researchers in their topic area, and we hope you enjoy and find this text useful as a "what to use" and "how to use it" guide to evidence-based treatments for children and adolescents.

REFERENCES

Chambless, D. L., & Hollon, S. D. (1998). Defining empirically supported therapies. *Journal of Consulting and Clinical Psychology, 66*(1), 7–18.

Chambless, D. L., & Ollendick, T. H. (2001). Empirically supported psychological interventions: Controversies and evidence. *Annual Review of Psychology, 52*, 685–716.

Glass, R. M. (2005). Fluoxetine, cognitive-behavioral therapy, and their combination for adolescents with depression: Treatment for Adolescents with Depression Study (TADS) randomized controlled trial. *Journal of Pediatrics, 146*(1), 145.

MTA Cooperative Group. (1999). A 14-month randomized clinical trial of treatment strategies for attention-deficit/hyperactivity disorder: Multimodal Treatment Study of Children with ADHD. *Archives of General Psychiatry, 56*(12), 1073–1086.

Southam-Gerow, M. A., & Prinstein, M. J. (2014). Evidence base updates: The evolution of the evaluation of psychological treatments for children and adolescents. *Journal of Clinical Child and Adolescent Psychology, 43*(1), 1–6.

Walkup, J. T., Albano, A. M., Piacentini, J., Birmaher, B., Compton, S. N., Sherrill, J. T., et al. (2008). Cognitive behavioral therapy, sertraline, or a combination in childhood anxiety. *New England Journal of Medicine, 359*(26), 2753–2766.

CHAPTER 2

Examining Developmental Considerations of Evidence-Based Practices for Youth

Elle Brennan, Yolanda E. Murphy,
and Christopher A. Flessner

A BRIEF HISTORY OF PEDIATRIC PSYCHOTHERAPY

Psychotherapy has taken numerous forms throughout its many centuries-long history. The more contemporary conceptualizations of psychotherapy as a science and a practice, however, can be traced back to more recent times (Freedheim et al., 1992), with Sigmund Freud commonly credited as the father of psychoanalytic theory, and well known for his work in the treatment of psychiatric maladies in adults. However, the movement toward the development of child psychotherapy in the 1920s was largely propelled by his daughter, Anna Freud, and her colleague Melanie Klein. As such, child psychotherapy really began as a relatively recent extension of prevailing adult therapeutic practices and concepts.

Prior to the modern era, children were often believed to experience a much more limited array of psychiatric issues (Achenbach & Edelbrock, 1978). Over time, and with a recent bloom in the 1980s, however, practice with children has begun to suggest that the young mind functions quite similarly to that of the adult in many respects. This trend has most recently been exemplified with the publication of the fifth edition of the *Diagnostic and Statistical Manual of Mental Disorders* (DSM-5; American Psychiatric Association, 2013), in which an empirically supported developmental approach has been adopted for many psychiatric disorders. Disorders previously thought to be present only in children are now extended into adulthood (e.g., separation anxiety disorder), and some whose previous formulations were based solely on research in adults (e.g., posttraumatic stress disorder) are now being better fitted to youth. Ideally, such shifts will encourage further

8

research and lead to better understanding of prevalence rates and symptom presentation for children with various psychiatric disorders.

What early evidence-based work was conducted regarding psychotherapy for children was largely anecdotal and conclusions that were drawn relied heavily on individual case studies. Levitt (1957, 1963) reviewed some of the earlier therapy literature, including a few treatment studies with adolescents or children that indicated psychotherapy was no more effective than the passage of time for the treatment of psychiatric distress in children. These reviews mapped on to similar findings by other authors, most notably Eysenck (1960). However, the treatment studies conducted at the time and included in the reviews were largely faulted with weak methodology, small sample sizes, and often unclear treatment practices. With the progression of the field over the past several decades has come substantially increased research effort characterized by greater rigor and regulation. Moreover, recent meta-analyses have suggested that psychotherapy for children and adolescents does indeed work (e.g., Weersing & Weisz, 2002). Alongside this objectivity has come improved understanding of the variety of maladies that children may experience, including emotional issues, social stressors, behavioral challenges, and *in vivo* risk factors, as well as more specific definitions for what constitutes an adequate evidence base for a given treatment to be considered top of the line.

DEFINING EVIDENCE-BASED PRACTICES

As such, several decades of work have contributed to the defining and regulation of what constitutes a sufficient evidence base for a given program of psychotherapy. This has been in line with a larger movement towards scientifically sound evidence-based medicinal practices (Sackett, Richardson, Rosenberg, & Haynes, 1997, 2000). The first formal report regarding the movement toward evidence-based practice for psychology was released in the early 1990s (Task Force on Promotion and Dissemination of Psychological Procedures, 1995) in an attempt to bring together professionals from a variety of training backgrounds to establish which psychotherapies from a wide array of theoretical foundations have recognized value. The Task Force categorized "empirically validated" treatments by three levels of empirical support in an attempt to better categorize the state of psychotherapy research at the time: well-established treatments, probably efficacious treatments, and experimental treatments (see Table 2.1).

Differentiation of the first two categories is based primarily on the number of research teams that have investigated a given treatment, the level to which a treatment has been proven superior (e.g., better than wait list, better than placebo), and how well the treatment procedures and participant information have been specified. Treatment outcomes must also be determined as not being due to chance or alternative confounds such as the passage of time or participant differences, in order to receive empirical validation. In contrast, experimental treatments are more broadly differentiated as they are generally unmanualized and have not yet been found to meet requirements for being probably efficacious. The use of such practices is often limited to clinical settings and tends to lack scientific testing. New untested treatments would also fall under this category; however, the standing of any specific treatment program may improve with further testing and improved consistency.

TABLE 2.1. Criteria for Evidenced-Based Practices

Category	Criteria
Well-established treatments	• Two or more good experiments with between-group designs demonstrating either (1) superiority (i.e. to pill, placebo, or additional treatment) or (2) equivalence to an already established treatment. or • Efficacy is demonstrated utilizing intervention comparisons in good multiple, single-case design experiments. • Experiments utilize treatment manuals or treatments methods are explicitly detailed. • Sample characteristics are explicitly detailed. • Treatment efficacy is demonstrated by at least two different investigators/teams.
Probably efficacious treatments	• Two experiments demonstrating significant superiority to wait-list control group. or • At least one experiment meets well-established criteria; however, all experiments have been conducted by one investigator/team. or • Three or more experiments of single-case design that meet well-established criteria.
Experimental treatments	• Treatments not yet meeting requirements for well-established or probably efficacious treatments.

Note. Adapted from Chambless et al. (1998). Copyright © 1998 the American Psychological Association. Adapted by permission.

Several areas of concern have been associated with the evidence-based treatment movement as well (e.g., Elliott, 1998; Kovacs, 1995; Norcross, 2001; Silverman, 1996). For instance, the requirement of manualization for well-established and probably efficacious treatments may be limited to certain theoretically driven treatment models (e.g., behavioral, cognitive-behavioral therapies), and may exclude those that are more dynamic or individually client-focused. As such, several commonly used psychotherapies have not been investigated for their effectiveness in such a structured manner. Often methods of treatment that have been found to be efficacious anecdotally also remain unknown to the greater psychological community and fail to be disseminated to a wider practice. Furthermore, psychotherapeutic approaches for children and adolescents are often tested for a specific malady alone or within a specific age range and not tested for a broader usage (for review, see David-Ferdon & Kaslow, 2008; Keel & Haedt, 2008). There is also a considerable amount of research that has compared and contrasted a specific psychotherapeutic program against "treatment as usual" (TAU), which is unfortunately often left unspecified in these reports and may involve a variety of practices with children and adolescents, often including poorly defined treatments such as play therapies, parent–child interaction therapies, and attachment therapies. This leaves a great deal of uncertainty as to the level at which a new treatment may actually perform. A greater push for transparency in descriptions of TAU and novel psychotherapeutic programs may aid in such comparisons, and may allow for greater ease in the manualization of such programs, with contingencies for needed flexibility.

Many factors must be considered in determining the efficacy of a treatment program, both with reference to the treatments to be tested and implemented, and the youth population to be served. As noted earlier, some of the concerns involving the treatments themselves through past criticisms and can also include factors such as the environment, assessment of a child's difficulties, and appropriate packaging (i.e., manualization) of an effective program. Furthermore, "childhood" as a concept is itself a moving target, with constant shifts in neurological growth, cognitive ability, regulatory skills, emotional literacy, and social demands. What constitutes a child versus an adolescent versus a young adult? Where do the defining lines get drawn and what does this mean for psychological assessment and treatment? Such factors create a need for treatments to be mindfully designed, tested, and applied in age-appropriate and, more generally, developmentally appropriate ways across childhood and across individual children. What follows is a discussion of such factors, as well as recommendations for defining and creating evidence-based practices that take into consideration the broad developmental needs of youth.

COGNITIVE, SOCIAL, AND EMOTIONAL DEVELOPMENT IN YOUTH

Several developmental domains (i.e., cognitive, social, and emotional) are of critical concern within pediatric psychointervention. While abnormalities in these domains are often noted for hypothesized roles in disorder etiology, normal development in such areas is equally important within youth intervention. As such, what follows is a discussion of the impact of normal youth development on pediatric treatment outcome.

Cognitive Development

Youth necessitating psychotherapy present with varying cognitive abilities associated with both normal developmental stages (e.g., Piaget's cognitive stages; Piaget, 1971) and pathologically induced abnormalities (e.g., misperceptions of ambiguous events as threating in anxious individuals, increased negative attributions in depressed individuals; Stallard, 2002). Normal cognitive differences may affect a youth's overall understanding of psychopathology and what is more may alter client insight into pertinent individual difficulties. Beyond this general understanding of psychopathology, cognitive developmental level is also likely to have a strong impact on youth's understanding and ability to engage within treatment. For example, compared to adolescent clients, young children may demonstrate limited comprehension of abstract concepts within cognitive-based therapies such as cognitive-behavioral therapy (CBT; Kuhn, 1999; Quakley, Coker, Palmer, & Reynolds, 2003). Additionally, among youth populations, differences in cognitive understanding may affect motivation for therapy. Weisz and Hawley (2002) summarized affected domains of motivational differences within adolescent client populations, including attentiveness, development of therapist–client alliance, skills acquisition, and application of learned skills outside of the clinical setting. Somewhat similarly, research has indicated a significant correlation between client motivation and treatment outcome, in which lower motivation is related to decreased treatment efficacy (Oliver, Stockdale, & Wormith, 2011).

As mentioned earlier, CBT is one of the most commonly utilized interventions among youth and adults, operating on the assumption of active participation of the client in the exploration of his or her thoughts (Grave & Blissett, 2004). As such, CBT is a plausible mechanism by which potential effects of cognitive level on treatment outcome may be hypothesized. Interestingly, the literature overall has indicated that CBT—when appropriately modified to developmental level—is an efficacious intervention for several youth disorders including, but not limited to, anxiety, obsessive–compulsive disorder (OCD), externalizing behaviors, and autism spectrum disorders (Cartwright-Hatton, Roberts, Chitsabesan, Fothergill, & Harrington, 2004; Freeman et al., 2007; Scarpa & Reyes, 2011), however research simultaneously demonstrates differences in intervention efficacy relative to client age group (McCart, Priester, Davies, & Azen, 2006; Sukhodolsky, Kassinove, & Gorman, 2004). For example, a 2000 meta-analysis examining CBT efficacy for antisocial behavior in youth demonstrated positive correlation between age and treatment effect size, suggesting increased efficacy among adolescents and older children compared to younger children (Bennett & Gibbons, 2000). Such findings were corroborated in a review examining developmental considerations in CBT, in which Grave and Blisset (2004) concluded that children age 11 years and over benefit more from CBT techniques than do children ages 5–11. Collectively, though cognitions have yet to be formally identified as the main change component within CBT, such findings suggest that cognitive-developmental level may play a critical mediating role in the efficacy of this intervention.

Social Development

A second factor related to youth treatment outcome is social development. Specifically, a youth's social-developmental level can affect critical treatment components, including the therapeutic alliance. For example, similarities and differences in social-developmental levels of both the client and therapist may affect both method (e.g., talking vs. playing) and amount of time (e.g., two sessions vs. several sessions) utilized to construct an alliance. As such, a therapist may find it easier building and maintaining a relationship with clients of one developmental level versus another. Notably, prior research highlights the therapeutic alliance as both a common component to therapies and a critical contributor to therapy outcome (Cummings et al., 2013; Lambert & Barley, 2001; Martin, Garske, & Davis, 2000).

Within the pediatric literature specifically, prior research indicates that while parent–therapist alliance remains a predictor of treatment outcome, so does child–therapist alliance. In particular, the child–therapist alliance has demonstrated a strong to modest correlation with treatment outcome, in which stronger alliances are associated with increased treatment efficacy (Karver, Handelsman, Fields, & Bickman, 2006; Kazdin, Marciano, & Whitley, 2005). What is more, such correlations have demonstrated consistency across developmental levels and various therapy types (Shirk & Karver, 2003). Considering these findings, rates in which the alliance is built or hindrance in alliance construction may have an important contribution (i.e., positive or negative) to youth treatment outcome.

Notably, social-developmental level of the client may also affect treatment outcome via social support (e.g., peer and family relationships). For instance, considering the critical role of family relationships as mechanisms of socialization among youth, social-developmental levels of these children must be assessed largely within the context of the family. Research assessing the influence of family relationships on treatment outcome in both child and adolescent populations indicate worse family functioning and parental support to be related to poor treatment outcome among youth exhibiting a range of symptoms including anxiety, obsessive–compulsive symptoms, antisocial behavior, and histories of sexual abuse (Cohen & Mannarino, 2000; Crawford & Manassis, 2001; Kazdin, 1995; Peris et al., 2012). Extending from the role of family relationships in young children, adolescence is highlighted as a period characterized by the formulation of critical peer relationships (Furman & Buhrmester, 1992). To the extent that these relationships are maintained throughout and subsequent to the therapeutic process, these may be considered either beneficial (e.g., peers promoting positive methods learned in therapy) or detrimental (e.g., peers promoting negative behaviors, noncompliance to treatment, lack of support) to treatment efficacy (Mrug et al., 2012; Weisz & Hawley, 2002). For example, Dadds and McHugh (1992) assessed the impact of social support in the outcome of child management and adjunctive ally training among children with conduct problems. Results demonstrated both interventions as efficacious and further showed that responders from either treatment reported higher levels of positive friend social support compared to nonresponders. Somewhat similarly, Dishion, Poulin, and Burraston (2001) examined utilization of group therapy in a sample of 130 youth with problem behaviors (e.g., smoking, teacher-reported delinquency). In brief, results indicated that deviancy training (i.e., extent to which youth received positive group attention for problem behaviors) was positively associated with increased delinquency. Collectively, such results demonstrate the potential impact of various mechanisms of socialization—depending on developmental level—on client behaviors and subsequently on treatment efficacy.

Emotional Development

Beyond previously discussed cognitive and social levels, emotional development similarly serves as an important contributor to youth treatment efficacy. In particular, the client's normal emotional developmental stages may affect his or her ability to recognize and sufficiently express and utilize emotions within therapy. Notably, past research with healthy youth populations has demonstrated improved performance in emotion matching tasks (i.e., fear and disgust; Herba, Landau, Russell, Ecker, & Phillips, 2006), emotion discrimination, and emotion regulation (Tottenham, Hare, & Casey, 2011) relative to participant age. Beyond these forms of research, studies have rarely considered the impact of normal emotional development on youth intervention; however, normal differences demonstrated do suggest that this may affect treatment engagement and pace (e.g., therapists may have to spend several sessions discussing emotions with clients at lower levels).

Collectively, cognitive, social, and emotional differences in youth development highlight critical areas of consideration for both general developmental stages and individual clients. As such, the following sections provide pertinent recommendations for therapists and researchers within the developmental and treatment domains.

DEVELOPMENTAL CONSIDERATIONS IN THE DESIGN OF PEDIATRIC EVIDENCE-BASED PRACTICES

The Issue of Assent

Another striking difference between the research and practice of psychotherapy for adults versus children is necessary ethical considerations. Informed consent, for example, provides an opportunity for institute-monitored self-protection in both research and clinical settings. However, those with diminished capacity to consent, such as children, are arguably the most vulnerable populations. With a general trend toward growth in research on children and adolescents, the importance and difficulty in defining what exactly is appropriate and necessary relative to informing minors about psychological research and treatment cannot be missed. Perhaps the most difficult hurdle of all is that, in many societies, children are largely powerless with regard to the decisions being made about them. This creates a dissonance between the intent to do meaningful work with children and the need to perceive children's views in an unadulterated way. Much controversy manifests, in that children are largely considered to be vulnerable, incompetent, and in need of protection from exploitation, which poses questions about whether they are capable of making decisions about their participation in psychotherapy, as well as contributing meaningfully to research.

The concept of "child" also largely points to a key relationship—that between the child and the parent (Morrow & Richards, 1996). While, ethically, parental consent is still required when children are involved in research and often for treatment, assent is also commonly documented. Parental consent serves the purpose of protecting the child from unjustified risks (Rossi, Reynolds, & Nelson, 2003), whereas assent essentially involves a child's voluntary agreement to participate, though it may be best understood in the context of parental permission (Denham & Nelson, 2002). Assent does, however, allow the child to express autonomy and to feel respected by the research process (Vitiello, 2008). The age at which assent should be sought is constantly under debate. Some find 7 years of age to be sufficient, though others advise that younger children tend to have poor understanding of programs they participate in and children over ages 11–15 tend to have a much greater understanding of research and clinical procedures (e.g., Rossi et al., 2003). This poses many methodological and ethical questions regarding the ability of young children to participate in programs researching and implementing novel treatments.

Researchers and clinicians might also argue that capacity for assent should be viewed as a continuum that is dependent on psychological age and cognitive ability, and that factors such as psychological state, physical age, and maturity level should be taken into account. For example, Lindeke, Hauck, and Tanner (2000) suggest that factors involved in appropriate understanding of the assent process are related to maturity and mental competence, and not solely based on biological age. Others argue that a model of autonomy is not the best way to conceptualize assent, and that a focus on cognitive ability should be further developed (Rossi et al., 2003). It is important to keep in mind that children's ability to provide assent may also become compromised by their tendency to trust adults as supportive and caring authority figures, or because they are afraid to disappoint or displease adults (Broome, 1999). Various studies have been conducted to determine the influential power that parents/guardians and researchers hold over children during the assent process; however, findings have been mixed (Rossi et al., 2003).

Moreover, while minors are protected under several codes and standards, regulations regarding the form and content of assent are also sorely lacking (e.g., Kimberly, Hoehn, Feudtner, Nelson, & Schreiner, 2006). The basic elements of informed consent have provided the central structure for the conceptualization of assent (information, comprehension, voluntariness). In contrast to the strict provisions set forth for documenting informed consent in adults, however, assent is not legally mandated in most states (Lindeke et al., 2000). The National Commission for the Protection of Human Subjects in Biomedical and Behavioral Research set forth initial guidelines for the practice of assent, but said guidelines were not incorporated into federal regulations (Rossi et al., 2003). This means the responsibility for determining when and how assent will be obtained, and what constitutes adequate documentation of assent, falls largely on individual institutions (Ungar, Joffe, & Kodish, 2006), allowing for significant variability in the breadth of information provided and the language used in assent documents between institutions and perhaps even sometimes within an institution. These are all important considerations to keep in mind when designing, piloting, and ultimately disseminating psychotherapy programs for pediatric samples.

Fortunately, work is being done to better standardize the practice of child assent in order to better protect clients and participants (Rossi et al., 2003). Despite this, more research is necessary to determine whether comprehension skills or other attributes are the best method to provide assent and to allow for greater consistency and comparability between studies, and whether assent needs to be a one-time concern or a starting point in a continuous process. Whether "age" brackets should be based on biological age or cognitive ability would also need to be determined. Ultimately, ethical and methodological considerations that apply to psychotherapy research in adults must also apply to that in children, with special considerations to be made in light of the population. Much of the research in this area has produced inconclusive findings, thus fueling the need for further research and development in the area of child assent procedures. Additional work toward designing, testing, and implementing programs in a flexible and ethical manner could ease some of the concerns associated with the Task Force's recommendations, adapting for both a wide range of ages and autonomy, as well as types of psychopathology.

What Constitutes Developmental Psychopathology?

The boundary between normal and abnormal is an ever mutable, highly derivative line that draws from current empirical findings, societal trends and expectations, as well as a given individual's context, developmental level, and experiences. Because the empirical study of developmental psychopathology is rather young (Achenbach & Edelbrock, 1978), it stands that many questions remain as to what does and does not constitute psychopathology in youth. Unfortunately, this lack of clarity can place significant limitations on the progression and implementation of adequate methods of treatment for youth. The distinction between normal and pathological with regard to psychological functioning can even be confused within specific symptoms (e.g., Cicchetti & Rogosch, 2002; Siegel & Scoville, 2000). This is partially due to normative changes and exploration, resulting in fluctuations in symptomatology based on age. Knowing the norms and developmental milestones (both positive and negative) that are expected of a given age group is often necessary to determine exactly what is and is not likely to be psychopathology in a child.

For example, substance use in a teenager may be representative of poor coping skills or addiction, or it may indicate more normative experimentation.

There is also evidence of some level of consistency in pediatric psychopathology, as approximately half of those disorders observed in adolescence have continued from earlier childhood (Rutter & Shaffer, 1980). It is not uncommon for a specific type of psychopathology to be exhibited differentially throughout the developmental process (e.g., disruptive behaviors); this is known as *heterotypic continuity* (Cicchetti & Rogosch, 2002). The importance of an understanding of heterotypic continuity for all psychologically minded professionals is further exemplified by the recent developmentally focused changes in DSM-5 (American Psychiatric Association, 2013). Fortunately, noting early trends in a child's behavior can often help to circumvent the development of more serious pathology later in childhood or adolescence, such as the potential transition from oppositional defiant disorder (ODD) to conduct disorder (CD). Biological differences between the sexes also come in to play during the child and adolescent years. Females become more likely than males to develop depression beginning in early adolescence, for example (Hankin et al., 1998; Nolen-Hoeskema & Girgus, 1994). While this particular difference appears to persist into adulthood (Kessler et al., 2003, 2005), the effects of puberty on the development of psychopathology are robust for both sexes (e.g., Gunnar, Wewerka, Frenn, Long, & Griggs, 2009; Hayward, Killen, Wilson, & Hammer, 1997; Lahey et al., 2006; Patton et al., 2004; Rudolph, Hammen, & Daley, 2006). Early detection of signs of risk (i.e., traumatic experiences, peer rejection) paired with adept intervention has also been found to be effective for many in staving off the development of psychological symptoms, or at least preventing the worsening of them.

Such children may benefit from either group or individual psychotherapy, and it is important to keep in mind that each child comes to psychotherapy with different experiences and a different understanding of those experiences. In the development and assessment of psychotherapy programs for pediatric samples, one must consider the variety of symptoms with which children may present, and how those symptoms may develop via multiple pathways. This is known as *equifinality*. Conversely, the same sort of experience in a group of children may result in a variety of outcomes, a concept known by the term *multifinality* (Cicchetti & Rogosch, 2002). Understanding both of these concepts can aid in the production of hypotheses regarding the course and presentation of psychopathology in a given child. Researchers and clinicians who seek to develop new methods or manuals for treating such psychopathology in youth must reflect on such factors as well. This is particularly important in treatment planning, or in determining how best to implement a program of treatment for youth with varying levels of functioning and symptom presentations.

Manualization of Psychosocial Treatments for Youth

Though the Task Force suggested well-established and probably efficacious treatments be manualized in an attempt to better define and disseminate those practices that are effective in psychotherapy, this requirement has been met with much controversy (e.g., Chambless & Ollendick, 2001). A psychotherapy manual is, after all, more or less an instruction guide for specific procedures associated with a specific approach to treatment. More recently, a broader emphasis on the principles underlying a given practice has been suggested, rather than a focus on the specific procedures involved (Chorpita, Daleiden, & Weisz, 2005). A too narrow focus on the detailed procedures of a treatment manual may cause need for constant revisions and retesting of these procedures, leading to confusion and wasted resources. For example, some manuals have been designed, written, and tested for very specific issues in children or adolescents only (e.g., attention-deficit/hyperactivity disorder [ADHD]), despite the fact that some aspects of such treatments may also prove beneficial in treating related or commonly comorbid disorders (e.g., ODD). These sorts of issues may leave clinicians at a loss, leading researchers and clinicians to instead seek to develop new and entirely untested interventions rather than adapt existing ones.

Interestingly, Chorpita and colleagues (2005) have proposed the creation of a type of psychotherapeutic practice inventory involving "practice elements." This method would devolve the seemingly effective aspects of treatment programs based on coding systems. Such a database could allow for broader application across a variety of ailments of those elements that have already proven effective in a specific usage. Concerns also exist regarding inflexibility of manualized programs relative to the particular needs of an individual client. Despite the fact that most manuals have been created with the expectation that liberties will be taken, such a database could allow clinicians to further utilize their clinical judgment and try out those aspects of an established therapy that appear most applicable for a given client. A particular strength of such a formally compiled manualized program, however, is that it helps keep therapists focused on specific goals and provides a timeline for therapy, both of which can be helpful when working with a complicated child case.

Many manualized therapies also involve both a therapist guide and a workbook for the client. While the individual of focus for a given therapy is of primary importance (i.e., parent vs. child), keeping any such workbook approachable for both parents and children of various ages may prove beneficial. Additionally, writing a manual broadly enough to encompass language and activities that will work with a variety of ages could allow for greater flexibility within a specific treatment approach. The manualized series created by Dr. Phillip Kendall to help youth deal with anxiety (i.e., Coping CAT, CAT Project—Kendall, Choudhury, Hudson, & Webb, 2002; Kendall & Hedtke, 2006) represents an excellent example of a specific approach to effective psychotherapy that has been broadened to work for a relatively inclusive age range (7–18 years old in this case). Similar success has been found with parenting interventions geared toward a variety of behavioral issues in youth (e.g., Positive Parenting Program [Triple P]—Sanders, Markie-Dadds, & Turner, 2001). Such adaptive multilevel programs factor in elements such as children's age and parenting requirements, for example, their autonomy versus independence. The concept of autonomy versus independence is particularly important when considering that many youth are brought to treatment, not always entirely willingly, by a consenting adult, bringing up the vital consideration of child assent in psychotherapy.

DEVELOPMENTAL CONSIDERATIONS WHEN IMPLEMENTING PEDIATRIC EVIDENCE-BASED PRACTICES

Identifying and Assessing Dysfunction

Psychopathology in youth may not always present in an overt fashion; rather, a child may suffer distress internally and give little external indication. The symptoms experienced by these youth are often quite common (e.g., fears, social timidity, or withdrawal). Conversely, some children and adolescents may present with more obvious emotional, developmental, or behavioral problems (e.g., lying, fighting, anhedonia). Many issues that are quite normative at one point in development (e.g., bedwetting) become abnormal and dysfunctional at another. The key is to discern at what point developmental norms persist into abnormality. To do this, one must have a solid knowledge of expectations for given periods of development, typical milestones, and general norms. Therapists must continually watch for instances of both positive symptoms (e.g., abnormal levels of worry) and negative ones (e.g., absence of an expected trait or age-appropriate achievement) across domains of social competence, cognitive abilities, emotional acuity, and physical growth. Additionally, therapists must be aware of a pediatric client's levels of autonomy and dependence when selecting, implementing, and individualizing a treatment program.

Mental illness in children is, after all, a moving target across developmental stages. Assessing dysfunction in youth, for example, might be dependent on reports from the child, parents, and even teachers. Parents and teachers may be more likely to provide consistent feedback; however, technically, they are external observers of the child's experience. Depending on the age of a child, self-reported symptoms and functioning may or may not be plausible. Young children, for instance, may have neither the necessary cognitive abilities to conceptualize their issues nor the linguistic skills to communicate their experiences. Generally, relying on multiple informants is likely to provide the best level of comprehension and assessment of a child's situation and experiences. Also important when choosing a specific manual or psychotherapeutic procedure for a given child or adolescent is determining what issue is most prominent, and most in need of treatment. Parents and teachers may report on observations regarding behavioral problems, whereas a child or adolescent may be more likely to report on his or her internal worry or depression. As youth often present with comorbid diagnoses (Caron & Rutter, 1991; Merikangas et al., 2011), the ability to best assess for primary concerns and to match an evidence-based practice to their needs is most necessary. This calls for a strong understanding of what psychotherapy is and what aspects of treatment best fit for a given symptom presentation for youth.

Defining Psychotherapy for Youth

Psychotherapy for children is primarily designated with the purpose of alleviating distress, reducing maladaptive behaviors, and/or increasing positive/adaptive behaviors. While often driven by differing theoretical models (Kendall, 2012), psychotherapy for children and adolescents commonly includes counseling and structured or planned interventions (Weisz, Weiss, Han, Granger, & Morton, 1995) with the overarching objective of improving interpersonal or intrapersonal functioning. Psychotherapy for youth is particularly unique as children are likely to have been brought to therapy per the will of another, such as a parent or caregiver. As such, children may more often present to treatment with more easily observable behavioral issues rather than emotional trouble. However, emotional turmoil may underlay behavioral expressions of dysregulation in some youth (Eisenberg et al., 2003).

Additionally, parents and children often note different problems (Yeh & Weisz, 2001). Parents may tend to perceive behavioral deficits as due to characteristics of the child, whereas children often attribute dysfunction to the context surrounding them (e.g., Jones & Nisbett, 1971; Malle, 2006). Parental report can also be influenced by personal psychopathology, marital discord, life stressors, and the availability of social support (De Los Reyes & Kazdin, 2005; Kazdin, 1994). Additionally, the goals of therapy are also a bit different with children and adolescents. Because it is often the parents/caregivers who are seeking some change, the child's "goals" (if these exist) might not match up with those set by the parent(s) and therapist. All of these factors must be considered when approaching psychotherapy for youth.

It is also extremely important when working with youth to consider who the client is in a given psychotherapy situation: the parent or child. It may often be the case that parents are bringing reluctant children to therapy who may reject aspects of, if not the treatment as a whole. This is particularly likely to be the case with treatment manuals that suggest more highly structured approaches to therapy. Especially with younger children, the therapist must carefully balance the importance of rapport with the child while focusing on the expectations of the parent, all the while bearing in mind what is best for the child and family. Though complications can ensue (Gvion & Bar, 2014), parents can play a variety of roles within treatment: acting as consultants, co-clients, and even collaborators (Kendall, 2012). In other cases, the therapist will work more directly with parents than with the child. Sometimes it is actually the "parenting" that is in need of treatment. Programs such as Triple P help to guide parents toward personal behaviors that can positively impact the behaviors and functioning of the child. Programs that involve token economies, for example, may prove beneficial across a variety of behavioral issues (e.g., inattention, disruptive behavior) and may be implemented by the parent or teacher following adequate training by a therapist. In group therapy setting for youth, some aspects of treatment may even be delivered by other children. Generally, treatment in children commonly includes parent, family, and teachers each in some manner (Kazdin, Siegel, & Bass, 1990; Koocher & Pedulla, 1977). Finding the right approach for a given child therapy case is an important step in implementing psychotherapy in an effective and efficacious way.

Determining the Appropriate Approach to Treatment

Some clinicians may seek to treat a child's symptoms, whereas others conceptualize a case by focusing on broader diagnoses. What is more, given frequent comorbidities among child clients, clinicians may approach treatment utilizing a problem-oriented perspective, during which treatment targets are prioritized based on relevant criteria (e.g., functional impairment of symptoms or diagnosis, symptom severity). For example, a child presenting with mild anxiety and severe attention difficulties (as a result of comorbid ADHD), may benefit from initial treatment of attention prior to addressing anxiety symptoms. Regardless of the conceptual approach utilized, however, several decisions must be made when determining the best method of treatment for a given child. Ultimately, the needs of the child and responsible adult must be considered in determining what treatment approach to choose and which skills are likely to be beneficial. For example, a program that incorporates increased monitoring may be most beneficial for parents of a child with conduct problems, while skills to aid in reduction of accommodation and vigilance may best benefit parents of an anxious child, and thus the child him or herself (e.g., Barmish

& Kendall, 2005). The age and developmental level of the child also need to be taken into consideration. For example, reduced monitoring may be appropriate for an 8-year-old child who has mastered a sense of danger regarding objects such as knives and scissors, but not for an unruly 4-year-old child.

Depending on the maturity level and presenting problems of a given child, various types of therapeutic interventions can be employed. Talking, playing, behavioral contingency and reward programs, as well as rehearsing skills and behaviors can be especially effective in youth. These methods are again impacted by a given child's previous experiences, level of comfort in treatment, communication style, ability to think abstractly, and environmental factors, all of which should again be taken into consideration.

Influence of the Environment and/or Context

Last, it is of utmost importance to consider the environmental and contextual factors at play with any pediatric client. Because youth, particularly young children, are largely dependent on their parents or caregivers, one can neither expect therapeutic change to occur within a vacuum nor expect a child to make vast changes on his or her own. External risk factors that influence child outcomes are often present prior to, throughout, and following treatment. Children also typically lack significant control of other influences, such as their familial dynamics, their home environment (including housing and neighborhood), their educational opportunities, and sometimes even their selected peer group. Children with unstable home environments (e.g., little parental supervision, domestic violence or disputes) may be less likely to benefit from the stability of the therapeutic environment because they continuously return to that initial instability. Low-income families might also involve parents who are constantly working, which disallows adequate parental involvement in daily life, as well as psychotherapy. Regardless of the reason, parents who are unable or unwilling to engage in psychotherapy for their child may also be less likely to bring their child, leading to poor attendance and attrition from treatment programs. For instance, 40–60% of children who start treatment terminate early, often against the advice of the clinician (Kazdin, 1996; Wierzbicki & Pekarik, 1993).

Some children, perhaps particularly adolescents, may be embarrassed or uncomfortable facing the risk of stigma from peers relating to psychiatric diagnoses and attending psychotherapy. It is possible that such children already are presenting with low social support and may thus disengage from therapy in fear of being ridiculed. In addition to poor social support, some children of underprivileged families may not have the resources to engage in therapy fully (e.g., payment for sessions, materials for rewards). Underfunded school systems may also be less likely to participate in treatment attempts for students who would benefit from the inclusion of teachers in therapy or monitoring. While many of these issues exist with adult psychotherapy clients as well, the degree to which children lack control over such contextual factors must be considered when implementing treatment programs for youth.

Ultimately, there are seemingly endless personal (e.g., social, cognitive) and treatment-based (e.g., assessment, direct implementation) factors to be taken into consideration with child psychotherapy, including those described earlier. The number and complexity of such factors may seem overwhelming and deter some psychologists from seeking to use or improve various psychotherapeutic modalities in the treatment of children and adolescents. However, with the guidance of the following recommendations, it is likely that any well-studied and -practiced researcher and/or clinician can effectively implement EBPs in his or her work.

RECOMMENDATIONS

For Therapists

Given the previously discussed considerations in treatment design and implementation (e.g., defining psychotherapy for youth, determining appropriate treatment approaches, addressing assent), appropriate communication among child, parent, and therapist is essential. As such, we recommend that initial therapy sessions include a formal discussion addressing treatment focus (e.g., child as the client, presenting symptoms, appropriate treatment goals, and planned treatment approach). Such a discussion may highlight important components of therapy and provide the family with a greater sense of involvement in the development of the child's treatment plan. These discussions should also address additional factors, including child assent (i.e., using age- and cognitively appropriate terminology and materials), and appropriate boundaries within information sharing (e.g., information may be disclosed to a parent at the discretion of the client). Initial discussion of these factors, as well as acknowledgment and processing of differing perspectives (e.g., appropriately addressing and processing when parent and child disagree in regard to treatment goals, reaching an agreement regarding information sharing), may decrease and potentially eliminate future conflicts and misconceptions between therapy participants. What is more, including children within this discussion (to an age-appropriate extent) and encouraging child assent may provide youth clients with an advantageous sense of autonomy and subsequently may increase motivation and participation in therapy.

The discussion presented herein further suggests that therapists must remain cognizant of normal developmental differences among age groups in general, as well as individual clients (e.g., individuals may also fall above or below their age developmental level). As discussed earlier, when such differences are measured accurately, they may facilitate proper assessment, as well as treatment implementation. The previously noted developmental differences also demonstrate the importance of flexibility within psychotherapeutic interventions with youth, advocating for the use of developmentally modified treatments. Unfortunately, early child-oriented interventions were constructed with little regard for developmental differences between adult and youth populations. Recognizing these past omissions, recent research has sought to examine the use of developmental modifications within current and novel treatments. For example, Choate-Summers and colleagues (2008) discussed the use of a developmentally modified family-based treatment program for children ages 5–8 with pediatric OCD. Specific modifications that differ from treatment with older children include providing both child and parent with techniques to understand, manage, and reduce OCD symptoms (vs. focusing on individual treatment with older children and adolescents), providing two sessions of psychoeducation to parents prior to child treatment (vs. providing techniques to the parent and child jointly), appropriately utilizing exposure within developmentally appropriate play (vs. repeated exposures without play), and incorporating formal parent training within therapy (vs. parents included at the discretion of the therapist). Preliminary evidence supported treatment suitability for young children, highlighting the beneficial use of developmentally sensitive treatments specifically within cognitive-behavioral therapies. Such results also corroborate additional research demonstrating the efficacy of developmentally modified treatments for youth (Hirshfeld-Becker et al., 2010; Luby, Lenze, & Tilman, 2012; Pincus, Eyberg, & Choate, 2005).

Several further recommendations are pertinent to additional, more person-centered developmental factors (i.e., social, emotional, environmental contexts). First, considering the previously discussed effects of social development on the therapeutic alliance, therapists may consider differential activities (e.g., discussing developmentally appropriate interests, play activities) based on developmental level to facilitate the formation of a beneficial relationship. In regard to the social domain, given the dependent nature of childhood (e.g., children depending on family for basic needs and support), family relationships are often recognized as an essential component to child development and treatment. For example, as discussed previously, family relationships are integral to understanding both a child's socialization and home environment. What is more, among child clients, families are often relied upon in part for a successful therapy experience (e.g., relying on families to bring the child to sessions, to ensure completion of homework, to provide external support, to engage in parent sessions). Therapists may consider further addressing and/or increasing family involvement for client's in which family domains hinder the therapeutic process (e.g., infrequent attendance due to additional parent engagements, parental behavior within the home contradictory to therapy tasks/goals) or become relevant to treatment goals (e.g., a goal may include improving family dynamics, working through family experiences, recognizing increased independence for an adolescent). Increased family involvement may be implemented through brief parent discussion (e.g., reserving time at the beginning or end of a session to discuss the importance of parental involvement and provide information on child's treatment progress and activities) and/or family focused sessions (i.e., parent and child attending sessions together or parents attending sessions individually) during which the importance of family involvement is discussed, critical family aspects are highlighted, and potential issues are addressed. Notably, given increased social interaction among adolescents and older clients, therapists may reserve additional time for the discussion of peer networks in addition to family relationships. Such modifications may also extend to issues regarding children's environmental context. For example, increased discussion of peer or family relationships may provide additional insight into a child's contextual factors and provide further opportunity to address such factors (e.g., modifying family components to therapy, addressing issues of stigma amongst peers, discovering alternative sources of social support).

Therapists may also modify treatments based on clients' emotional stages. For example, considering the variability in emotional literacy and expression in children, therapists may wish to utilize elementary methods (e.g., using a face chart to identify emotions) among clients at lower developmental levels versus more complex methods (e.g., relating feelings to thoughts and behaviors, challenging clients' thoughts) with emotionally advanced individuals. In addition to normal differences among clients, therapists should also maintain knowledge of current research advances within domains of abnormal development, pathology, and intervention research. Maintaining up-to-date knowledge across domains of abnormal development (in combination with factors such as clients' characteristics, culture, experiences, etc.) may further facilitate accurate differentiation between normal child development and pathology. In relation to intervention, though research in this domain has increased, literature indicates a significant gap between research findings and clinical practice (Ollendick & Davis, 2004; Weisz, 2000). Increased communication (e.g., increased publication dissemination between disciplines, conferences attendance, brief newsletters with research and clinical updates, Web-based dissemination of evidence-based practices) between researchers and clinicians may provide additional insight into the overall effectiveness of laboratory interventions and further influence future research endeavors.

For Researchers

Consideration of developmental levels in evidence-based intervention with youth similarly raises several critical recommendations for researchers. First, and perhaps most obvious in this domain, further research is necessary to examine the impact of specific normal developmental levels on child psychotherapy outcomes, particularly in relation to emotional development. Such research may wish to utilize diverse samples with respect to demographic variables (e.g., age, ethnicity, socioeconomic status) and treatment interventions (i.e., cognitive treatments, emotion regulation treatments). What is more, future research should consider increased utilization of longitudinal methods in the examination of etiological and maintenance factors of pediatric pathology, as well as mechanisms that might mediate treatment outcome. Further classification of etiological and maintainance factors may also provide increased insight into the development of various pediatric disorders and further enable differentiation between normal and pathological developmental differences. Similarly, examination of mediating mechanisms in treatment outcome can help identify critical target areas for future treatment modifications (e.g., increasing emphasis on peer relationships within treatments). Similarly, further research examining change mechanisms within pediatric intervention is warranted and may contribute to science's understanding of the treatment process, as well as psychopathology overall.

Last, researchers must also consider further investigation in the effectiveness and efficacy of current child psychotherapy interventions, as well as novel developmentally modified treatments. The extant literature indicates that while current treatments have demonstrated efficacy within laboratory settings, effectiveness research within clinical settings is scant (van de Wiel, Matthys, Cohen-Kettenis, & van Engeland, 2002). Such discrepancies limit true understanding of intervention success within clinical versus academic settings. Furthermore, as previously discussed, numerous interventions utilized among disordered youth have neglected to account for developmental differences between youth populations and original adult samples in which these treatments were utilized. Identification of critical areas in which current treatments lack and may be further improved through developmentally appropriate modifications are essential to optimal treatment efficacy in youth. What is more, research in these domains may help identify aspects of interventions that are detrimental and/or most suitable for particular developmental levels, potentially easing therapy selection for clinicians and decreasing the occurrence of nonresponse to child psychotherapeutic treatment.

CONCLUSION

Collectively, the discussion topics presented in this chapter demonstrate the importance of developmental considerations within pediatric evidence-based treatments. Specifically, such considerations are critical to treatment design, selection, implementation, and outcome. While the recommendations presented herein provide several potential methods of tackling and researching developmental differences in treatment among youth, additional methods targeting these domains are equally plausible. Furthermore, an improved understanding within these areas may contribute to the formation of more efficacious interventions, as well as increased understanding of pediatric psychopathology overall.

REFERENCES

Achenbach, T. M., & Edelbrock, C. S. (1978). The classification of child psychopathology: A review and analysis of empirical efforts. *Psychological Bullentin, 85*(6), 1275–1301.

American Psychiatric Association. (2013). *Diagnostic and statistical manual of mental disorders* (5th ed.). Arlington, VA: Author.

Barmish, A. J., & Kendall, P. C. (2005). Should parents be co-clients in cognitive behavioral therapy for anxious youth? *Journal of Clinical Child and Adolescent Psychology, 34*(3), 569–581.

Bennett, D. S., & Gibbons, T. A. (2000). Efficacy of child cognitive-behavioral interventions for antisocial behavior: A meta-analysis. *Child and Family Behavior Therapy, 22*(1), 1–15.

Broome, M. E. (1999). Consent (assent) for research with pediatric patients. *Seminars in Oncology Nursing, 15*(2), 96–103.

Caron, C., & Rutter, M. (1991). Comorbidity in child psychopathology: Concepts, issues and research strategies. *Journal of Child Psychology and Psychiatry, 32*(7), 1063–1080.

Cartwright-Hatton, S., Roberts, C., Chitsabesan, P., Fothergill, C., & Harrington, R. (2004). Systematic review of the efficacy of cognitive behavior therapies for childhood and anxiety disorders. *British Journal of Clinical Psychology, 43*(4), 421–436.

Chambless, D. L., Baker, M. J., Baucom, D. H., Beutler, L. E., Calhoun, K. S., & Crits-Christoph, P. (1998). Update on empirically validated therapies: II. *Clinical Psychologist, 51*(1), 3–16.

Chambless, D. L., & Ollendick, T. H. (2001). Empirically supported psychological interventions: Controversies and evidence. *Annual Review of Psychology, 52*, 685–716.

Choate-Summers, M. L., Freeman, J. B., Garcia, A. M., Coyne, L., Przeworski, A., & Leonard, H. L. (2008). Clinical considerations when tailoring cognitive behavioral treatment for young children with obsessive compulsive disorder. *Education and Treatment of Children, 31*(3), 395–416.

Chorpita, B. F., Daleiden, E. L., & Weisz, J. R. (2005). Identifying and selecting the common elements of evidence based interventions: A distillation and matching model. *Mental Health Services Research, 7*(1), 5–20.

Cicchetti, D., & Rogosch, F. A. (2002). A developmental psychopathology perspective on adolescence. *Journal of Consulting and Clinical Psychology, 70*(1), 6–20.

Cohen, J. A., & Mannarino, A. P. (2000). Predictors of treatment outcome in sexually abused children. *Child Abuse and Neglect, 24*(7), 983–994.

Crawford, A. M., & Manassis, K. (2001). Familial predictors of treatment outcome in childhood anxiety disorders. *Journal of the American Academy of Child and Adolescent Psychiatry, 40*(10), 1182–1189.

Cummings, C. M., Caporino, N. E., Settipani, C. A., Read, K. L., Compton, S. N., March, J., et al. (2013). The therapeutic relationship in cognitive-behavioral therapy and pharmacotherapy for anxious youth. *Journal of Consulting and Clinical Psychology, 81*, 859–864.

Dadds, M. R., & McHugh, T. A. (1992). Social support and treatment outcome in behavioral family therapy for child conduct problems. *Journal of Consulting and Clinical Psychology, 60*(2), 252–259.

David-Ferdon, C., & Kaslow, N. J. (2008). Evidence-based psychosocial treatments for child and adolescent depression. *Journal of Clinical Child and Adolescent Psychology, 37*(1), 62–104.

De Los Reyes, A., & Kazdin, A. E. (2005). Informant discrepancies in the assessment of childhood psychopathology: A critical review, theoretical framework, and recommendations for further study. *Psychological Bulletin, 131*(4), 483–509.

Denham, E. J., & Nelson, R. M. (2002). Self-determination is not an appropriate model for understanding parental permission and child assent. *Anesthesiology Analogs, 94,* 1049–1051.

Dishion, T. J., Poulin, F., & Burraston, B. (2001). Peer group dynamics associated with iatrogenic effects in group interventions with high-risk young adolescents. *New Directions for Child and Adolescent Development, 91,* 79–92.

Eisenberg, N., Cumberland, A., Spinrad, T. L., Fabes, R. A., Shepard, S. A., Reiser, M., et al. (2003). The relations of regulation and emotionality to children's externalizing and internalizing problem behavior. *Child Development, 72*(4), 1112–1134.

Elliott, R. E. (1998). Editor's introduction: A guide to the empirically supported treatments controversy. *Psychotherapy Research, 8,* 115–125.

Eysenck, H. J. (1960). Personality and behaviour therapy. *Proceedings of the Royal Society of Medicine, 53*(7), 504–508.

Freedheim, D. K., Freudenberger, H. J., Kessler, J. W., Messer, S. B., Peterson, D. R., Strupp, H. H., et al. (1992). *History of psychotherapy: A century of change.* Washington, DC: American Psychological Association.

Freeman, J. B., Choate-Summers, M. L., Moore, P. S., Garcia, A. M., Sapyta, J. J., Leonard, H. L., et al. (2007). Cognitive behavioral treatment for young children with obsessive compulsive disorder. *Biological Psychiatry, 61*(3), 337–343.

Furman, W., & Buhrmester, D. (1992). Age and sex differences in perceptions of networks of personal relationships. *Child Development, 63*(1), 103–115.

Grave, J., & Blissett, J. (2004). Is cognitive behavior therapy developmentally appropriate for young children?: A critical review of the evidence. *Clinical Psychology Review, 24,* 399–420.

Gunnar, M. R., Wewerka, S., Frenn, K., Long, J. D., & Griggs, C. (2009). Developmental changes in HPA activity over the transition to adolescence: Normative changes and associations with puberty. *Development and Psychopathology, 21,* 69–85.

Gvion, Y., & Bar, N. (2014). Sliding doors: Some reflection on the parent–child–therapist triangle in parent work–child psychotherapy. *Journal of Child Psychotherapy, 41*(1), 58–72.

Hankin, B. L., Abramson, L. Y., Moffitt, T. E., Silva, P. A., McGee, R., & Angell, K. A. (1998). Development of depression from preadolescence to young adulthood: Emerging gender differences in a 10 year longitudinal study. *Journal of Abnormal Psychology, 107,* 128–141.

Hayward, C., Killen, J. D., Wilson, D. M., & Hammer, L. D. (1997). Psychiatric risk associated with early puberty in adolescent girls. *Journal of the American Academy for Child and Adolescent Psychiatry, 36,* 255–262.

Herba, C. M., Landau, S., Russell, T., Ecker, C., & Phillips, M. L. (2006). The development of emotion-processing in children: Effects of age, emotion, and intensity. *Journal of Child Psychology and Psychiatry, 47*(11), 1098–1106.

Hirshfeld-Becker, D. R., Masek, B., Henin, A., Blakely, L. R., Pollock-Wurman, R. A., McQuade J., et al. (2010). Cognitive behavioral therapy for 4- to 7-year-old children with anxiety disorders: A randomized clinical trial. *Journal of Consulting and Clinical Psychology, 78*(4), 498-510.

Jones, E. E., & Nisbett, R. E. (1971). The actor and the observer: Divergent perceptions of the causes of behavior. In E. E. Jones, D. E. Kanouse, H. H. Kelly, R. E. Nisbett, S. Valins, & B. Weiner (Eds.), *Attribution: Perceiving the causes of behavior* (pp. 79–94). Morristown, NJ: General Learning Press.

Karver, M. S., Handelsman, J. B., Fields, S., & Bickman, L. (2006). Meta-analysis of therapeutic relationship variables in youth and family therapy: The evidence for different relationship variables in the child and adolescent treatment outcome literature. *Clinical Psychology Review, 26*(1), 50–65.

Kazdin, A. E. (1994). Informant variability in the assessment of childhood depression. In W. M. Reynolds & H. F. Johnston (Eds.), *Handbook of depression in children and adolescents* (pp. 249–271). New York: Springer.

Kazdin, A. E. (1995). Child, parent and family dysfunction as predictors of outcome in cognitive-behavioral treatment of antisocial children. *Behaviour Research and Therapy, 33*(3), 271–281.

Kazdin, A. E. (1996). Dropping out of child psychotherapy: Issues for research and implications for practice. *Clinical Child Psychology and Psychiatry, 1*(1), 133–156.

Kazdin, A. E., Marciano, P. L., & Whitley, M. K. (2005). The therapeutic alliance in cognitive-behavioral treatment of children referred for oppositional, aggressive, and antisocial behavior. *Journal of Consulting and Clinical Psychology, 73*(4), 726–730.

Kazdin, A. E., Siegel, T. C., & Bass, D. (1990). Drawing on clinical practice to inform research on child and adolescent psychotherapy: Survey of practitioners. *Professional Psychology: Research and Practice, 21*(3), 189–198.

Keel, P. K., & Haedt, A. (2008). Evidence-based psychosocial treatments for eating problems and eating disorders. *Journal of Clinical Child and Adolescent Psychology, 37*(1), 39–61.

Kendall, P. C. (2012). Guiding theory for therapy with children and adolescents. In P. C. Kendall (Ed.), *Child and adolescent therapy: Cognitive-behavioral procedures* (4th ed., pp. 3–24). New York: Guilford Press.

Kendall, P. C., Choudhury, M., Hudson, J., & Webb, A. (2002). *"The C.A.T Project" manual for the cognitive behavioral treatment of anxious adolescents*. Ardmore, PA: Workbook.

Kendall, P. C., & Hedtke, K. A. (2006). *Cognitive-behavioral therapy for anxious children: Therapist manual* (3rd ed.). Ardmore, PA: Workbook.

Kessler, R. C., Berglund, P., Demler, O., Jin, R., Koretz, D., Merikangas, K. R., et al. (2003). The epidemiology of major depressive disorder: Results from the National Comorbidity Survey Replication (NCS-R). *Journal of the American Medical Association, 289*, 3095–4105.

Kessler, R. C., Berglund, P., Demler, O., Jin, R., Merikangas, K. R., Walters, E. E. (2005). Lifetime prevalence and age-of-onset distributions of DSM-IV disorders in the National Comorbidity Survey Replication. *Archives of General Psychiatry, 62*, 593–602.

Kimberly, M. B., Hoehn, K. S., Feudtner, C., Nelson, R. M., & Schreiner, M. (2006). Variation in standards of research compensation and child assent practices: A comparison of 69 institutional review board-approved informed permission and assent forms for 3 multicenter pediatric clinical trials. *Journal of Pediatrics, 117*, 1706–1711.

Koocher, G. P., & Pedulla, B. M. (1977). Current practices in child psychotherapy. *Professional Psychology, 8*(3), 275–287.

Kovacs, A. L. (1995). We have met the enemy and he is us! *Independent Practitioner, 15*(3), 135–137.

Kuhn, D. (1999). A developmental model of critical thinking. *Educational Researcher, 28*(2), 16–46.

Lahey, B. B., Van Hulle, C. A., Waldman, I. D., Rodgers, J. L., D'Onofrio, B. M., Pedlow, S., et al. (2006). Testing descriptive hypotheses regarding sex differences in the development of conduct problems and delinquency. *Journal of Abnormal Child Psychology, 34*, 737–755.

Lambert, M. J., & Barley, D. E. (2001). Research summary on the therapeutic relationship and psychotherapy outcome. *Psychotherapy: Theory, Research, Practice, Training, 38*(4), 357–361.

Levitt, E. E. (1957). The results of psychotherapy with children: An evaluation. *Journal of Consulting Psychology, 21*(3), 189–196.

Levitt, E. E. (1963). Psychotherapy with children: A further evaluation. *Behaviour Research and Therapy, 1*(1), 45–51.

Lindeke, L. L., Hauck, M. R., & Tanner, M. (2000). Practical issues in obtaining child assent for research. *Journal of Pediatric Nursing, 15*(2), 99–104.

Luby, J., Lenze, S., & Tilman, R. (2012). A novel early intervention for preschool depression: Findings from a pilot randomized controlled trial. *Journal of Child Psychology and Psychiatry, 53*(3), 313–322.

Malle, B. F. (2006). The actor–observer asymmetry in attribution: A (surprising) meta-analysis. *Psychological Bulletin, 132*(6), 895–919.

Martin, D. J., Garske, J. P., & Davis, M. K. (2000). Relation of the therapeutic alliance with outcome and other variables: A meta-analytic review. *Journal of Consulting and Clinical Psychology, 68*(3), 438–450.

McCart, M. R., Priester, P. E., Davies, W. H., & Azen, R. (2006). Differential effectiveness of behavioral parent-training and cognitive-behavioral therapy for antisocial youth: A meta-analysis. *Journal of Abnormal Child Psychology, 34*(4), 525–541.

Merikangas, K. R., He, J. P., Burstein, M., Swendsen, J., Avenevoli, S., Case, B., et al. (2011). Service utilization for lifetime mental disorders in US adolescents: Results of the National Comorbidity Survey–Adolescent Supplement (NCS-A). *Journal of the American Academy of Child and Adolescent Psychiatry, 50*(1), 32–45.

Morrow, V., & Richards, M. (1996). The ethics of social research with children: An overview. *Children and Society, 10*, 90–105.

Mrug, S., Molina, B. S. G., Hoza, B., Gerdes, A. C., Hinshaw, S. P. Hechtman, L., et al. (2012). Peer rejection and friendships in children with attention-deficit/hyperactivity disorder: Contributions to long term outcomes. *Journal of Abnormal Child Psychology, 40*, 1013–1026.

Nolen-Hoeksema, S., & Girgus, J. S. (1994). The emergence of gender differences in depression during adolescence. *Psychological Bulletin, 115*(3), 424–443.

Norcross, J. C. (2001). Purposes, processes and products of the task force on empirically supported therapy relationships. *Psychotherapy: Theory, Research, Practice, Training, 38*(4), 345–356.

Oliver, M. E., Stockdale, K. C., & Wormith, J. S. (2011). A meta-analysis of predictors of offender treatment attrition and its relationship to recidivism. *Journal of Consulting and Clinical Psychology, 79*(1), 6–21.

Ollendick, T. H., & Davis, T. E., III. (2004). Empirically supported treatments for children and adolescents: Where to from here? *Clinical Psychology: Science and Practice, 11*(3), 289–294.

Patton, G. C., McMorris, B. J., Toumbourou, J. W., Hemphill, S. A., Donath, S., & Catlano, R. F. (2004). Puberty and the onset of substance use and abuse. *Pediatrics, 114*, 300–306.

Peris, T. S., Sugar, C. A., Bergman, R. L., Chang, S., Langley, A., & Piacentini, J. (2012). Family factors predict treatment outcome for pediatric obsessive–compulsive disorder. *Journal of Consulting and Clinical Psychology, 80*(2), 255–263.

Piaget, J. (1971). The theory of stages in cognitive development. In D. R. Green, M. P. Ford, & G. B. Flamer (Eds.), *Measurement and Piaget* (pp. 1–111). New York: McGraw-Hill.

Pincus, D. B., Eyberg, S. M., & Choate, M. L. (2005). Adapting parent–child interaction therapy for young children with separation anxiety disorder. *Education and Treatment of Children, 28*(2), 163–181.

Quakely, S., Coker, S., Pamer, K., & Reynolds, S. (2003). Can children distinguish between thoughts and behaviors? *Behavioral and Cognitive Psychotherapy, 31*(2), 159–168.

Rossi, W. C., Reynolds, W., & Nelson, R. M. (2003). Child assent and parental permission in pediatric research. *Theoretical Medicine, 24*, 131–148.

Rudolph, K. D., Hammen, C., & Daley, S. E. (2006). Mood disorders. In D. A. Wolfe & E. J. Mash (Eds.), *Behavioral and emotional disorders in adolescents: Nature, assessment, and treatment* (pp. 300–342). New York: Guilford Press.

Rutter, M., & Shaffer, D. (1980). DSM-III: A step forward or back in terms of the classification of child psychiatric disorders? *Journal of the American Academy of Child Psychiatry, 19*(3), 371–394.

Sackett, D. L., Richardson, W. S., Rosenberg, W., & Haynes, R. B. (1997). *How to practice and teach evidence based medicine.* New York: Churchill Livingstone.

Sackett, D. L., Richardson, W. S., Rosenberg, W., & Haynes, R. B. (2000). *Evidence-based medicine: How to practice and teach* (2nd ed.). Edinburgh, UK: Churchill Livingstone.

Sanders, M. R., Markie-Dadds, C., & Turner, K. M. T. (2001). *Practitioner's manual for Standard Triple P.* Brisbane, Australia: Families International.

Scarpa, A., & Reyes, N. M. (2011). Improving emotion regulation with CBT in young children with high functioning autism spectrum disorders: A pilot study. *Behavioural and Cognitive Psychotherapy, 39*(4), 495–500.

Shirk, S. R., & Karver, M. (2003). Prediction of treatment outcome from relationship variables in child and adolescent therapy: A meta-analytic review. *Journal of Consulting and Clinical Psychology, 71*(3), 452–464.

Siegel, A. W., & Scovill, L. C. (2000). Problem behavior: The double symptom of adolescence. *Development and Psychopathology, 12,* 763–793.

Silverman, W. H. (1996). Cookbooks, manuals, and paint-by-numbers: Psychotherapy in the 90's. *Psychotherapy: Theory, Research, Practice, Training, 33,* 207–215.

Stallard, P. (2002). Cognitive behavior therapy with children and young people: A selective review of key issues. *Behavioural and Cognitive Psychotherapy, 30,* 297–309.

Sukhodolsky, D. G., Kassinove, H., & Gorman, B. S. (2004). Cognitive-behavioral therapy for anger in children and adolescents: A meta-analysis. *Aggression and Violent Behavior, 9*(3), 247–269.

Task Force on Promotion and Dissemination of Psychological Procedures. (1995). Training in and dissemination of empirically-validated psychological treatments: Report and recommendations. *Clinical Psychologist, 48,* 3–23.

Tottenham, N., Hare, T. A., & Casey, B. J. (2011). Behavioral assessment of emotion discrimination, emotion regulation, and cognitive control in childhood, adolescence, and adulthood. *Frontiers in Psychology, 2*(39), 1–9.

Ungar, D., Joffe, S., & Kodish, E. (2006). Children are not small adults: Documentation of assent for research involving children. *Journal of Pediatrics, 4,* S32–S33.

van de Wiel, N., Matthys, W., Cohen-Kettenis, P. C., & van Engeland, H. (2002). Effective treatments of school-aged conduct disordered children: Recommendations for changing clinical and research practices. *European Child and Adolescent Psychiatry, 11*(2), 79–84.

Vitiello, B. (2008). Effectively obtaining informed consent for child and adolescent participation in mental health research. *Ethics and Behavior, 18*(2–3), 182–198.

Weersing, V. R., & Weisz, J. (2002). Mechanisms of action in youth psychotherapy. *Journal of Child Psychology and Psychiatry, 43*(1), 3–29.

Weisz, J. R. (2000). Agenda for child and adolescent psychotherapy research: On the need to put science into practice. *Archives of General Psychiatry, 57,* 837–838.

Weisz, J. R., & Hawley, K. M. (2002). Developmental factors in the treatment of adolescents. *Journal of Consulting and Clinical Psychology, 70*(1), 21–43.

Weisz, J. R., Weiss, B., Han, S. S., Granger, D. A., & Morton, T. (1995). Effects of psychotherapy with children and adolescents revisited: A meta-analysis of treatment outcome studies. *Psychological Bulletin, 117*(3), 450–468.

Wierzbicki, M., & Pekarik, G. (1993). A meta-analysis of psychotherapy dropout. *Professional Psychology: Research and Practice, 24*(2), 190–195.

Yeh, M., & Weisz, J. R. (2001). Why are we here at the clinic?: Parent–child (dis)agreement on referral problems at outpatient entry. *Journal of Consulting and Clinical Psychology, 69*(6), 1018–1025.

CHAPTER 3

Evidence-Based Assessment and Case Formulation

Katharina Manassis

THE GOALS OF ASSESSMENT

There are many possible goals for psychological assessment of children, from determining intelligence and educational abilities to evaluating various neuropsychiatric functions, to exploring vocational interests and beyond. This chapter, however, focuses on assessment that is helpful in preparation for evidence-based treatment of children. When other types of assessment are indicated, the reader may refer to comprehensive texts (e.g., Vance, 1997) or consult colleagues with expertise in relevant areas.

Regardless of the focus of assessment, certain best practices have been emphasized in the field, including adherence to the highest ethical standards when assessing children, selecting instruments that are psychometrically sound and developmentally appropriate, developing a collaborative relationship with the child's family, cultural sensitivity and freedom from cultural bias in one's assessment, and awareness of the role of one's own emotions in the assessment process (Vance, 1997). Those best practices that are particularly salient when assessing children prior to treatment are discussed further in this chapter.

The first essential goal of a treatment-focused assessment is to engage the child and family in a collaborative relationship that aims to discover the best way(s) to alleviate the child's symptoms. Without such a collaborative relationship, the family is unlikely to engage in treatment, and the child's symptoms will probably continue. Ensuring that the assessment venue is comfortable for everyone, engaging in some brief but relevant casual conversation (e.g., how the traffic was on the way to the appointment, how the child is reacting to missing school for the appointment), explaining the structure of the visit (e.g., who will be interviewed first, when any questionnaires used will be administered), making empathic comments, and finding out what the child and family are hoping to learn by the end of the assessment are all ways of making the clinician seem humane and building rapport at the beginning of the assessment visit. I usually conclude these introductory remarks by asking for the family's reaction to the assessment plan (e.g., "How does that sound to you?"), in order to determine any modifications the family members might find helpful. For example, allowing a parent to leave briefly to put money into a parking meter sometimes does more to build rapport than multiple empathic comments. When the assessment is focused on an adolescent, giving the youth the option of being interviewed alone first is sometimes a helpful gesture that acknowledges the value adolescents place on autonomy from their parents. When time is short, it is sometimes tempting to forego the initial, rapport-building conversation, but doing so often results in disappointed clients and limited treatment engagement.

A second goal of assessment is to ascertain the child's main difficulties and factors contributing to these in order to plan treatment. Diagnosis and case formulation usually complement each other in meeting this goal. Most evidence-based treatments are focused on particular diagnostic groups, so a clear diagnosis is important. Diagnoses also make it easier for professionals to communicate about cases, may sometimes be used to support children's access to resources, and are relatively objective because they are based on phenomenology (i.e., a description of symptoms) and therefore involve little speculation on the clinician's part. However, although a diagnosis often provides a useful picture of current symptoms, it does not provide information on how those symptoms developed, what factors may be maintaining them (and might therefore undermine treatment), or what factors (apart from the proposed treatment) might help ameliorate them. A case formulation, on the other hand, offers a testable set of hypotheses about factors that are germane to the development, maintenance, and amelioration of symptoms (reviewed in Manassis, 2014), and is discussed further in the section on synthesizing information. Although more speculative than a diagnosis, a case formulation avoids the problem of "lumping" dissimilar children under the same diagnostic label, considers historical and contextual information that may suggest ways of tailoring treatment to the individual child, and is sometimes less stigmatizing than a diagnosis.

In addition to diagnosis and case formulation, functional analysis and the use of baselines can be helpful in planning treatment. A functional analysis is a detailed description of the main situations in which symptoms occur, focusing on the antecedents of the child's symptoms or behavior and the subsequent consequences the child experiences (Waguespack, Vaccaro, & Continere, 2006; Wightman, Julio, & Virues-Ortega, 2014). This description allows clinicians to identify common triggers for symptoms and people in the child's environment to identify common patterns of response that may or may not be helpful. It can be incorporated into the overall case formulation or be seen as a separate "miniformulation" of specific situations that warrant attention in treatment. To identify situations that merit functional analysis, it is often useful to ask parents about a typical day in the child's life (e.g., events before, during, and after school, and in the evening before bedtime), and report more details about situations where symptoms are evident. "If I had a video camera at your house (or your child's school) at this time, what would I see?" is sometimes a fruitful question to elicit further details about relevant situations.

A baseline is useful to quantify the main problems prior to treatment in order to allow monitoring over time (Manassis, 2009). Symptom frequency, duration, intensity, interference with usual activities, and the degree of control the child feels over the symptoms can all be quantified for situations that occur regularly (usually weekly or more), then checked every few weeks to detect progress or lack of progress. Small positive changes can then be used to encourage further effort in treatment, and lack of progress may signal a need to modify treatment. Repeated administration of standardized questionnaires (e.g., the Children's Depression Inventory [Kovacs, 2004] or the Multidimensional Anxiety Scale for Children [March, 2004]) is also used to monitor progress in some cases.

Some authors have suggested also including measures of treatment readiness in the assessment (Manassis, 2009; Prochaska & DiClemente, 1984). The client's motivation to pursue treatment is an important aspect of readiness (Prochaska & DiClemente, 1984), and often becomes evident when spelling out treatment expectations. Parents who disagree about the child's need for treatment, who are engaged in a high-conflict divorce or custody dispute, or who encounter frequent crises in their lives (e.g., unstable employment or living situation) may have difficulty successfully engaging in treatment. Parents who are unsure whether they can bring the child consistently every week, participate in some sessions (or a part of every session, depending on one's treatment model), and support the child's work between sessions may also have this difficulty. Similar motivational considerations apply to adolescents who are considering psychotherapy. Younger children with limited treatment motivation often engage if their parents are committed to their treatment. Some types of evidence-based treatment have additional requirements. Successful cognitive-behavioral therapy, for example, requires children to have certain cognitive and attentional abilities (Manassis, 2009). Therapists can minimize some of these requirements (e.g., help with reading and writing; provide frequent redirection; and break sessions into short segments to reduce the need for sustained attention), but the child must still be able to understand the concepts being taught. By briefly showing the child a simple exercise from the manual or program proposed, the clinician may be able to evaluate this understanding. The amount of help a child needs when completing a standardized questionnaire is also sometimes indicative of the degree of support he or she will need in a cognitively based therapy.

Finally, the assessment must proceed in an organized and developmentally sensitive manner that allows adequate time for feedback and treatment-focused discussion with the child and family (Morris, 2004). Usually, an organized assessment includes both structured and unstructured elements. Structured elements (e.g., structured or semistructured interviews, questionnaires) ensure that relevant information is obtained systematically to avoid missing important facts. Unstructured elements (e.g., having a young child play with figures that resemble family members; observing family interactions as the family is interviewed or as members separate for individual interviews) often provide clues to treatment-relevant feelings and relationship issues that are not always acknowledged when children and parents respond to specific questions. In the section "How to Gather Information" I discuss these issues in more detail. *Developmental sensitivity* refers to the need to use age-appropriate language with children, and to tailor the assessment to their developmental abilities. For example, a preschooler may not be able to attend throughout a lengthy family interview, and may be anxious about being interviewed without a parent present. A common compromise is to allow the child to play with toys in the office during most of the family interview but set aside a short time to engage with the child while the parents sit quietly in the background. By contrast, a school-age child is usually invited to engage in the family interview and is expected to tolerate his or her parents leaving the office to allow for an individual interview, unless there is significant separation anxiety. As I mentioned earlier, an adolescent may elect to be interviewed alone before the therapist sees the parents. Flessner (Chapter 2, this volume) discusses developmental considerations in more detail. Providing feedback and discussing treatment options with children and families is discussed further in the section "Communicating Findings and Feedback."

Below are further descriptions on how to gather assessment information, what information to gather, and how to synthesize information and provide feedback.

HOW TO GATHER INFORMATION

The treatment-focused assessment generally consists of interviews, standardized measures, and collateral information from people outside the family. Each of these modalities has strengths and limitations, as summarized in Table 3.1. Therefore, they should be thought of as complementary tools in the assessment process. Assessment requires the presence of the child or adolescent and at least one parent, though it is ideal if all custodial parents can attend because treatment decisions cannot be made without agreement among them. Any nonattending custodial parents should, at minimum, be interviewed by telephone. Some clinicians prefer to see all family members to gain a better perspective on family interactions. As mentioned earlier, it is important to take some time to set the child and family at ease and develop a collaborative relationship with them. Next, the clinician must clearly spell out the order of interviews and administration of measures. If collateral information is to be obtained, most jurisdictions require the parents' written permission to do so and, in the case of older adolescents, the youth's permission as well.

Interviews

When interviewing, the clinician gathers information from two sources: the verbal responses of the interviewee(s) and observations. The nature of the interviews used varies somewhat depending on the child's developmental level, the nature of the presenting problems, and the usual procedures in one's clinic. It is important, however, to have the opportunity to interview children and parents both together and separately. The former allows the clinician to observe typical parent–child and parent–parent interactions. For example, some parents immediately speak for the child, others encourage the child to speak but offer help if the child struggles with a question, and still others order the child to speak and provide little support if he or she is unable to answer a question. Some families do not take turns speaking at all and interrupt each other or become argumentative. Each of these approaches to the family interview reflects different relationship styles that may be relevant to treatment success. Separate interviews are important because perceptions of children's difficulties are known to vary widely by informant (reviewed in Miller, Martinez, Shumka, & Baker, 2014), and some sensitive information is disclosed more readily in private. For example, adolescents are more likely to answer questions about sexuality or substance abuse honestly when their parents are not present; young children

TABLE 3.1. Strengths and Limitations of Various Assessment Modalities

Modality	Strengths	Limitations
Clinical interview	• May reveal treatment motivation, family dynamics, and other issues not necessarily revealed in response to specific questions.	• Not systematic, so risk of missing important facts. • Risk of less vocal members being neglected in family interviews.
Structured/ semistructured interview	• Systematic and thorough, so low risk of missing important facts.	• Can seem rigid or tedious to some interviewees, jeopardizing rapport.
Questionnaires	• Efficient way of screening for, collecting data on, or monitoring targeted symptoms. • Quantifying symptoms allows comparison to norms.	• Differences among informants are common and may make results challenging to interpret.
Behavioral observations	• Provide important information on child's mental status. • May reveal treatment motivation, family dynamics, and other issues not necessarily revealed in response to specific questions.	• One should not assume that observation at a single time point necessarily reflects typical behavior for that child/family.
Collateral information	• Provides environment-specific reports on child behavior. • Facilitates coordination of care among professionals.	• Gathering such information requires family and (in older teens) youth permission.

are more likely to disclose being abused or bullied or witnessing domestic violence when seen individually; parents are more likely to reveal family secrets, marital problems, or personal mental health problems when their child is not present.

As mentioned earlier, the order of interviews is somewhat age-dependent. Adolescents sometimes prefer to be interviewed alone first, although there are exceptions, so it is always worth asking about this preference. Younger children are often interviewed with their parents first and alone later, with the clinician recognizing that the child's participation in the family interview may be limited in very young children. In this case, the child may become tired of talking and play with toys in the office while the clinician interviews the parents. However, this fact should be relayed to the child (i.e., "I will be asking your parents some more questions about you, and you are welcome to play if you like"), so that it is clear that the child is not being deliberately ignored. The clinician may elect to start with the parent interview if the child is very upset or resistant to coming into the office, or if the parent requests it (usually because of a desire to avoid answering certain questions in front of the child).

Parents may have implicit hopes or expectations regarding the outcome of the assessment that are worth exploring at the outset. One could ask, for example, "What do you hope will happen after today's meeting?" or "What do you think would be most helpful for your child?" The answers can help clarify parents' expectations of mental health care and readiness to engage in treatment. Some parents are seeking recommendations rather than ongoing therapy for their child; others expect therapy; and still others bring their child expecting a specific type of treatment. For example, in my own practice, I often see parents who insist that their child needs cognitive-behavioral therapy, even if the child is not a good candidate for this treatment. Talking about these issues openly early in the assessment can often avoid hurt feelings at its conclusion.

There are a number of standardized interviews that address common diagnoses in children, and the choice often depends on the focus of one's clinic (e.g., anxiety clinics often use the Anxiety Disorders Interview Schedule [Silverman & Albano, 2004]; depression-focused clinics may use the Schedule for Affective Disorders and Schizophrenia for School-Age Children [K-SADS; Kaufman, Birmaher, & Brent, 1997]), time constraints, and clinician familiarity with a particular interview, as well as psychometric considerations. In any case, if a structured diagnostic interview is used, it is important to explain the nature of this interview at the outset. For example, the clinician can say, "I will ask you a series of specific questions about problems you may have observed in your child. Later, there will be time to discuss your concerns about (child's name) more generally, but for now please answer only the questions asked." Without such an explanation, the interview process can seem rather cold or lacking in empathy. If an unstructured interview is used, the clinician generally starts with open-ended questions about each person's concerns, then moves on to more specific questions based on their responses. It is important to engage everyone in the room in this process, to avoid neglecting less vocal family members.

In addition to clarifying the diagnosis, interviewers should inquire about risk and protective factors in relation to the child's symptoms, as these will eventually be synthesized into a case formulation. A useful framework for exploring these systematically is provided by George Engel's biopsychosocial model (Engel, 1977), which has recently been broadened to include a fourth, cultural/spiritual dimension (Skinner, 2009). One wants to explore each of the four aspects of the model, its relationship to the child's difficulties, and its evolution over the child's lifetime. Each aspect is discussed further (see the section "Key Information to Gather").

Observations of the child are used to evaluate his or her mental status (reviewed in Tomb, 2008). For example, one can note abnormal movements (e.g., tics); unusual mannerisms (e.g., stereotypies that commonly occur in autism); tense or relaxed facial expression and body posture; and restlessness (common in attention-deficit/hyperactivity disorder [ADHD] and some forms of anxiety) or very slow movements (common in depression). The rate, prosody, and clarity of speech are also important. For example, tone of voice may be unusual in children on the autistic spectrum, mood disorders can slow or accelerate the rate of speech, and articulation problems may result in embarrassment or teasing of the child at school. The child's vocabulary may provide a clue as to cognitive functioning, but it can also reflect shyness, the education level of family members, struggling with a new language, or (in the case of stilted or precocious vocabulary) a lack of awareness of social norms. The child's responses to open-ended questions can vary from silence (in children who are defensive or overly self-conscious) to very detailed, circumstantial descriptions (in children who are either unfocused or anxious to include a lot of information). Losing track of questions entirely or talking about unrelated matters is a very concerning sign, as it may indicate thought disorder. Some defiant children, however, can also provide unusual answers or deliberately avoid answering questions. Distraction by noises or objects in the office is common in children with ADHD; distraction by internal stimuli is common in some children with autism. No single observation is diagnostic, but taken together the observations provide clues to the nature of the child's difficulties.

The emotions expressed during an interview are often worth noting as well. For example, a child may say that something is not upsetting but avert his or her gaze, or shift uncomfortably in his or her chair when asked about the issue. In this case, the child's body language is more informative than his or her words. The predominant emotion and variations in emotional expression are also important. For example, persistent sad or irritable mood may be a sign of depression; mood lability may indicate mania. However, children's emotional reactions to the clinician may also mirror their typical reactions to their parents. Thus, children raised by critical parents may try to appease the clinician; those in conflicted parent–child relationships may be defiant.

One's own emotional reactions to children or parents can also be informative. Although these reactions may relate to personal biases, some children and parents consistently elicit certain reactions from those around them. It is often worth asking oneself, "How would I react if I were the teacher, parent, or peer of this child?"; "How would I react if I had to live with this person as my parent or my spouse?"; or "How would I react if I were a teacher dealing with this parent?" The answers sometimes elucidate interpersonal processes that can contribute to children's problems or ameliorate them.

When two or more people are interviewed together, the clinician may observe interactions among them that reflect aspects of their interpersonal relationships. Such observations may include small gestures that indicate like or dislike of another person, signs of deference to another person, and various communication styles. From these observations, clinicians can learn about family factors relevant to the child's difficulties or to the chances of successful treatment. For example, they may learn about the degree of power various people exert in the family, closeness and trust in family relationships, the ability of family members to respect others' psychological boundaries and points of view, the degree of structure versus flexibility that is usual in the family, people's usual way of handling strong feelings, and the overall problem-solving style of the family. There are many different styles of family interaction that can support or interfere with children's healthy development (reviewed in Skinner, Steinhauer, & Santa Barbara, 1983), and support or interfere with successful treatment. One cautionary note about behavioral observations: All children and families occasionally have an "off day" on which their behavior is atypical. Thus, observations at a single time point may not necessarily reflect usual behavior.

Questionnaires

Questionnaires are often an efficient way to gain structured, normative data about targeted child symptoms and functioning. Measures providing the greatest evidence base for specific disorders and problems (e.g., child anxiety, depression) are described in greater detail in other chapters in this text. If questionnaires are to be part of the assessment, it is helpful to indicate when there will be time to complete them. Usually, parents have time to complete questionnaires during the child interview, and children have time during the parent interview. Young children may need assistance with completion, though, because they may struggle with reading the questions or with understanding some of the concepts, so having a clinician available to clarify questions for them is advisable.

Needless to say, there should be a clear purpose for administering every questionnaire used. When large packages of questionnaires are administered routinely, they can become tiring for children and families, sometimes resulting in invalid responses or adverse effects on the therapeutic relationship. To choose the best questionnaire for a particular situation, consider its main purpose, as well as its psychometric properties and age- and cultural appropriateness. That purpose may include screening for problems when there is limited time to explore these during interviews (e.g., broad-spectrum questionnaires such as the Child Behavior Checklist [Achenbach, 2012] or the Strengths and Difficulties Questionnaire [Goodman, 1997]), augmenting interview information (e.g., some children are reluctant to disclose certain information to interviewers but reveal it on questionnaires), quantifying the degree of difficulty a child experiences in a particular area relative to established norms (e.g., the Multidimensional Anxiety Scale for Children [March, 2004]; the Children's Depression Inventory [Kovacs, 2004]), monitoring change in a particular area over time (and sometimes in relation to treatment), and measuring or comparing symptoms across different environments (e.g., administering an ADHD-specific questionnaire to parents regarding the home environment, and to teachers regarding the school environment).

Questionnaire results must be interpreted in the context of other assessment information, and one cannot make a diagnosis based solely on questionnaires. For example, some defiant or emotionally unaware children deny their symptoms, yet show considerable impairment based on parent or teacher report. In this case, the child may meet diagnostic criteria despite a subclinical questionnaire score. Conversely, an anxious child may endorse many symptoms on a standardized anxiety questionnaire but show little or no impairment in relation to these symptoms. In this case, the child may not meet diagnostic criteria despite scoring in the clinical range on the questionnaire.

When parents and children both complete questionnaires, discrepancies between parent and child report are the rule rather than the exception (reviewed in Miller et al., 2014). Reasons for these discrepancies may include children's or parents' difficulty reading or comprehending the questions (hence possibly the need to assist with completion); children's minimization or exaggeration of their symptoms (because of defensiveness, oppositionality, anxiety, or a desire to avoid or obtain help); parents' minimization or exaggeration of their children's symptoms (for similar reasons); parents' difficulty evaluating certain symptoms because they pertain to the child's inner world; and children's difficulty evaluating certain symptoms because they pertain to others' perceptions of their behavior. Sometimes these discrepancies can be informative. For example, a high level of symptoms by child report relative to parent report can indicate a highly distressed child, a lack of parental empathy for the child's distress, or both. A low level of symptoms by child report relative to parent report can indicate a defensive or oppositional child, an overly anxious parent, or both.

Collateral Information

Information from sources outside the child's immediate family is often important in mental health assessment. One reason for this is that children's behaviors may differ depending on the child's environment. Thus, a child could be quite well mannered at school but difficult to manage at home. Alternatively, some children exhibit abilities in the home environment (where they typically feel safe) that they do not exhibit at school (where they may be more inhibited). Still other children appear competent or even mature when assessed by adults but may struggle with peer interactions. Therefore, it is important to obtain information about the child's functioning at home, at school, and with peers. Teacher observations of the child, both in the classroom and during lunch or break times, are often especially helpful in assessing the impact of a child's mental health problems on academic and social functioning. Attendance records and report cards can provide further information on the child's school functioning. Not all clinicians are able to leave the office to observe children directly in class or on the playground, but if available this opportunity should be pursued in addition to the previously decribed sources of information.

A second reason to obtain collateral information is to coordinate care across multiple professionals. At minimum, it is important to obtain information from the family doctor or pediatrician to ensure that medical etiologies for the child's problems have been ruled out. These physicians may also have valuable insights regarding the child's development or family functioning, often having followed the child for a number of years. If the child's symptoms had a sudden or unusual onset, medical information is particularly important because this pattern may indicate an organic etiology or traumatic event. The new onset of psychotic symptoms always warrants detailed medical investigations.

Talking to previous mental health practitioners is also important to avoid duplicating services and to determine past obstacles to treatment success, so these can be avoided in future. Discussions with current mental health practitioners often avoid "many cooks spoiling the broth" and ensure that the child and family receive consistent messages about how to address problems. Response to past developmental interventions (e.g., occupational therapy, speech therapy) is often relevant to mental health care, so reports about these are important to obtain as well. Developmental problems may also affect self-esteem, academic functioning, and peer relationships, so it is important to gauge their severity and impact on the child's life. Regardless of the professional in question, however, the parents (and, in older adolescents, the teen as well) must consent to one's communication with the other practitioner.

KEY INFORMATION TO GATHER

Information is gathered in order to further the goals of assessment. Therefore, the clinician gathers diagnostic information, and information relevant to case formulation and functional analysis and baselines. Gathering information relevant to diagnosis, functional analysis, and baselines was described earlier, so in this section I describe information needed for a comprehensive case formulation. Since first described by Engel (1977), the biopsychosocial approach to case formulation has been widely used in medicine and mental health care. This model advocates examining a variety of biological, psychological, and social factors that might contribute to the client's presentation or ameliorate symptoms, as well as the interactions among these factors. In the last decade or so, many authors have advocated adding a fourth, cultural/spiritual dimension to this model

(Skinner, 2009). I now describe key information pertaining to each dimension, which is summarized in Table 3.2. Then, I provide an example to illustrate the process of case formulation. A more detailed description of case formulation with children and adolescents can be found in my book *Case Formulation with Children and Adolescents* (2014).

Biological Information

Biological risk and protective factors can be constitutional, related to the effects of illness or substances on the brain, related to the psychological effects of illness, or related to lifestyle.

Constitutional factors may include a family history of mental illness, child temperament, and common genetic or chromosomal differences that affect the developing brain. When inquiring about family history, one should distinguish between psychological problems in the immediate versus extended family. In the immediate family, it is important to determine when the problems occurred in relation to the child's development, in order to assess their impact. For example, maternal depression during a child's infancy may result in disturbances in parent–child attachment (Rutter, 1995), whereas during adolescence, it may result in the child being given developmentally inappropriate responsibilities in the family. Information on the extended family is useful when evaluating the child's risk for specific disorders, and it may also reveal parental fears about the child's future. For example, a parent may fear that a child is "just like his or her schizophrenic aunt/uncle" and will suffer the same fate, and be reassured when provided with accurate information about this risk. Information regarding the child's early temperament may predict risk of certain disorders (e.g., behaviorally inhibited temperament increases risk of social anxiety; reviewed in Cremers & Roelofs, 2016) and also help identify mismatches between parent and child temperament. For instance, an active, rambunctious child might be perceived as difficult and unruly in a family of intellectuals but be perceived in a more positive light in a family in which the parents also have a high activity level. Finally, there are several genetic or chromosomal syndromes that can affect children's psychological development. Down syndrome (also called trisomy 21), fragile X syndrome, and DiGeorge syndrome (also called 22q11.2 deletion syndrome) are common culprits (Skuse & Seigal, 2010), though there are many more. When psychological problems occur in the context of delayed cognitive development, concurrent medical problems, or unusual facial features, these syndromes should be suspected and investigated through genetic consultation. Furthermore, the role of gene–environment interactions in mental health has received research attention recently and will likely be of increasing relevance to case formulation in future. Because of these interactions, some genetic variants are only considered risk factors in the presence of certain environmental risks. For example, the short allele of the serotonin transporter gene is considered a risk factor for depression only in the presence of child maltreatment (Dodge & Rutter, 2011).

When evaluating possible effects of illness or substances on the brain, it is important to obtain both prenatal and postnatal information on the child's health. Inquire about the child's health at birth, pregnancy or birth complications, and exposure to substances during pregnancy (e.g., alcohol, tobacco, street drugs). Fetal alcohol effects are, unfortunately, a particularly common factor contributing to cognitive and behavioral difficulties in children and youth (Ethen, Ramadhani, & Scheuerle, 2008). Delays in early

TABLE 3.2. Common Topics of Inquiry in Case Formulation

<u>Biological aspects</u>

- Family history of mental illness
- Child temperament
- Genetic or chromosomal abnormality (only if cognitive delay, facial difference, concurrent medical problem[s])
- Pregnancy or birth complications
- Substance use during pregnancy
- Developmental delays
- Illnesses or accidents requiring hospitalization (esp. head injury)
- Medications taken regularly
- Substance abuse
- Rapid or atypical onset of psychological symptoms
- Chronic illnesses or medical conditions (e.g., anaphylaxis)
- Disability and age of onset
- Management of illness or disability
- Eating, sleeping, exercise, and media routines
- Aptitudes, abilities, and perceived strengths

<u>Psychological aspects</u>

- Pregnancy planned or unplanned
- Early parent–child attachment, including parental trauma/psychiatric history
- Extended separation(s) from parent/foster care
- Development of independence from parents (e.g., day care, kindergarten)
- Adjustment to sibling(s)
- Peer relationships (preschool to present)
- Self-regulation (preschool to present)
- Adaptation to school entry
- Current cognitive development relative to peers
- Current psychosocial development relative to peers
- Coping style when stressed
- Psychological strengths

<u>Social aspects</u>

- Stressful events preceding symptoms
- Major life changes
- Child relationship with each parent
- Sibling relationships and how managed
- Family conflict
- Parental psychopathology
- Parenting style of each parent, including cultural norms
- Previous parental attempts to help child, including circular interactions
- Previous parental experiences with child mental health professionals
- Child and family activities outside of school; community connections
- Family financial status
- Family experiences of discrimination or other social disadvantage
- Child's daily school experience
- Child's academic performance and school attendance
- Friendships and how close
- Popularity among peers

(continued)

TABLE 3.2. (*continued*)

- Bullying, including cyberbullying
- Home and school communication, and key school personnel
- School supports

Cultural/spiritual aspects

- Family identification with any particular cultural or spiritual tradition
- Parents' understanding of child symptoms in cultural/spiritual context
- Parents' treatment expectations in cultural/spiritual context
- Child agreement–disagreement with parents' understanding and treatment expectations
- Culture-bound syndromes (only if atypical presentation)
- Spiritual/cultural coping practices

---

motor or verbal development are another important clue to possible neurological problems impacting the child's presentation. To screen for current medical problems affecting the child's presentation, inquire about illnesses requiring hospitalization, medications the child requires on a regular basis, substance abuse, and significant head injuries. Also, suspect such problems if psychological symptoms have abrupt onset, associated medical symptoms, an atypical presentation (i.e., one that is inconsistent with previous temperament or developmental course), are unresponsive to environmental change, or occur at night while the child is sleeping (reviewed in Tomb, 2008). For example, a rapid onset of depression in the absence of psychosocial stresses may relate to anemia, low thyroid levels, or infectious mononucleosis; sudden anxiety in a previously well-adjusted child may indicate exposure to a new medication or drug (e.g., certain asthma medications; energy drinks containing caffeine), high thyroid levels, or exposure to a traumatic event.

The psychological effects of illness vary depending on whether illness is acute or chronic, the degree and timing of associated disability, and its predictability. Acute illnesses that are serious and unpredictable are often very anxiety provoking. For example, anaphylactic reactions, asthmatic attacks, and seizures often result in anxious avoidance of situations associated with the event, even if these are low risk (Monga & Manassis, 2006). Disabling conditions have different effects on children depending on when they occur during development (reviewed in Simeonsson & Rosenthal, 2001). Congenital or early-onset disabilities may drastically alter children's developmental course and families' perceptions of their potential, but emotional adaptation to new disabilities can be very challenging for older children. Chronic illness management often becomes a source of stress for families, particularly as children enter adolescence, when they may assert their autonomy by becoming noncompliant with illness management routines.

In some cases, illnesses affect the brain directly but also have psychological sequelae. For instance, a significant head injury may have an adverse effect on a child's ability to regulate emotions and to do schoolwork (direct effects). However, the need to adapt to decreased academic performance may adversely affect self-esteem, and parental attempts to protect the child from further injury may result in parent–child conflict (psychological sequelae).

Lifestyle factors such as eating, sleeping, exercise, and media exposure habits may all contribute to psychological well-being or ill health, so these are worth assessing. If there has been a recent loss of weight or failure to gain weight appropriate to growth, specific questions about eating disorders are also indicated. Mild forms of some psychological problems (e.g., mild anxiety, mild irritability or low mood) may respond to improvements in lifestyle, and such improvements often prevent further physical problems as well. For example, limiting "screen time" and increasing aerobic exercise may improve mood and also decrease the risk of childhood obesity. Thus, assessing lifestyle factors routinely allows clinicians to make recommendations that may improve children's mental and physical health.

Constitutional and lifestyle factors may also represent a source of strength or resilience for some children. Specific talents or abilities, a pleasant appearance, intelligence, being seen as good-natured or easygoing, sociability, or being a desired child can all contribute positively to psychological development, as can a healthy, athletic lifestyle.

Psychological Information

Normative psychological development was discussed by Flessner (Chapter 2, this volume), so the following is a relatively brief overview that is pertinent to assessment.

There are many different theories about children's cognitive and emotional development, but they generally agree that young children are highly dependent on their family environment to support healthy psychological growth. As children mature, school influences, peer influences, and the larger social environment become increasingly salient, but family influences predominate initially. Therefore, inquiring about early family experiences is essential to a thorough assessment. Beginning with prenatal factors, clinicians can ask whether the child was the product of a planned pregnancy, as unplanned pregnancy can both contribute to parent–child relationship difficulty and cause financial, logistical, and emotional problems in the family. Parent–child attachment has been linked to many psychological outcomes (reviewed in Rutter, 1995), so it is worth asking about this factor. Children with suboptimal attachment styles also may have difficulty trusting adults, potentially affecting the therapeutic relationship in treatment. Asking about the parents' experience with the child as an infant and toddler (e.g., "What sort of baby was he or she? How did he or she make you feel as a parent?") is often a good way to broach the subject of attachment. More detailed inquiry is indicated with parents who suffered from psychological problems when the child was young, or who have a personal history of trauma or abuse because these factors often relate to disorganized or suboptimal attachment. Foster care placement(s) in the early years can also adversely affect attachment.

Beyond infancy, children are expected to develop a number of emotional and interpersonal abilities. The ability to cope autonomously when separated from parents, to play both independently and with peers, to adapt to the arrival of a sibling, to follow rules and routines, and to manage transitions and changes in routine are some common preschool challenges. At school age, the need to meet academic requirements and to tolerate comparisons with one's peers during tests and other performance situations is added to this list. A host of cognitive and emotion regulation abilities contribute to school performance. In adolescence, expectations increase further as youth try to develop greater autonomy from their families, develop unique identities, and begin to venture into romantic relationships. Brief questions that may elicit information relevant to psychological development from parents include the following: "Is there anything your child can't or won't do that other children of the same age do?"; "Are there any things you believe your child should be able to do but is not doing?" Sometimes these questions also prompt helpful discussions of realistic or unrealistic parental expectations at different ages. For example, expecting a preschooler consistently to refrain from teasing his or her sibling is probably not realistic. To elicit strengths, one can ask: "What does your child do well or take pride in?"; "What do you admire about your child?"; "What do you like about your child?"; "What do your child's teachers or friends like about your child?"; "What does your child enjoy?"; "What do you enjoy doing with your child?"; "What does your child enjoy doing without you?"

Cognitive development interacts with emotional development, and often aids one's understanding of children's emotional difficulties. For example, a preschooler may not be able to work on a particular behavior daily to obtain a reward on the weekend given his or her limited understanding of time; the recognition that death is permanent occurs around age 8 and sometimes triggers separation anxiety; being ahead or behind one's peers cognitively can affect academic performance and therefore self-esteem. Further details on expected cognitive milestones are reviewed in a book by Berk (2012).

Constitutional factors, cognitive development, and emotional development further interact as children develop styles of coping with adversity or negative emotion. Coping and emotion regulation have been identified as important transdiagnostic elements of assessment (reviewed in Compas, Watson, Reising, & Dunbar, 2014). Modifying coping styles or expanding a child's repertoire of coping strategies is also a common focus of intervention, so some initial assessment of coping style is often worthwhile. For example, anxious children typically engage in avoidant coping, which exacerbates their anxiety; depressed youth often withdraw from social interactions resulting in isolation, which further exacerbates their low mood. Parental responses to the child's attempts to cope may also merit attention, as these responses may affect coping style and amplify or reduce distress. For example, parents of anxious children often inadvertently reinforce avoidant coping (Barrett, Rapee, Dadds, & Ryan, 1996), reducing child distress in the short term but perpetuating avoidant coping, resulting in increased child anxiety over time. Recent findings suggest that disengagement coping (cognitive and behavioral avoidance, denial, wishful thinking) is generally less adaptive than other styles and may therefore merit particular attention (Compas et al., 2014).

In summary, cognitive, emotional, and interpersonal factors, and the interactions among them, can all contribute to children's psychological difficulties, and can all represent sources of psychological strength. It is important to assess these in the context of the child's environment and his or her development.

Social Information

There are myriad social factors that can influence child development, but to succinctly and systematically assess these, it is often helpful to ask about children's home life, school life, peer relationships, activities outside of school, and stressful events. Stressful events include those events that occurred just prior to the onset of symptoms, and events at any point in the child's life that were either perceived as traumatic or represented significant life changes (e.g., a household move, change of school, parental separation, parents' remarriage). I now discuss key points regarding home, school, and peer environments.

Children and parents each provide different perspectives on the home environment. Children are often less guarded than parents about disclosing family conflict and other negative family interactions, as parents may "put their best foot forward" when speaking to the assessing clinician. Asking children about their level of comfort talking to each parent can introduce a discussion of parent–child relationships, including any aspects of parents' behavior that may be frightening or abusive. Conversely, asking about activities the child enjoys with each parent or with the family can introduce a discussion of positive aspects of home life. Most children acknowledge some sibling rivalry, but it is worth inquiring about its extent (e.g., whether any sibling has been significantly hurt) and the parents' typical response (e.g., even-handed vs. blaming one child consistently).

Parents can provide valuable information about factors influencing behavior toward their children, and about challenges the family may be facing within the community and society at large. Elicit information about parental psychopathology (or "trouble with nerves" or "emotional issues" in layman's terms), aspects of parenting perceived to be difficult (both in general and specifically with this child), cultural norms for parental behavior, and similarities or differences between spouses in parenting style. Asking about previous parental attempts to help the child with his or her difficulties often reveals further information about parenting challenges.

With respect to child psychopathology, some typical parenting patterns identified include neglectful/punishing parenting associated with child delinquency (Hoeve et al., 2008); overprotective or overly controlling parenting associated with childhood anxiety disorders (Hudson & Rapee, 2001); and parental rejection or lack of warmth associated with childhood depression (Magaro & Weisz, 2006). However, these patterns do not necessarily originate entirely with parents. Rather, circular interactions often occur in which parent and child behavior become mutually reinforcing. For example, anxious children may appear more vulnerable than the average, eliciting protective behavior from parents, which in turn prevents the child from facing feared situations, resulting in further child anxiety. Identifying such patterns so that alternative behaviors can be found is usually more helpful than blaming either parents or children. Because parents are not always aware of these patterns, they must sometimes be identified through clinician observation rather than questioning (see the earlier section on interviews).

Parental experiences with previous child mental health professionals are often worth exploring. Asking about these experiences can elicit family patterns of help seeking or help rejecting, identify the need to rebuild trust in cases in which a previous professional was perceived as unhelpful or even harmful, and identify other professionals who may still be involved in the child's care. Communicating with current mental health providers is essential to ensuring coordinated care, so clinicians should obtain family permission to do so. If families are reluctant to permit interprofessional communication, their wishes must be respected, but the reasons should be discussed.

Finally, parents can provide valuable information about the family's connection to its community, and about societal influences on the child's mental health. Asking about child and family activities outside school hours can reveal the family's degree of connection to supports such as extended family, religious organizations, the local neighborhood, and recreation programs, as well as adverse circumstances the family faces. For example, some children do not participate in recreation programs because the family cannot afford these, or because it is not safe to walk through the neighborhood to a recreation facility.

Although it is a sensitive topic, asking about family financial circumstances routinely is usually a helpful practice given the strong links between poverty and child mental and physical ill health (Cheng, Johnson, & Goodman, 2016), and the fact that financial problems can interfere with child treatment. It is also important to discuss families' experiences of further social disadvantages due to discrimination because these may influence both the child's presentation and treatment engagement.

Asking children about their experiences at school provides a much richer description of school factors contributing to their presentation than merely perusing a report card. In addition to academic skills, success at school requires abilities such as separating from the home environment without distress; remaining seated and attending to an adult for long periods of time; adapting to the teaching style of different educators; interacting and working cooperatively with diverse peers; maintaining one's composure in a large, possibly noisy classroom; navigating around a large school building (including, in high school, maintaining an organized locker and using a combination lock); eating and using the bathroom outside the home; and knowing and following the rules of common games. The query, "Take me through a regular day at school, starting when you arrive in the morning" is often a helpful way to elicit school-relevant information from children.

Interactions with peers, particularly when starting a new school or new grade, are often a source of worry for children. Ask about both positive and negative aspects of these: Does the child have friends or acquaintances who are supportive? Does the child see friends outside of school, and does the family encourage or restrict such contact? How does the child communicate with friends (e.g., texting, social media, telephone)? Does the child feel well liked or popular? Does the child have peers who are mean or engage in bullying? Also, ask specifically about bullies who use electronic media (i.e., cyberbullying). Children who are socially isolated are more likely to be victimized than others (Crawford & Manassis, 2011), so bullying should be suspected in such children even though they may be reluctant to disclose it during an initial interview.

Last, discussing home and school communication with parents can be very informative. When parents value education and perceive their child's school as supportive, mental health difficulties in the school setting can often be readily addressed. When parents are unhappy with their child's school, this process becomes much more difficult. Asking whether there is one person at the school whom the parents trust is often helpful, as this "point person" may be able to facilitate home and school communication. Also ask about school supports for the child (e.g., access to a school social worker or school nurse when the child is distressed; assistive technology for children with motor or learning difficulties), as enhancing these may improve both the child's school experience and the parents' impression of the school.

Cultural/Spiritual Information

Although often relevant to children's mental health, eliciting cultural/spiritual information can be challenging because clinicians may fear offending families if the discussion is awkward. Some practitioners routinely talk to children and families about the fact that biological, psychological, social, and cultural or spiritual factors are all important to understanding the child's difficulties and will therefore all be discussed. Then, they ask open-ended questions about the cultural/spiritual area, such as "What aspects of your culture or spirituality do you feel connected to?" or "What do you value/not value about the culture you were raised in?" or "What do you find meaningful in your life?" or "What is your spiritual orientation?" Most authors in this field advocate using such open-ended questions to elicit information (Aten, O'Grady, & Worthington, 2012), rather than following a specific line of questioning.

A second way to introduce a discussion of cultural or spiritual factors is to relate them to the presenting problem. In this case, the clinician asks parents to describe their understanding of the child's symptoms based on their culture or spiritual tradition. By showing respectful curiosity about their worldview, the clinician thus increases parents' comfort with talking about cultural or spiritual matters. Then, he or she can explore ideas about causes of symptoms, possible treatments, the role of the child in treatment, the role of the parents in treatment, and the role of the clinician and/or traditional healers, all within the parents' frame of reference. It may also be helpful to clarify the child and family's goals for treatment by asking: "In your culture, how do people think a child should be functioning at this age?" and "In your culture, how do people think a family should be functioning with a child of this age?"

During the individual child interview, inquire about the child's agreement or disagreement with the parents' views. Children can be distressed when torn between traditional and North American worldviews and expectations. Disagreement with parental views is particularly common in adolescence, and may be more tolerated in some cultures than others.

Awareness of cultural concepts of distress (also termed *culture-specific syndromes*) is sometimes helpful. These syndromes are listed in the DSM-5 Appendix (American Psychiatric Association, 2013), together with related DSM-5 conditions and comprise a combination of psychiatric and somatic symptoms that are considered to be a recognizable disease only within a specific culture. They usually have no biochemical basis but may have a specific folk remedy. Inquiring about such syndromes is helpful when a child presents with a cluster of psychiatric and somatic symptoms that are not typical of any particular diagnosis. *Susto* ("fright" or "soul loss" in Central America), *Shenjing Shuairuo* ("weakness of the nervous system" in Mandarin Chinese), and *Kufungisisa* ("thinking too much" in Zimbabwe) are some examples cited in DSM-5.

On the other hand, some children benefit from coping strategies that emerge from their cultural or spiritual backgrounds. Pargament, Koenig, and Perez (2000) have summarized key coping strategies that emerge from spiritual or religious worldviews. These include benevolent reappraisal (the stressor has benefits in a spiritual context); collaborative religious coping (problem solving with God); seeking support from God or one's religious community; religious rituals to purify oneself or mark important life transitions; providing spiritual support to others; and using belief to help one forgive oneself or others. In addition, practices such as prayer and meditation are perceived as helpful in many traditions. Cross-cultural spiritual values such as compassion, gratitude, forgiveness, and hope can also contribute to mental health.

SYNTHESIZING INFORMATION TO DEVELOP A CASE FORMULATION

Parry, Roth, and Fonagy (2005) suggest that evidence-based practice be based on clinical practice guidelines and applied using clinical judgment that is based on a clear case formulation. The case formulation is a dynamic set of hypotheses that provide one possible explanation for the child's difficulties (the "explanatory model"), which can be tested and revised (reviewed in Manassis, 2014). Treatment response or lack of response tests these hypotheses, supporting or disconfirming them. Hypotheses can also be updated as a result of obtaining new information about the child, changes in the child's environment, and developmental changes. In addition to providing testable hypotheses, the case formulation can also enrich one's understanding of the child's difficulties, and aid engagement with the child and family when this understanding is shared.

The process of case formulation usually begins with a table listing risk and protective factors in each of the four content areas described earlier (biological, psychological, social, cultural/spiritual), organized chronologically (see Table 3.3). Factors in the remote past are listed first, followed by those in the recent past (often including events or changes that may have triggered the current presentation), and finally those affecting the child presently. Present factors merit particular attention, as these factors may support or interfere with treatment.

Next, the table of risk and protective factors must be converted into a coherent story of how the child's difficulties developed. This is done by thinking about which risk and protective factors may be linked, both within and between content areas. For example, within the social content area, parents who are very protective (a potential risk factor for anxiety disorders) may limit their children's access to peer situations outside the family, resulting in social isolation (a further social risk factor for internalizing problems). If

TABLE 3.3. Risk and Protective Factors for S

Content area	Biological	Psychological	Social	Cultural/spiritual
Remote past	• Good physical health Cautious temperament • Maternal depression	• Father distant • Insecure mother–child attachment	• Product of unplanned pregnancy • Witnessing domestic violence	• Family isolation from community supports
Recent past	• Intelligence • Medical investigations reinforce sick role	• Enmeshed/caregiving relationship with mother • Somatizing negative emotion ("stomachaches") • Shyness/anxious traits	• Academic success Isolation from peers • One close friend	"
Present	"	• Further somatization • Perception of self as "sick" becoming entrenched	• Friend moves away • Bullying • School avoidance • Maternal attention to "sickness" reinforces it	"

social isolation is severe, it may also interfere with the development of age-appropriate social skills (a psychological risk factor). If a family receives support from its religious community (a cultural/spiritual factor), and this support results in reduced parenting stress and improved parent–child relationships (a social factor), this is an example of linked protective factors.

It is important to consider which links among factors are very likely, and which ones are more speculative. For instance, when a child performs poorly at school due to inattention and there is a history of ADHD in the immediate family, the family history (biological risk factor) and the school failure (social risk factor) are probably linked. On the other hand, if an adolescent girl shows cognitive distortions that suggest depressive thinking (psychological risk factor) shortly after entering puberty (biological risk factor), pubertal hormones are not necessarily causing her depression, although this possibility may be considered among other hypotheses.

Finally, the case formulation "story" must be written in a manner that makes sense to the clinician, and sometimes edited for presentation to various audiences (see the section on communicating findings and feedback). Table 3.3 shows an example of how to list risk and protective factors for an anxious 10-year-old girl, and the corresponding case formulation is provided below:

S was a bright and healthy albeit cautious child. She was born into a troubled marriage that had been prompted by her unplanned arrival. Her father was distant and her parents often fought, sometimes resulting in violence. Witnessing domestic violence may have predisposed S to subsequent anxiety. Her mother struggled with significant depression. Her depression coupled with the unplanned nature of the pregnancy probably resulted in an insecure attachment relationship with S.

As she grew older, S provided her mother with emotional support. This "caregiving" pattern is common with insecure attachment, but the fact that the family was isolated from the community (leaving her mother with nobody else to confide in) probably contributed as well. Given her temperament, history of witnessed violence, and inability to obtain comfort from either parent, S became increasingly anxious and developed stomachaches when she was emotionally upset. She had a series of medical investigations for these stomachaches, potentially reinforcing her perception of herself as "sick," but all results were within normal limits.

At school, S did well academically but was shy around peers (given her anxious tendencies). She had one close friend but became the target of bullies after her friend moved away (isolated, anxious children are easily victimized; Crawford & Manassis, 2011). Likely in response to this stress, S's stomach pains returned and were worse than ever. She began avoiding school because of these pains and stayed at home with her mother, who insisted that her daughter had an undiagnosed medical problem. Her mother's attention to the symptoms and support of her daughter's belief that they were caused by a medical problem likely reinforced S's perception of herself as "sick," perpetuating her tendency to show somatic symptoms in response to anxiety and other distress.

Interestingly, a quick review limited to S's current difficulties might lead to the simplistic conclusion: "This child is avoiding school because she was bullied." The resulting bullying-focused intervention would be unlikely to succeed in returning S to school and to healthy, age-appropriate functioning. Case formulation reveals a more complex developmental picture and the need for a more detailed plan of intervention.

COMMUNICATING FINDINGS AND FEEDBACK

Communicating assessment results to families effectively takes time. Usually, a verbal feedback session occurs and a written report follows. Some clinicians send the written report only to the referring professional, not to the family. However, by the end of a long assessment appointment, many children and families are fatigued and emotionally stressed, so verbal feedback is often forgotten. Providing a written report to families, or at least a written summary of key recommendations, is therefore advisable. I discuss verbal and written feedback in turn.

Verbal feedback must be presented in language that is understandable to everyone in the room. In young children, providing information separately in child-friendly language may therefore be helpful. Older children can participate in feedback sessions with their parents, though it is important to ask specifically for the child's reaction to what is said in order to avoid focusing exclusively on the adults in the room. Adolescents sometimes prefer to know ahead of time what their parents will be told to ensure that certain issues will remain confidential, and as long as there is no risk of harm from doing so (e.g., failing to disclose suicidal ideation cannot be condoned) this wish can be respected.

Importantly, the feedback session should be a dialogue. In other words, the clinician presents his or her impressions of the problems and appropriate treatment, then invites the child and family to respond to these ideas. Responses may include asking clarifying questions, providing additional information that was not previously considered relevant, challenging the clinician's interpretation of the problems, or expressing views on various treatments. The clinician should take the time to address all issues raised, even if an additional appointment is required to do so. Rushing the feedback session can result in misunderstandings that undermine subsequent treatment.

Families are sometimes reluctant to challenge "experts," resulting in low participation in the feedback session. In this case, it is sometimes helpful to get them to summarize what they have heard in order to determine comprehension and to look for any signs of discomfort. Signs of discomfort may reflect hidden disagreement with the clinician. Routinely asking, "Is there anything that I have missed or misunderstood?" is another helpful practice that often clarifies families' perceptions of what the clinician has said.

Verbal feedback by clinicians usually includes a restatement of the presenting problem(s), an attempt to link the presenting problem(s) to one or more diagnoses or treatable conditions (e.g., negative, attention-seeking behavior is not a diagnosis, but it can certainly be treated with behavior modification), a case formulation, and an attempt to link the diagnoses and case formulation to an evidence-based treatment plan. If the assessing clinician will also be providing treatment, a discussion of treatment expectations may also be included (e.g., goals of treatment, time frame, what happens when treatment ends, expectations of change, role of child/parent/therapist in treatment, logistics of appointments). Finally, a discussion of how the findings will be documented includes asking about any nonessential details the family does not want included in the report, and communication with other professionals involved in the child's mental health care. Permission forms may also need to be signed to allow for such communication.

It is often helpful to think ahead of time about how best to organize and present all of this information, so that the presentation is both coherent and respectful of child and family perspectives. Emphasizing the multifactorial nature of most mental health problems reduces the chances of families feeling blamed for the child's difficulties. Emphasizing the child's and family's strengths encourages a hopeful attitude toward treatment. Providing a rationale for treatment, including the evidence for and against various treatment options, is educational and encourages frank discussion. If families do not agree with the treatment(s) proposed, the assessing clinician can then explore reasons for this disagreement and help the family evaluate alternatives.

Written reports can be sent to both families and referring professionals if they are worded clearly and avoid discipline-specific jargon. Alternatively, some clinicians send summaries of recommendations to families and more thorough reports to referring professionals. In either case, reports should avoid language that might be seen as pejorative, provide clear diagnostic information, and emphasize elements of the case formulation that are relevant to treatment and for which there is strong evidence.

Busy referring professionals sometimes skip to the last page of the report to view recommendations, so it is particularly important that these be clear. Lengthy descriptions of possible interventions can be difficult to interpret and implement, so a concise list is often helpful. This list should spell out recommendations for the child, the parent(s), and the referring professional, as well as describe the treatment proposed by the clinician. For example, in an anxious child, cognitive-behavioral therapy may be the evidence-based treatment recommended, but before starting, the child may be asked to write down his or her worries or anxious situations, while the parents are asked to read a relevant parenting book and the referring professional is asked to rule out hyperthyroidism as a contributing factor.

USING FINDINGS TO PLAN TREATMENT

Treatment planning for various disorders is discussed in detail in subsequent chapters of this volume, but principles that relate to assessment and cut across diagnoses are outlined here.

Diagnoses usually direct clinicians to corresponding evidence-based treatments. Case formulations and functional analyses, on the other hand, often help clinicians identify factors likely to moderate the success of those treatments and therefore require additional clinical attention. For example, a functional analysis of parent–child interactions in the early morning may reveal factors likely to interfere with the evidence-based treatment of anxiety-related school avoidance. Conversely, protective factors identified in the case formulation (e.g., athletic ability, academic success, positive peer relationships, trusting relationship with at least one adult, absence of significant family conflict) may enhance the benefits of evidence-based treatment.

Many children present with several diagnoses or mental health problems, so several interventions may need to be planned. Urgent issues such as bullying or abuse usually need to be addressed before safe, effective evidence-based treatment can occur. Other issues can be addressed either sequentially or concurrently. Modular treatments and transdiagnostic approaches are increasingly allowing concurrent treatment of several issues (reviewed in Ehrenreich-May & Chu, 2014; see Harvey, Chapter 17, this volume). When planning interventions for various problems, it is often helpful to consider:

- Which problem is causing the most impairment?
- Which problem is easiest/most feasible to start with?
- Which problems can be addressed concurrently?
- Which problem is the child motivated to start with?
- Which problem are the parents motivated to start with?
- Which protective factors could be strengthened?

Highly impairing problems need to be addressed at some point but may be challenging to start with. When problems are addressed concurrently, it is important to make sure that children and families are not overburdened with multiple interventions. When children and parents are motivated to work on different problems, it is important to discuss the differences, so that a compromise can be reached and both parties' priority problems are addressed eventually. Protective factors are often neglected, but they may be important in enhancing treatment gains and/or maintaining children's and parents' optimism during a course of treatment. For example, a depressed teen who cannot focus on schoolwork but still can contribute to a school club or activity and be recognized for that contribution may retain some hope of improvement.

Finally, it is important to remember that assessment results are hypotheses about the case, and may need to be revised in future. This does not mean that the initial assessment was inadequate. Rather, new information may emerge that was not disclosed initially, circumstances of the child's life may change, unexpected responses to intervention may suggest a need to reconceptualize the case, or developmental change may alter a child's symptoms or level of functioning over time. Astute clinicians revisit baselines periodically to monitor children's progress after assessment and are willing to reevaluate their ideas about a case when unexpected changes occur. Thus, they progressively develop a more accurate and meaningful understanding of their young clients' difficulties over time.

REFERENCES

Achenbach, T. (2012). Child Behavior Checklist (for 6–18). Available at *www.aseba.org*.
American Psychiatric Association. (2013). *Diagnostic and statistical manual of mental disorders* (5th ed.). Arlington, VA: Author.
Aten, J. D., O'Grady, K. A., & Worthington, E. L., Jr. (Eds.). (2012). *The psychology of religion and spirituality for clinicians: Using research in your practice.* New York: Routledge.
Barrett, P. M., Rapee, R. M., Dadds, M. M., & Ryan, S. M. (1996). Family enhancement of cognitive style in anxious and aggressive children. *Journal of Abnormal Child Psychology, 24*(2), 187–203.
Berk, L. E. (2012). *Child development.* London: Pearson.
Cheng, T. L., Johnson, S. B., & Goodman, E. (2016). Breaking the intergenerational cycle of disadvantage: The three generation approach. *Pediatrics, 137*(6, Pt. 2), e20152467.
Compas, B. E., Watson, K. H., Reising, M. M., & Dunbar, J. P. (2014). Stress and coping in child and adolescent psychopathology. In J. Ehrenreich-May & B. C. Chu (Eds.), *Transdiagnostic treatments for children and adolescents: Principles and practice* (pp. 35–58). New York: Guilford Press.

Crawford, M., & Manassis, K. (2011). Anxiety, social skills, friendship quality, and peer victimization: An integrated model. *Journal of Anxiety Disorders, 25,* 924–931.

Cremers, H. R., & Roelofs, K. (2016). Social anxiety disorder: A critical overview of neurocognitive research. *WIREs Cognitive Science, 7*(4), 218–232.

Dodge, K. A., & Rutter, M. (Eds.). (2011). *Gene–environment interactions in developmental psychopathology.* New York: Guilford Press.

Ehrenreich-May, J., & Chu, B. C. (Eds.). (2014). *Transdiagnostic treatments for children and adolescents: Principles and practice.* New York: Guilford Press.

Engel, G. L. (1977). The need for a new medical model: A challenge for biomedicine. *Science, 196,* 129–136.

Ethen, M. K., Ramadhani, T. A., & Scheuerle, A. E. (2008). Alcohol consumption by women before and during pregnancy. *Maternal and Child Health Journal, 13*(2), 274–285.

Goodman, R. (1997). The Strengths and Difficulties Questionnaire: A research note. *Journal of Child Psychology and Psychiatry, 38,* 581–586.

Hoeve, M., Blokland, A., Dubas, J. S., Loeber, R., Gerris, J. R. M., & van der Laan, P. H. (2008). Trajectories of delinquency and parenting styles. *Journal of Abnormal Child Psychology, 36*(2), 223–235.

Hudson, J. L., & Rapee, R. M. (2001). Parent–child interactions and the anxiety disorders: An observational analysis. *Behaviour Research and Therapy, 39,* 1411–1427.

Kaufman, J., Birmaher, B., & Brent, D. (1997). Schedule for Affective Disorders and Schizophrenia for School-Age Children—Present and Lifetime Version (K-SADS-PL): Initial reliability and validity data. *Journal of the American Academy of Child and Adolescent Psychiatry, 36,* 980–988.

Kovacs, M. (2004). *Children's Depression Inventory 2.* Toronto, ON, Canada: Multi-Health Systems.

Magaro, M. M., & Weisz, J. R. (2006). Perceived control mediates the relation between parental rejection and youth depression. *Journal of Abnormal Child Psychology, 34,* 867–876.

Manassis, K. (2009). *Cognitive behavioral therapy with children: A guide for the community practitioner.* New York: Routledge.

Manassis, K. (2014). *Case formulation with children and adolescents.* New York: Guilford Press.

March, J. S. (2004). *Multidimensional Anxiety Scale for Children.* Toronto, ON, Canada: Multi-Health Systems.

Miller, L. D., Martinez, Y. J., Shumka, E., & Baker, H. (2014). Multiple informant agreement of child, parent, and teacher ratings of child anxiety within community samples. *Canadian Journal of Psychiatry, 59*(1), 34–39.

Monga, S., & Manassis, K. (2006). Treating childhood anxiety in the presence of life-threatening anaphylactic conditions. *Journal of the American Academy of Child and Adolescent Psychiatry, 45,* 1007–1010.

Morris, T. L. (2004). Developmentally sensitive assessment of social anxiety. *Cognitive and Behavioral Practice, 11,* 13–28.

Pargament, K. I., Koenig, H. G., & Perez, L. M. (2000). The many methods of religious coping: Development and initial validation of the RCOPE. *Journal of Clinical Psychology, 56,* 519–543.

Parry, G., Roth, A., & Fonagy, P. (2005). Psychotherapy research, health policy, and service provision. In A. Roth & P. Fonagy (Eds.), *What works for whom?: A critical review of psychotherapy research* (2nd ed., pp. 43–65). New York: Guilford Press.

Prochaska, J. O., & DiClemente, C. C. (1984). Self change processes, self efficacy and decisional balance across five stages of smoking cessation. *Progress in Clinical Biological Research, 56,* 131–140.

Rutter, M. (1995). Clinical implications of attachment concepts: Retrospect and prospect. *Journal of Child Psychology and Psychiatry, 36*(4), 549–571.

Silverman, W. K., & Albano, A. M. (2004). *Anxiety Disorders Interview Schedule (ADIS-IV) Child/parent clinician manual*. Boulder, CO: Graywind.

Simeonsson, R. J., & Rosenthal, S. L. (Eds.). (2001). *Psychological and developmental assessment: Children with disabilities and chronic conditions*. New York: Guilford Press.

Skinner, H. A., Steinhauer, P. D., & Santa Barbara, J. (1983). The Family Assessment Measure. *Canadian Journal of Community Mental Health, 2*, 91–105.

Skinner, W. (2009). Approaching concurrent disorders. In *Treating concurrent disorders: A guide for counsellors* (pp. xi–xvii). Toronto, ON, Canada: Centre for Addiction and Mental Health.

Skuse, D., & Seigal, A. (2010). Behavioral phenotypes and chromosomal disorders. In M. Rutter, D. Bishop, D. Pine, S. Scott, J. S. Stevenson, E. A. Taylor, & A. Thapar (Eds.), *Rutter's child and adolescent psychiatry* (5th ed.). New York: Wiley-Blackwell.

Tomb, D. A. (2008). *Psychiatry* (7th ed.). Philadelphia: Lippincott, Williams & Wilkins.

Vance, H. B. (1997). *Psychological assessment of children: Best practices for school and clinical settings* (2nd ed.). New York: Wiley.

Waguespack, A., Vaccaro, T., & Continere, L. (2006). Functional behavioral assessment and intervention with emotional/behaviorally disordered students: In pursuit of state of the art. *International Journal of Behavioral Consultation and Therapy, 4*(2), 463–474.

Wightman, J., Julio, F., & Virues-Ortega, J. (2014). Advances in the indirect, descriptive, and experimental approaches to the functional analysis of problem behavior. *Psicothema, 26*(2), 186–192.

PART II

PSYCHOLOGICAL DISORDERS IN YOUTH

Depression and Suicidality

Jennifer Wolff, Elisabeth Frazier, Stephanie Davis,
Rachel D. Freed, Christianne Esposito-Smythers,
Richard Liu, and Anthony Spirito

D epression is one of the most common youth psychiatric conditions in the United States (Copeland, Shanahan, Costello, & Angold, 2011; Kessler et al., 2012; Merikangas et al., 2010). The past 30 years of research indicate that depression can be effectively treated with psychotherapy. While there are a number of psychotherapy treatment options available, cognitive-behavioral therapy (CBT) is the most widely researched approach to treating depression in youth. In this chapter, we provide an overview of the diagnosis of depression and the rationale underlying the use of CBT for the treatment of depression and *suicidality* (defined as suicidal thoughts and suicide attempts) in youth. We then briefly review the literature on assessment and treatment of depressed and suicidal youth, and finally outline a description of the core cognitive, affective, and behavioral techniques used in CBT treatment for this population.

THE DSM-5 DEFINITION OF DEPRESSION

According to the fifth edition of the *Diagnostic and Statistical Manual of Mental Disorders* (DSM-5; American Psychiatric Asssociation, 2013), major depressive disorder (MDD) in children and adolescents is characterized by five or more of the following symptoms most of the day, nearly every day, for at least 2 weeks: depressed or irritable mood; loss of interest or pleasure in activities; appetite disturbance; sleep disturbance; psychomotor agitation or retardation; fatigue or loss of energy; poor concentration or difficulty making decisions; feelings of worthlessness or excessive guilt; and recurrent thoughts of death, suicidal ideation, or a suicide attempt. At least one of the five symptoms must be depressed or irritable mood, or loss of interest or pleasure in activities, and the symptoms must cause clinically significant distress or impairment.

DSM-5 also includes a new category, persistent depressive disorder. which encompasses more chronic forms of depression, including chronic major depression and what was previously referred to as dysthymia in DSM-IV (American Psychiatric Association, 2000). Persistent depressive disorder in youth is characterized by a depressed mood occurring for most of the day, more days than not, for at least 1 year (2 years for adults). Patients may not have had any periods lasting longer than 2 months in which they were depression-free and must have two or more of the following: appetite disturbance, sleep disturbance, fatigue or loss of energy, poor concentration or difficulty making decisions, low self-esteem, or feelings of hopelessness. Henceforth, we use the term *depression* to refer to MDD and persistent depressive disorder.

PREVALENCE AND COURSE

Depression affects approximately 3% of youth under age 13, and rates increase as youth enter adolescence (Costello, Copeland, & Angold, 2011; Costello, Erkanli, & Angold, 2006). Among adolescents surveyed in the National Comorbidity Survey–Adolescent Supplement, 11.7% met lifetime criteria for depression, and the 12-month and 30-day prevalence rates were 8.2 and 2.6%, respectively (Costello, Mustillo, Erkanli, Keeler, & Angold, 2003; Kessler et al., 2012). Beginning around age 13, girls become twice as likely as boys to experience depression, and this gender gap persists throughout adulthood (Hankin & Abramson, 2001; Merikangas et al., 2010).

The average depressive episode in youth is 7–9 months (Birmaher et al., 1996). In the Treatment for Adolescents with Depression Study (TADS; TADS Team, 2005), among treatment-seeking adolescents, median episode duration was about 10 months. High rates of relapse are observed in both treated and untreated youth populations, with 34–75% experiencing relapse 1–5 years after a first episode (Kennard, Emslie, Mayes, & Hughes, 2006).

Epidemiological studies show that as many as 75% of adolescents with lifetime depression experience severe impairment and/or distress (Merikangas et al., 2010). Youth-onset depression also tends to continue past adolescence and is associated with elevated risk of psychosocial impairment in adulthood (Birmaher, Arbelaez, & Brent, 2002; Harrington, Fudge, Rutter, Pickles, & Hill, 1990; Lewinsohn, Rohde, Klein, & Seeley, 1999; Weissman, Wolk, Goldstein, et al., 1999). Childhood onset is associated with a particularly pernicious course, including higher morbidity, severity, and impairment, compared to adolescent onset (Korczak & Goldstein, 2009; Weissman, Wolk, Wickramaratne, et al., 1999). Almost one-fourth (24%) of chronically depressed adolescents endorse a history of suicide attempts (Asarnow et al., 2011). The risk for suicide appears to persist into adulthood, such that more than 25% of individuals with prepubertal-onset depression, and 50% of individuals with adolescent-onset depression, endorsed at least one suicide attempt when followed up over 10–15 years (Weissman, Wolk, Goldstein, et al., 1999; Weissman, Wolk, Wickramaratne, et al., 1999).

COMMON COMORBID CONDITIONS

Youth with depression often also have one or more comorbid conditions (Angold, Costello, & Erkanli, 1999; TADS Team, 2005). The most common comorbid disorders are anxiety, disruptive behavior (i.e., conduct and oppositional defiant disorders), substance use, and attention-deficit/hyperactivity disorders (Biederman, Faraone, Mick, & Lelon, 1995; Rohde, Lewinsohn, & Seeley, 1991; TADS Team, 2005). The presence of comorbid disorder(s) is associated with higher recurrence, longer episode duration, worse treatment response, poorer functioning, and higher rates of suicide attempts (Birmaher et al., 1996; Lewinsohn, Rohde, & Seeley, 1995).

ETIOLOGICAL/CONCEPTUAL MODEL(S) OF DEPRESSION

Twin and adoption studies provide evidence that genetic factors account for 31–42% of the variance in the transmission of depression (Sullivan, Neale, & Kendler, 2000). Nonetheless, the etiology of depression is widely acknowledged as a complex interplay of biological and psychosocial factors.

Stress plays an important role in the onset and maintenance of depression (Hammen, 2009), and depressive episodes in adults and youth are often preceded by stressful life events (Grant et al., 2006). Interpersonal stressors may be especially salient, particularly among girls (Rudolph & Hammen, 1999; Rudolph et al., 2000); and early loss or maltreatment is strongly associated with the development and course of depression (Kendler, Gardner, & Prescott, 2002). However, the link between stress and depression appears to be moderated by certain (interrelated) vulnerabilities, including biological (e.g., genetic, neuroendocrine, hormonal), cognitive (e.g., dysfunctional attitudes, negative cognitive style, ruminative response style), personal (e.g., poor coping and affect regulation skills, temperament), and interpersonal (e.g., insufficient support, poor attachment, family conflict) factors. A full review of these factors is beyond the scope of this chapter, but we highlight some relevant findings below.

First, genetic association studies have implicated particular gene variations (e.g., serotonin transporter gene and brain-derived neurotrophic factor polymorphisms) that may interact with negative environmental factors to influence the expression of depression (Brown & Harris, 2008), likely via effects on stress response (Levinson, 2006). Other biological mechanisms related to abnormalities in stress response (e.g., increased hypothalamic–pituitary–adrenal [HPA] axis reactivity, altered autonomic nervous system functioning) also show associations with depression in the context of negative events (Pariante & Lightman, 2008; Rottenberg, 2007). Finally, researchers have identified certain anomalies in brain structure (e.g., brain asymmetry, cortical thinning—Peterson et al., 2009; Rao et al., 2010; Tomarken, Dichter, Garber, & Simien, 2004) and function (e.g., disruptions in the processing of reward and loss—Forbes & Dahl, 2012; Gotlib et al., 2010) associated with depression vulnerability.

Second, cognitive vulnerability factors, particularly in interaction with negative events, also play a salient role in the development and maintenance of depression (Abela & Hankin, 2008; Lakdawalla, Hankin, & Mermelstein, 2007). Cognitive theories propose that maladaptive thinking patterns influence the ways in which individuals attend to, interpret, and respond to negative life events. Indeed, the association between stress and negative cognitions predict both depression onset and increases in symptoms in youth (Carter & Garber, 2011), particularly among adolescents (Lakdawalla et al., 2007).

Third, individual differences in temperament and personality are related to the emergence of depression (Compas, Connor-Smith, Saltzman, Thomsen, & Wadsworth, 2001; Kovacs & Yaroslavsky, 2014). Both depressed youth and those at risk may be less successful at regulating negative arousal, such that they have more limited repertoires of emotion regulation strategies, use less effective strategies, or fail to use strategies within their repertoires, and have lower self-efficacy regarding the effectiveness of these strategies and their ability to implement them (see Compas et al., 2001; Yap, Allen, & Sheeber, 2007). Studies further suggest that use of adaptive coping strategies (e.g., strategies aimed at problem solving or increasing positive emotions) may buffer the effects of stress, thereby offering protection against the onset of depression, whereas the use of maladaptive strategies (e.g., avoidance, self-blame, isolation) in the face of stress may hasten depressive symptoms (Compas et al., 2001).

Fourth, interpersonal processes have been shown to impact onset and maintenance of depression in youth. For example, research shows that low peer acceptance and peer victimization are associated with, and may contribute to, the development of youth depression (Platt, Cohen Kadosh, & Lau, 2013). Abundant evidence links youth depression with exposure to adverse family environments characterized by conflict/hostility, criticism, harsh discipline, poor communication, and limited support, warmth, attachment, and validation from caregivers (McLeod, Weisz, & Wood, 2007; Sheeber, Hops, & Davis, 2001). In fact, disruptions in family environment are often cited as an important mechanism of intergenerational transmission of depression (e.g., Goodman & Gotlib, 1999). Adolescence may be a time in which interpersonal/social relationships are particularly salient, especially for girls, which may partly explain the emergent sex differences during the transition to adolescence (Cyranowski, Frank, Young, & Shear, 2000; Prinstein, Borelli, Cheah, Simon, & Aikins, 2005).

EVIDENCE-BASED TREATMENTS FOR DEPRESSION IN CHILDREN AND ADOLESCENTS

The Society of Clinical Child and Adolescent Psychology (APA Division 53) reviews effective treatments for youth, categorizes them into various levels of empirical support (Southam-Gerow & Prinstein, 2014; see *www.effectivechildtherapy.com*). The overall effect size of psychotherapy for youth depression is estimated at 0.34 (Weisz, McCarty, & Valeri, 2006) and both CBT and interpersonal psychotherapy (IPT) are considered well-established treatments that have the most empirical support for treating depressed youth. Table 4.1 provides a summary of treatment studies in youth with depressive spectrum disorders.

Cognitive-Behavioral Therapy

CBT emphasizes the relationship between thoughts, feelings, and behaviors, with the premise that modifying one's thoughts and/or behaviors can improve one's mood. CBT

TABLE 4.1. Overview of Interventions for Depressed Adolescents Tested in Randomized Clinical Trials

Study	Sample	Demographics	Therapists and fidelity	Treatment conditions	Depression variables	Depression results	Level
Individual CBT							
			Stand-alone interventions				
Brent et al. (1997)	United States; recruited from psychiatric clinic; 100% MDD	N = 107 Age: 13–16 Gender: 75.7% female Race: 83.2% white	CBT: master's-level therapists with median of 10 years experience; sessions videotaped; weekly supervision; therapy sessions rated for fidelity	CBT (n = 37) Sessions: M = 12.1 (SD = 3.6) SBFT (n = 35) Sessions: M = 10.7 (SD = 4.7) NST (n = 35) Sessions: M = 11.2 (SD = 4.2)	Self: BDI Clinician: KSADS-P/E; C-GAS	CBT showed a lower rate of MDD at the end of treatment compared to NST and higher rate of remission/more rapid rate of relief compared to SBFT and NST.	I
Group CBT							
Clarke et al. (1999)	United States; recruited through announcements to health professionals and school counselors and through advertisements; 76% MDD, 12.5% DD, 11.5% comorbid MDD and DD	N = 96 Age: 14–18 Gender: 71% female Race: no data presented	CBT: advanced graduate psychology or social work students, master's or doctoral-level clinicians; weekly supervision; sessions videotaped; sessions randomly selected and rated for compliance by experienced group leader	CBT (n = 37) Sessions: M = 14.1 (SD = 1.7) CBT + parent (n = 32) Sessions: Mothers = 7.9 (range = 6–9) Fathers = 5.8 (range = 3–8) WL (n = 27)	Self: BDI Parent: CBCL Clinician: HAM-D, K-SADS, LIFE, GAF	CBT with and without parent intervention showed improvements in depression per youth, but not parent report; mixed findings per clinician report. CBT-only group showed significant improvements in global functioning per clinician report. No significant effect from addition of parent group.	I
Clarke et al. (2002)	United States; recruited from hospital records; 93% MDD; 3% DD	N = 88 Age: 13–18 Gender: 69% female Race: 9% minority	CBT + HMO: master's-level therapists; all sessions audiotaped; fidelity ratings completed by senior supervisor	CBT + HMO (n = 71) Sessions: M = 10.1 (SD not reported) HMO only (n = 47)	CES-D; HAM-D; K-SADS-PL; GAF; CBCL	No significant differences between CBT and usual HMO case per self-, parent, and clinician report.	II

(continued)

TABLE 4.1. *(continued)*

Study	Sample	Demographics	Therapists and fidelity	Treatment conditions	Depression variables	Depression results	Level
Rohde et al. (2004)	United States; recruited from county juvenile justice department; 100% MDD + CD	N = 93 Age: 13–17 Gender: 48% female Race: 80.6% white, 1.1% AA, 3.2% Native American, 1.1% Asian, 4.3% Hispanic, 9.7% other ethnicity	CBT: master's-level or higher mental health provider and college/ high school student assistant LS: high school teachers and adult assistants Fidelity: all sessions videotaped; sessions randomly selected and rated for adherence and competence by authors	CBT (n = 45) Sessions: M = 8.4 (SD = 5.7) LS (n = 48) Sessions: M = 7.6 (SD = 5.7)	Self: BDI-II, SAS-SR Clinician: HAM-D, KSADS-E, LIFE	CWD-A showed significantly higher depression recovery rates (39 vs. 19%) per self- but not parent report. Mixed results based on clinician ratings.	I
IPT–A							
Mufson et al. (1999)	United States; recruited from depression psychiatric clinic; 100% MDD	N = 48 Age: 12–18 Gender: 73% female Race: 71% Hispanic	IPT-A: Licensed clinical psychologist, child psychiatrists, master's-level psychologists with 10 years experience; all training and study sessions videotaped; weekly supervision; fidelity ratings completed	IPT-A (n = 24) Sessions: M = 9.8 (SD not reported) TAU (n = 24) Sessions: M = 2.8 (SD not reported)	BDI; SAS-SR; C-GAS; DISC; HAM-D; K-SADS-E	Compared to control, IPT-A group showed more significant decreases in depression and improved functioning (per self- and clinician report); IPT-A group showed significantly more recovery than control (IPT-A: 74%; control: 46%)	I
Mufson et al. (2004)	United States; referred for mental health services; 100% MDD	N = 63 Age: 12–18 Gender: 84% female Race: 71% Hispanic	IPT-A: doctoral-level psychologist and school-based social workers; weekly supervision; treatment adherence and competence checklists completed by supervisors	IPT-A (n = 34) Sessions: M = 10.5 (SD not reported) TAU (n = 29) Sessions: M = 7.9 (SD not reported)	BDI; HAM-D; CGI; C-GAS	Compared to control, IPT-A group showed fewer depressive symptoms per clinician ratings and self-report. IPT-A group showed better global functioning per clinician	I

Study	Sample	Therapist/intervention	Conditions (n)	Measures	Results	Level
Roselló & Bernal (1999)	Puerto Rico; recruited from school systems; 3.9% MDD; 76.1% MDD + DD	N = 71 Age: 13–18 Gender: 54% female Nationality: 100% Puerto Rican	CBT and IPT: clinical psychology doctoral students; all therapy sessions videotaped and rated for fidelity	CBT (n = 25) Session attendance not reported IPT (n = 23) Session attendance not reported WL (n = 23) Session attendance not reported	Self: CDI Parent: CBCL	ratings and better general and social functioning per self-report. Based on self- but not parent-report, CBT and IPT showed significantly fewer depressive symptoms than control. No differences between CBT and IPT.	I
PCIT–ED						
Luby et al. (2012)	United States; recruited from primary care; 100% MDD	N = 54 Age: 3–7 Gender: 37.2% female Race: 86% white, 9.3% black, 4.7% other	PCIT-ED: master's- or doctoral-level clinicians; sessions videotaped and reviewed in weekly supervision sessions; tapes rated for fidelity DEPI: master's-level clinician or licensed clinical psychologist; no mention of fidelity	PCIT-ED (n = 25) 96% of completers (n = 19) attended all 14 sessions DEPI (n = 18) 80% of completers (n = 10) attended all 12 sessions	Clinician: PAPA Parent: PFC-S	Significant improvement shown in both groups, with PCIT-ED showing significance in more domains.	III
Brent et al. (2008)	United States; recruited from clinical sources and advertisements; 100% MDD and clinical depressive symptoms despite 8-week treatment with SSRIs	N = 334 Age: 12–18 Gender: 70% female Race: 82% white	CBT: therapists with at least a master's degree in mental health field and previous CBT training; 2-day training at the beginning and midpoint of study; audiotapes reviewed for pharmacotherapy sessions (92.8%	CBT + medication CBT + change to venlafaxine (n = 83) Change to venlafaxine (n = 83) CBT + change to another SSRI (n = 83) Change to another SSRI (n = 85)	Interview: CDRS-R, CGI, C-GAS	A higher proportion of participants in the CBT groups (no difference between CBT and medication group) compared to the medication-only groups showed an adequate clinical response.	I

(continued)

TABLE 4.1. (continued)

Study	Sample	Demographics	Therapists and fidelity	Treatment conditions	Depression variables	Depression results	Level
			acceptable quality assessed by Pharmacotherapy Rating Scale) and CBT sessions (93.9–94.9% acceptable quality assessed by Cognitive Therapy Rating Scale)	CBT sessions (both groups): $M = 8.3$ (SD not reported) Medication sessions = 3			
Clarke et al. (2005)	United States; recruited from HMO; all participants prescribed an SSRI by a primary care physician; 100% MDD	$N = 152$ Age: 12–18 Gender: 78% female Race: not reported	CBT: All master's-level therapists; intervention sessions were videotaped and 57 sessions were randomly selected and rated by a senior supervisor on a CBT protocol adherence scale ($M = 82.7\%$ adherence, $SD = 11.6$)	CBT + SSRI ($n = 77$) Sessions: $M = 5.3$ ($SD = 2.9$) SSRI ($n = 75$)	Self-report: CES-D, HRSD, YSR Parent: CBCL Interview: K-SADS; C-GAS; Social Adjustment Scale for Youth	No significant advantages of CBT + SSRI over the SSRI condition. No significant group differences in depression recovery at 6-, 12-, 26-, and 52-week follow-ups. CBT + SSRI showed significantly greater improvement on Short-Form 12, number of visits, and medication days.	II
Goodyer et al. (2007)	United Kingdom; recruited from six specialist services; 100% MDD	$N = 208$ Age: 11–17 Gender: 74% female Race: not reported	CBT: psychiatrists, experienced therapists, and trained therapists (had previous training, attended 3-hour training, and had to deliver supervised CBT to at least three patients at an agreed competence level)	CBT + SSRI ($n = 105$) Sessions: $M = 10.6$ ($SD = 5.7$) SSRI only ($n = 103$) Sessions: $M = 6.5$ ($SD = 4$)	Interview: K-SADS, Health of the Nation Outcome Scales for Children and Adolescents Self/parent report: CDRS-R, CGI, Mood and Feelings Questionnaire	Both groups showed improvement in depression, functioning and mood. No significant advantage of combined group over medication only.	I

Study	Setting	Sample	Therapist	Groups	Measures	Results	
Melvin et al. (2006)	Australia; referred for assessment of depression; 60.3% MDD, 23.3% DD, 16.4% DDNOS	$N = 73$ Age: 12–18 Gender: 66% female Race: not reported	CBT: registered and supervised probationary psychologists, general medical practitioners, and social workers; all have 1–5 years experience in CBT; weekly/biweekly supervision with expert therapist and weekly supervision with peers	CBT only ($n = 22$) Sessions: $M = 10.91$ (SD not reported) Sertraline only ($n = 26$) Med appointments $= 6.92$ (SD not reported) Combined ($n = 25$) Sessions: $M = 11.32$ (SD not reported)	Interview: K-SADS, GAF, GARFS Self-report: RADS	CBT-only had significantly lower odds of a depressive disorder than medication-only, but combined group did not significantly differ from either the CBT- or medication-only groups. All group showed significant improvement on self-report measures of depression but no between-group differences.	I
TADS Team (2004)	United States; recruited from clinics, ads, physicians, clinicians, and schools, and juvenile justice facilities at 13 academic and community clinics; 100% MDD	$N = 439$ Age: 12–17 Gender: 54.4% female Race: 73.8% white, 12.5% AA, 8.9% Hispanic	CBT: therapists trained and supervised by project developers; psychiatrists for adolescents also trained and supervised by project developers	CBT only ($n = 111$) Fluoxetine only ($n = 109$) Placebo ($n = 112$) CBT + fluoxetine ($n = 107$) CBT sessions (both groups): $M = 11$ (SD not reported)	Interview: CDRS-R, CGI Self-report: RADS	Combined treatment was more effective in reducing depressive symptoms and overall psychological difficulties than all other treatment groups. Fluoxetine-only was better than CBT-only. *Follow-up data indicate that participants in all three active treatment groups ($n = 243$) did not significantly differ in depressive symptoms at 36 weeks. Treatment effects persisted at a 1-year follow-up (TADS, 2007; TADS et al., 2009).	I

Note. AA, African American; BDI, Brief Depression Inventory; CBCL, Child Behavior Checklist; CBT, cognitive-behavioral therapy; CDI, Children's Depression Inventory; CDRS-R, Children Depression Rating Scale—Revised; CES-D, Center for Epidemiological Studies–Depression Scale; C-GAS, Children's Global Assessment Scale; DD, dysthymic disorder; DDNOS, depressive disorder not otherwise specified; DEPI, Developmental Education and Parenting Intervention; DISC, Diagnostic Interview Schedule for Children; GAF, Global Assessment of Functioning; HAM-D, Hamilton Depression Rating Scale; HMO, health maintenance organization; IPT-A, interpersonal psychotherapy for depressed adolescents; K-SADS, Schedule for Affective Disorders and Schizophrenia for School-Age Children; LIFE, Longitudinal Interval Follow-Up Evaluation; LS, life skills/tutoring; MDD, major depressive disorder; NST, nondirective supportive treatment; PAPA, Preschool Age Psychiatric Assessment; PCIT-ED, parent–child interaction therapy emotion development; PFC-S, Preschool Feelings Checklist—Scale Version; RADS, Reynolds Adolescent Depression Scale; SAS-SR, Social Adjustment Scale–Self-Report Version; SBFT, systemic behavior family therapy; SSRI, selective serotonin reuptake inhibitor; TAU, treatment as usual; WL, wait list; YSR, Youth Self-Report.

for adolescents generally consists of affect monitoring, pleasant activities scheduling, cognitive restructuring, communication, and conflict resolution. CBT for children places greater emphasis on parenting skills and responses to emotion. For adolescents, group CBT, without a parent component, is a "well-established" treatment, and individual CBT, with or without a parent/family component, and group CBT with a parent component are considered "probably efficacious." For children, group CBT, with or without a parent/family component, is considered "well established." Recent meta-analyses show moderate effect sizes posttreatment ($d = 0.53$—Klein, Jacobs, & Reinecke, 2007) and at follow-up ($d = 0.59$—Klein et al., 2007) for the various modalities of CBT (discussed below).

Individual CBT

In one of the earliest studies of CBT efficacy, Brent and colleagues (1997) found that adolescents who received individual CBT reported improvement in depressive symptoms more quickly, as well as greater rates of remission, compared to adolescents who received family therapy or nondirective supportive therapy. The largest randomized controlled trial (RCT) of CBT, TADS, compared treatment outcomes for 12- to 17-year-olds who received CBT only, fluoxetine only, combined CBT and fluoxetine, and placebo. Posttreatment (Week 12) depression scores were significantly lower in the combined CBT and medication group than in the CBT only and the fluoxetine only groups (March et al., 2004). Additionally, youth in the medication-only group had significantly lower depression scores than youth in the CBT-only group. However, the CBT-only and medication-only groups no longer had significant differences in depression scores at 18 weeks, and both groups had equivalent outcomes to the combined CBT and medication group by 24 weeks (March et al., 2007) and 1 year naturalistic follow-up (TADS Team et al., 2009).

Group CBT

In addition to individual CBT, researchers have examined the efficacy of group CBT. Adolescents who participated in the Coping with Depression in Adolescence (CWD-A) program, with and without parent intervention, demonstrated greater symptom improvement and higher remission rates than youth in a wait-list control group (Clarke, Rohde, Lewinsohn, Hops, & Seeley, 1999; Lewinsohn, Clarke, Hops, & Andrews, 1990). Additionally, group CBT is as effective at reducing depressive symptoms as usual mental health care and a life skills training/academic tutoring group (Clarke et al., 2002; Rohde, Clarke, Mace, Jorgensen, & Seeley, 2004).

Interpersonal Psychotherapy

IPT focuses on the interrelationship between depressive symptoms and interpersonal functioning. IPT-A is an adaptation specifically for depressed adolescents that incorporates parents in treatment and modifies treatment goals to be developmentally appropriate (i.e., increasing independence; Mufson & Sills, 2006). Individual IPT-A is considered a "well-established" treatment.

To date, the handful of RCTs that have examined the efficacy of IPT-A in both clinic samples and school-based clinics have demonstrated a greater reduction in depressive symptoms and greater improvements in interpersonal functioning for youth receiving IPT-A than youth receiving clinical monitoring or treatment as usual (Mufson et al., 2004; Mufson, Weissman, Moreau, & Garfinkel, 1999). Additionally, youth who received IPT-A displayed comparable reductions in depression symptoms as youth who received CBT, with both treatments showing moderate effects compared to a wait-list control condition (Rosselló & Bernal, 1999).

Promising Interventions

Several treatments targeting child depression are considered "experimental." For example, Luby, Lenze, and Tillman (2012) modified parent–child interaction therapy to target increasing emotion recognition and regulation (PCIT-ED) and found that PCIT-ED was associated with reductions in depressive symptoms in 3- to 7-year-olds. Similarly, Kovacs and colleagues (2007) created contextual emotion regulation therapy (CERT), a developmentally appropriate treatment that focuses on emotion regulation of sadness. In an open trial of CERT, 7- to 12-year-olds demonstrated significant reductions in depressive symptoms across treatment, with 53% no longer meeting criteria for dysthymia (Kovacs et al., 2007). Furthermore, reductions in depressive symptoms were maintained at 6- and 12-month follow-up. These treatment approaches are promising, with large-scale RCTs under way.

Additionally, third-wave approaches, including mindfulness training and acceptance and commitment therapy (ACT), have gained increasing attention in recent years. Hilt and Pollak (2012) demonstrated that brief interventions teaching distraction or mindfulness successfully reduced rumination following a negative mood induction in 9- to 14-year-olds. Further evaluation is needed to determine the efficacy of mindfulness-based interventions as a means to treat depression in youth.

Technology has also been incorporated into newer interventions. For example, Nelson, Barnard, and Cain (2003) demonstrated that CBT remains effective in reducing depressive symptoms when delivered via videoconferencing with the therapist. Relatedly, Merry and colleagues (2012) developed a computerized version of CBT (SPARX, Smart, Positive, Active, Realistic, X-factor thoughts). In an RCT of adolescents with mild to moderate depression, those in the SPARX condition had comparable reduction in depression scores to that of youth receiving treatment as usual (TAU; mainly counseling).

Pharmacological Interventions

Along with therapy, medication has proven effective in treating depression in youth. Currently, selective serotonin reuptake inhibitors (SSRIs) are the primary pharmacological intervention for child and adolescent depression, with fluoxetine and escitalopram approved by the U.S. Food and Drug Administration (FDA; Centers for Medicare and Medicaid Services, 2013). Combined treatment with medication and therapy has been shown to be more effective than either treatment alone (Brent et al., 2008; Clarke et al., 2005; March et al., 2007). Therapy and medication appear to complement each other, with medication allowing quicker symptom alleviation in youth, and CBT bolstering coping skills for more positive long-term effects, and potential for reduced risk of suicidal ideation and behavior (March et al., 2004).

Predictors of Treatment Outcomes

Several factors have been shown to moderate treatment response. For example, youth with more severe symptoms evidence poorer response to treatment (Barbe, Bridge, Birmaher, Kolko, & Brent, 2004). Similarly, greater family conflict portends poorer treatment outcome (Brent & Maloof, 2009; Curry et al., 2006). Additionally, youth who had more negative cognitions prior to treatment responded better to the combination of therapy and medication, compared to medication alone (Curry et al., 2006). In contrast, CBT has been shown to be less effective for depressed youth with a history of trauma (Barbe et al., 2004).

TREATMENTS FOR SUICIDAL BEHAVIOR IN CHILDREN AND ADOLESCENTS

As we discussed earlier, it is common for depressed youth to experience suicidal thoughts or engage in suicidal behaviors (Asarnow et al., 2008, 2011). While it is evident that such symptoms require treatment, there is some debate over how best to target these distressing thoughts and behaviors. Some clinical researchers have postulated that by adequately treating the underlying depressive disorder, suicidal ideation and behavior will remit along with the other symptoms. However, some evidence suggests that this is not the case (Linehan, 1997). That is, suicidal thoughts and behaviors must be addressed directly if these problems are to improve.

According to American Psychological Association Division 53 criteria, there are no "well-established" treatments for adolescent suicidality, but CBT with individual, family, *and* parent training sessions, as well as attachment-based family therapy have been designated as "probably efficacious" (Glenn, Franklin, & Nock, 2014). Table 4.2 includes a list of treatments that (1) are solely designed for adolescents with suicidal ideation (SI) or a recent suicide attempt; (2) have been tested in an RCT; and (3) examine suicide outcomes independent of nonsuicidal self-injury. These interventions are briefly reviewed below, along with a few promising approaches.

Individual CBT

Individual CBT was compared to supportive relational therapy (SRT) in a 10-week protocol for adolescents who made a suicide attempt (SA; Donaldson, Spirito, & Esposito-Smythers, 2005). One therapist provided individual therapy plus one family session throughout two treatment phases (weekly 3-month active, monthly 3-month maintenance). Up to two additional family and crisis sessions could be delivered as needed. CBT and SRT were associated with equivalent reductions in SI at midtreatment (3 months) and treatment end (6 months). Only 5% of adolescents reattempted suicide over the course of 6 months, with no differences across conditions. Individual CBT has been designated as an "experimental" intervention for adolescent SI (Glenn et al., 2014).

Individual, Parent, and Family CBT

One study tested an integrated CBT (I-CBT) to address adolescent suicidality (SI and/or SA) and substance use disorders (SUDs; Esposito-Smythers, Spirito, Kahler, Hunt,

TABLE 4.2. Overview of Interventions for Suicidal Adolescents Tested in Randomized Clinical Trials

Study	Sample	Demographics	Therapists and fidelity	Treatment conditions	Suicide variables	Suicide results	Level
Individual CBT			Stand-alone interventions				
Donaldson et al. (2005)	United States; recruited from emergency department and inpatient psychiatric unit; 100% SA	N = 39 Age: 12–17 Gender: 82% female Race: 85% white, 10% Hispanic, 5% AA	CBT & SRT: master's- and doctoral-level psychologists; trained by author; weekly supervision and audiotape review; fidelity ratings completed	CBT (n = 15); Sessions = 9.7 (SD = 2.4) SRT (n = 16) Sessions = 9.5 (SD = 1.3)	SI: Suicidal Ideation Questionnaire–Senior. SA: Structured Follow-up Interview	Equivalent reductions in SI at mid and end of tx (3 and 6 months postbaseline) across CBT and SRT groups. No difference in SA.	II
Individual + parent + family CBT							
Esposito-Smythers et al. (2011)	United States; recruited from inpatient psychiatric unit; 75% SA, 100% SI, 100% SUD 63.9% alcohol, 83.3% cannabis	N = 36 Age: 13–17 Gender: 67% female Race: 88.9% white, 13.8% Hispanic	CBT-I: master's- and doctoral-level psychologists; trained by author, weekly supervision and audiotape review; fidelity ratings completed	CBT-I (n = 19) Sessions: M = 45.7 (SD = 15.7) TAU (n = 17) Session: M = 24.6 (SD = 13.2)	SI: Suicidal Ideation Questionnaire–Senior. SA: K-SADS-PL Other: Child and Adolescent Services Assessment	CBT-I had fewer SAs, psychiatric hospitalizations, and emergency department visits at 6-month follow-up (18 months postbaseline). No difference in SI.	II
Individual + parent + family multisystemic therapy							
Huey et al. (2004)	United States; recruited adolescents evaluated for inpatient psychiatric hospitalization; 51% SI, suicide plan, and/or SA	N = 156 Age: 10–17 Gender: 45% female Race: 33% white, 65% AA, 1% other	MST: master's-level clinicians; three times per week to daily supervision by psychiatrist; family sessions audiotaped and reviewed for fidelity, and supervision by MST experts on weekly	MST (n = 57) M = 123 days (SD = 29) and 97.1 (SD = 57.1) contact hours + 44% hospitalized Inpatient + TAU	SI: Two items from the Brief Symptom Inventory and one from the Youth Risk Behavior Survey SA: One item from Child	MST had greater rate of reduction in adolescent reported SAs at 1-year follow-up (18 months postbaseline) than inpatient hospitalization + TAU. No difference in parent-reported SAs or adolescent-reported SIs. *(continued)*	II

TABLE 4.2. (continued)

Study	Sample	Demographics	Therapists and fidelity	Treatment conditions	Suicide variables	Suicide results	Level
			basis; parents completed adherence checklists	(n = 56) 100% inpatient, approx. 26% out-of-home placement (range 31–78 days), 75% outpatient (M = 8.5 sessions)	Behavior Checklist and one from the Youth Risk Behavior Survey		

Individual + parent + family attachment-based family therapy

Study	Sample	Demographics	Therapists and fidelity	Treatment conditions	Suicide variables	Suicide results	Level
Diamond et al. (2010)	United States; recruited from primary care and emergency department; 100% clinically significant SI and depressive symptoms, 62% history of SA	N = 66 Age: 12–17 Gender: 83% female Race: 26% white, 74% AA	ABFT: master's-level social workers and doctoral-level psychologists; trained, certified, and supervised by authors; fidelity monitored through weekly case discussion, live supervision, and audiotape review	ABFT (n = 35) Session attendance not reported TAU (n = 31) Sessions attendance not reported	SI: Suicidal Ideation Questionnaire–Junior and Scale for Suicidal Ideation SA: not reported	Greater rate of improvement in SI for both self-report and clinician-rated measures during tx period (baseline to 3 months) but not 3-month follow-up (baseline to 6 months). Greater amount of improvement in SI during treatment and follow-up on both SI measures. Greater recovery from clinically significant SI across time points in favor of ABFT. No analyses conducted to examine differences in SAs.	II

Note. AA, African American; ABFT, attachment-based family therapy; CBT, cognitive-behavioral therapy; DISC, Diagnostic Interview Schedule for Children; K-SADS-PL, Schedule for Affective Disorders and Schizophrenia for School-Age Children—Present and Lifetime Versions; MST, multisystemic therapy; SA, suicide attempt; SI, suicidal ideation; SRT, supportive relational therapy; SUD, substance use disorder; TAU = treatment as usual; tx, treatment.

& Monti, 2011). Adolescents were recruited from a psychiatric inpatient unit and randomized to I-CBT or TAU by providers in the community. The I-CBT protocol included three treatment phases (weekly 6-month active, biweekly 3-month continuation, monthly 3-month maintenance). Two therapists (one for the adolescent and one for parents) delivered individual, parent training, and family therapy sessions. Medication management was provided, as needed, across conditions with the study child psychiatrist. I-CBT was associated with fewer SAs (5 vs. 35%), psychiatric hospitalizations, heavy drinking days, and days of cannabis use relative to TAU at 6-month follow-up (18 months postbaseline). Comparable reductions were evident across groups in SI and drinking days. CBT with individual, family, and parent training sessions has been designated as a "probably efficacious" intervention for adolescent suicidal behavior (Glenn et al., 2014).

Individual, Parent, and Family Multisystemic Therapy

One study tested a version of multisystemic therapy (MST; Henggeler et al., 1999) adapted for youth with psychiatric emergencies (Huey et al., 2004). Adolescents evaluated for psychiatric inpatient hospitalization were randomized to MST or to inpatient psychiatric hospitalization + TAU (INPT+TAU). MST was delivered in home, school, and/or community settings and included frequent (daily when needed) but time-limited (3–6 months), individual, parent, and family sessions, with a focus on behavioral parent training. At 18 months postbaseline, the two groups showed comparable reductions in SI. MST was associated with a lower rate of youth, but not parent, reported SAs relative to INPT+TAU after controlling for baseline differences in SAs. MST, also referred to as *family-based ecological treatment,* has been designated as a "possibly efficacious" intervention for adolescent SI (Glenn et al., 2014).

Attachment-Based Family Therapy

One study compared attachment-based family therapy (ABFT) for adolescents with clinically significant SI and depressive symptoms to TAU (Diamond et al., 2010). ABFT is an emotional-focused, process oriented intervention that employs cognitive-behavioral and psychoeducational techniques. ABFT was associated with a faster rate of improvement in SI during the treatment period (baseline to 3 months) but not follow-up (3–6 months) relative to TAU. ABFT was also associated with greater declines in SI at treatment end and at follow-up. Analyses were not conducted to examine differences in rates of SAs (ABFT = 11%, TAU = 22%) due to the small number of cases. ABFT has been designated as a "probably efficacious" intervention for adolescent SI (Glenn et al., 2014).

Integrated Pharmacotherapy and Psychotherapy

One study, the Treatment of Adolescent Suicide Attempters (TASA) project (Brent et al., 2009), tested pharmacotherapy alone and in combination with CBT for adolescents with an SA. A total of 124 depressed adolescents with a recent SA were entered in one of three conditions: SSRI ($n = 15$), CBT for suicide prevention (CBT-SP; $n = 18$), or combination therapy ($n = 93$). Because many families would not accept randomization at the start of the trial, most participants (84%) chose their treatment assignment. CBT-SP included up to 22 sessions (individual and family) over 6 months. All participants showed a significant decrease in SI from baseline to the end of treatment. Approximately 12% of participants reattempted suicide, and 19% had a suicidal event (SA, completion, suicide plan, or clinically significant SI). CBT with individual and family sessions has been designated as an "experimental" intervention for adolescent SI and events (Glenn et al., 2014).

Promising Interventions

Dialectical behavior therapy (DBT), a promising new therapy for suicidal adolescents based on quasi-experimental and open pilot trials, is a primarily skills-based approach designed to improve mindfulness, distress tolerance, emotional regulation, and interpersonal effectiveness through weekly individual therapy, weekly multifamily skills training, and regular telephone consultation with therapists. Rathus and Miller (2002) tested a 12-week outpatient DBT protocol with 111 adolescents who engaged in self-harm (SA and/or nonsuicidal self-injury [NSSI]) with borderline features. DBT was compared to TAU (12 weeks of psychodynamic and supportive individual and family therapy) using a quasi-experimental design. The DBT group had fewer psychiatric hospitalizations than did the TAU group. Approximately 7% made an SA during the course of treatment, with no differences across groups (3.4% DBT vs. 8.6% TAU). Furthermore, adolescents in the DBT group reported significant reductions in SI pre- to posttreatment. DBT has been designated as an "experimental" intervention for adolescent SI and self-harm (Glenn et al., 2014).

EVIDENCE-BASED ASSESSMENT
OF DEPRESSION IN CHILDREN AND ADOLESCENTS

There are several important points to consider in determining the appropriate instrument to use in clinical and research settings. In particular, it is essential to determine the degree of training required to achieve reliability and validity in the administration of the measure, the amount of time available for conducting the assessment, and the primary purpose of the assessment (e.g., screening to provide differential diagnosis, treatment monitoring). What follows is a brief and selective overview of some of the most commonly used, empirically supported assessment measures for depression in adolescents.

Structured and Semistructured Diagnostic Interviews

The Kiddie-Schedule for Affective Disorders and Schizophrenia for School-Age Children—Present and Lifetime Versions (K-SADS-PL; Kaufman et al., 1997) is a semistructured diagnostic interview that includes an assessment of current and past psychopathology, including episodes of major depression, in youth ages 6–18. An initial screener determines whether the full mood module is administered. Final diagnostic determinations are based on interviews conducted separately with parent and child, using data from both interviews to arrive at a consensus diagnosis. In forming consensus, more weight is generally given to adolescent-reported internalizing and parent-reported externalizing symptoms, following procedures recommended to maximize detection of adolescent psychopathology (Kaufman et al., 1997). As the K-SADS-PL has been widely used in clinical research, there has been substantial empirical support for its use (Kaufman et al., 1997). When rigorous diagnostic assessment is required, particularly when differential diagnosis is of interest, the use of the K-SADS-PL may be appropriate. Its strength lies in large part in its reliance on trained assessors using clinical judgment to ascertain whether endorsed symptoms meet clinical threshold and to determine whether a symptom common to several disorders is better accounted for by one syndrome than another (e.g., whether loss of weight specifically occurs within the context of a depressive episode or is a more accurately characterized as a manifestation of an eating disorder). This greater accuracy, however, requires a longer administration time compared to other interviews (average administration time is 35 minutes, when no psychopathology is present, to 75 minutes, in the case of psychiatric respondents; Nezu, Ronan, Meadows, & McClure, 2000). The Diagnostic Interview Schedule for Children (DISC; Shaffer, Fisher, Lucas, Hisenroth, & Segal, 2004) is another commonly used, more highly structured interview.

Clinician Rating Scales

One clinician rating scale that is often used as a screening instrument and to index depressive symptom severity is the Children's Depression Rating Scale-Revised (CDRS-R; Poznanski, Freeman, & Mokros, 1985), a brief, 17-item semistructured interview encompassing DSM-IV depression symptoms. Rating of 14 items is based on verbal responses to interview questions, and rating of three items (i.e., depressed facial affect, listless speech, and hypoactivity) is based on behavioral observation. The reliability and validity of this instrument are adequate (Poznanski & Mokros, 1996; Poznanski et al., 1985). The CDRS-R takes 20–30 minutes to administer and score. Although some training and clinical experience is required for reliable and valid administration, these demands are much lower than in the case of the K-SADS, in part because the CDRS-R solely focuses on depression rather than multiple disorders.

Self-Report Measures

The Children's Depression Inventory 2 (CDI 2; Kovacs, 2010) is a commonly used and empirically supported self-report measure of depressive symptoms in children and adolescents ages 7–17 years. The CDI 2 consists of 28 items that assess how the respondent has been feeling over the past 2 weeks, with higher total scores reflecting greater depressive symptom severity. The CDI 2 generally takes up to 15 minutes to complete and has demonstrated high test–retest reliability and internal consistency (Kovacs, 2010). Although the CDI 2 exhibits relatively high sensitivity (i.e., ability to accurately detect cases of depression) and specificity (i.e., ability to accurately identify individuals without depression), it is generally recommended for use as a screening or treatment-monitoring tool rather than as a diagnostic instrument (Kovacs, 2010).

For adolescents age 13 years or older, another widely used self-report measure of depressive symptoms, the Beck Depression Inventory–II (BDI-II; Beck, Steer, & Brown, 1996), is an appropriate alternative. This measure has 21 items, with higher total scores indicating greater symptom severity, usually takes 5 to 10 minutes to complete, and has sound psychometric properties (Beck et al., 1996). As with the CDI 2, it may function better as a screening instrument than for diagnostic determinations. Other commonly used self-report depressive symptom measures include the Depression Self-Rating Scale for Children (DSRS; Birleson, 1981) and the Center for Epidemiological Studies of Depression Scale for Children (CES-DC; Weissman, Orvaschel, & Padian, 1980).

Computer Adaptive Testing

A relatively recent development in the assessment of depressive symptoms in children and adolescents is the National Institutes of Health–initiated Patient-Reported Outcomes Measurement Information System (PROMIS) pediatric depressive symptoms scale (Irwin et al., 2010). An objective of the PROMIS is to design instruments that are efficient, precise, and thereby suitable for use in clinical research settings. The PROMIS pediatric depressive symptoms scale is designed for use with children ages 8–17. It is also unique among self-report measures in utilizing modern statistical techniques for scale development, particularly item response theory, rather than classical test theory (Ravens-Sieberer et al., 2006; for more information, see DeWalt, Rothrock, Yount, & Stone, 2007; Irwin et al., 2010). There are currently two versions of this measure: a static (i.e., fixed length), 8-item short form and a larger, 14-item bank designed for use with computer adaptive testing. This measure showed reasonable reliability in an outpatient pediatric sample (Varni et al., 2014).

ASSESSMENT OF YOUTH SI AND BEHAVIOR

Because of the risk for suicidality in depressed youth, suicidal thoughts and behaviors should be assessed on a regular basis. If clinically significant suicidal thoughts or recent suicidal behavior are reported, a comprehensive suicide risk assessment is essential. There are numerous instruments available to assess SI and behavior, particularly in adolescents (see Goldston, 2003). Below we review a few of the most commonly used interviews and self-report measures that have been validated for use in clinical and community-based youth samples.

Clinician Rating Scales

The Columbia–Suicide Severity Rating Scale (pediatric version) (C-SSRS; Posner et al., 2011) is a brief structured interview that asks about adolescent SI/behavior and NSSI. The C-SSRS comes in three versions: lifetime, current (previous 6 months), and recent (since the prior visit). The C-SSRS website (*www.cssrs.columbia.edu*) contains information on the tool, as well as training in its use.

The Self-Injurious Thoughts and Behaviors Interview (SITBI; Nock, Holmberg, Photos, & Michel, 2007) is a structured interview, in short and long versions, used to assess SI and behavior, as well as NSSI over the past week, month, year, and lifetime. Follow-up questions assess the frequency and strength of thoughts or urges, multiple details surrounding suicidal acts, and the likelihood of engaging in the same behaviors in the future.

Self-Report Measures

The Suicidal Ideation Questionnaire (SIQ; Reynolds, 1985) is a self-report measure that assesses severity of SI over the last month in middle school (SIQ-Junior; 15 items) and high school (SIQ-Senior; 30 items) youth. Adolescents rate items on a 7-point Likert scale ranging from *never* to *almost every day,* and critical items as well as cutoff scores for clinically significant SI to help guide risk assessment.

If unable to acquire one of these (or other) validated assessment instruments, the therapist can ask questions that tap the frequency of suicidal thought (e.g., "How frequent are your current suicidal thoughts—once a week, a few days a week, daily? How long do they last—a few minutes, a few hours, most of the day?"), disclosure ("Have you told anyone about your suicidal thoughts? Who did you tell? When?"), duration ("How long ago did you first start to have these thoughts?"), and specificity of any suicidal plans ("Did you make a suicide plan? How and when did you plan to attempt suicide? Have you made any preparations such as a suicide note or giving away belongings?"). It is also important to assess the availability of means for a future suicide attempt (e.g., pills, firearms) and steps taken to remove these means from the home until the episode resolves.

EVIDENCE-BASED TREATMENT IN PRACTICE

Because CBT has the most evidence as a treatment for children and adolescents with depression, whether it is provided in individual, group, or with additional family component modalities, we focus in this section on the details of this approach. CBT treatments for depressed youth place varying emphasis on the cognitive and behavioral components of care. The behavioral component of treatments for depression emphasizes various skills deficits in the domains of coping skills, interpersonal relationships, and participation in pleasant activities. The cognitive component typically focuses on social problem-solving skills and identifying and challenging schemas, automatic thoughts, and cognitive distortions that cast experiences in an overly negative manner. In all, CBT for depressed youth addresses lagging cognitive and behavioral skills that are needed to create and maintain supportive relationships and to regulate emotion.

Assessment information guides treatment is several ways. First, this information is used to consider comorbid conditions and tailoring of the treatment to emphasize other internalizing or externalizing problems. For example, youth who have comorbid behavior problems may benefit from an emphasis on problem solving and parent sessions aimed at contingency management. Second, assessment results are used to prioritize modules. For instance, if assessment results indicate a large number of cognitive distortions, cognitive restructuring may be introduced and practiced earlier and more regularly in treatment. Similarly, assessment results that identify issues in the family environment may suggest a need for greater treatment emphasis on family communication and problem solving.

The following information explains the standard skills taught to youth and to their parents, when applicable, in CBT for depression. In addition, since depressed youth may have comorbid conduct and substance use problems, as well as deficits in communication and social skills, several supplemental skills are described and should be applied as needed based on the presenting problems of the patient. Within the sections below, we include sample dialogue between a patient and therapist that is based on a composite of actual therapy sessions.

General Session Outline

Sessions are 60 minutes in duration, with the exception of the introductory session, which usually takes 90 minutes. Typically, treatment occurs weekly for the first 6 months, then is tapered to biweekly or monthly for months 7–12. In a recently completed trial, the number of sessions ranged from 11 to 48 (Esposito-Smythers et al., 2011). All sessions, except for the initial introduction session, begin with the child/adolescent completing an assessment of past week's mood (i.e., average and highest ratings on a scale from 1 to 10 of happy, angry, sad, and anxious) and the frequency, intensity, and duration of suicidal thoughts and acts. Urges and acts of NSSI, medication adherence, and substance use are also monitored. These written ratings are reviewed verbally by the therapist and often tracked as a line graph to provide feedback over the course of treatment. If parents are participating in therapy, which is recommended, this information should also be gathered from the parents' perspective each week.

As noted earlier, when suicidality and/or NSSI are endorsed, clinicians should discuss the frequency, intensity, and duration of these symptoms, and conduct a risk assessment as needed. Clinicians and patients should collaboratively review the trigger(s) and chain of events leading up to unsafe thoughts and behaviors, the consequences of such behaviors, and make a plan for how to deal with these triggers in the future with health coping strategies. This is an excellent time to review the patient's coping plan, reasons for living, and pros and cons of unsafe behaviors, and update these items as needed. Parents should also be informed of any unsafe behaviors, and parental monitoring and access to potential dangerous materials should be reviewed.

Next, the clinician and patient work together to set an agenda for the current session. The clinician encourages the patient to identify something he or she would like to discuss, and the clinician adds suggestions about important topics. This works best as a collaborative process, valuing and incorporating the patient's ideas and perspective, to build rapport and engagement throughout the session. Any safety issues should be placed first on the agenda, and clinicians should try to relate any agenda items to skills the patient already possesses or that will be introduced later in the session.

In order to encourage generalization of the skills learned in CBT for depression, patients are asked to complete weekly assignments to practice CBT skills in real-life situations throughout the week. The clinician and patient review the homework from the previous session together, identify any barriers to completing the assignment, problem-solve how to improve skills usage, and praise all efforts related to applying skills outside of session. It is important to follow up on homework when it is given to emphasize commitment to treatment and the importance of practicing skills outside of session.

Then, the session moves into introducing a new CBT skill or practicing a skill that has already been taught. The clinician provides a rationale for the skill and discusses with the patient how the skill may be helpful in relation to his or her presenting problems. Socratic questioning is used, in addition to didactics, to help the patient identify uses for the skill and to understand the steps involved in practicing the skill. The clinician and patient work collaboratively to complete worksheets related to the skill, identify how this skill can be applied in the patient's life, and address any questions about the skill. Homework is assigned, and barriers to completing the homework are discussed.

At the end of the session, the clinician and patient address any remaining agenda item(s) that were not already covered in the context of the skill. Then, if applicable, a family check-in is conducted. Whenever the parent(s) and child are brought together in session, it is helpful to begin by having each person give a positive comment to the other. These should be prepared ahead of time during the individual session to ensure the content of the comment is appropriate and helps set a positive tone and model positive communication. Next, the child/adolescent and the parent share an overview with each other of what they learned in session and how they will practice the skill before the next session. Any agenda items that require a family discussion are presented and addressed or added to the agenda for the next session.

Sessions are designed to be flexible, in that they can be used to target a wide variety of presenting problems. Also, individual sessions can be completed with the child/adolescent and/or with the parent(s), so that all who participate in therapy learn a common language and skills set that they can apply to their own difficulties, as well as problems that affect the family as a whole (see Table 4.3). When teaching skills CBT, the core principles of psychotherapy should also be observed by clinicians, and these can be evaluated and monitored using the Cognitive Therapy Rating Scale (CTRS; Young & Beck, 1980) or a similar measure, which can be completed by the therapist and/or supervisor.

Standard CBT Skills for Depressed Youth

Introduction to Treatment

In this session, unlike other sessions, the parent and child/adolescent meet with the clinician together for the majority of the session. To begin, the clinician reviews the limits of confidentiality and makes very clear to the family when information about suicidality, NSSI, and substance use will be shared or not shared. Next, the clinician explains the structure of sessions, the use of skills and homework assignments, and the importance of parental involvement (if applicable). The introduction to treatment continues with a review of the family's expectations for treatment, troubleshooting barriers to treatment, and providing an overview of the goals of treatment based in empirical evidence for the efficacy of CBT for depression in youth.

The session then moves into an introduction to CBT and the interrelatedness of thoughts, feelings, and behaviors. Examples are given about how different interpretations about a situation or behaviors in a situation can lead to different emotions and outcomes. This concept is then used to explain how intervening with CBT skills can alter the way a person thinks about and acts in upsetting situations, which may improve the associated emotion reaction and lead to better decision making.

Next, pragmatic information regarding safety is reviewed. This includes discussing appropriate parental monitoring, as well as securing a commitment from the family to remove or lock up all sharp objects, guns, weapons, medications, and substances in the home to remove access from the depressed youth, if necessary. Such steps are especially crucial when a patient is expressing suicidality and/or NSSI.

TABLE 4.3. Treatment Protocol Outline

Name of session	Type of session	Objective
Introduction to treatment	Family	Orient to treatment program and conduct safety planning
Behavioral activation	Teen, parent	Decrease sedentary behavior and increase the frequency of healthy pleasant activities
Problem solving	Teen, parent, family	Learn how to generate and evaluate options to problems, and identify the most effective solution
Cognitive restructuring	Teen, parent	Become aware of the link between thoughts and feelings, and identify thinking mistakes that contribute to negative emotions and behaviors
Affect regulation	Teen, parent	Become aware of triggers and signs (physiological, cognitive, and behavioral) of affect arousal and develop coping plan
Skills practice	Teen, parent, family	Practice applying previously learned skills to current problems
Emotion coaching	Parent	Identify and respond empathically to teen's feelings
Contingency management	Parent, family	Identify appropriate limits and set up rewards and consequences to help change teen behavior
Family communication	Family	Learn and practice positive communication skills
Distress tolerance	Teen, parent	Develop safe, effective coping skills to help tolerate situations that trigger significant negative emotions
Relaxation	Teen, parent	Decrease stress through the use of deep breathing, muscle relaxation, and the use of imagination
Behavioral chain	Teen, parent	Identify and address the sequence of thoughts, feelings, and behaviors that culminate in risky behaviors and poor parenting choices
Increasing social support	Teen	Identify supporters, learn how to increase support from current support system and add new supporters
Relapse Prevention	Family	Review treatment progress, recommendations, and prevention plan, and conclude treatment

After this introductory material is presented, each family member is asked to identify goals for treatment. These include individual, family, school/work, peer, and any other goals the patient and parent(s) would like to address in therapy. Each family member shares his or her goals, and the clinician helps identify how they might be addressed using CBT. Next, the clinician meets individually with the child/adolescent to build rapport and create a safety plan. The safety plan includes listing reasons for living, identifying triggers for unsafe behaviors, and creating lists of (1) ways to help keep the patient's environment safe, (2) warning signs that the patient may become unsafe, (3) coping strategies the patient can employ on his or her own to stay safe, (4) other people who can help distract the patient if he or she is feeling unsafe, and (5) several options of people the patient can contact (i.e., parent, therapist, trusted family friend, school counselor) in case of a psychiatric emergency. Safety plans should be written out and regularly revisited and updated throughout therapy. It is helpful to make copies of the safety plan and to enter the information into the teen's and parent's cell phones if available.

Behavioral Activation

The goal of this session is to help the youth (and parent) decrease sedentary behavior and increase the frequency of pleasant activities to improve youth mood and parental self-care. The clinician begins by providing a rationale for how behavioral activation helps maintain positive thoughts and emotions. By increasing the number of healthy positive activities, individuals spend less time isolating themselves and engaging in behaviors that result in negative consequences; instead, they spend more time focusing on things other than their mood, and engaging in activities that bring them pleasure and enjoyment. Patients are provided with an extensive list of potential healthy, pleasant activities and are asked to generate some of their own. When identifying activities, it is important to keep in mind that the activities should be enjoyable to the patient, something the patient can do frequently, something the patient has control over and to which the parents will not object, and activities that are relatively inexpensive and healthy.

The clinician and patient then fill out a schedule for the week, including the activities identified, and set a goal to increase the number and/or duration of daily pleasant, healthy activities beyond the patient's current level of activity. If the patient already has a busy schedule, the focus can be on how to improve the activities in which the patient currently participates to make them more enjoyable. At least some activities that involve other family members should be included in the schedule to help increase the frequency of family members' pleasant times together and effective communication to improve family relationships. Patients may also identify additional activities they would like to do in the future, typically, special events that may cost more money or that cannot be done on a daily basis. The patient reviews the new plan with his or her parent(s) during the family check-in to make sure all activities are approved, and the family members problem-solve around any barriers to completing the activities identified.

Problem Solving

The goal of this session is to help the child–parent generate novel ways of dealing with triggers that lead to conflict and affect arousal, and systematically evaluate options to identify the most effective solution. We use the acronym "SOLVE" (Donaldson & Lam, 2004) to cover the basic steps in problem solving. Each letter in the word SOLVE stands for a different step of the problem-solving process: "Select a problem," "generate Options," rate the "Likely outcome" of each option, choose the "Very best option," and "Evaluate" how well each option worked.

The clinician begins by helping the youth generate a list of triggers for the problem behavior (e.g., NSSI, SI, distressed mood), typically, two to five events. Next, the clinician provides a rationale for the use of problem solving, explaining how people may feel stuck if they do not have different options for how to resolve difficult situations, which may result in unsafe coping strategies such as NSSI, substance use, or SAs. The patient and clinician then work together to identify the triggers of the patient's primary presenting problem and begin to methodically go through the SOLVE system, beginning with identifying a specific, clearly defined problem.

> THERAPIST: Now let's go back to your Triggers Worksheet and select one of these triggers to work on using the SOLVE exercise. Which one would you like to work on today?
>
> PATIENT: Fights with my boyfriend. When he gets mad and stops responding to my calls and texts I just get more and more upset. I keep calling, texting, and leaving him messages that make everything worse.
>
> THERAPIST: So should we define the problem as "How to cope when my boyfriend is mad"?
>
> PATIENT: That sounds good.

Next, the clinician assists the patient in identifying all possible options he or she can think of to address the identified problem. This is simply a brainstorming exercise, and the clinician should remind the patient not to evaluate the options at this stage, only to generate as many options as possible. For patients who have a history of NSSI, substance use, or suicidality, these options may be listed along with other options the patient has tried in the past, especially early in treatment.

> THERAPIST: Let's start by listing all the things you can think of that might solve this problem. What are some of the ideas that come to mind?
>
> PATIENT: I can ignore him, tell him I want to break up, or call his friends to see if they can get him to call. I could also just give him some space and try again tomorrow.
>
> THERAPIST: Is there anything else you can think of?
>
> PATIENT: No.
>
> THERAPIST: Can I make a suggestion? From what you've told me before, it seems like it sometimes helps to talk to your aunt. Is that an option we should consider in this situation?
>
> PATIENT: Yeah, if she's around she can be a big help.
>
> THERAPIST: Does this situation ever lead to thoughts of suicide or cutting?

PATIENT: Yeah, it's one of the things that led up to being in the hospital. I just wanted to feel better and I ended up cutting myself and taking some pills.

THERAPIST: I can see how sometimes the situation becomes so overwhelming that it doesn't seem like there are other options to feel better in the moment. Let's write those things down and we'll talk about the pros and cons of those options.

The next step is to evaluate the pros and cons of each option to determine if it will likely lead to a positive, negative, or neutral outcome. High-risk behaviors (e.g., NSSI, substance use, or suicidality) should be fleshed out in detail to ensure that the patient thinks through the pros and cons of these options, guiding the patient to see how the cons outweigh the pros for these behaviors. After weighing all the likely outcomes, the clinician helps guide the patient to the best option(s) using Socratic questioning. The patient forecasts how well the chosen option will work to solve the identified problem, and the clinician helps the patient determine if there are any ways to make the solution even more effective.

THERAPIST: OK, so now let's go through and consider the pros and cons of each option. How about the option of hurting yourself? What might happen if you choose that?

PATIENT: Well, I might feel better in the moment, but then I start worrying about people seeing the marks and getting mad at me. I also worry about the scars and what people at school are going to say. It's also part of how I ended up in the hospital before, which I don't want to happen again.

THERAPIST: So in the short-term, you might feel better, and in the long-term, there might be other consequences.

PATIENT: I guess so. I always get stuck on feeling better right away and it's hard to remember all the other things that might happen.

THERAPIST: So does that mean it's a negative overall?

PATIENT: Yes.

THERAPIST: Let's consider the other options. What are the pros and cons of talking to your aunt?

PATIENT: Well, she seems to understand me and can help to calm me down, but sometimes she's busy with her friends. I think it would mostly be a positive.

After considering all the pros and cons, the patient and therapist choose the best option, work collaboratively to troubleshoot any potential barriers to carrying out the identified plan, and revisit it at the following session to see how well it worked. If it worked well, the patient has identified a successful solution to his or her problem. If it did not work well, the patient returns to the list of options and identifies a new strategy to try to address the problem.

THERAPIST: So overall, what do you think the best option would be?

PATIENT: Talking to my aunt.

THERAPIST: Great. What if she is busy? What could you do in that situation?

PATIENT: Well, I could text her and ask if she had a few minutes to talk.

THERAPIST: Great!

The therapist may need to model the skills necessary to progress through the problem-solving steps. The typical depressed adolescent will have difficulties generating "options" but usually improves with practice. A simpler version of problem solving is to ask the adolescent to list the pros and cons of an action, such as breaking up with a boyfriend/girlfriend.

Cognitive Restructuring

The goal of this session is to help the youth become more aware of the link between his or her thoughts and feelings, to identify common thinking mistakes that may contribute to negative emotions or poor parenting behaviors, and develop disputes for these thinking mistakes to identify more helpful ways of thinking. The therapist begins by reviewing how thoughts, feelings, and behaviors are all connected and generates examples with the patient of how he or she can interpret the same situation in different ways to lead to different emotional and behavioral responses. The main message is that it is not the situation that makes a person feel a certain emotion, but rather the way the person thinks about or interprets the situation.

Next, the clinician introduces the patient to a list of various types of thinking mistakes and identifies which thinking mistakes may be commonly used by the patient, reassuring the patient that these thinking mistakes are normal and happen to everyone. Common thinking mistakes reviewed include the following:

1. *Black-and-white thinking.* You view a situation or person as all good or all bad, without noticing any points in between.

2. *Predicting the worst.* You predict the future negatively without considering other more likely outcomes.

3. *Missing the positive.* You focus on the negatives and fail to recognize your positive experiences and qualities.

4. *Feelings as facts.* You think something must be true because you "feel" it so strongly, ignoring evidence to the contrary.

5. *Jumping to conclusions.* You decide that things are bad, without any definite evidence either through *mindreading* (assuming that you know what others are thinking without asking) or through *fortune telling* (predicting things will turn out badly).

6. *Assuming control.* You assume that you can control how others behave in situations where you really don't have any control

7. *Expecting perfection.* You believe that you (or others) should be perfect in the things that you (or others) say or do.

Then, the therapist guides the patient through identifying an activating event, the emotion the patient felt during that event, and the automatic thoughts that the patient generated in response. We call our techniques the "ABCDE method" and introduce this method as a skill that helps adolescents deal with maladaptive beliefs or thoughts. Each letter of the ABCDE method stands for a different step in the cognitive restructuring process. The first step in changing a maladaptive thought is to identify the *A*, activating event, that is associated with thought. In teaching the ABCDE method, the letter *C* (consequences) is described next as the consequences or feelings related to the activating event. Next, the adolescent is taught that the *B* in the ABCDE method stands for beliefs, and that it is one's beliefs that lead to negative affect. The adolescent then learns that feeling better involves modifying these maladaptive beliefs or *D*, disputing them. The last step begins with an *E* and stands for effect. The adolescent is taught that he or she may not be able to change the fact that a negative activating event happened but he or she can change the beliefs and feelings surrounding the event and affect the decisions he or she makes.

During step *B*, it is normal for the patient to start with surface-level thoughts (e.g., when describing automatic thoughts after the breakup of a romantic relationship, a teen might identify thinking, "What did I do wrong? Why is this happening to me? What's wrong with me?"), and it may be necessary for the clinician to guide the patient to deeper, core thoughts (e.g., "Nobody loves me. I am unlovable. I will always be alone"). Core thoughts tend to be broad, generalized judgments the patient makes about him- or herself or the world. In the example of a romantic breakup, a patient may make a generalized judgment that he or she is unlovable and will always be alone based on that one relationship ending. Once the automatic and core thoughts are identified, the clinician and patient identify which types of thinking mistakes these thoughts represent.

THERAPIST: So let's give the ABCDE method a try using the fight with your boyfriend as the "activating event." Then let's skip the second step for a minute and go to the third step. The 3rd step is to identify "consequences or feelings" related to the "activating event." How did you feel after the fight with your boyfriend?

PATIENT: Hopeless.

THERAPIST: OK, let's write this feeling down next to "consequences." Now, let's go back to the second step, which is to identify "beliefs." What were you thinking after the fight with your boyfriend that led you to feel hopeless?

PATIENT: I hate my life.

THERAPIST: OK, let's write that down as your first belief. What else?

PATIENT: No one cares about me.

THERAPIST: OK, let's write that down, too.

Next, the clinician helps the patient identify disputes for the inaccurate, and/or unhelpful thoughts preciously identified. The clinician and youth must be careful not to use a dispute that is the exact opposite of the automatic thought because this will likely be difficult for the patient to believe in and may not be accurate. For example, if a patient identifies "I'm a failure" as an automatic thought after failing a math test, it is unlikely that he or she will believe the dispute, "I am not a failure. I can get an 'A' next time." However, it may be more accurate and believable to use a dispute such as "I may not be good at math, but I am a great athlete and do well in biology." The disputes are the most important step of cognitive restructuring because they help argue against negative, unhelpful beliefs and allow the patient to look at situations in a different way. If the patient has difficulty generating disputes, he or she can be prompted to question whether the automatic thought is true, and if so, whether it is helpful. Socratic questioning can also be used to help guide a patient to developing effective dispute. Such questions may include "What is the evidence for or against this belief? Does this belief help you feel the way that you want? What would your friend say if he/she heard this belief? Is there another explanation for this event?" Finally, once disputes are generated, the therapist helps the patient evaluate the effect or outcome of changing the maladaptive automatic beliefs the patient originally identified. The goal is not to make the patient feel completely happy about a difficult situation, but rather to ease some of the negative emotion the patient feels and allow him or her to have a more realistic viewpoint of the situation.

> THERAPIST: Now, the next step is to take a look at these beliefs and dispute them if needed. I want you to ask yourself two questions as you evaluate them. The questions are (1) Is this belief true? And if it is true, (2) is this belief helpful? If the answer is "no" to either of these questions, then it is important to dispute them. So, let's get started. Is it true that you hate your life?
>
> PATIENT: Yes, it is true.
>
> THERAPIST: So, you hate everything about your life including your sister, your friends, and everything else?
>
> PATIENT: Well, maybe not everything. I like spending time with some people.
>
> THERAPIST: So what is a more accurate statement?
>
> PATIENT: I don't hate everything about my life?
>
> THERAPIST: OK, that is better. But what was it that you really disliked in the moment?
>
> PATIENT: Fighting with my boyfriend?
>
> THERAPIST: Right, so a more accurate statement may be "I don't like fighting with my boyfriend, but there are other people and things I enjoy." Why don't you go ahead and write that down? And what about your next thought. "No one cares about me." Is that true?
>
> PATIENT: It feels that way.
>
> THERAPIST: OK, let's think about the "evidence for the belief" and "evidence against the belief." What is some evidence you have that no one cares about you?
>
> PATIENT: My boyfriend and I are always fighting and he's never there for me.
>
> THERAPIST: OK, now, what about "evidence against" this belief? Can you think of any?
>
> PATIENT: No, not really.

THERAPIST: Well, do you think that your parents would bring you here if they did not care about you?

PATIENT: Probably not.

THERAPIST: OK, so let's write down, "My parents help when I need it." Now, you told me that you were on the swim team last semester. Who would come to your meets?

PATIENT: My parents, sister, and boyfriend all came.

THERAPIST: Would they do that if they did not care about you?

PATIENT: Probably not.

THERAPIST: OK, so let's write that down, too. Now, let's take a look at the things that you have listed under your "evidence for belief" column. Is it true that *no one* cares about you?

PATIENT: No, I guess not.

THERAPIST: OK, and is it common for people to have disagreements in relationships?

PATIENT: Well, yes.

THERAPIST: OK, so is it possible that arguing is something that occurs in all relationships and it does not necessarily mean no one cares about you?

PATIENT: Yes, it is possible.

THERAPIST: OK, so why don't you write down "All relationships have ups and downs" under the "evidence against belief" column.

PATIENT: Yes, it is possible.

THERAPIST: Now, let's take a look at your two columns. Taking into account all of this information, is it really true that no one cares about you?

PATIENT: No, I guess not, but it feels that way.

THERAPIST: OK, so what is a more accurate belief?

PATIENT: People in my life do care about me but they don't always show it?

THERAPIST: OK, that is much better. Let's write that down under your disputes.

Affect Regulation

The goal of this session is to help the child or parent become more aware of triggers and signs (physiological, cognitive, and behavioral) of emotional arousal and develop appropriate coping skills to regulate this arousal. The therapist begins by explaining that when negative activating events trigger negative, maladaptive, or untrue beliefs, these beliefs can cause depressed mood and anger. These negative feelings can also cause the body to start to feel out of control, which can be experienced as muscle tightness, a faster heart rate, sweating, shortness of breath, and other physiological symptoms. The more one's body feels out of control, the harder it is to use problem solving or cognitive restructuring skills. Therefore, it is important to be aware of physiological signs that indicate emotional arousal and learn ways to keep negative affect under control.

Next, the therapist asks the patient to describe how he or she was feeling during a recent activating event. With suicidal adolescents, it is useful to focus on events that resulted in SI or suicidal behavior. Then, the therapist presents the patient with a list of physiological and behavioral symptoms associated with negative affect, referred to as "body talk," and asks the patient to identify the symptoms he or she experienced when in the stressful situation. The patient and therapist work together to complete the "feelings thermometer" worksheet that includes an image of a thermometer with numbers listed in order beside it, ranging from 1 to 10. Beside the bottom of the thermometer is a rating "1," which stands for *calm and cool,* and beside the top is the rating "10," which stands for *extremely upset,* or the highest level possible of the feeling the patient identified (e.g., anger) during the activating event. The patient assigns each physiological and behavioral symptom previously identified, as well as notable cognitions, to the numbers indicating increasing intensities of the thermometer.

> THERAPIST: Okay, so you have selected "hopeless" as the main feeling that you experienced at the time of your suicide attempt. So let's list "hopelessness" at the top of your emotions thermometer above the number "10." Now, what I would like you to do is to fill in the lines by each rating on the feelings thermometer with the "body talk" you circled on your worksheet. "Body talk" symptoms do not occur all at once but successively, like a set of dominos falling. So, I want you to think back to the night of your fight with your parents. Of all of the body talk that you circled, what was the first body talk symptom that you noticed?
>
> PATIENT: I started to crack my knuckles.
>
> THERAPIST: OK, good, so why don't you write this on the line by "1." What next?
>
> PATIENT: I started to yell at my boyfriend.
>
> THERAPIST: OK, so where would that fall on the thermometer?
>
> PATIENT: Probably around "3."
>
> THERAPIST: Good. Then what?
>
> PATIENT: I hung up the phone and then started sending him lots of mean text messages.
>
> THERAPIST: OK, where should that go?
>
> PATIENT: Probably around "7."
>
> THERAPIST: Then what?
>
> PATIENT: I started to cry.
>
> THERAPIST: OK, when did that occur?
>
> PATIENT: Around "9."
>
> THERAPIST: Now, what I would like you to do next is to list negative beliefs that you might have had on the feelings thermometer. Can you think of any negative beliefs that you might have experienced when you first started to argue with your boyfriend?
>
> PATIENT: "It's not fair."

THERAPIST: Good, where should that go?

PATIENT: Around "4."

THERAPIST: What else?

PATIENT: "No one cares about me."

THERAPIST: OK, please write that in on the appropriate line. What else?

PATIENT: "I hate my life."

THERAPIST: And where should that go?

PATIENT: That was probably around "8."

Next, the patient indicates his or her personal "danger zone" on the thermometer, meaning the point of emotional arousal at which his or her body spirals so far out of control that he or she is at risk for unsafe or suicidal behavior. Finally, the patient and therapist work collaboratively to create a "stay cool" plan to use when patient begins to notice early "body talk" and negative beliefs to prevent him or her from reaching the "danger zone" and point of "extreme upset" and unsafe behavior. Relaxation training is often taught as a means of managing physiological arousal, including paced breathing and guided imagery.

THERAPIST: OK, now the next step is to identify your personal danger zone—that is the point on your thermometer where your body spirals so far out of control that it is hard to calm back down, leaving you at risk for unsafe or suicidal behavior. Where would that be?

PATIENT: Probably when I start thinking about how much I hate my life.

THERAPIST: Good, so what I would like you to do is to begin to recognize the early "body talk" that precedes this thought so that you can work on decreasing it before you hit your danger zone. You can do this by creating a "stay cool" plan to use when you begin to notice early "body talk" and negative beliefs. This includes things that you can do and things that you can say to yourself to help yourself calm down. So let's go ahead and work on a "stay cool" plan. Let's try to list at least three things that you can do when you begin to notice your early body talk.

PATIENT: I can walk away when I start to get upset, listen to my music, maybe take a walk, or go online.

THERAPIST: Yes, those are all good things that can help you keep your cool. And what about things that you can tell yourself? You can use the disputes that we came up with last week if that would be helpful.

PATIENT: I can remind myself that there are good things about my life and things will get better.

THERAPIST: Great, what else?

PATIENT: I can remind myself that we've worked things out before.

THERAPIST: Those are two great beliefs. Why don't you write down both of them?

Finally, before the adolescent leaves the session, parents are briefed on the session content so that they are aware of the child's coping plan and can provide support.

CBT Skills for Parents of Depressed Youth

The core CBT skills we described in detail earlier were initially developed for the child/adolescent. However, they can also be applied to the parent(s) in relation to their child's behavior, their own affect arousal, and various parenting issues. Basic parenting skills such as monitoring, attending to positive behavior, and contingency management are included in many treatment plans.

Other family-based CBT skills for depressed adolescents focus on improving communication and support while reducing conflict. A building block for teaching better communication is to help parents identify and respond empathically to their child's feelings, which is sometimes called *emotion coaching*. Its goal is to increase the child's experience of empathy and validation from parents, which is a crucial building block to behavior change.

Additional Skills

In addition to the core skills outlined earlier, several useful supplemental skills can be used to enhance basic CBT. For example, a functional analysis or chain analysis of target behaviors can help identify patterns of behavior and times when patients can utilize skills rather than engage in destructive behaviors. Distress tolerance can help patients tolerate uncomfortable emotions and enhance affect regulation strategies (Linehan, 1993).

Skills Practice

Skills practice sessions are used to help the youth/parent/family implement previously learned skills for current problems. Patients and family members should be learning to implement these skills more independently as time progresses. These skills practice sessions are particularly useful when crises are brought into session or the youth/parent/family needs more practice with a particular skill.

Relapse Prevention

Finally, as patients near the end of treatment, it is helpful to review the progress made, the skills learned, and future goals that need continued work. As part of this process, it is important to conduct a relapse prevention session to prepare the patient to become his or her own therapist and use the skills learned in therapy in daily life moving forward. In this session, the clinician, youth, and family work together to identify potential triggers and warning signs of a future lapse, and plan how the youth will use skills learned to cope with such issues, as well as how the family will support him or her in this process.

CONCLUSIONS

Considerable progress has been made over the past several decades in the treatment of depression and suicidality in adolescence. Although the number of efficacy studies for depression has increased, there is still a need for data indicating how these treatments work, as well as how to increase and improve the use of evidence-based practices such as CBT in community settings. Future trials are necessary to inform best practices in treating depressed children and adolescents.

REFERENCES

Abela, J. R. Z., & Hankin, B. L. (2008). Cognitive vulnerability to depression in children and adolescents: A developmental psychopathology perspective. In J. R. Z. Abela & B. L. Hankin (Eds.), *Handbook of depression in children and adolescents* (pp. 35–78). New York: Guilford Press.

American Psychiatric Association. (2000). *Diagnostic and statistical manual of mental disorders* (4th ed., text rev.). Washington, DC: Author.

American Psychiatric Association. (2013). *Diagnostic and statistical manual of mental disorders* (5th ed.). Washington, DC: Author.

Angold, A., Costello, E. J., & Erkanli, A. (1999). Comorbidity. *Journal of Child Psychology and Psychiatry, 40*(1), 57–87.

Asarnow, J. R., Baraff, L. J., Berk, M., Grob, C., Devich-Navarro, M., Suddath, R., et al. (2008). Pediatric emergency department suicidal patients: Two-site evaluation of suicide ideators, single attempters, and repeat attempters. *Journal of the American Academy of Child and Adolescent Psychiatry, 47*(8), 958–966.

Asarnow, J. R., Porta, G., Spirito, A., Emslie, G., Clarke, G., Wagner, K. D., et al. (2011). Suicide attempts and nonsuicidal self-injury in the Treatment of Resistant Depression in Adolescents: Findings from the TORDIA study. *Journal of the American Academy of Child and Adolescent Psychiatry, 50*(8), 772–781.

Barbe, R. P., Bridge, J. A., Birmaher, B., Kolko, D. J., & Brent, D. A. (2004). Lifetime history of sexual abuse, clinical presentation, and outcome in a clinical trial for adolescent depression. *Journal of Clinical Psychiatry, 65*(1), 77–83.

Beck, A., Steer, R., & Brown, G. (1996). *Manual for the Beck Depression Inventory–II*. San Antonio, TX: Psychological Corporation.

Biederman, J., Faraone, S., Mick, E., & Lelon, E. (1995). Psychiatric comorbidity among referred juveniles with major depression: Fact or artifact? *Journal of the American Academy of Child and Adolescent Psychiatry, 34*(5), 579–590.

Birleson, P. (1981). The validity of depressive disorder in childhood and the development of a self-rating scale: A research report. *Journal of Child Psychology and Psychiatry, 22*, 73–88.

Birmaher, B., Arbelaez, C., & Brent, D. (2002). Course and outcome of child and adolescent major depressive disorder. *Child and Adolescent Psychiatric Clinics of North America, 11*(3), 619–637.

Birmaher, B., Ryan, N. D., Williamson, D. E., Brent, D. A., Kaufman, J., Dahl, R. E., et al. (1996). Childhood and adolescent depression: A review of the past 10 years. Part I. *Journal of the American Academy of Child and Adolescent Psychiatry, 35*(11), 1427–1439.

Brent, D., Emslie, G., Clarke, G., Wagner, K. D., Asarnow, J. R., Keller, M., et al. (2008). Switching to another SSRI or to venlafaxine with or without cognitive behavioral therapy for adolescents with SSRI-resistant depression: The TORDIA randomized controlled trial. *Journal of the American Medical Association, 299*(8), 901–913.

Brent, D. A., Greenhill, L. L., Compton, S., Emslie, G., Wells, K., Walkup, J. T., et al. (2009). The Treatment of Adolescent Suicide Attempters Study (TASA): Predictors of suicidal events in an open treatment trial. *Journal of the American Academy of Child and Adolescent Psychiatry, 48*(10), 987–996.

Brent, D. A., Holder, D., Kolko, D., Birmaher, B., Baugher, M., Roth, C., et al. (1997). A clinical psychotherapy trial for adolescent depression comparing cognitive, family, and supportive therapy. *Archives of General Psychiatry, 54*(9), 877–885.

Brent, D. A., & Maloof, F. T. (2009). Pediatric depression: Is there evidence to improve evidenced based treatments? *Journal of Child Psychology and Psychiatry, 50,* 142–152.

Brown, G. W., & Harris, T. O. (2008). Depression and the serotonin transporter 5-HTTLPR polymorphism: A review and a hypothesis concerning gene–environment interaction. *Journal of Affective Disorders, 111*(1), 1–12.

Carter, J. S., & Garber, J. (2011). Predictors of the first onset of a major depressive episode and changes in depressive symptoms across adolescence: Stress and negative cognitions. *Journal of Abnormal Psychology, 120*(4), 779–796.

Centers for Medicare and Medicaid Services. (2013). *Antidepressant medications: Use in pediatric patients.* Washington, DC: U.S. Department of Health and Human Services.

Clarke, G. N., Debar, L., Lynch, F., Powell, J., Gale, J., O'Conner E., et al. (2005). A randomized effectiveness trial of brief cognitive-behavioral therapy for depressed adolescents receiving antidepressant medication. *Journal of the American Academy of Child and Adolescent Psychiatry, 44,* 888–898.

Clarke, G. N., Hornbrook, M., Lynch, F., Polen, M., Gale, J., O'Connor, E., et al. (2002). Group cognitive-behavioral treatment for depressed adolescent offspring of depressed parents in a health maintenance organization. *Journal of the American Academy of Child and Adolescent Psychiatry, 41*(3), 305–313.

Clarke, G. N., Rohde, P., Lewinsohn, P. M., Hops, H., & Seeley, J. R. (1999). Cognitive-behavioral treatment of adolescent depression: Efficacy of acute treatment and booster sessions. *Journal of the American Academy of Child and Adolescent Psychiatry, 38,* 272–279.

Compas, B. E., Connor-Smith, J. K., Saltzman, H., Thomsen, A. H., & Wadsworth, M. E. (2001). Coping with stress during childhood and adolescence: Problems, progress, and potential in theory and research. *Psychological Bulletin, 127*(1), 87–127.

Copeland, W., Shanahan, L., Costello, E. J., & Angold, A. (2011). Cumulative prevalence of psychiatric disorders by young adulthood: A prospective cohort analysis from the Great Smoky Mountains Study. *Journal of American Academy of Child and Adolescent Psychiatry, 50*(3), 252–261.

Costello, E. J., Copeland, W., & Angold, A. (2011). Trends in psychopathology across the adolescent years: What changes when children become adolescents, and when adolescents become adults? *Journal of Child Psychology and Psychiatry, 52*(10), 1015–1025.

Costello, E. J., Erkanli, A., & Angold, A. (2006). Is there an epidemic of child or adolescent depression? *Journal of Child Psychology and Psychiatry, 47*(12), 1263–1271.

Costello, E. J., Mustillo, S., Erkanli, A., Keeler, G., & Angold, A. (2003). Prevalence and development of psychiatric disorders in childhood and adolescence. *Archives of General Psychiatry, 60*(8), 837–844.

Curry, J., Rohde, P., Simons, A., Silva, S., Vitiello, B., Kratochvil, C., et al. (2006). Predictors and moderators of acute outcome in the Treatment for Adolescents with Depression Study (TADS). *Journal of the American Academy of Child and Adolescent Psychiatry, 45,* 1427–1439.

Cyranowski, J. M., Frank, E., Young, E., & Shear, M. K. (2000). Adolescent onset of the gender difference in lifetime rates of major depression: A theoretical model. *Archives of General Psychiatry, 57*(1), 21–27.

DeWalt, D., Rothrock, N., Yount, S., & Stone, A. A. (2007). PROMIS cooperative group: Evaluation of item candidates: The PROMIS qualitative item review. *Medical Care, 45,* S12–S21.

Diamond, G. S., Wintersteen, M. B., Brown, G. K., Diamond, G. M., Gallop, R., Shelef, K., et al. (2010). Attachment-based family therapy for adolescents with suicidal ideation: A randomized controlled trial. *Journal of the American Academy of Child and Adolescent Psychiatry, 49*(2), 122–131.

Donaldson, C., & Lam, D. (2004). Rumination, mood and social problem-solving in major depression. *Psychological Medicine, 34*(7), 1309–1318.

Donaldson, D., Spirito, A., & Esposito-Smythers, C. (2005). Treatment for adolescents following a suicide attempt: Results of a pilot trial. *Journal of the American Academy of Child and Adolescent Psychiatry, 44*(2), 113–120.

Esposito-Smythers, C., Spirito, A., Kahler, C. W., Hunt, J., & Monti, P. (2011). Treatment of co-occurring substance abuse and suicidality among adolescents: A randomized clinical trial. *Journal of Consulting and Clinical Psychology, 79*(6), 728–739.

Forbes, E. E., & Dahl, R. E. (2012). Research review: Altered reward function in adolescent depression: What, when and how? *Journal of Child Psychology and Psychiatry, 53*(1), 3–15.

Glenn, C. R., Franklin, J. C., & Nock, M. K. (2014). Evidence-based psychosocial treatments for self-injurious thoughts and behaviors in youth. *Journal of Clinical Child and Adolescent Psychology, 44*(1), 1–29.

Goldston, D. (2003). *Measuring suicidal behaviors and risk among children and adolescents.* Washington, DC: American Psychological Press.

Goodman, S. H., & Gotlib, I. H. (1999). Risk for psychopathology in the children of depressed mothers: A developmental model for understanding mechanisms of transmission. *Psychological Review, 106*(3), 458–490.

Goodyer, I., Dubicka, B., Wilkinson, P., Kelvin, R., Roberts, C., Byford, S., et al. (2007). Selective serotonin reuptake inhibitors (SSRIs) and routine specialist care with and without cognitive behaviour therapy in adolescents with major depression: Randomised controlled trial. *British Medical Journal, 335*, 106–107.

Gotlib, I. H., Hamilton, J. P., Cooney, R. E., Singh, M. K., Henry, M. L., & Joormann, J. (2010). Neural processing of reward and loss in girls at risk for major depression. *Archives of General Psychiatry, 67*(4), 380–387.

Grant, K. E., Compas, B. E., Thurm, A. E., McMahon, S. D., Gipson, P. Y., Campbell, A. J., et al. (2006). Stressors and child and adolescent psychopathology: Evidence of moderating and mediating effects. *Clinical Psychology Review, 26*(3), 257–283.

Hammen, C. (2009). Adolescent depression: Stressful interpersonal contexts and risk for recurrence. *Current Directions in Psycholical Science, 18*(4), 200–204.

Hankin, B. L., & Abramson, L. Y. (2001). Development of gender differences in depression: An elaborated cognitive vulnerability-transactional stress theory. *Psychological Bulletin, 127*(6), 773–796.

Harrington, R., Fudge, H., Rutter, M., Pickles, A., & Hill, J. (1990). Adult outcomes of childhood and adolescent depression: I. Psychiatric status. *Archives of General Psychiatry, 47*(5), 465–473.

Henggeler, S. W., Rowland, M. D., Randall. J., Ward, D. M., Pickrel, S. G., Cunningham, P. B., et al. (1999). Home-based multisystemic therapy as an alternative to the hospitalization of youths in psychiatric crisis: Clinical outcomes. *Journal of the American Academy of Child and Adolescent Psychiatry, 38*, 1331–1339.

Hilt, L. M., & Pollak, S. D. (2012). Getting out of rumination: Comparison of three brief interventions in a sample of youth. *Journal of Abnormal Child Psychology, 40*, 1157–1165.

Huey, S. J., Jr., Henggeler, S. W., Rowland, M. D., Halliday-Boykins, C. A., Cunningham, P. B., Pickrel, S. G., et al. (2004). Multisystemic therapy effects on attempted suicide by youths presenting psychiatric emergencies. *Journal of the American Academy of Child and Adolescent Psychiatry, 43*(2), 183–190.

Irwin, D. E., Stucky, B., Langer, M. M., Thissen, D., DeWitt, E. M., Lai, J.-S., et al. (2010). An item response analysis of the pediatric PROMIS anxiety and depressive symptoms scales. *Quality of Life Research: International Journal of Quality of Life Aspects of Treatment, Care and Rehabilitation, 19*(4), 595–607.

Kaufman, J., Birmaher, B., Brent, D., Rao, U., Flynn, C., Moreci, P., et al. (1997). Schedule for affective disorders and schizophrenia for school-age children–present and lifetime version (K-SADS-PL): Initial reliability and validity data. *Journal of the American Academy of Child and Adolescent Psychiatry, 36*(7), 980–988.

Kendler, K. S., Gardner, C. O., & Prescott, C. A. (2002). Toward a comprehensive developmental model for major depression in women. *American Journal of Psychiatry, 159*(7), 1133–1145.

Kennard, B. D., Emslie, G. J., Mayes, T. L., & Hughes, J. L. (2006). Relapse and recurrence in pediatric depression. *Child and Adolescent Psychiatric Clinics of North America, 15*(4), 1057–1079, xi.

Kessler, R. C., Avenevoli, S., Costello, E. J., Georgiades, K., Green, J. G., Gruber, M. J., et al. (2012). Prevalence, persistence, and sociodemographic correlates of DSM-IV disorders in the National Comorbidity Survey Replication Adolescent Supplement. *Archives of General Psychiatry, 69*(4), 372–380.

Klein, J. B., Jacobs, R. H., & Reinecke, M. A. (2007). Cognitive-behavioral therapy for adolescent depression: A meta-analytic investigation of changes in effect-size estimates. *Journal of the American Academy of Child and Adolescent Psychiatry, 46,* 1403–1413.

Korczak, D. J., & Goldstein, B. I. (2009). Childhood onset major depressive disorder: Course of illness and psychiatric comorbidity in a community sample. *Journal of Pediatrics, 155*(1), 118–123.

Kovacs, M. (2010). *Children's Depression Inventory–Second Edition (CDI-2) manual.* North Tonawanda, NY: Multi-Health.

Kovacs, M., Sherrill, J., George, C. J., Pollock, M., Tumuluru, R. V., & Ho, V. (2007). Contextual ermotion-regulation therapy for childhood depression: Description and pilot testing of a new intervention. *Journal of the American Academy of Child and Adolescent Psychiatry, 45,* 892–903.

Kovacs, M., & Yaroslavsky, I. (2014). Practitioner Review: Dysphoria and its regulation in child and adolescent depression. *Journal of Child Psychology and Psychiatry, 55*(7), 741–757.

Lakdawalla, Z., Hankin, B. L., & Mermelstein, R. (2007). Cognitive theories of depression in children and adolescents: A conceptual and quantitative review. *Clinical Child and Family Psychology Review, 10*(1), 1–24.

Levinson, D. F. (2006). The genetics of depression: A review. *Biological Psychiatry, 60*(2), 84–92.

Lewinsohn, P. M., Clarke, G. N., Hops, H., & Andrews, J. (1990). Cognitive-behavioral treatment for depressed adolescents. *Behavior Therapy, 21,* 385–401.

Lewinsohn, P. M., Rohde, P., Klein, D. N., & Seeley, J. R. (1999). Natural course of adolescent major depressive disorder: I. Continuity into young adulthood. *Journal of the American Academy of Child and Adolescent Psychiatry, 38*(1), 56–63.

Lewinsohn, P. M., Rohde, P., & Seeley, J. R. (1995). Adolescent psychopathology: III. The clinical consequences of comorbidity. *Journal of the American Academy of Child and Adolescent Psychiatry, 34*(4), 510–519.

Linehan, M. M. (1993). *Cognitive-behavioral treatment of borderline personality disorder.* New York: Guilford Press.

Linehan, M. (1997). Behavioral treatments of suicidal behaviors and definitional obfuscation and treatment outcomes. *Annals of the New York Academy of Sciences, 836,* 302–328.

Luby, J., Lenze, S., & Tillman, R. (2012). A novel early intervention for preschool depression: Findings from a pilot randomized controlled trial. *Journal of Child Psychology and Psychiatry, 53,* 313–322.

March, J., Silva, S., Petrycki, S., Curry, J., Wells, K., Fairbank, J., et al. (2004). Fluoxetine, cognitive-behavioral therapy, and their combination for adolescents with depression: Treatment for Adolescents With Depression Study (TADS) randomized controlled trial. *Journal of the American Medical Association, 292*(7), 807–820.

March, J. S., Silva, S., Petrycki, S., Curry, J., Wells, K., Fairbank, J., et al. (2007). The Treatment for Adolescents With Depression Study (TADS): Long-term effectiveness and safety outcomes. *Archives of General Psychiatry, 64,* 1132–1143.

McLeod, B. D., Weisz, J. R., & Wood, J. J. (2007). Examining the association between parenting and childhood depression: A meta-analysis. *Clinical Psychology Review, 27*(8), 986–1003.

Melvin, G. A., Tonge, B. J., King, N. J., Heyne, D., Gordon, M. S., & Klimkeit, E. (2006). A comparison of cognitive-behavioral therapy, sertraline, and their combination for adolescent depression. *Journal of the American Academy of Child and Adolescent Psychiatry, 45,* 1151–1161.

Merikangas, K. R., He, J. P., Burstein, M., Swanson, S. A., Avenevoli, S., Cui, L., et al. (2010). Lifetime prevalence of mental disorders in U.S. adolescents: Results from the National Comorbidity Survey Replication—Adolescent Supplement (NCS-A). *Journal of the American Academy of Child and Adolescent Psychiatry, 49*(10), 980–989.

Merry, S. N., Stasiak, K., Shepherd, M., Frampton, C., Fleming, T., & Lucassen, M. F. G. (2012). The effectiveness of SPARX, a computerised self help intervention for adolescents seeking help for depression: Randomised controlled non-inferiority trial. *British Medical Journal, 344,* 1–16.

Mufson, L., Dorta, K. P., Wickramaratne, P., Nomura, Y., Olfson, M., & Weissman, M. M. (2004). A randomized effectiveness trial of interpersonal psychotherapy for depressed adolescents. *Archives of General Psychiatry, 61,* 577–584.

Mufson, L., & Sills, R. (2006). Interpersonal psychotherapy for depressed adolescents (IPT-A): An overview. *Nordic Journal of Psychiatry, 60,* 431–437.

Mufson, L., Weissman, M. M., Moreau, D., & Garfinkel, R. (1999). Efficacy of interpersonal psychotherapy for depressed adolescents. *Archives of General Psychiatry, 56,* 573–579.

Nelson, E., Barnard, M., & Cain, S. (2003). Treating childhood depression over videoconferencing. *Telemedicine Journal and e-Health, 9,* 49–55.

Nezu, A., Ronan, G., Meadows, E., & McClure, K. (2000). *Practitioners' guide to empirically based measures of depression.* New York: Kluwer/Academic.

Nock, M. K., Holmberg, E. B., Photos, V. I., & Michel, B. D. (2007). The Self-Injurious Thoughts and Behaviors Interview: Development, reliability, and validity in an adolescent sample. *Psychological Assessment, 19*(3), 309–317.

Pariante, C. M., & Lightman, S. L. (2008). The HPA axis in major depression: Classical theories and new developments. *Trends in Neurosciences, 31*(9), 464–468.

Peterson, B. S., Warner, V., Bansal, R., Zhu, H., Hao, X., Liu, J., et al. (2009). Cortical thinning in persons at increased familial risk for major depression. *Proceedings of the National Academy of Sciences of USA, 106*(15), 6273–6278.

Platt, B., Cohen Kadosh, K., & Lau, J. Y. (2013). The role of peer rejection in adolescent depression. *Depression and Anxiety, 30*(9), 809–821.

Posner, K., Brown, G. K., Stanley, B., Brent, D. A., Yershova, K. V., Oquendo, M. A., et al. (2011). The Columbia–Suicide Severity Rating Scale: Initial validity and internal consistency findings from three multisite studies with adolescents and adults. *American Journal of Psychiatry, 168*(12), 1266–1277.

Poznanski, E., Freeman, L., & Mokros, H. (1984). Children's Depression Rating Scale–Revised. *Psychopharmacology Bulletin, 21,* 979–989.

Poznanski, E., & Mokros, H. (1996). *Children's Depression Rating Scale–Revised.* Los Angeles: Western Psychological Services.

Prinstein, M. J., Borelli, J. L., Cheah, C. S., Simon, V. A., & Aikins, J. W. (2005). Adolescent girls' interpersonal vulnerability to depressive symptoms: A longitudinal examination of reassurance-seeking and peer relationships. *Journal of Abnormal Psychology, 114*(4), 676–688.

Rao, U., Chen, L.-A., Bidesi, A. S., Shad, M. U., Thomas, M. A., & Hammen, C. L. (2010). Hippocampal changes associated with early-life adversity and vulnerability to depression. *Biological Psychiatry, 67*(4), 357–364.

Rathus, J., & Miller, A. (2002). Dialectical behavior therapy adapted for suicidal adolescents. *Suicide and Life-Threatening Behavior, 32,* 146–157.

Ravens-Sieberer, U., Erhart, M., Wille, N., Wetzel, R., Nickel, J., & Bullinger, M. (2006). Generic health-related quality-of-life assessment in children and adolescents: Methodological considerations. *Pharmacoeconomics, 24,* 1199–1220.

Reynolds, W. M. (1985). *Suicidal Ideation Questionnaire.* Odessa, FL: Psychological Assessment Resources.

Rohde, P., Clarke, G. N., Mace, D. E., Jorgensen, J. S., & Seeley, J. R. (2004). An efficacy/effectiveness study of cognitive-behavioral treatment for adolescents with comorbid major depression and conduct disorder. *Journal of the American Academy of Child and Adolescent Psychiatry, 43*(6), 660–668.

Rohde, P., Lewinsohn, P. M., & Seeley, J. R. (1991). Comorbidity of unipolar depression: II. Comorbidity with other mental disorders in adolescents and adults. *Journal of Abnormal Psychology, 100*(2), 214–222.

Rosselló, J., & Bernal, G. (1999). The efficacy of cognitive-behavioral and interpersonal treatments for depression in Puerto Rican adolescents. *Journal of Consulting and Clinical Psychology, 67,* 734–745.

Rottenberg, J. (2007). Cardiac vagal control in depression: A critical analysis. *Biological Psychology, 74*(2), 200–211.

Rudolph, K. D., & Hammen, C. (1999). Age and gender as determinants of stress exposure, generation, and reactions in youngsters: A transactional perspective. *Child Development, 70*(3), 660–677.

Rudolph, K. D., Hammen, C., Burge, D., Lindberg, N., Herzberg, D., & Daley, S. E. (2000). Toward an interpersonal life-stress model of depression: The developmental context of stress generation. *Development and Psychopathology, 12*(2), 215–234.

Shaffer, D., Fisher, P., Lucas, C., Hisenroth, M. J., & Segal, D. L. (2004). The Diagnostic Interview Schedule for Children (DISC). In M. J. Hilsenroth & D. L. Segal (Eds.), *Comprehensive handbook of psychological assessment: Vol. 2. Personality assessment* (pp. 256–270). Hoboken, NJ: Wiley.

Sheeber, L., Hops, H., & Davis, B. (2001). Family processes in adolescent depression. *Clinical Child and Family Psychology Review, 4*(1), 19–35.

Southam-Gerow, M. A., & Prinstein, M. J. (2014). Evidence base updates: The evolution of the evaluation of psychological treatments for children and adolescents. *Journal of Clinical Child and Adolescent Psychology, 43*(1), 1–6.

Sullivan, P. F., Neale, M. C., & Kendler, K. S. (2000). Genetic epidemiology of major depression: Review and meta-analysis. *American Journal of Psychiatry, 157*(10), 1552–1562.

TADS Team. (2004). Fluoxetine, cognitive behavioral therapy, and their combination for adolescents with depression: Treatment for adolescents with depression study (TADS) randomized controlled trial. *Journal of the American Medical Association, 292,* 807–820.

TADS Team. (2005). The Treatment for Adolescents With Depression Study (TADS): Demographic and clinical characteristics. *Journal of the American Academy of Child and Adolescent Psychiatry, 44*(1), 28–40.

TADS Team, March, J., Silva, S., Curry, J., Wells, K., Fairbank, J., et al. (2009). The Treatment for Adolescents With Depression Study (TADS): Outcomes over 1 year of naturalistic follow-up. *American Journal of Psychiatry, 166*(10), 1141–1149.

Tomarken, A. J., Dichter, G. S., Garber, J., & Simien, C. (2004). Resting frontal brain activity: Linkages to maternal depression and socio-economic status among adolescents. *Biological Psychology, 67*(1–2), 77–102.

Varni, J. W., Magnus, B., Stucky, B. D., Liu, Y., Quinn, H., Thissen, D., et al. (2014). Psychometric properties of the PROMIS® Pediatric Scales: Precision, stability, and comparison of different scoring and administration options. *Quality of Life Research: International Journal of Quality of Life Aspects of Treatment, Care and Rehabilitation, 23*(4), 1233–1243.

Weissman, M. M., Orvaschel, H., & Padian, N. (1980). Children's symptom and social functioning self-report scales: Comparison of mothers' and children's reports. *Journal of Nervous and Mental Disease, 168*(12), 736–740.

Weissman, M. M., Wolk, S., Goldstein, R. B., Moreau, D., Adams, P., Greenwald, S., et al. (1999). Depressed adolescents grown up. *Journal of the American Medical Association, 281*(18), 1707–1713.

Weissman, M. M., Wolk, S., Wickramaratne, P., Goldstein, R. B., Adams, P., Greenwald, S., et al. (1999). Children with prepubertal-onset major depressive disorder and anxiety grown up. *Archives of General Psychiatry, 56*(9), 794–801.

Weisz, J. R., McCarty, C. A., & Valeri, S. M. (2006). Effects of psychotherapy for depression in children and adolescents: A meta-analysis. *Psychological Bulletin, 132*(1), 132–149.

Yap, M. B., Allen, N. B., & Sheeber, L. (2007). Using an emotion regulation framework to understand the role of temperament and family processes in risk for adolescent depressive disorders. *Clinical Child and Family Psychology Review, 10*(2), 180–196.

Young, J., & Beck, A. T. (1980). *Cognitive Therapy Scale rating manual*. Philadelphia: University of Pennsylvania.

CHAPTER 5

Bipolar Disorder

Amy E. West and Sally M. Weinstein

THE DSM-5 DEFINITION OF BIPOLAR DISORDER

Bipolar disorder (BD) in children and adolescents, a chronic and debilitating disorder, has been diagnosed with substantially greater frequency over the past 20 years (Washburn, West, & Heil, 2011). Pediatric bipolar disorder (PBD) is currently diagnosed using the fifth edition of the *Diagnostic and Statistical Manual of Mental Disorders* (DSM-5; American Psychiatric Association, 2013), although there is considerable debate regarding the accurate characterization of BD in children and adolescents. Bipolar I disorder is diagnosed if the patient has met full criteria for a manic episode, and commonly has met full criteria for major depressive disorder (MDD) or a mixed mood episode (co-occurring symptoms of mania and depression). Bipolar II disorder is diagnosed if full criteria have been met for past/present MDD and past/present hypomania. Cyclothymia is diagnosed if there is a history of at least 2 years of numerous periods of hypomanic symptoms and numerous periods of depressive symptoms that do not meet full criteria for MDD or mania. Unspecified BD is diagnosed if there is a history of significant symptoms of mania and depression that do not meet intensity, duration, or frequency thresholds for a full mood episode by DSM criteria. Diagnosis of a manic episode is based on the presence of episodes of either extreme irritability or elevated, expansive mood in combination with at least five of the following symptoms: grandiosity, decreased need for sleep, hypersexuality, racing thoughts, pressured speech, distractibility, and impulsive behavior. The episode must represent a change from previous behavior and last for at least 2 weeks. An MDD diagnosis is based on the presence of depressed or irritable mood or loss of interest or pleasure and at least five other symptoms, including sleep problems, fatigue, difficulty concentrating, weight or appetite changes, feelings of guilt or worthlessness, changes in psychomotor activity, and suicidal ideation. Symptoms must persist over 2 weeks and represent a substantial change from baseline.

A growing literature suggests that PBD presents differently in children and adolescents than in those with onset in adulthood. Youth onset is associated with less defined and shorter cycles (e.g., ultradian cycling), prominent irritability, chronic interepisode subsyndromal symptoms, recurrent subsyndromal episodes, mixed mood episodes, and high rates of comorbid conditions, such as attention-deficit/hyperactivity disorder (ADHD) and oppositional defiant disorder (ODD) (Biederman, 1995; Leibenluft, Charney, Towbin, Bhangoo, & Pine, 2003). Thus, many children and adolescents are diagnosed with unspecified BD because their episodes are shorter and/or too rapidly fluctuating to meet the duration criteria specified for both adults and youth. The term *broad phenotype* (Brotman et al., 2006) is often used to describe these youth who experience either (1) symptoms of mania and depression that are episodic but do not meet duration criteria or (2) chronic, severe mood dysregulation and hyperarousal that is extremely impairing, but for whom discrete episodes are not evident. There remains debate in the literature as to the inclusion of the "broad" phenotype in the bipolar spectrum (e.g., unspecified BD) or as a distinct diagnostic category (e.g., severe mood dysregulation or disruptive mood dysregulation disorder [DMDD]) (American Psychiatric Association, 2000; Brotman et al., 2007; McClellan, Kowatch, Findling, & Work Group on Quality, 2007).

Even with a standardized definition of PBD, challenges to diagnosis remain (Danner et al., 2009; Youngstrom, Freeman, & Jenkins, 2009). Differentiating between normative development and bipolar symptoms can be difficult, requiring sensitivity to and expertise in the developmental manifestation of mania and depression symptoms in youth. Accurate diagnosis is further complicated by the overlap of symptoms, as well as the co-occurrence of BD with other disorders (e.g., ADHD, disruptive behavior disorders). Discrete moods can be difficult to isolate due to rapid cycling and mixed mood symptoms. Finally, the variability in symptom presentation across mood states can lead to misdiagnosis, especially when there is limited access to multiple raters (i.e., both parents, teachers, self). For example, without an accurate history, bipolar symptoms may be misdiagnosed as severe ADHD or as MDD.

PREVALENCE AND COURSE

There are limited data available to inform prevalence rates for PBD. Current epidemiological data suggest that PBD occurs in approximately 1–2% of the population worldwide (Van Meter, Moreira, & Youngstrom, 2011), with some estimates for the "broad" phenotype as high as 3.3% (Brotman et al., 2006). There are few longitudinal studies on the course of BD across the lifespan, especially with regard to the transition from adolescence to adulthood. Retrospective studies of adults with BD indicate that as many as 60% of affected adults experienced symptoms of BD before age 20; 10–20% reported symptoms before age 10 (Egeland, Hostetter, Pauls, & Sussex, 2000; Lish, Dime-Meenan, Whybrow, Price, & Hirschfeld, 1994; Loranger & Levine, 1978). It remains unclear whether those children and adolescents diagnosed with PBD will demonstrate continuity of their childhood presentation of symptoms into adulthood.

The course of PBD across childhood and adolescence is chronic and severe. Results from the Course and Outcome of Bipolar Youth study indicate that 80% of youth ages 7–17 with bipolar spectrum disorders fully recover about 2.5 years after their index episode (the episode that brought them to treatment); however, approximately 60% subsequently have at least one recurrence within 1.5 years after recovery (Birmaher et al., 2009). The chronicity and recurrence of symptoms results in significant impairments in all domains of psychosocial functioning—individual, family, peer, and school/community. Compared to their peers, children with PBD demonstrate higher rates of math and reading problems (Henin et al., 2007; Pavuluri, O'Connor, Harral, Moss, & Sweeney, 2006) and disruptive school behavior (Geller, Zimerman, et al., 2002), as well as limited peer networks, bullying, and poor social skills (Geller, Craney, et al., 2002; Wilens et al., 2003). Poor family functioning complicates symptom management and coping. Individuals with PBD often experience strained sibling and parent relationships (Geller et al., 2000; Wilens et al., 2003), characterized by less warmth, affection, and intimacy, and more fighting, forceful punishment, and conflict (Schenkel, West, Harral, Patel, & Pavuluri, 2008). These negative experiences take their toll on development; not surprisingly, adolescents with PBD exhibit low self-esteem, hopelessness, external locus of control, maladaptive coping strategies (Rucklidge, 2006), poor social functioning (T. R. Goldstein, Miklowitz, & Mullen, 2006), high expressed emotion, and chronic stress in their family life (Kim, Miklowitz, Biuckians, & Mullen, 2007), as well as overall lower levels of family adaptability and cohesion (Keenan-Miller, Peris, Axelson, Kowatch, & Miklowitz, 2012). Youth with PBD are also at high risk for suicide attempts, with as many as 44% of adolescents with BD attempting suicide before age 18 (Lewinsohn, Seeley, & Klein, 2003). In adulthood, these patients demonstrate greater mental health care utilization, elevated rates of other chronic disease and health conditions, lower rates of school graduation, and loss of career productivity (Kessler et al., 2006; Kupfer, 2005; Lewinsohn, Olino, & Klein, 2005). Thus, PBD places a considerable burden on educational, occupational, and health care systems.

COMMON COMORBID CONDITIONS

Rates of comorbidity in PBD are high. A review of the major PBD phenomenology studies to date (Axelson et al., 2006) suggested significant rates of comorbid psychiatric disorders: ADHD, 69–87%; ODD, 46–86%; conduct disorder (CD), 12–41%; axiety disorders, 14–54%, and substance use disorder, 0–7% (average age of these samples ranged from 10 to 11 years). In the past, clinicians looked to the unique symptoms of mania (e.g., expansive mood, hypersexuality, racing thoughts, decreased need for sleep) to help differentiate bipolar from other conditions. However, recent research has challenged the sole reliance on mania symptoms for differential diagnosis. In the Longitudinal Assessment of Manic Symptoms study, Findling and colleagues (2010) found that whereas youth with elevated symptoms of mania demonstrated increased risk for PBD, 75% of these youth did not have PBD and were diagnosed with other disorders (e.g., ADHD, ODD, CD). These authors suggested that elevated mania may be a better indicator of severe psychopathology rather than a specific marker for PBD. Increased knowledge of the underlying physiology and the brain mechanisms impaired in PBD and other disorders may ultimately enable a better understanding of true comorbidity versus overlapping brain dysfunction that are common across diagnostic categories. For example, Youngstrom, Arnold, and Frazier (2010) have proposed that, especially with regard to ADHD comorbidity, high rates might reflect problems with our categorical diagnostic system; these researchers suggest that a dimensional understanding of symptoms and a focus on overlapping underlying biological substrates may yield more useful and accurate information.

ETIOLOGICAL/CONCEPTUAL MODELS OF PBD

The symptoms and psychosocial impairments in PBD likely persist because of the complex interplay of biological vulnerabilities, learned behaviors, and maladaptive interpersonal interactions that reinforce cognitive distortions and disruptive behavioral patterns. The symptoms of PBD are associated with profound psychosocial impairments across domains of social, academic, and family function (T. R. Goldstein et al., 2009; West & Pavuluri, 2009). These impairments may be not only a function of the symptoms but also may create a context of stressors that increase risk for onset and exacerbation. Youth with PBD demonstrate disruptive school behavior (Geller, Zimerman, et al., 2002), and their social functioning is marred my limited peer networks, peer victimization, and poor social skills (Geller, Craney, et al., 2002; T. R. Goldstein et al., 2006; Wilens et al., 2003). Families of youth with PBD may experience frequent sibling and parental conflict (Geller et al., 2000; Wilens et al., 2003); lower levels of warmth, family adaptability, and cohesion (T. R. Goldstein et al., 2009; Keenan-Miller et al., 2012; Schenkel et al., 2008); and chronic stress in family life (Kim et al., 2007). These difficulties may extend to the intrapersonal sphere, with youth with PBD exhibiting low self-esteem, hopelessness, external locus of control, and maladaptive coping strategies (T. R. Goldstein et al., 2009; Rucklidge, 2006).

Although the psychosocial manifestations of PBD symptoms are well documented and understood, only recently has research investigated the neurological underpinnings of the various symptoms and functional impairments observed in PBD. Preliminary findings have indicated that children with PBD demonstrate impairments in cognitive domains associated with learning, problem solving, and cognitive–emotional modulation, including attention, working memory, executive function, verbal memory, and processing speed, relative to healthy controls and in some cases, children with other psychiatric disorders (Bearden et al., 2006; Dickstein et al., 2004, 2007; Doyle et al., 2005; Henin et al., 2007; McClure et al., 2005; Pavuluri, Schenkel, et al., 2006). These neurocognitive impairments appear to persist over time (Pavuluri, West, Hill, Jindal, & Sweeney, 2009) and occur independent of mood state (Pavuluri, Schenkel, et al., 2006). Recently, Passarotti and Pavuluri (2011) summarized neuroscientific findings in PBD to propose an integrated neurobiological model involving altered functioning of the brain circuits responsible for response inhibition, reward, and executive functioning that underlie the affect dysregulation, low frustration tolerance, impulsivity, and maladaptive reward seeking experienced by youth with PBD. This model also differentiates the pathogenesis of symptoms and impairments in PBD from common co-occurring disorders such as ADHD (Passarotti & Pavuluri, 2011).

Research utilizing various genetic methods consistently demonstrates the importance of a genetic contribution to BD, with genetic factors explaining 60–85% of the variance in risk (Smoller & Finn, 2003). For example, studies examining monozygotic versus dizygotic twins indicate concordance estimates ranging from .33 to .75 for mono-zygotic twins and from zero to .13 for dizygotic twins (Kieseppa, Partonen, Haukka, Kaprio, & Lonnqvist, 2004). The genetic etiology of PBD is complex, and research is only beginning to identify specific genes that may elevate risk for BD (Barnett & Smoller, 2009; Kennedy, Cullen, DeYoung, & Klimes-Dougan, 2015). In addition, recent evidence suggests a pathophysiological relationship between immune system–mediated inflamma-tion and psychiatric disorders. This innovative model for understanding mood disorders submits that chronic, low-grade systemic inflammation (a complex reaction involving the immune and central nervous systems) may cause changes in brain structure and func-tion that inclines people toward mood dysregulation (Coppen, 1967; Schildkraut, 1965). Furthermore, inflammatory processes may interact with many other pathophysiological domains implicated in mood disorders, including neurotransmitter metabolism, neuro-endocrine function, synaptic plasticity, epigenetics, and behavior (Maes et al., 2009; Rai-son, Capuron, & Miller, 2006). While evidence supporting the pathogenic link between neuroendocrine/inflammatory markers and psychiatric disorders is strongest among adults with MDD (Dowlati et al., 2010), accumulating evidence suggests a similar ele-vated inflammatory signature in BD, and may be involved in mood dysregulation among youth as well (Berk et al., 2011).

Research on the neurocognitive and/or neurobiological circuits that underlie PBD symptoms is advancing quickly; new knowledge will not only help researchers more accurately characterize the pathogenesis of the disorder but also inform more targeted treatment approaches that operate on the specific mechanisms of illness. However, while knowledge is accumulating, the fact remains that PBD confers a very poor prognosis for those it affects and represents a substantial psychiatric burden. There is a clear need for high-quality, evidence-based pharmacological and psychosocial treatment methods to treat acute symptoms, improve psychosocial functioning, enhance quality of life, and optimize the chance for long-term remission of PBD symptoms.

EVIDENCE-BASED TREATMENTS FOR PBD

This section provides an overview of evidence-based psychosocial interventions designed for adjunctive use with pharmacotherapy to target PBD. A recent review (Fristad & MacPherson, 2014) evaluated existing psychosocial treatments for PBD following guide-lines provided by the Task Force on the Promotion and Dissemination of Psychological Procedures (Chambless et al., 1996, 1998; Chambless & Hollon, 1998; Chambless & Ollendick, 2001; Southam-Gerow & Prinstein, 2014) We present the treatments below in order of current evidence base, as identified by Fristad and MacPherson (2014) but updated to include recent research.

Well-Established and Probably Efficacious Treatments

"Well-established" treatments include those with support in at least two rigorous ran-domized controlled trials (RCTs), with active controls conducted by two independent research teams. Currently, there are no well-established treatments for PBD. How-ever, several existing interventions meet criteria for "probably efficacious" treatments, requiring either superiority to active control in at least one well-conducted RCT or two experiments demonstrating superiority to wait-list controls: child- and family-focused cognitive-behavioral therapy (CFF-CBT), family-focused therapy (FFT) for adolescents, and multifamily psychoeducational psychotherapy (MF-PEP).

CFF-CBT: The RAINBOW Program

To our knowledge, CFF-CBT is the only adaptation of CBT specific to school-age youth with BD that has been developed and tested. CFF-CBT is a family-focused CBT intervention for children ages 7–13 with PBD (West & Weinstein, 2012). The psychotherapeutic methods used in CFF-CBT are driven by three areas of research evidence: (1) affective circuitry brain dysfunction in PBD (e.g., poor problem solving during affective stimulation because of underactivity in the dorsolateral prefrontal cortex); (2) developmentally specific symptoms of PBD (e.g., rapid cycling, mixed mood states, comorbid disorders); and (3) the impact of PBD on psychosocial and interpersonal functioning (e.g., poor social functioning, family stress). Based on the scientific findings in these areas, the core concepts and initial CFF-CBT curricula were developed. Interventions in CFF-CBT integrate cognitive-behavioral approaches with psychoeducation, interpersonal psychotherapy, mindfulness, and positive psychology techniques, and are employed across multiple domains—individual, family, peer, and school. In practice, CFF-CBT is delivered through 12 weekly 60- to 90-minute sessions (equally divided among child-only, parent-only, and family sessions). The key components of CFF-CBT are captured by the acronym RAINBOW: Routine; Affect regulation; I can do it (self-efficacy boosting); No negative thoughts and live in the now; Be a good friend and Balanced lifestyles for parents; Oh, how can we solve this problem; and Ways to get social support. The range of topics covered includes establishing a predictable routine, mood monitoring, teaching behavioral management, increasing parent and child self-efficacy, decreasing negative cognitions, improving social functioning, engaging in collaborative problem solving, and increasing social support (see Table 5.1). Open-trial data support the efficacy of CFF-CBT in individual (Pavuluri et al., 2004), group (Pavuluri et al., 2009), and maintenance models (West, Henry, & Pavuluri, 2007). In addition, a recent RCT ($N = 69$) of youth with BD (ages 7–13, mean = 9 years) indicated efficacy for adjunctive (to medication) CFF-CBT in improving mania, depression, and global functioning compared to a control group receiving dose-matched psychotherapy as usual (West et al., 2014).

FFT for Adolescents

Miklowitz and colleagues (2004) adapted FFT for adults with BD to adolescents (FFT-A). The goal of FFT-A is to reduce symptoms and increase psychosocial functioning through an increased understanding about the disorder, decreased family conflict, and improved family communication, coping, and problem solving. FFT-A is delivered in 21 individual sessions over the course of 9 months and is organized into three components: psychoeducation (e.g., developing an understanding of the symptoms, etiology, and course of the disorder), communication enhancement training (e.g., active listening skills, role playing, and offering feedback), and problem solving (e.g., identifying problems and generating effective solutions). The efficacy of FFT-A as an adjunct to pharmacotherapy was

TABLE 5.1. Outline of CFF-CBT Treatment Protocol

Session	Participants	CFF-CBT components and topics covered
1	Child and parents together	• Orientation to treatment/goal setting • Engagement and relationship building with child and parents
2	Child and parents together	• *A: Affect regulation* • Psychoeducation about PBD • Mood charting via daily mood calendar (Figure 5.1)
3	Parents only	• *R: Routine; A: Affect regulation* • Affect regulation skills: establishing routines and anger management • Identifying and acknowledging parents' difficult feelings
4	Child only; parent check-in	• *A: Affect regulation* • Affect regulation skills • Labeling emotions; recognizing difficult feelings; triggers of anger and sadness
5	Child only; parent check-in	• *I: I can do it!; N: No negative thoughts and live in the now* • Problem solving and positive thinking • Cognitive and behavioral ("think" and "do") coping skills
6	Parents only	• *I: I can do it!; N: No negative thoughts and live in the now* • Identifying and promoting positive qualities in child • Positive thinking and mantras; reframing negative thoughts; mindfulness strategies
7	Child only; parent check-in	• *Be a good friend* • Communication skills and interpersonal problem solving
8	Parents only	• *B: Be a good friend and balanced lifestyle for parents* • Promoting child's social competence • Behavior management strategies • Balanced lifestyle for parents and enhancing self-care
9	Parents, child, siblings	• *O: Oh, how do we solve this problem?* • Psychoeducation about PBD provided to siblings • Family coping and problem-solving
10	Child and parents together	• *W: Ways to find support* • Identifying and enhancing access of social support networks
11	Child and parents together	• Reflection on RAINBOW experience • Review of RAINBOW skills, creation of RAINBOW binder to internalize and consolidate therapy tools
12	Child and parents together	• Celebration; follow-up/maintenance plan

examined in a two-site RCT with 58 adolescents (ages 12–17, mean = 14.5) with bipolar spectrum disorders and their families (Miklowitz et al., 2008). All participants received pharmacotherapy and were randomized to receive either FFT-A or "enhanced care" (three weekly family sessions focused on psychoeducation and relapse prevention). Results indicated that FFT-A youth experienced shorter time to recovery from depression, less time in depressive episodes, and lower depression severity scores over the 2-year study period than did those in the control condition. A recent RCT of FFT-A conducted with a larger sample (N = 145) of adolescents with BD (ages 12–18, mean = 15.6 years) indicated that those who participated in the treatment did not differ from an enhanced care control condition (three psychoeducation sessions) on time to recovery or recurrence, or weeks ill during follow-up. However, secondary analyses did reveal that participants in FFT-A had less severe manic symptoms during Year 2 (follow-up period) than controls (Miklowitz et al., 2014). FFT-A was recently adapted for youth who may be at risk for BD by virtue of (1) a diagnosis of BD not otherwise specified, MDD, or cyclothymic disorder and (2) having a first-degree relative with the diagnosis of BD I or II and active mood symptoms. Data from a small randomized trial of FFT-A (N = 40) for at-risk youth (ages 9–17, mean = 12.3 years) indicated more rapid recovery from initial mood symptoms, more weeks in remission, and a more favorable trajectory of mania symptoms over 1 year compared to youth in enhanced care (Miklowitz et al., 2013).

Psychoeducation

Fristad and colleagues (Fristad, Goldberg-Arnold, & Gavazzi, 2002; Fristad, Verducci, Walters, & Young, 2009) developed an adjunctive MF-PEP for children ages 8–12 with BD or depressive spectrum disorders and their parents. This treatment was originally developed to be delivered across eight multifamily group sessions. The goals of MF-PEP are to educate parents and children about the child's illness (either depression or BD), available treatment approaches, strategies for symptom management, problem-solving and communication skills, and coping skills, and to provide support for the parents. An RCT (N = 165) of adjunctive MF-PEP in youth (ages 8–12, mean = 10 years) with unipolar depression or BD demonstrated efficacy in reducing mood symptoms (Fristad et al., 2009) compared to a wait-list control group. Fristad and colleagues also adapted the treatment into an individual format (IF-PEP) delivered across 24 individual sessions and demonstrated preliminary efficacy for this intervention versus wait-list control in a small RCT (Fristad, 2006).

Possibly Efficacious Treatments

Dialectical behavior therapy (DBT) was adapted by T. R. Goldstein, Axelson, Birmaher, and Brent (2007) for adolescents with BD. DBT was originally developed for adults with borderline personality disorder to target emotional instability by combining standard cognitive-behavioral techniques for emotion regulation with concepts of distress tolerance, acceptance, and mindfulness (Linehan et al., 2006). DBT for adolescents with BD is delivered over the course of 1 year and comprises two modalities: family skills training (delivered to the whole family) and individual psychotherapy for the adolescent. The acute treatment phase lasts 6 months and includes 24 weekly sessions that alternate between individual and family therapy. The continuation treatment is 12 additional sessions that taper in frequency over the rest of the year. DBT has been evaluated in two studies, including a small open trial (T. R. Goldstein et al., 2007) and a pilot randomized trial (T. R. Goldstein et al., 2015) thus meeting criteria for a "possibly efficacious treatment" (i.e., at least two rigorous clinical studies demonstrating efficacy). The preliminary open trial of DBT for adolescents with BD was conducted with 10 youth, ages 14–18. Findings demonstrated significant decreases in suicidality, nonsuicidal self-injurious behavior, emotional dysregulation, and depression symptoms after the 1-year intervention (T. R. Goldstein et al., 2007). Additionally, a recent pilot RCT compared DBT (n = 14) to psychosocial treatment as usual (TAU; n = 6) in adolescents ages 12–18 with BD. Findings indicated improvement in depression symptoms and suicidal ideation at posttreatment for those receiving DBT compared to TAU (T. R. Goldstein et al., 2015).

Experimental Treatments

Hlastala and colleagues adapted *interpersonal and social rhythm therapy* (IPSRT; Frank et al., 2005) for adolescents with BD (IPSRT-A; Hlastala & Frank, 2006). IPSRT-A is in an earlier stage of development and is therefore classified as an *experimental treatment* (i.e., not yet tested in an RCT). IPSRT is an evidence-based psychotherapy for adults with BD that targets instability in circadian rhythms and neurotransmitter systems because of their known vulnerability as a precipitant for mood episodes. IPSRT aims to stabilize social and sleep routines, and to address interpersonal precipitants to dysregulation such as interpersonal conflict, role transitions, and interpersonal functioning deficits. IPSRT is primarily an individual treatment, but this adaptation to adolescents does incorporate brief family psychotherapy. A pilot open trial of IPSRT-A in 12 adolescents (mean age = 16.5) with BD indicated decreased symptoms and improved functioning from pre- to posttreatment (Hlastala, Kotler, McClellan, & McCauley, 2010).

Pharmacological Interventions

Historically, pharmacology has been the front-line treatment for PBD, and medications indicated for BD in adults are increasingly being used for children and adolescents. Most pharmacological treatment trials on PBD have focused on the treatment of bipolar mania (Hamrin & Iennaco, 2010). The agents typically used to treat mania in children and adolescents include lithium, antiepileptic drugs with mood-stabilizing effects, and second-generation antipsychotic (SGA) medications. Few large-scale, prospective studies have examined pharmacological treatment for PBD; thus, many of these medications are used without specific U.S. Food and Drug Administration (FDA) approval for PBD (Washburn et al., 2011). Although evidence supporting the effectiveness of these medications is increasing, significant gaps remain, and extant research suggests questionable efficacy of medications to fully address the disorder experience. In general, pharmacotherapy for PBD is complicated by low response rates and poor tolerability (B. I. Goldstein, Sassi, & Diler, 2012), and is not sufficient to address the range of PBD symptoms and functional impairments. For example, medication does not address important psychosocial domains such as understanding and accepting PBD, coping and problem-solving, and family support and communication. Thus, adjunctive psychosocial treatment is considered an essential component of effective treatment for PBD (McClellan et al., 2007) to address broader domains of functioning.

Predictors of Treatment Response

Few studies have examined predictors or moderators of psychosocial interventions in youth with PBD, but existing research highlights child and parent/family factors that influence treatment outcomes. In a recent examination of 165 youth with depression or bipolar spectrum disorders, nonresponse to psychosocial treatment was predicted by better baseline child global functioning, lower levels of stress/trauma history, and presence of personality disorder symptoms in parents (MacPherson, Algorta, Mendenhall, Fields, & Fristad, 2014). Moreover, children with moderately impaired functioning responded better to group psychoeducation relative to a wait-list control, while children with less impairment responded similarly in both conditions. Similarly, families characterized as high in expressed emotion (EE; i.e., overinvolvement and criticism) showed greater symptom improvement in response to FFT-A compared to a brief educational control, whereas low-EE families responded equally to the treatment conditions (D. J. Miklowitz et al., 2009). Our group recently examined treatment moderators of CFF-CBT in the randomized trial of 69 youth with PBD and their parents/caregivers (Weinstein, Henry, Katz, Peters, & West, 2015). Findings highlighted parent functioning as a moderator of child symptom response to CFF-CBT versus an enhanced TAU: Children of parents with higher depressive symptoms showed significantly greater improvement in their own depressive symptoms and, marginally, overall reduction in psychiatric severity across the course of CFF-CBT versus TAU. These findings suggest that parental depressive symptoms, even at subthreshold levels, interfered with treatment in TAU, and therefore converge with findings in the PBD literature suggesting that the effects of specialized treatment for PBD may be greatest for the higher-risk youth and families that these treatments are designed to target.

EVIDENCE-BASED ASSESSMENT AND TREATMENT IN PRACTICE

Assessment

The appropriate treatment of BD in children and adolescent is predicated on an accurate diagnosis. To improve the interrater reliability of PBD diagnoses, Youngstrom, Findling, Youngstrom, and Calabrese (2005) developed an evidence-based assessment protocol that incorporates existing approaches to the assessment of PBD for a variety of complex clinical presentations. This diagnostic protocol includes five steps: (1) screening for mania; (2) establishing an actuarial estimate of the likelihood of PBD; (3) evaluating diagnostic criteria with high specificity to PBD; (4) obtaining evidence of episodes; and (5) extending the window of assessment.

The first step involves screening for the presence of mania symptoms. The protocol recommends the use of the parent version of the Child Mania Rating Scale (CMRS), which is the first rating scale designed and tested specifically to screen for PBD (Pavuluri, Henry, Devineni, Carbray, & Birmaher, 2006). The CMRS includes 21 developmentally specific items that correspond to DSM criteria for BD. It has demonstrated strong psychometric properties indicating interrater reliability, concurrent validity with the Young Mania Rating Scale (YMRS), and sensitivity to symptom change across treatment (Pavuluri, Henry, et al., 2006; West, Celio, Henry, & Pavuluri, 2011).

In the second step of the protocol, the results of the screening measure and additional information (e.g., family history of BD) are used to obtain a probability estimate of PBD. This estimate is obtained through the use of a nomogram, which uses Bayes' theorem to estimate the probability of a diagnosis based on test findings or clinical observations (Youngstrom et al., 2005; Youngstrom & Youngstrom, 2005). The nomogram functions like a probability "slide rule" and allows the clinician to combine information about risk without having to rely on mathematical calculations. A detailed description of how to use the nomogram to obtain a probability estimate of PBD is available elsewhere (Jenkins, Youngstrom, Washburn, & Youngstrom, 2011).

The third step in the protocol involves evaluating symptoms to determine eligibility for a mood episode. This evidence-based protocol recommends that clinicians focus on those criteria that are highly specific to BD rather than focusing on criteria that overlap with other disorders, including (1) *decreased need for sleep* (e.g., a child may refuse to go to bed, or play, sing, or watch television late into the evening/early morning but deny feeling tired in the morning); (2) *unstable self-esteem and grandiosity* (e.g., the child or adolescent may make unsubstantiated statements that indicate inflated self-esteem or grandiosity beyond what is considered developmentally appropriate and that demonstrates mood congruency); (3) *hypersexuality* (e.g., pleasure-focused sexual behavior that is either developmentally atypical or unusual and uncharacteristic of the child—masturbating in public, touching strangers inappropriately); (4) *elated mood* (e.g., excessive and developmentally inappropriate excitability, silliness, and giddiness, uncontrollable laughter and joking); (5) *pressured speech and racing thoughts* (e.g., child reports that his or her mind is going so fast that he or she cannot stop it and his or her mouth cannot keep up); and (6) *goal-directed activity* (e.g., constantly fiddling with everything at home, playing games, or fighting with siblings, with inability to stop or slow down). Structured diagnostic interviews such as the Washington University in St. Louis Kiddie Schedule for Affective Disorders and Schizophrenia (WASH-U-KSADS; Geller et al., 2001) or the Schedule for Affective Disorders and Schizophrenia for School-Age Children—Present and Lifetime Versions (KSADS-PL; Kaufman et al., 1997) can be helpful instruments to assess these core symptom domains; the WASH-U-KSADS in particular includes suggested questions and probes to assess developmentally specific manifestations of mania and depressive symptoms.

The fourth step in the protocol involves obtaining evidence of episodes. A formal diagnosis of BD based on DSM criteria requires the identification of an index episode, be it a major depressive episode, dysthymic episode, manic episode, hypomanic episode, or mixed episode. The assessment of episodes requires information about both current and past symptoms; assessment tools such as the National Institute of Mental Health (NIMH) Life Chart Method (Denicoff et al., 2000) can be helpful in documenting lifetime mood episodes.

The final step in this evidence-based approach is to extend the window of assessment, particularly when the evidence for episodes is unclear or the clinician is not fully confident about the diagnosis. For the most accurate diagnosis, it is recommended that the window of assessment be extended, both retrospectively and prospectively, to clearly delineate changes in mood episodes (Youngstrom et al., 2005). The diagnosis of PBD is complex; as mentioned previously, the developmentally-specific manifestations of mania in children and adolescents can be challenging to assess and differential diagnosis often difficult. Additional expert guidance for diagnosing PBD can be found in the literature (Youngstrom, Birmaher, & Findling, 2008; Youngstrom et al., 2005, 2009). Although complex and the subject of some controversy, determining an accurate diagnosis of PBD is critical to the provision of effective treatment.

Treatment: CFF-CBT

Overview of Key Treatment Components

As reviewed previously in this chapter, PBD involves a combination of neurological underpinnings and both innate and learned patterns of emotional responses, thoughts, and behaviors. Neuroscientific research suggests that youth with PBD experience disturbances in the neural systems responsible for processing and modulating emotions (Pavuluri, O'Connor, Harral, & Sweeney, 2007), and therefore have difficulty regulating their emotions because they may experience a shutdown of emotional and cognitive control systems in the presence of affectively charged stimuli. CBT aims to address these impairments in affective circuitry, as well as impairments in social and family functioning, through various techniques at both the child and family levels. The integration of theory and psychosocial treatment research to date suggests several core components of CBT for youth with PBD. A primary component is *psychoeducation* to build the family's understanding of the symptoms, etiology, and typical course of PBD. Psychoeducation is the core parent- and family-level intervention and serves as the foundation for subsequent skills-building interventions. Important targets for psychoeducation include parental education about mood symptoms, the nature of mood episodes, risk factors and comorbidity, the role of medications and psychosocial treatment, and how to navigate mental health care and educational systems (Fristad et al., 2002).

CBT for PBD also focuses on the development of *affect regulatory strategies* to address impairments in emotion regulation at the child level, as well as to enhance parent self-regulation. Child-focused strategies include instruction and practice in the self-monitoring of mood states, recognizing and labeling feelings, and coping skills to manage expansive, negative, and irritable moods. Parents also benefit from interventions aimed at increasing their own affect regulation to boost parenting efficacy, particularly with regard to their management of rage episodes, as well as other behavioral management and coping strategies. All current evidence-based models for PBD incorporate affect and behavioral regulation strategies at the family level into their treatment model (Fristad et al., 2002; Miklowitz, 2012; West & Weinstein, 2012). As part of this work, youth and parents may learn *cognitive restructuring techniques* to reduce negative thought patterns (e.g., thought stopping, reframing situations positively, modifying thoughts, and use of positive self-talk/mantras during difficult situations). In addition, *mindfulness skills* can help parents manage their own difficult emotions and maintain equanimity in the face of their child's mood swings, rage episodes, or behavioral misconduct.

Parent training in *behavioral management strategies* can target the rage episodes common in PBD to help families prevent and cope with affective "storms." For example, many parents have previously incorporated behavioral management techniques developed for children with disruptive behavior disorders, which emphasize immediate contingency enforcement, redirection, and the swift implementation of consequences. Unfortunately, in youth with PBD, these methods often result in escalation of negative emotions given that the child's rage is understood as a neurobiologically mediated loss of control over emotional responses, rather than deliberate or manipulative behavior. As such, parents are instructed to use calming tones and to modulate their own responses so as not to model negative emotional reactivity. They are encouraged to focus on defusing the situation, keeping everyone safe, and using an empathic, collaborative problem-solving approach. Consequences and limits, if necessary, can be implemented later, when the child is calm. This approach is far more effective than more traditional behavioral management approaches in addressing affective outbursts that are common in PBD. Other behavioral strategies for regulating youth mood include establishing simple and predictable routines, minimizing the number of transitions, emphasizing the timing and tone of interactions during mood episodes, and using positive reinforcement. Youth and parents also engage in *problem-solving skills training* to target interpersonal and family difficulties, as well as to enhance self-efficacy related to coping with the disorder. Similarly, *social skills training* for youth focuses on role play, listening and communication skills, and increasing capacity for empathy to improve the interpersonal difficulties associated with PBD. Finally, parents are encouraged to engage in *self-care*—nourishing and relaxing activities—and to utilize their social support networks to help cope with the demands of caring for a child with PBD. Together, these cognitive-behavioral interventions help address the range of cognitive, social, and interpersonal impairments that are typical of PBD and provide families with a set of tools and skills to buffer against the negative impact of symptoms and improve their quality of life.

Parents also need support in coping with the burden of managing their child's illness. To achieve this goal, family-based interventions often have parent-focused sessions, designed to provide parents with space to process difficult feelings, learn the importance of good self-care, and connect to positive social supports. For example, CFF-CBT involves intensive work with the parents to address their own therapeutic needs and help them develop more effective parenting strategies for their child (West & Weinstein, 2012). Similarly, the content covered in the parent-only MF-PEP group sessions provides parents specific strategies to cope with the variety of challenges associated with their child's illness (Fristad et al., 2002). Although FFT-A does not typically involve individual work with the parents, it addresses the therapeutic needs of family members by working with the patient and family members together to decrease family conflict and enhance family communication (Miklowitz, 2012). Parents also may need assistance in advocating for their child's educational needs. Most children with PBD require adaptations to the academic environment to help them function appropriately and succeed both academically and socially; many have structured educational and social interventions as part of an individualized educational plan (IEP) (West & Peters, 2014).

Table 5.1 is a session-by-session outline of the CFF-CBT treatment protocol.

Key Measures/Tools Used during Treatment

CFF-CBT is a manual-based treatment. The manual includes a conceptual overview, session-by-session content, a clinician's guide, and all supplementary materials. The treatment materials include numerous weekly handouts and worksheets to aid in psycho-education and skills development. For example, a weekly mood monitoring worksheet (see Figure 5.1) helps children track their moods three times per day by coloring in how they feel. A feelings poster helps children identify and label how they are feeling. A "My Bugs" worksheet (see Figure 5.2) helps children identify and list their greatest triggers for anger, sadness, and other negative mood states. A "Think and Do" worksheet helps children identify alternative thoughts and actions in difficult situations. These worksheets, some of which are completed in session and others for homework, are compiled at the end of treatment into a CFF-CBT/RAINBOW binder to serve as a resource for children as they navigate mood regulation posttreatment. Parents are provided with summary worksheets at each child session reviewing the RAINBOW skills learned in that session and tasks to practice at home. To track treatment-related changes, clinicians are encouraged to administer measures of mania, depression, and psychosocial functioning over the course of treatment, such as the CMRS (Pavuluri, Henry, et al., 2006), the Children's Depression Inventory (CDI; Kovacs, 1992, 2014); and the Children's Global Assessment Scale (CGAS; Shaffer et al., 1983).

Case Example

Kelly B,* a 10-year-old, white female who lived at home with her biological parents and 14-year-old sister, was initially evaluated for the stabilization of her symptoms with medication. The psychiatrist diagnosed her with bipolar I disorder, carefully evaluated her medication needs, and prescribed a mood stabilizer. However, after a few months of medication management, though her acute symptoms improved somewhat, it became clear that substantial residual symptoms and psychosocial difficulties were not addressed by medication. To further improve her functioning, her psychiatrist referred her to a psychologist within the program for therapy. Kelly appeared to be a potential candidate for CFF-CBT/RAINBOW therapy, an approach developed to treat youth ages 7–13 with bipolar spectrum disorders and their families. At the time of her initial therapy appointment, Kelly was stable on medication and continued to attend regular follow-up appointments with her psychiatrist. The initial assessment with the psychologist was conducted via a structured clinical interview and mood symptoms rating scales (parent, child, and clinician reports). These measures indicated that Kelly did indeed met criteria for bipolar I disorder. She was experiencing frequent irritability, mood lability, and intense periods of anger or "rage attacks." During these episodes, Kelly became physically and verbally aggressive, destructive (e.g., knocking over chairs with such force that they occasionally broke), and made impulsive or risky decisions (e.g., running "away" from home without shoes). During her rage episodes, she was typically inconsolable. Despite her parents' best efforts to intervene, often they found that they had to "wait it out." In the meantime,

---

*This fictionalized case is based on the integration of information from multiple cases. Name and disorder characteristics do not identify a particular patient.

Name: _____   **Month:** _____

Color in the square using a color that best described your overall mood for each part of the day.
Key:
Blue = Sad
Red = Angry/Explosive
Gray = Crabby/Irritable
Yellow = Happy
Orange = Silly
Green = Neutral/Fair
Purple = Worried

Week 1:   **Date:** _____ to _____

	Sunday	Monday	Tuesday	Wednesday	Thursday	Friday	Saturday
Morning							
Afternoon							
Evening							

Week 2:   **Date:** _____ to _____

	Sunday	Monday	Tuesday	Wednesday	Thursday	Friday	Saturday
Morning							
Afternoon							
Evening							

FIGURE 5.1. Daily mood calendar.

Kelly would often scream and cry so hard that she made herself vomit, or bang on her parents' door. Her parents feared for her health and safety during these episodes, as well as the health and safety of her sister. These episodes occurred several times per week, and had decreased somewhat in frequency and intensity since initiating medication. Although the irritability and rage were the most concerning symptoms for the family, Kelly also had a history of periods of elated and giddy moods with increased energy, increased activity in several areas, motor hyperactivity, reduced sleep, and racing thoughts. For example, Kelly's parents would come downstairs in the morning to find that she had been play-ing on the computer since 2:00 A.M., and did not seem particularly fatigued. During

What Are My Bugs???

1) _____

2) _____

3) _____

4) _____

5) _____

6) _____

7) _____

8) _____

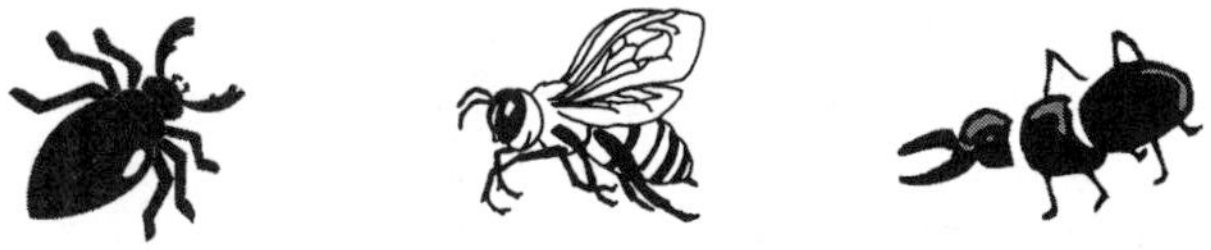

FIGURE 5.2. "My Bugs" worksheet.

these times, she often became obsessively involved in multiple activities (e.g., art projects, singing, video games) or extremely focused on play dates with peers, and pursued these activities with extreme intensity and focus. These periods of elated mood were often followed by an increase in irritability and depressed mood, rage, tearfulness, and feelings of worthlessness. During these periods, Kelly would express extreme remorse for her rage episodes, and state that she hated herself and wanted to die. Kelly's parents reported that she would often cycle between periods of euphoria and depressed/angry mood within the same day, sometimes multiple times per day. They expressed feeling utterly exhausted, hopeless, and at a loss for how to help her. They stated that her behavior had "wreaked havoc" on their family environment and that they all felt like they had to "walk on eggshells" around her, and their interactions as a family were ridden with tension and fear. Her sister was reluctant to invite friends to their home, for fear of witnessing a rage episode, and her parents also refrained from socializing in general. Both her mother and father felt helpless and isolated, and stated that her behavior had put a strain on their own relationship and self-care. They reported feeling so exhausted that they often reacted to her with either their own extreme anger/irritability or despair and withdrawal, both of which seemed to make things worse.

Kelly attended treatment sessions with her mother; her father attended parent-only and family sessions when he could. Below is a session-by-session illustration of treatment with Kelly and her family.

SESSIONS 1 AND 2: INTRODUCTION, TREATMENT OVERVIEW, AND PSYCHOEDUCATION

The first phase of treatment focused on orienting the family to the treatment model, engaging the family in the treatment process, and problem-solving barriers to adherence and identifying therapy goals. The therapist described the theoretical underpinnings of the treatment and how it could be helpful for Kelly and her family.

> "RAINBOW is a psychosocial treatment for parents and children developed to address factors associated with the bipolar disorder in children that might make the illness worse, such as lack of self-esteem, overstressed parents, coping skills that don't work, or poor peer relationships. The foundation of RAINBOW is the *vulnerability–stress* model, which means that psychosocial *stressors* interact with the child's individual *genetic* and *biological predisposition* to make symptoms worse. We cannot change genetics, but we can help change the psychosocial functioning of the child and family to make symptoms better and help everybody function better—in relationships, at home, and in school."

In this session, the clinician assessed and addressed Mrs. B's understanding and agreement with the treatment model. The therapist explained that there are several thoughts or feelings Mr. and Mrs. B might have regarding their involvement in treatment. Because of the "biological" and "genetic" underpinnings of PBD, the therapist acknowledged that Kelly's parents might not understand the importance of psychosocial interventions beyond medication intervention. She explained that this is why it is important to address engagement and expectations for treatment.

> "This treatment works best when everyone—Kelly, Mom, Dad, me—are all actively involved. There is no 'magic bullet.' The idea is to work together—some things may work, others may not. Change takes time. You have had years of interacting with each other a certain way, and it will take time for everyone to learn new skills and ways of acting. Things may even get worse before they get better, but it doesn't mean we are not making progress."

In the second session, the clinician provided Kelly and her parents with psychoeducation about PBD, including symptoms, neurobiological underpinnings, and medication.

> "We are much better at dealing with things that we understand. Pediatric bipolar disorder is complex, and there is a lot of misinformation out there. So, today we are going to talk about what bipolar disorder looks like in kids, what the course is, and how this all applies to you."

Kelly's core symptoms were identified and discussed in the context of scientific findings about differences in brain functioning. This was done to emphasize that PBD is a brain disorder and to help reduce attributions of blame associated with symptoms. Kelly and her mother also developed a common language for her symptoms (e.g., rage episodes were named "volcanoes" and Kelly's anger was described as "lava"). This process enabled Kelly to distance herself from her symptoms and to recognize that they were something that affected her but did not define her. The importance of medication was also discussed within the context of Kelly's experience of PBD symptoms. Finally, Mrs. B and Kelly were instructed to monitor Kelly's daily mood states and triggers for any mood fluctuations via a structured mood calendar (see Figure 5.1).

"Often, we don't know how we are feeling, or how it affects the way we act. But, if we pay attention, we may start to notice patterns in our moods—certain people, places, or times we feel a certain way. If we know these things, we can learn ways to decrease difficult feelings, and increase pleasant feelings. Let's start to pay attention to your moods during the week with this calendar."

SESSIONS 4–6: AFFECT REGULATION FOR THE CHILD AND PARENTS

The second phase of treatment focused on Kelly's affect dysregulation and the management of rage episodes. However, before implementing any changes, the therapist worked individually with Mrs. B to help her acknowledge and begin to accept her own difficult feelings about parenting a child with BD.

THERAPIST: Before we talk about how to improve Kelly's moods, let's focus on you. What has this experience been like for you?

MRS. B: It's been . . . difficult. But she's my daughter.

THERAPIST: A lot of times parents tell me that they feel a huge range of emotions—anger, resentment, shame.

MRS. B: Well . . . this isn't the life I planned on. I was so excited to have two girls—I couldn't wait to do things all together as she got older, talk, share. But we can't do anything together, or with anyone! It's exhausting, and sometimes, I just don't know how we are going to make it. Or how she is going to make it to 18 without winding up in jail, or something worse. And I can't help but blame my husband sometimes because mood disorders run in *his* family. But then I feel so guilty for thinking this way about Kelly, and her dad. (*Becomes tearful.*)

THERAPIST: Parenting is a daunting task at best—these feelings are not only completely understandable, but expected. Negative feelings about your child do not make you a bad parent. But with time, we can work on accepting Kelly for who she is—rather than what you expected her to be. This is not an easy process! However, thinking about her behaviors as something that she can't always control, rather than as deliberate negative behaviors, may help you begin to see her in a new light.

In addition to processing these difficult feelings, the therapist worked with Kelly's parents to implement consistent routines to improve two identified areas of difficulty: bedtime and transitions. In the morning, Mrs. B agreed to help Kelly implement a soothing and consistent bedtime routine that included a bath, quiet one-on-one time or reading with her mother or father in her bed, 15 minutes of reading for pleasure, and lights out. All electronic devices were off-limits during the bedtime routine, and Kelly drew and decorated a picture chart of this routine. To help ease other transitions, Mrs. B committed to providing ample warnings and posting the daily schedule around the house to help Kelly anticipate and prepare for transitions. Parent sessions during this phase also focused on helping them to manage Kelly's anger outbursts as a family. The analogy of "putting out a fire" was used to facilitate Mr. and Mrs. B's ability to remain neutral and calm while defusing the situation, versus engaging in the episode and exacerbating Kelly's distress. Coping plans were developed to help prevent these episodes and to manage them if they did occur. Coping strategies included having Mrs. B use self-statements/mantras to remind herself that she had a plan to cope with and to modulate her own responses to Kelly's intense emotion, and mindfulness-based techniques to remain focused on the present moment and increase her ability to stay calm and empathic. In addition, the plan included reaching out to Kelly's father or other family members for support, implementing soothing activities to help Kelly deescalate her anger, and using appropriate consequences for target negative behaviors (e.g., physical or verbal aggression) only after everyone involved was feeling calm and emotionally stabilized. Mr. and Mrs. B were instructed in specific cognitive and mindfulness-based techniques to use during difficult situations (e.g., reframing Kelly's behavior in the context of her neurocircuitry to foster greater empathy and focusing on breathing in the present moment to avoid feeling overwhelmed).

Child sessions during this phase primarily focused on helping Kelly to identify and express her feelings and to better understand the triggers for difficult emotions and negative moods—which were called her "bugs." The therapist employed games, worksheets, drawings, songs, and role play to help Kelly practice cognitive and behavioral skills for coping with future "bugs" and the negative emotions they evoked. The physiological warning signs, or "clues," of anger were identified to facilitate use of coping skills.

THERAPIST: When we first feel angry, we usually get a warning sign—or an "anger clue." This may be in our body—like clenching our teeth or making a fist. When we lose control, it's like a volcano exploding. Our anger is kind of like the lava bubbling up inside of us. But we have clues in our body that can help us stop the volcano from exploding. Let's figure out where you feel anger in your body.

KELLY: Well, my feet want to kick something.

THERAPIST: Do you notice anything else changing in your body—like a feeling in your hands, stomach, or even your face?

KELLY: My face gets all hot, and I guess my hand gets balled into a fist, ready to hit.

THERAPIST: Now we've identified your anger clues. When you feel these sensations in your body, you know your anger is bubbling up and it's time to take action. We're going to help you figure out what you can do to stop the lava bubbles from turning into an exploding volcano.

After identifying her "bugs," the child sessions in this phase covered the development of various coping strategies, including the use of "think and do" skills to brainstorm ways of responding to triggers at home and school, and drawing on positive thinking and mantras to provide confidence when dealing with tough emotions or situations. The therapist helped Kelly to identify her many positive qualities and discuss how she could use these strengths and positive qualities to cope with her "bugs." The therapist helped

Kelly to understand that these qualities comprised the core of her identity and that BD was just one small part of who she was. Finally, the therapist helped to normalize feelings of frustration, sadness, and other negative emotions that occurred when Kelly was triggered and found it difficult to employ her coping strategies. The therapist helped Kelly develop scripts to use in these situations that fostered self-compassion rather than self-criticism and blame.

SESSIONS 7–10: SOCIAL SKILLS AND PROBLEM SOLVING

As Kelly's family became better able to prevent and manage affect dysregulation and rage episodes, the third phase of treatment focused on developing social skills, and understanding and managing family and environmental stressors that contributed to stress and poor coping. The child session in this phase focused on improving Kelly's social skills. She learned the difference between verbal and nonverbal communication, what defined respectful communication, and communication skills such as BEME skills (Back straight, Eye contact, Mouth to speak clearly, Ears to listen), and "I" messages. She practiced engaging in appropriate conversations with the therapist and parents in sessions, and given the homework of practicing with peers.

THERAPIST: What does the word "respect" mean?

KELLY: I don't really know. Maybe it means to be nice and not be mean.

THERAPIST: That's a great answer! Let's think more about what that means in practice and how it relates to being respectful of other people. If you are trying to be nice, maybe you might try to be considerate of other people's feelings and treat others how you would like to be treated. You might also try to be accepting of what other people think or believe and try to be kind to others. Can you give me some examples of ways in which you show respect to your parents?

KELLY: Last night I helped my mom do the dishes even though she didn't ask me. Also I paid attention to my dad when he said it was time to go to bed and I didn't fight him. And I gave him a big hug and a kiss good night.

THERAPIST: Those are great examples of ways in which you were considerate of your parent's feelings and acted in a loving way toward them. That was respectful behavior.

The therapist asked Kelly for examples of both respectful and disrespectful behavior, and they discussed the consequences of both for Kelly.

Parent sessions in this phase focused on building Kelly's social competence through supervised playdates with peers, and advocating for her social needs at school. Mrs. B was encouraged to be a social skills coach for Kelly, and she and the therapist discussed different ways that she could help Kelly problem-solve and cope in difficult interpersonal situations. In addition, behavioral management for rage episodes was a major focus of this phase of treatment. The therapist discussed with Mrs. B what methods she currently used to address Kelly's behavioral outbursts. Mrs. B reported that she had read a lot of parenting books that emphasized immediate contingency enforcement, redirection, and the swift implementation of consequences. The therapist educated her about the fact that many of these techniques were developed for children with a disruptive behavior disorder and that, unfortunately, in youth with PBD, these methods can backfire. The therapist normalized the fact that many parents are left puzzled as to why these strategies only seem to make the episodes worse and feel very demoralized. The therapist emphasized that children whose rage is rooted in a loss of control over emotional responses (rather than a purposeful, manipulative behavior) will not respond to limit setting in the moment; in fact, this will only exacerbate their negative emotions. Rather, she instructed Mrs. B to use calming tones and try to modulate her own responses so as not to model negative emotional reactivity. Mrs. B was encouraged to focus on defusing the situation, keeping everyone safe, and using an empathic, collaborative problem-solving approach. She and the therapist discussed how consequences and limits, if necessary, could be implemented later when Kelly was calm. Another focus of the parent work in this phase of treatment was an emphasis on Mrs. B's well-being and balance between self-care and parenting responsibilities to avoid "burnout." For example, Mrs. B was encouraged to schedule one yoga class and one friend outing (two important self-care activities she identified) and she and Mr. B committed to one date night every 2 weeks to nurture their relationship.

Finally, this session included a session attended by all family members. This session was attended by Kelly, her sister, and her parents. The therapist provided education on PBD and suggested strategies to improve family interactions through family problem solving. Family members were prompted to identify their strengths as well as familywide "bugs" and to develop coping plans for managing their "bugs" as a team. Kelly's family also agreed on ways to increase positive family interactions (e.g., planned family outings).

THERAPIST: We know that sometimes Kelly gets really angry and feels like she can't help it. Let's talk about how each member of the family feels in these situations and how they respond. Kelly, we'll start with you.

KELLY: I feel bad. And I can't control it. I start crying and screaming and sometimes slam my door.

MRS. B: Sometimes I feel like I don't know what to do. I don't know how to help her. And I'm scared for my other daughter's safety because sometimes she gets violent. And I just get really frustrated that nothing seems to help. I often end up screaming myself, and I know that doesn't help.

MR. B: I hate seeing my little girl like that. I just don't understand why she can't calm down, but I'm starting to understand better now. Usually when she gets like that I try to reason with her or talk to her.

SISTER: It scares me. She gets really mean and seems like a different sister, not my sister. I feel like she is going to hurt someone, like I need to protect my mom.

THERAPIST: Thank you all for sharing so honestly. It's really important that you all talk to each other about how you feel. We know that Kelly often cannot control her feelings in these situations and that it is really hard to know what to do to help her, so it's nobody's fault that sometimes things get out of control. We are going to talk about ways you can work together as a family to express your feelings to each other, cope with these situations, and problem-solve solutions. Together we're going to come up with a family coping plan so you can work together as a team!

SESSIONS 11 AND 12: AFFECT REGULATION FOR CHILD AND PARENTS

The final treatment phase focused on preparing for the transition from weekly therapy to monthly maintenance sessions. Kelly created a binder of therapy exercises to help her remember and use these therapy tools. The therapist discussed with Mrs. B and Kelly ways to continue to implement therapy strategies at home and how to problem-solve challenges or barriers that arose. Positive changes in the family across treatment were reviewed and celebrated, including Kelly's increased awareness of her moods and triggers, and a reduction in her episodes from daily outbursts to less frequent and less intense episodes.

OUTCOMES OF TREATMENT

Over the course of treatment, Kelly demonstrated greater insight into her symptoms, improved self-esteem and a sense of efficacy in coping, and the ability cognitively to reframe her angry thoughts (e.g., "Nobody loves me"). She was increasingly able to use her coping skills independently and prevent her anger from escalating. Kelly responded well to the presentation of therapy material in a nonthreatening, creative, and engaging manner, and also benefited from the therapist's work to help her recognize her many positive qualities. Kelly's parents became increasingly proficient in their ability to recognize warning signs of distress and either disengage or help to soothe Kelly early on to prevent further escalation. As a result of these changes at the individual and family levels, Kelly's anger episodes decreased in intensity, frequency, and duration. Mrs. B also reported great improvement in her self-efficacy as a parent and her attention to her own self-care, and improved family relationships. Objective measures at the conclusion of the treatment indicated significant improvement in Kelly's mania and depression symptoms, family cohesion, and overall global functioning.

CONCLUSION

PBD is a complex and multifaceted disorder that demonstrates a unique clinical presentation and developmentally specific symptoms compared to adult-onset BD. The heterogeneous symptoms and psychosocial impairments associated with PBD confer an extremely poor prognosis and represent a significant public health burden. Although psychopharmacology to stabilize mood is often a first-line treatment approach, psychosocial intervention is considered essential to address broader domains of functioning, such as self-concept, peer relationships, and family communication. Several psychosocial treatment models have been developed for children and adolescents, and various levels of evidence support their efficacy. Intervention approaches that may be beneficial for PBD include affect regulation strategies, cognitive restructuring, behavior management, problem solving, and social skills training. In addition, it is imperative that interventions involve intensive work with parents to address their own cognitive and emotional functioning and to increase self-care and social support. At the family level, intervention must address family communication, coping, and problem solving. Finally, effective treatment incorporates advocacy for success in the school environment.

REFERENCES

American Psychiatric Association. (2000). *Diagnostic and statistical manual of mental disorders* (4th ed., text rev.). Washington, DC: Author.

American Psychiatric Association. (2013). *Diagnostic and statistical manual of mental disorders* (5th ed.). Arlington, VA: Author.

Axelson, D., Birmaher, B., Strober, M., Gill, M. K., Valeri, S., Chiappetta, L., et al. (2006). Phenomenology of children and adolescents with bipolar spectrum disorders. *Archives of General Psychiatry, 63*(10), 1139–1148.

Barnett, J. H., & Smoller, J. W. (2009). The genetics of bipolar disorder. *Neuroscience, 164*(1), 331–343.

Bearden, C. E., Glahn, D. C., Monkul, E. S., Barrett, J., Najt, P., Kaur, S., et al. (2006). Sources of declarative memory impairment in bipolar disorder: Mnemonic processes and clinical features. *Journal of Psychiatric Research, 40*(1), 47–58.

Berk, M., Kapczinski, F., Andreazza, A., Dean, O., Giorlando, F., Maes, M., et al. (2011). Pathways underlying neuroprogression in bipolar disorder: Focus on inflammation, oxidative stress and neurotrophic factors. *Neuroscience and Biobehavioral Reviews, 35*(3), 804–817.

Biederman, J. (1995). Developmental subtypes of juvenile bipolar disorder. *Harvard Review of Psychiatry, 3*(4), 227–230.

Birmaher, B., Axelson, D., Goldstein, B., Strober, M., Gill, M. K., Hunt, J., et al. (2009). Four-year longitudinal course of children and adolescents with bipolar spectrum disorders: The Course and Outcome of Bipolar Youth (COBY) study. *American Journal of Psychiatry, 166*(7), 795–804.

Brotman, M. A., Kassem, L., Reising, M. M., Guyer, A. E., Dickstein, D. P., Rich, B. A., et al. (2007). Parental diagnoses in youth with narrow phenotype bipolar disorder or severe mood dysregulation. *American Journal of Psychiatry, 164*(8), 1238–1241.

Brotman, M. A., Schmajuk, M., Rich, B. A., Dickstein, D. P., Guyer, A. E., Costello, E. J., et al. (2006). Prevalence, clinical correlates, and longitudinal course of severe mood dysregulation in children. *Biological Psychiatry, 60*(9), 991–997.

Chambless, D. L., Baker, M. J., Baucom, D. H., Beutler, L. E., Calhoun, K. S., Crits-Christoph, P., et al. (1998). Update on empirically validated therapies: II. *Clinical Psychologist, 51*(1), 3–16.

Chambless, D. L., & Hollon, S. D. (1998). Defining empirically supported therapies. *Journal of Consulting and Clinical Psychology, 66*(1), 7–18.

Chambless, D. L., & Ollendick, T. H. (2001). Empirically supported psychological interventions: Controversies and evidence. *Annual Review of Psychology, 52*(1), 685–716.

Chambless, D. L., Sanderson, W. C., Shoham, V., Bennett Johnson, S., Pope, K. S., Crits-Christoph, P., et al. (1996). An update on empirically validated therapies. *Clinical Psychologist, 49*, 5–18.

Coppen, A. (1967). The biochemistry of affective disorders. *British Journal of Psychiatry, 113*(504), 1237–1264.

Danner, S., Fristad, M. A., Arnold, L. E., Youngstrom, E. A., Birmaher, B., Horwitz, S. M., et al. (2009). Early-onset bipolar spectrum disorders: Diagnostic issues. *Clinical Child and Family Psychology Review, 12*(3), 271–293.

Denicoff, K. D., Leverich, G. S., Nolen, W. A., Rush, A. J., McElroy, S. L., Keck, P. E., et al. (2000). Validation of the prospective NIMH-Life-Chart Method (NIMH-LCM-p) for longitudinal assessment of bipolar illness. *Psychological Medicine, 30*(6), 1391–1397.

Dickstein, D. P., Nelson, E. E., McClure, E. B., Grimley, M. E., Knopf, L., Brotman, M. A., et al. (2007). Cognitive flexibility in phenotypes of pediatric bipolar disorder. *Journal of the American Academy of Child and Adolescent Psychiatry, 46*(3), 341–355.

Dickstein, D. P., Treland, J. E., Snow, J., McClure, E. B., Mehta, M. S., Towbin, K. E., et al. (2004). Neuropsychological performance in pediatric bipolar disorder. *Biological Psychiatry, 55*(1), 32–39.

Dowlati, Y., Herrmann, N., Swardfager, W., Liu, H., Sham, L., Reim, E. K., & Lanctot, K. L. (2010). A meta-analysis of cytokines in major depression. *Biological Psychiatry, 67*(5), 446–457.

Doyle, A. E., Wilens, T. E., Kwon, A., Seidman, L. J., Faraone, S. V., Fried, R., et al. (2005). Neuropsychological functioning in youth with bipolar disorder. *Biological Psychiatry, 58*(7), 540–548.

Egeland, J. A., Hostetter, A. M., Pauls, D. L., & Sussex, J. N. (2000). Prodromal symptoms before onset of manic–depressive disorder suggested by first hospital admission histories. *Journal of the American Academy of Child and Adolescent Psychiatry, 39*(10), 1245–1252.

Findling, R. L., Youngstrom, E. A., Fristad, M. A., Birmaher, B., Kowatch, R. A., Arnold, L. E., et al. (2010). Characteristics of children with elevated symptoms of mania: The Longitudinal Assessment of Manic Symptoms (LAMS) study. *Journal of Clinical Psychiatry, 71*(12), 1664–1672.

Frank, E., Kupfer, D. J., Thase, M. E., Mallinger, A. G., Swartz, H. A., Fagiolini, A. M., et al. (2005). Two-year outcomes for interpersonal and social rhythm therapy in individuals with bipolar I disorder. *Archives of General Psychiatry, 62*(9), 996–1004.

Fristad, M. A. (2006). Psychoeducational treatment for school-aged children with bipolar disorder. *Development and Psychopathology, 18*(4), 1289–1306.

Fristad, M. A., Goldberg-Arnold, J. S., & Gavazzi, S. M. (2002). Multifamily psychoeducation groups (MFPG) for families of children with bipolar disorder. *Bipolar Disorder, 4*(4), 254–262.

Fristad, M. A., & MacPherson, H. A. (2014). Evidence-based psychosocial treatments for child and adolescent bipolar spectrum disorders. *Journal of Clinical Child and Adolescent Psychology, 43*(3), 339–355.

Fristad, M. A., Verducci, J. S., Walters, K., & Young, M. E. (2009). Impact of multifamily psychoeducational psychotherapy in treating children aged 8 to 12 years with mood disorders. *Archives of General Psychiatry, 66*(9), 1013–1021.

Geller, B., Bolhofner, K., Craney, J. L., Williams, M., DelBello, M. P., & Gundersen, K. (2000). Psychosocial functioning in a prepubertal and early adolescent bipolar disorder phenotype. *Journal of the American Academy of Child and Adolescent Psychiatry, 39*(12), 1543–1548.

Geller, B., Craney, J. L., Bolhofner, K., Nickelsburg, M. J., Williams, M., & Zimerman, B. (2002). Two-year prospective follow-up of children with a prepubertal and early adolescent bipolar disorder phenotype. *American Journal of Psychiatry, 159*(6), 927–933.

Geller, B., Zimerman, B., Williams, M., Bolhofner, K., Craney, J. L., DelBello, M. P., et al. (2001). Reliability of the Washington University in St. Louis Kiddie Schedule for Affective Disorders and Schizophrenia (WASH-U-KSADS) mania and rapid cycling sections. *Journal of the American Academy of Child and Adolescent Psychiatry, 40*(4), 450–455.

Geller, B., Zimerman, B., Williams, M., Delbello, M. P., Frazier, J., & Beringer, L. (2002). Phenomenology of prepubertal and early adolescent bipolar disorder: examples of elated mood, grandiose behaviors, decreased need for sleep, racing thoughts and hypersexuality. *Journal of Child and Adolescent Psychopharmacology, 12*(1), 3–9.

Goldstein, B. I., Sassi, R., & Diler, R. S. (2012). Pharmacologic treatment of bipolar disorder in children and adolescents. *Child and Adolescent Psychiatric Clinics of North America, 21*(4), 911–939.

Goldstein, T. R., Axelson, D. A., Birmaher, B., & Brent, D. A. (2007). Dialectical behavior therapy for adolescents with bipolar disorder: A 1-year open trial. *Journal of the American Academy of Child and Adolescent Psychiatry, 46*(7), 820–830.

Goldstein, T. R., Birmaher, B., Axelson, D., Goldstein, B. I., Gill, M. K., Esposito-Smythers, C., et al. (2009). Psychosocial functioning among bipolar youth. *Journal of Affective Disorders, 114*(1), 174–183.

Goldstein, T. R., Fersch-Podrat, R. K., Rivera, M., Axelson, D. A., Merranko, J., Yu, H., et al. (2015). Dialectical behavior therapy for adolescents with bipolar disorder: Results from a pilot randomized trial. *Journal of Child and Adolescent Psychopharmacology, 25*(2), 140–149.

Goldstein, T. R., Miklowitz, D. J., & Mullen, K. L. (2006). Social skills knowledge and performance among adolescents with bipolar disorder. *Bipolar Disorder, 8*(4), 350–361.

Hamrin, V., & Iennaco, J. D. (2010). Psychopharmacology of pediatric bipolar disorder. *Expert Review of Neurotherapeutics, 10*(7), 1053–1088.

Henin, A., Mick, E., Biederman, J., Fried, R., Wozniak, J., Faraone, S. V., et al. (2007). Can bipolar disorder-specific neuropsychological impairments in children be identified? *Journal of Consulting and Clinical Psychology, 75*(2), 210–220.

Hlastala, S. A., & Frank, E. (2006). Adapting interpersonal and social rhythm therapy to the developmental needs of adolescents with bipolar disorder. *Development and Psychopathology, 18*(4), 1267–1288.

Hlastala, S. A., Kotler, J. S., McClellan, J. M., & McCauley, E. A. (2010). Interpersonal and social rhythm therapy for adolescents with bipolar disorder: Treatment development and results from an open trial. *Depression and Anxiety, 27*(5), 457–464.

Jenkins, M. M., Youngstrom, E. A., Washburn, J. J., & Youngstrom, J. K. (2011). Evidence-based strategies improve assessment of pediatric bipolar disorder by community practitioners. *Professional Psychology: Research and Practice, 42*(2), 121–129.

Kaufman, J., Birmaher, B., Brent, D., Rao, U., Flynn, C., Moreci, P., et al. (1997). Schedule for Affective Disorders and Schizophrenia for School-Age Children—Present and Lifetime Version (K-SADS-PL): Initial reliability and validity data. *Journal of the American Academy of Child and Adolescent Psychiatry, 36*(7), 980–988.

Keenan-Miller, D., Peris, T., Axelson, D., Kowatch, R. A., & Miklowitz, D. J. (2012). Family functioning, social impairment, and symptoms among adolescents with bipolar disorder. *Journal of the American Academy of Child and Adolescent Psychiatry, 51*(10), 1085–1094.

Kennedy, K. P., Cullen, K. R., DeYoung, C. G., & Klimes-Dougan, B. (2015). The genetics of early-onset bipolar disorder: A systematic review. *Journal of Affective Disorders, 184*, 1–12.

Kessler, R. C., Akiskal, H. S., Ames, M., Birnbaum, H., Greenberg, P., Hirschfeld, R. M., et al. (2006). Prevalence and effects of mood disorders on work performance in a nationally representative sample of U.S. workers. *American Journal of Psychiatry, 163*(9), 1561–1568.

Kieseppa, T., Partonen, T., Haukka, J., Kaprio, J., & Lonnqvist, J. (2004). High concordance of bipolar I disorder in a nationwide sample of twins. *American Journal of Psychiatry, 161*(10), 1814–1821.

Kim, E. Y., Miklowitz, D. J., Biuckians, A., & Mullen, K. (2007). Life stress and the course of early-onset bipolar disorder. *Journal of Affective Disorders, 99*(1–3), 37–44.

Kovacs, M. (1992). *Children's Depression Inventory*. North Tonawanda, NY: Multi-Health Systems.

Kovacs, M. (2014). *Children's Depression Inventory 2*. North Tonawanda, NY: Multi-Health Systems.

Kupfer, D. J. (2005). The increasing medical burden in bipolar disorder. *Journal of the American Medical Association, 293*(20), 2528–2530.

Leibenluft, E., Charney, D. S., Towbin, K. E., Bhangoo, R. K., & Pine, D. S. (2003). Defining clinical phenotypes of juvenile mania. *American Journal of Psychiatry, 160*(3), 430–437.

Lewinsohn, P. M., Olino, T. M., & Klein, D. N. (2005). Psychosocial impairment in offspring of depressed parents. *Psychological Medicine, 35*(10), 1493–1503.

Lewinsohn, P. M., Seeley, J. R., & Klein, D. N. (2003). *Bipolar disorder in adolescents: Epidemiology and suicidal behavior*. New York: Guilford Press.

Linehan, M. M., Comtois, K. A., Murray, A. M., Brown, M. Z., Gallop, R. J., Heard, H. L., et al. (2006). Two-year randomized controlled trial and follow-up of dialectical behavior therapy vs therapy by experts for suicidal behaviors and borderline personality disorder. *Archives of General Psychiatry, 63*(7), 757–766.

Lish, J. D., Dime-Meenan, S., Whybrow, P. C., Price, R. A., & Hirschfeld, R. M. (1994). The

National Depressive and Manic–Depressive Association (DMDA) survey of bipolar members. *Journal of Affective Disorders, 31*(4), 281–294.

Loranger, A. W., & Levine, P. M. (1978). Age at onset of bipolar affective illness. *Archives of General Psychiatry, 35*(11), 1345–1348.

MacPherson, H. A., Algorta, G. P., Mendenhall, A. N., Fields, B. W., & Fristad, M. A. (2014). Predictors and moderators in the randomized trial of multifamily psychoeducational psychotherapy for childhood mood disorders. *Journal of Clinical Child and Adolescent Psychology, 43*(3), 459–472.

Maes, M., Yirmyia, R., Noraberg, J., Brene, S., Hibbeln, J., Perini, G., et al. (2009). The inflammatory and neurodegenerative (I&ND) hypothesis of depression: Leads for future research and new drug developments in depression. *Metabolic Brain Disease, 24*(1), 27–53.

McClellan, J., Kowatch, R., Findling, R. L., & Work Group on Quality, I. (2007). Practice parameter for the assessment and treatment of children and adolescents with bipolar disorder. *Journal of the American Academy of Child and Adolescent Psychiatry, 46*(1), 107–125.

McClure, E. B., Treland, J. E., Snow, J., Schmajuk, M., Dickstein, D. P., Towbin, K. E., et al. (2005). Deficits in social cognition and response flexibility in pediatric bipolar disorder. *American Journal of Psychiatry, 162*(9), 1644–1651.

Miklowitz, D. J. (2012). Family-focused treatment for children and adolescents with bipolar disorder. *Israel Journal of Psychiatry and Related Sciences, 49*(2), 95–101.

Miklowitz, D. J., Axelson, D. A., Birmaher, B., George, E. L., Taylor, D. O., Schneck, C. D., et al. (2008). Family-focused treatment for adolescents with bipolar disorder: Results of a 2-year randomized trial. *Archives of General Psychiatry, 65*(9), 1053–1061.

Miklowitz, D. J., Axelson, D. A., George, E. L., Taylor, D. O., Schneck, C. D., Sullivan, A. E., et al. (2009). Expressed emotion moderates the effects of family-focused treatment for bipolar adolescents. *Journal of the American Academy of Child and Adolescent Psychiatry, 48*(6), 643–651.

Miklowitz, D. J., George, E. L., Axelson, D. A., Kim, E. Y., Birmaher, B., Schneck, C., et al. (2004). Family-focused treatment for adolescents with bipolar disorder. *Journal of Affective Disorders, 82*(Suppl. 1), S113–S128.

Miklowitz, D. J., Schneck, C. D., George, E. L., Taylor, D. O., Sugar, C. A., Birmaher, B., et al. (2014). Pharmacotherapy and family-focused treatment for adolescents with bipolar I and II disorders: A 2-year randomized trial. *American Journal of Psychiatry, 171*(6), 658–667.

Miklowitz, D. J., Schneck, C. D., Singh, M. K., Taylor, D. O., George, E. L., Cosgrove, V. E., et al. (2013). Early intervention for symptomatic youth at risk for bipolar disorder: A randomized trial of family-focused therapy. *Journal of the American Academy of Child and Adolescent Psychiatry, 52*(2), 121–131.

Passarotti, A. M., & Pavuluri, M. N. (2011). Brain functional domains inform therapeutic interventions in attention-deficit/hyperactivity disorder and pediatric bipolar disorder. *Expert Review of Neurotherapeutics, 11*(6), 897–914.

Pavuluri, M. N., Graczyk, P. A., Henry, D. B., Carbray, J. A., Heidenreich, J., & Miklowitz, D. J. (2004). Child- and family-focused cognitive-behavioral therapy for pediatric bipolar disorder: Development and preliminary results. *Journal of the American Academy of Child and Adolescent Psychiatry, 43*(5), 528–537.

Pavuluri, M. N., Henry, D. B., Devineni, B., Carbray, J. A., & Birmaher, B. (2006). Child mania rating scale: Development, reliability, and validity. *Journal of the American Academy of Child and Adolescent Psychiatry, 45*(5), 550–560.

Pavuluri, M. N., O'Connor, M. M., Harral, E. M., Moss, M., & Sweeney, J. A. (2006). Impact of neurocognitive function on academic difficulties in pediatric bipolar disorder: A clinical translation. *Biological Psychiatry, 60*(9), 951–956.

Pavuluri, M. N., O'Connor, M. M., Harral, E., & Sweeney, J. A. (2007). Affective neural circuitry during facial emotion processing in pediatric bipolar disorder. *Biological Psychiatry, 62*(2), 158–167.

Pavuluri, M. N., Schenkel, L. S., Aryal, S., Harral, E. M., Hill, S. K., Herbener, E. S., et al. (2006). Neurocognitive function in unmedicated manic and medicated euthymic pediatric bipolar patients. *American Journal of Psychiatry, 163*(2), 286–293.

Pavuluri, M. N., West, A., Hill, S. K., Jindal, K., & Sweeney, J. A. (2009). Neurocognitive function in pediatric bipolar disorder: 3-year follow-up shows cognitive development lagging behind healthy youths. *Journal of the American Academy of Child and Adolescent Psychiatry, 48*(3), 299–307.

Raison, C. L., Capuron, L., & Miller, A. H. (2006). Cytokines sing the blues: Inflammation and the pathogenesis of depression. *Trends in Immunology, 27*(1), 24–31.

Rucklidge, J. J. (2006). Psychosocial functioning of adolescents with and without paediatric bipolar disorder. *Journal of Affective Disorders, 91*(2–3), 181–188.

Schenkel, L. S., West, A. E., Harral, E. M., Patel, N. B., & Pavuluri, M. N. (2008). Parent–child interactions in pediatric bipolar disorder. *Journal of Clinical Psychology, 64*(4), 422–437.

Schildkraut, J. J. (1965). The catecholamine hypothesis of affective disorders: A review of supporting evidence. *American Journal of Psychiatry, 122*(5), 509–522.

Shaffer, D., Gould, M. S., Brasic, J., Ambrosini, P., Fisher, P., Bird, H., et al. (1983). A children's global assessment scale (CGAS). *Archives of General Psychiatry, 40*(11), 1228–1231.

Smoller, J. W., & Finn, C. T. (2003). Family, twin, and adoption studies of bipolar disorder. *American Journal of Medical Genetics C: Seminars in Medical Genetics, 123*, 48–58.

Southam-Gerow, M. A., & Prinstein, M. J. (2014). Evidence base updates: The evolution of the evaluation of psychological treatments for children and adolescents. *Journal of Clinical Child and Adolescent Psychology, 43*(1), 1–6.

Van Meter, A. R., Moreira, A. L., & Youngstrom, E. A. (2011). Meta-analysis of epidemiologic studies of pediatric bipolar disorder. *Journal of Clinical Psychiatry, 72*(9), 1250–1256.

Washburn, J. J., West, A. E., & Heil, J. A. (2011). Treatment of pediatric bipolar disorder: A review. *Minerva Psichiatrica, 52*(1), 21–35.

Weinstein, S. M., Henry, D. B., Katz, A. C., Peters, A. T., & West, A. E. (2015). Treatment moderators of child- and family-focused cognitive-behavioral therapy for pediatric bipolar disorder. *Journal of the American Academy of Child and Adolescent Psychiatry, 54*(2), 116–125.

West, A. E., Celio, C. I., Henry, D. B., & Pavuluri, M. N. (2011). Child Mania Rating Scale—Parent Version: A valid measure of symptom change due to pharmacotherapy. *Journal of Affective Disorders, 128*(1), 112–119.

West, A. E., Henry, D. B., & Pavuluri, M. N. (2007). Maintenance model of integrated psychosocial treatment in pediatric bipolar disorder: A pilot feasibility study. *Journal of the American Academy of Child and Adolescent Psychiatry, 46*(2), 205–212.

West, A. E., & Pavuluri, M. N. (2009). Psychosocial treatments for childhood and adolescent bipolar disorder. *Child and Adolescent Psychiatric Clinics of North America, 18*(2), 471–482.

West, A. E., & Peters, A. T. (2014). Bipolar disorders. In C. Alfano & D. Beidel (Eds.), *Comprehensive evidence-based interventions for school-aged children and adolescents* (pp. 163–175). Hoboken, NJ: Wiley.

West, A. E., & Weinstein, S. M. (2012). A family-based psychosocial treatment model. *Israel Journal of Psychiatry and Related Sciences, 49*(2), 86–93.

West, A. E., Weinstein, S. M., Peters, A. T., Katz, A. C., Henry, D. B., Cruz, R. A., et al. (2014). Child-and family-focused cognitive-behavioral therapy for pediatric bipolar disorder: A randomized clinical trial. *Journal of the American Academy of Child and Adolescent Psychiatry, 53*(11), 1168–1178.

Wilens, T. E., Biederman, J., Forkner, P., Ditterline, J., Morris, M., Moore, H., et al. (2003). Patterns of comorbidity and dysfunction in clinically referred preschool and school-age children with bipolar disorder. *Journal of Child and Adolescent Psychopharmacology, 13*(4), 495–505.

Youngstrom, E. A., Arnold, L. E., & Frazier, T. W. (2010). Bipolar and ADHD comorbidity: Both artifact and outgrowth of shared mechanisms. *Clinical Psychology (New York), 17*(4), 350–359.

Youngstrom, E. A., Birmaher, B., & Findling, R. L. (2008). Pediatric bipolar disorder: Validity, phenomenology, and recommendations for diagnosis. *Bipolar Disorder, 10*(1, Pt. 2), 194–214.

Youngstrom, E. A., Findling, R. L., Youngstrom, J. K., & Calabrese, J. R. (2005). Toward an evidence-based assessment of pediatric bipolar disorder. *Journal of Clinical Child and Adolescent Psychology, 34*(3), 433–448.

Youngstrom, E. A., Freeman, A. J., & Jenkins, M. M. (2009). The assessment of children and adolescents with bipolar disorder. *Child and Adolescent Psychiatric Clinics of North America, 18*(2), 353–390, viii–ix.

Youngstrom, E. A., & Youngstrom, J. K. (2005). Evidence-based assessment of pediatric bipolar disorder, Part II: Incorporating information from behavior checklists. *Journal of the American Academy of Child and Adolescent Psychiatry, 44*(8), 823–828.

CHAPTER 6

Anxiety Disorders

Sarah M. Kennedy, Jamie A. Mash,
Saneya H. Tawfik, and Jill Ehrenreich-May

THE DSM-5 DEFINITION OF ANXIETY DISORDERS

Anxiety disorders, as defined in the fifth edition of the *Diagnostic and Statistical Manual of Mental Disorders* (DSM-5; American Psychiatric Association, 2013), feature fears and worries that are excessive and accompanied by related behavioral disturbances, such as avoidance and extreme distress. These disorders share common clinical processes that include impairing fear of real or perceived threats posed by stimuli or situations, as well as anticipation of future threats. Although anxiety disorders can be highly comorbid with other emotional disorders, the situations that are feared or avoided, as well as the cognitions associated with the anxiety, often differentiate the disorders. One important change in DSM-5 is its developmental approach and examination of anxiety disorders across the lifespan, which helps differentiate between typical fears that develop during childhood and adolescence, and disorders that require treatment (American Psychiatric Association, 2013). Although normative age-related experiences can cause typical fears during childhood and adolescence (e.g., fears associated with beginning preschool, parent separation, attending parties or social events during adolescence), anxiety disorders differ from typical fears by the persistent and excessive worry, fear, and/or avoidance displayed.

In addition to DSM-5's developmental approach, several diagnostic changes have occurred. Selective mutism is now classified as an anxiety disorder due to its high comorbidity with anxiety (Manassis et al., 2003; Yeganeh, Beidel, Turner, Pina, & Silverman, 2003). In addition, panic disorder and agoraphobia are no longer linked in DSM-5 due to findings suggesting that individuals with Agoraphobia do not always experience panic symptoms (Wittchen et al., 2008). Furthermore, posttraumatic stress disorder and obsessive–compulsive disorder are no longer found in the DSM-5 chapter on anxiety disorders due to neuroimaging and genetic studies demonstrating that there are differences among these disorders in terms of risk factors, heritability, treatment, and course (for reviews, see Friedman et al., 2011; Storch, Abramowitz, & Goodman, 2008). Instead, they are arranged sequentially after anxiety disorders in different DSM-5 chapters and are discussed, respectively, by Keller, Burton, and Feeny (Chapter 9) and Peris and Schneider (Chapter 10) in this volume. The prevalent anxiety disorders now found in DSM-5 include separation anxiety disorder (SAD), specific phobia, social anxiety disorder (SocAD), panic disorder, agoraphobia, and generalized anxiety disorder (GAD). Specific phobias and panic disorders are discussed, respectively, by Oar, Farrell, Byrne, and Ollendick (Chapter 7) and Pincus, Korn, and DiFonte (Chapter 8) in this volume; therefore, they are not included in this chapter. The prevalent DSM-5 subtypes reviewed in this chapter are SAD, SocAD, and GAD.

Before discussing the prevalence, course, and etiology of SAD, SocAD, and GAD, we briefly review diagnostic criteria for these anxiety disorders. SAD refers to developmentally inappropriate anxiety or excessive fear about separation from home or attachment figures (American Psychiatric Association, 2013). This fear or anxiety must be present for at least 4 weeks (e.g., not simply at the beginning of the school year for children), and must cause clinically significant distress and/or impairment in social or academic areas. SocAD describes extreme fear or anxiety about potential negative evaluation by others in at least one social situation (American Psychiatric Association, 2013). Children with SocAD often fear that others will think them stupid, that they will do something to embarrass themselves in social situations, or that others will laugh at or make fun of them. To meet criteria for SocAD, fear of social evaluation must persist for at least 6 months, lead to avoidance of social situations, and cause clinically significant impairment in important areas of a child's functioning. Finally, GAD is often described as a "free-floating" type of anxiety involving excessive anxiety or worry about a number of events or activities (American Psychiatric Association , 2013). As with SocAD, anxiety or worry in GAD must be present for at least 6 months, must be difficult to control, and must result in at least one physical symptom such as sleep disturbance, fatigue, muscle aches, irritability, or poor concentration.

PREVALENCE AND COURSE

Anxiety disorders are the most common mental disorders among children and adolescents (Beesdo, Knappe, & Pine, 2009; Silverman & Ollendick, 2008). Although some changes have occurred between DSM-IV-TR and DSM-5, core criteria for the anxiety disorders covered in this chapter have not changed significantly; thus, similarity in prevalence rates between the two DSM editions is assumed. It should be noted that community prevalence rates vary due to factors such as differences in assessment scales used, age groups studied, and multiple sources of information (e.g., parent and teacher reports, self-reports). Estimates of lifetime prevalence of anxiety disorders in children and adolescents range from 15 to 20% (Beesdo, Knappe, & Pine, 2009). For adolescents, approximately 1 in 5 meet criteria for a mental disorder and experience severe impairment across their lifetimes (Merikangas et al., 2010). Rates for specific anxiety disorders among adolescents vary from 2.2% for GAD to 7.6% for SAD and 9.1% for SocAD (Merikangas et al.,

2010). In one of the first comprehensive summaries on the prevalence of anxiety disorders using the DSM-5 format, Kessler, Petukhova, Sampson, Zaslavsky, and Wittchen (2012) reconfirmed previous epidemiological findings (e.g., Costello, Egger, & Angold, 2004) that one of the most common disorders among youth is SocAD (approximately 7.4%). All anxiety disorders occur more frequently in females than in males, and females are up to two times as likely to develop anxiety disorders (Costello, Mustillo, Erkanli, Keeler, & Angold, 2003; Zahn-Waxler, Shirtcliff, & Marceau, 2008). Gender differences occur as early as childhood and increase with age (Zahn-Waxler et al., 2008).

The onset of anxiety disorders is often early (Egger & Angold, 2006), and prevalence increases throughout childhood and adolescence (Beesdo et al., 2007; Bongers, Koot, Van der Ende, & Verhulst, 2003). The median age of onset of all emotional and behavioral problems is earliest for anxiety disorders (Merikangas et al., 2010). In fact, anxiety disorders are relatively common among preschool-age children. Recent evidence suggests that the onset of anxiety disorders may occur as early as age 3, and up to 9% of preschoolers experience an anxiety disorder (Egger & Angold, 2006; Luby, 2013). Early-onset anxiety disorders are risk factors for the development of other emotional disorders later in life, including depressive disorders in adolescence and adulthood (Beesdo et al., 2007). Thus, early identification and treatment of anxiety may be key to impacting what could otherwise be a stable or worsening trajectory over the lifespan.

In fact, the course of childhood anxiety disorders is often chronic and can impair adaptive functioning, social relationships, and academic achievement in children and adolescents (La Greca & Lopez, 1998; Silverman & Ollendick, 2008; Van Ameringen, Mancini, & Farvolden, 2003). While SAD is typically thought of as a disorder of early childhood, the prevalence of GAD and SocAD increases with age among children (Beesdo et al., 2009) and during adolescence (Costello, Copeland, & Angold, 2011). In a nationally representative sample among U.S. adolescents, lifetime prevalence of anxiety disorders was found to be as high as 31.9% (Meringkas et al., 2010). If left untreated, the relatively stable trajectory of childhood anxiety can increase the risk for adult anxiety, depressive disorders, substance abuse, and suicide attempts (Beesdo et al., 2007; Bittner et al., 2007; Boden, Fergusson, & Horwood, 2007; Gregory et al., 2007; Pine, Cohen, Gurley, Brook, & Ma, 1998).

COMMON COMORBID CONDITIONS

Anxiety disorders in childhood and adolescence commonly co-occur with other DSM-5 disorders, including other anxiety disorders, depressive disorders, and disruptive, impulse control, and conduct disorders. When discussing comorbid conditions, it is useful to distinguish between *concurrent comorbidity* (comorbid disorders occurring at the same time) and *sequential comorbidity* (one disorder temporally preceding another). Typically, concurrent comorbidity is assessed via cross-sectional designs, while sequential comorbidity is assessed either via longitudinal designs or cross-sectional designs involving retrospective reporting of past psychological history. Comorbidity estimates vary depending on sample characteristics (e.g., clinic vs. community samples), assessment methods (e.g., structured interviews vs. self-report of symptoms), and reporters (e.g., youth only or parent only vs. youth and parents).

In general, the majority of children and adolescents with an anxiety disorder have one or more comorbid psychological disorders. As many as two-thirds of clinic-referred youth with a primary anxiety disorder receive an additional diagnosis (Leyfer, Gallo, Cooper-Vince, & Pincus, 2013), with other anxiety disorders being the most common comorbid conditions (Angold, Costello, & Erkanli, 1999). GAD and SocAD appear to be particularly comorbid, with approximately one-third of youth with GAD also being diagnosed with SocAD, and just under a one-third of youth with SocAD also being diagnosed with GAD in a clinical sample (Leyfer, Gallo, Cooper-Vince, & Pincus, 2013). Depressive disorders are also common in youth with anxiety disorders. Concurrent comorbidity between depression and anxiety has been observed to be as high as 75% in some clinical samples (Weersing, Gonzalez, Campo, & Lucas, 2008), although a number of studies indicate that anxiety comorbidity is much more common in youth with primary depression than is depression comorbidity in youth with primary anxiety (e.g., Axelson & Birmaher, 2001; Garber & Weersing, 2010; Ollendick, Jarrett, Grills-Taquechel, Hovey, & Wolff, 2008). In general, evidence suggests that anxiety disorders typically precede the onset of depressive disorders in cases with sequential comorbidity (e.g., Brady & Kendall, 1992; Keenan & Hipwell, 2005). However, Cummings, Caporino, and Kendall (2014) have proposed that there may be multiple pathways leading to anxiety, depression, and their comorbidity, with anxiety-related impairment leading to depression in some cases, depression-related impairment leading to anxiety in other cases, and a shared diathesis for anxiety and depression expressed in different ways in still other cases, depending on environmental or developmental factors.

In addition to comorbidity with other internalizing disorders, anxiety disorders are often comorbid with externalizing disorders. Comorbidity of anxiety symptoms and attention-deficit/hyperactivity disorder (ADHD) is three times greater than that expected by chance (Angold, Costello, & Erkanli, 1999), with rates of co-occurrence ranging widely from 8 to 40% (Halldorsdottir & Ollendick, 2014; Larson, Russ, Kahn, & Halfon, 2011). The co-occurrence of oppositional defiance disorder (ODD) and anxiety disorders in youth is estimated to be about 10–15% (Verduin & Kendall, 2003), also three times greater than what would be expected by chance (Angold et al., 1999). Comorbidity of anxiety disorders and ODD/conduct problems is especially pronounced in boys and in youth with an early onset of conduct problems (Barker, Oliver, & Maughan, 2010; Verduin & Kendall, 2003).

ETIOLOGICAL/CONCEPTUAL MODELS OF ANXIETY DISORDERS

A number of theoretical models have been proposed to help explain the development of anxiety disorders in youth. Barlow (2000, 2002) proposed the triple vulnerability model of emotional disorders, whereby biological vulnerability (e.g., temperament), general psychological vulnerability resulting from early life experiences, and disorder-specific psychological vulnerability interact to increase the likelihood of developing an anxiety or related emotional disorder over time. This model provides a useful framework for discussing our current understanding of the etiology of anxiety in general, as well as vulnerabilities uniquely related to the development of SAD, SocAD, and GAD. The model is also consistent with the idea of "goodness of fit" between an at-risk youth and his or her environment, which suggests that environmental factors may either temper or exacerbate biological vulnerability, depending on whether the environment provides a good or poor match with child temperament (Thomas & Chess, 1977). Given the centrality of the triple vulnerability model to etiological conceptions of core anxiety disorders in youth, all three types of vulnerabilities are reviewed in this section.

Biological Vulnerabilities

It is now well established that having a parent with an anxiety disorder significantly increases a child's likelihood of receiving an anxiety disorder diagnosis (e.g., Beidel & Turner, 1997; Hudson, Dodd, Lyneham, & Bovopoulous, 2011). Twin studies have consistently indicated that genetic factors account for a moderate amount (e.g., around 30%) of the variance in child anxiety (Drake & Ginsburg, 2012; Nolte, Guiney, Fonagy, Mayes, & Luyten, 2011), with separation anxiety features generally evidencing a lower degree of heritability than features of other core anxiety disorders (e.g., shyness/inhibition; Eley et al., 2003). Genetic factors may confer risk for anxiety disorders through *endophenotypes,* or heritable traits that are stable over time and associated with disease development (Gottesman & Gould, 2003). *Behavioral inhibition* (BI), which refers to increased reactivity and negative emotionality in response to novelty, is a stable temperament factor that affects up to 15% of typically developing children and may be one such endophenotype implicated in anxiety (Fox, Henderson, Marshall, Nichols, & Ghera, 2005). BI is evident in infancy and is associated with physiological abnormalities such as increased autonomic reactivity, elevated level of morning cortisol, heightened startle response, more vigilant attention styles, and greater amygdala activation in response to threatening stimuli (for a review, see Degnan, Almas, & Fox, 2010). Longitudinal studies indicate that BI in early childhood increases risk for the development of anxiety disorders in later childhood, adolescence, and adulthood (Altman, Sommer, & McGoey, 2009; Muris, Van Brakel, Arntz, & Schouten, 2011; Pahl, Barrett, & Gullo, 2012). Other neurobiological and neuroendocrine factors, such as variations in the serotonin transporter gene (Perez-Edgar et al., 2010) and alterations in the set point of the hypothalamic–pituitary–adrenal (HPA) axis (Nolte et al., 2011) have been implicated as biological vulnerabilities for anxiety.

General Psychological Vulnerabilities

A number of general psychological vulnerabilities, including attachment quality, parenting and family factors, and cognitive biases, have been linked to the development of anxiety disorders in youth. Such factors may "mediate" the relationship between biological vulnerabilities and anxiety (i.e., be *caused by* biological vulnerability) or may "moderate" this relationship (i.e., be preexisting factors that *interact with* biological vulnerability). Insecure attachment styles, particularly an anxious attachment style, predict the development of later anxiety much more strongly than do secure attachment styles (Warren, Huston, Egeland, & Sroufe, 1997) and are moderately associated with child anxiety symptoms (Drake & Ginsburg, 2012). Insecure attachment may moderate the relationship between BI and anxiety, as research has shown that children with high levels of BI who were also insecurely attached displayed the highest levels of anxiety over time (Muris et al., 2011). With regard to parenting factors, parental overcontrol or over-protection has been consistently linked with youth anxiety (Drake & Ginsburg, 2012; Ginsburg, Siqueland, Masia-Warner, & Hedtke, 2005), perhaps because consistent provision of overprotection facilitates youth avoidance, limits access to novelty, and prevents the development of self-efficacy. It is possible that youth with temperament styles that may be considered anxious or inhibited may encourage or facilitate overprotective or overinvolved parenting (i.e., a meditational relationship), or there may be an interaction between child temperament and parenting characteristics (i.e., a moderating relationship). Other parenting and family factors, such as rejection or criticism, low warmth, modeling of anxious behaviors, and high conflict, have also been associated with vulnerability for anxiety, although not as strongly (Drake & Ginsburg, 2012). Finally, a number of information-processing biases, such as selective attention to threat, a tendency to interpret ambiguous scenarios as threatening, and a tendency to recall threat-related memory content selectively, have been associated with anxiety in youth (Barrett, Rapee, Dadds, & Ryan, 1996; Creswell & O'Connor, 2011; Field & Field, 2013).

Disorder-Specific Psychological Vulnerabilities

In addition to the previously discussed general risk factors implicated in the etiology of anxiety, a number of disorder-specific vulnerabilities have been identified for SAD, SocAD, and GAD. With regard to SAD, studies have indicated that CO_2 hypersensitivity may be a specific risk factor for both SAD and adult-onset panic disorder, which demonstrate high heterotypic continuity across the lifespan (Battaglia et al., 2009; Roberson-Nay et al., 2010). Early parental loss or separation has also been related to the development of SAD (Battaglia et al., 2009; Cronk, Slutske, Madden, Bucholz, & Heath, 2004). With regard to SocAD, although behavioral inhibition has been linked to the development of a variety of anxiety disorders, recent evidence from longitudinal studies suggests that chronic, high behavioral inhibition is associated most strongly or even uniquely with the development of SocAD (e.g., Muris et al., 2011; Rapee, 2014). Additionally, interpersonal factors such as low perceived peer acceptance, lack of social support, and lower friendship quality may play a role in the etiology of SocAD (Festa & Ginsburg, 2011; La Greca & Lopez, 1998; La Greca & Stone, 1993). In the case of GAD, adult etiological models have identified a number of cognitive risk factors for the development of the disorder, such as positive beliefs about the usefulness of worry, negative beliefs about the dangers of worry, cognitive monitoring, and intolerance of uncertainty (see Kertz & Woodruff-Borden, 2011, for a review). Such models have not been adequately tested in youth, but there is evidence to suggest that intolerance of uncertainty and a high degree of cognitive monitoring are specifically associated with symptoms of GAD in youth (Bacow, May, Brody, & Pincus, 2010; Read, Comer, & Kendall, 2013).

We have reviewed in the preceding sections the prevalence and course of anxiety disorders in youth, their comorbidities, and etiological models. In general, anxiety disorders are common in youth, onset early, increase in prevalence throughout childhood and adolescence, and often co-occur with other anxiety disorders, depressive disorders, and externalizing disorders. Anxiety disorders "run in families" and are moderately heritable. The most well-supported risk factors for anxiety include BI and parental overcontrol/overprotection, although additional parenting characteristics, biological and cognitive vulnerabilities, and social factors also play a role. Evidence-based treatments for children and adolescents (discussed in the following section) are thought to target these and other risk factors for anxiety.

EVIDENCE-BASED TREATMENTS FOR ANXIETY DISORDERS IN CHILDREN AND ADOLESCENTS

The evidence-based treatment movement has led to the identification of a number of interventions for child and adolescent anxiety disorders, with varying levels of empirical support. Chambless and Hollon (1998) initially proposed a scheme for determining when psychological treatments should be considered evidence-based treatments for various psychiatric disorders. Efficacy trials were given the greatest weight, followed by research on effectiveness in routine care settings and cost-effectiveness research. According to Chambless and Hollon, a good between-group experimental design includes 25–30 patients within each treatment condition, and compares the treatment being tested for efficacy to a control treatment (wait-list control or placebo treatment/pill) or to another, already established treatment. Additionally, clinical profiles of clients enrolled in treatment studies should be evaluated in a structured way (i.e., by clinical interview), and reliable and valid outcome measures should be used. Since it is difficult to define what is clinically significant in terms of overall effect size of a treatment for a given group, guidelines involving effect size are somewhat flexible, but studies should provide data suggesting that proposed evidence-based treatments produce statistically significant changes in symptoms from baseline, and are at least equal in efficacy to an already established treatment (Chambless & Hollon, 1998). Since the establishment of these criteria for determining treatment efficacy, well-established and possibly efficacious treatments have been identified for the treatment of children and adolescents with anxiety disorders, including SAD, SocAD, and GAD.

To date, several reviews have evaluated whether currently available psychosocial treatments for anxiety disorders in youth meet the guidelines established by the American Psychological Association's Division 12 Task Force for determining empirically supported treatments (Chambless & Ollendick, 2001; James, James, Cowdrey, Soler, & Choke, 2013; Silverman & Ollendick, 2008). Existent well-established treatments for pediatric anxiety disorders may be composed of either individual cognitive-behavioral therapy techniques (components of CBT) such as exposure or psychoeducation, or multiple CBT techniques, such as exposure, cognitive restructuring, and relaxation training, all presented within one multicomponent CBT package (Higa-McMillan, Francis, Rith-Najarian, & Chorpita, 2016). Well-established treatments include such multicomponent CBT packages (in group or individual format), CBT packages with parent involvement, CBT packages plus medication, or more focused presentations of individual components of CBT for anxiety, such as exposure, or psychoeducation, presented independently. All but three probably efficacious treatments are CBT packages. Although basic skills and therapeutic techniques differ between variants of CBT, exposure is the most commonly occurring treatment technique among well-established treatments. It has been used in 124 of the 165 study groups (87.9%) reviewed by Higa-McMillan and colleagues (2016). Cognitive techniques are also commonly implemented across well-established treatments, and have been integrated into 102 out of 165 studies (61.8%) reviewed by Higa-McMillan and colleagues. Relaxation techniques have been employed in 89 of 165 studies (53.9%), anxiety or emotion-focused psychoeducation for children has been included in 70 of 165 studies (42%), and modeling has been incorporated into treatment in 56 out of 165 studies (33.9%).

CBT and exposure-based treatments are the most supported interventions for child and adolescent anxiety. Evidence from numerous studies supports improvement in both symptoms and global functioning post-CBT, with CBT being the only treatment to meet well-established intervention criteria based on treatment-based changes in global functioning (Chorpita et al., 2011; Ishikawa, Okajima, Matsuoka, & Sakano, 2007; James et al., 2013; Rapp, Dodds, Walkup, & Rynn, 2013; Silverman, Pina, & Viswesvaran, 2008). Furthermore, CBT is the only treatment with demonstrated effects on quality of life (Hofmann, Wu, & Boettcher, 2014). Additionally, CBT and exposure-based therapies produce the largest effect sizes of psychosocial treatments, with effects also lasting at least 1-year posttreatment (Compton et al., 2014; Kendall et al., 1997). Evidence also supports CBT's efficacy when applied in different treatment formats (i.e., with or without parental involvement, individual and group formats) and settings (Chorpita et al., 2011; Ginsburg, Drake, Winegrad, Fothergill, & Wissow, 2016; Higa-McMillan et al., 2015; Ishikawa et al., 2007; James et al., 2013; Rapp et al., 2013; Silverman et al., 2008). Both individual and group CBT are efficacious, producing similar effect sizes, while Internet-delivered programs produce weaker effect sizes (Higa-McMillan et al., 2016; Khanna & Kendall, 2010; Rapp et al., 2013; Rooksby, Elouafkaoui, Humphris, Clarkson, & Freeman, 2015). See Table 6.1 for a summary of evidence-based psychosocial treatments for pediatric anxiety disorders.

In addition to CBT and exposure-based therapies, promising new, probably efficacious treatments include acceptance and commitment therapy (ACT; which might also be considered a form of behavior therapy), attention only, hypnosis, and cultural storytelling (Burckhardt, Manicavasagar, Batterham, & Hadzi-Pavlovic, 2016; Costantino & Malgady, 1994; Hancock et al., 2016; Manassis et al., 2010; Stanton, 1994). Such treatments have primarily been evaluated in subclinical and/or specific cultural groups (i.e., subclinical high-anxious primary school children in attention only; subclinical Hispanic youth for cultural storytelling; and subclinical test-anxious white males for hypnosis), with the exception of acceptance and commitment therapy. The latter has been compared to CBT in one randomized controlled trial (RCT), evidencing similar outcomes (Hancock et al., 2016). However, the goals of ACT are similar to those of CBT, with the primary focus of treatment being the use of learned skills to manage uncomfortable emotional experiences and cope with anxious thoughts and resultant behaviors. Thus, it is difficult to draw a clear distinction between the two treatments at this stage.

Promising New Behavioral Treatments

Several novel behavioral interventions also show promise as potential new evidence-based therapies for anxiety disorders. Such interventions, including attention bias modification (ABM) and cognitive bias modification (CBM), have been developed based on evidence from neuroscience studies that implicate specific brain regions in the pathophysiology of anxiety disorders (Bar-Haim, 2010; Bar-Haim, Lamy, Pergamin,

TABLE 6.1. Evidence-Supported Treatments for Pediatric Anxiety Disorders Based on Symptom Reduction

Level 1: Well-established treatments	Level 2: Probably efficacious treatments	Level 3: Possibly efficacious treatments	Level 4: Experimental treatments	Level 5: Treatments of questionable efficacy
CBT (individual or group format)	Family psychoeducation (CBT foundation)	Contingency management[a]	Biofeedback	Assessment/ monitoring
Exposure (CBT foundation)	Relaxation (CBT foundation)	Group therapy[a]	CBT with parents only	Attachment therapy
CBT with parents	Assertiveness training (CBT foundation)		Play therapy	Client-centered therapy
Education (CBT foundation)	Stress inoculation (CBT foundation)		Psychodynamic therapy	Eye movement desensitization and reprocessing
CBT plus medication	CBT for child and parent (CBT foundation)		Rational emotive therapy	Peer pairing
	Cultural storytelling[a]		Social skills training	Psychoeducation (CBT foundation)
	Hypnosis[a]			Relationship counseling
	Attention[a]			Teacher psychotherapy

Note. Based on Higa-McMillan, Francis, Rith-Najarian, and Chropita (2016).
[a]Tested only in a subclinical population.

Bakermans-Kranenburg, & van IJzendoorn, 2007; Beard, 2011; Beard & Amir, 2009; Pine, 2007). Recent research shows that individuals with anxiety disorders possess automatic attentional biases toward threatening stimuli and a tendency to interpret ambiguous stimuli in the environment as threatening (Amin, Foa, & Coles, 1998; Bar-Haim et al., 2007; Beard & Amir, 2009; Rozenman, Amir, & Weersing, 2014). Accordingly, computer-based ABM and CBM programs retrain anxious individuals' attention away from threat or prevent individuals from interpreting ambiguous situations as threatening, respectively. Theoretically, such modification of threat-related attention and interpretation biases should reduce symptoms of anxiety in clinical populations of adults and youth (Bar-Haim, 2010; Bar-Haim et al., 2007; Beard, 2011; Beard & Amir, 2009; Pine, 2007).

Research support for such interventions is just beginning to surface. Several studies have provided support for ABM as an adjunctive treatment that enhances CBT efficacy in clinically anxious youth (Britton et al., 2013; Shechner et al., 2014), and recent research provides preliminary support for CBM as an adjunctive treatment for high anxious youth (Sportel, de Hullu, de Jong, & Nauta, 2013). Research also supports the use of ABM as a stand-alone treatment for treating high-anxious (Bar-Haim, 2010; Bar-Haim, Morag, & Glickman, 2011) and clinically anxious youth possessing an attention bias toward threat or away from positive stimuli prior to treatment (Eldar et al., 2012; Waters, Pittaway, Mogg, Bradley, & Pine, 2013), as well as the use of CBM as a stand-alone treatment for high-anxious (Lau, Molyneaux, Telman, & Belli, 2011; Vassilopoulos, Banerjee, & Prantzalou, 2009; Vassilopoulos, Blackwell, Misailidi, Kyritsi, & Ayfanti, 2014) and clinically anxious youth (Lau, Pettit, & Creswell, 2013). However, effect sizes of such treatments are generally smaller than those observed in CBT trials (Bar-Haim, 2010) and, to date, research comparing ABM or CBM directly to CBT in a clinical population is nonexistent. Future research may shed light on whether computer-based behavioral interventions such as ABM and CBM might serve as alternatives to CBT.

Pharmacological Interventions

A substantial body of evidence supports the use of pharmacological treatments for SAD, SocAD, and GAD, both alone and in combination with CBT. Overall, selective serotonin reuptake inhibitors (SSRIs) such as sertraline, fluvoxamine, and fluoxetine have amassed the largest research support and are considered the first-line pharmacological treatment for anxiety disorders in youth (Keeton & Ginsburg, 2008). Placebo-controlled studies of SSRIs have found large mean effect sizes (ESs) for social anxiety symptoms following 8–16 weeks of treatment (ES = 1.30, range = 1.07–1.85; Segool & Carlson, 2008) and have resulted in treatment response in 60–90% of youth across anxiety diagnoses (Keeton & Ginsburg, 2008; Seidel & Walkup, 2006). Furthermore, results from the Child–Adolescent Anxiety Multimodal Study (CAMS) have supported acute and long-term benefits of SSRI use in anxious youth, both as a monotherapy and in combination with CBT. After 12 weeks of treatment, anxious youth who received a combination of CBT + sertraline achieved the largest reduction in anxiety symptoms and benefited significantly more from treatment than did youth receiving CBT monotherapy, sertraline monotherapy, or pill placebo (ES = 0.86, $p < .001$; Walkup et al., 2008). Sertraline monotherapy (ES = 0.45) and CBT monotherapy (ES = 0.31) were equally effective and superior to pill placebo ($p < .001$; Walkup et al., 2008). Combination therapy largely maintained this advantage over CBT and sertraline monotherapies at 24 and 36 weeks postrandomization, although this advantage decreased over time, and all conditions maintained superiority over pill placebo (Piacentini et al., 2014). However, by the time of a long-term follow-up 6 years after randomization, treatment condition no longer predicted diagnostic remission of anxiety severity, perhaps because as many as 50% of youth received both medication and therapy at some point following treatment termination (Ginsburg et al., 2014).

Despite the efficacy of SSRIs in treating youth anxiety disorders, concerns have been raised about their side effects and safety when used in this population. Placebo-controlled trials have reported increased gastrointestinal distress, insomnia, vomiting, and loss of appetite with SSRIs compared to pill placebo, and increased risk of suicidality (about 2% higher compared to placebo) has also been observed (for a review, see Compton, Kratochvil, & March, 2007). However, results from the CAMS trial indicated that there were no statistical differences in adverse events (including suicidality) between sertraline and placebo conditions (Mohatt, Bennett, & Walkup, 2014). In summary, there have been mixed findings with regard to increased side effects or adverse events associated with SSRI use, but available evidence does not indicate significant safety concerns (Mohatt et al., 2014). SSRI therapy may in fact confer several benefits, especially in cases of more severe anxiety and when used early in treatment. SSRIs may result in more rapid improvement than CBT alone, possibly as soon as 3–4 weeks into treatment (Keeton & Ginsburg, 2008). These early benefits may increase youths' motivation and ability to engage in therapy, especially in cases of more severe anxiety.

Predictors, Mediators, and Moderators of Treatment Response

As discussed in previous sections, several interventions for youth anxiety have now accumulated sufficient research evidence to be considered empirically supported treatments. While such treatments are efficacious for many anxious youth, up to 50% of youth still meet criteria for their principal anxiety disorder at posttreatment (Hudson et al., 2009; Kendall, Hudson, Gosch, Flannery-Schroeder, & Suveg, 2008; Walkup at al., 2008), and as many as 40% continue to meet criteria at follow-up (Hudson et al., 2009; Kendall, Hudson, Gosch, Flannery-Schroeder, & Suveg, 2008). Improving response and remission rates for evidence-based therapies requires that we understand for whom treatments work (predictors), for whom and under what conditions treatments work (moderators), and why treatments work (mediators). *Predictors* of treatment response are defined as preexisting youth characteristics (e.g., demographic characteristics, family factors, clinical severity) that influence treatment response, whereas *moderators* are pretreatment characteristics that interact with treatment condition to determine response (Kraemer, Wilson, Fairburn, & Agras, 2002). *Mediators,* on the other hand, are factors affected by treatment that temporally precede and play a causal role in treatment response (Kazdin, 2007). Predictors, moderators, and mediators of response to interventions for youth anxiety are reviewed in this section.

Data on predictors and moderators of treatment response have been somewhat mixed, but, in general, few consistent predictors and moderators have emerged. Although younger age might be thought to predict poorer treatment response due to young children's limited ability to engage with the cognitive components of CBT, most studies have not found age to be a significant predictor or moderator of treatment response (Alfano et al., 2009; Kendall et al., 2008; Nilsen, Eisemann, & Kvernmo, 2013). Similarly, neither child gender nor ethnicity is a consistent predictor or treatment outcome, although there is some evidence that family involvement in therapy may improve treatment response for girls but not boys (for a review, see Nilsen, Eisemann, & Kvernmo, 2013). It has been suggested that parental psychopathology may predict or moderate treatment response, as parents with internalizing problems may undermine treatment by modeling anxious or avoidant coping styles. While several studies have indeed found that parental psychopathology predicts poorer response to CBT (e.g., Southam-Gerow, Kendall, & Weersing, 2001) other studies have found no relationship (Ginsburg et al., 2011; Kley, Heinrichs, Bender, & Tuschen-Caffier, 2012). There is also some evidence that parental anxiety may moderate treatment outcomes. Family CBT has been found to outperform individual CBT when both parents have an anxiety disorder (Kendall et al., 2008), and recent research suggests that parental anxiety may actually predict more rapid and greater response to treatment with sertraline (Gonzalez et al., 2015).

With respect to baseline psychopathology, including symptom severity and comorbidity, findings have also been inconsistent. Several studies have found that higher baseline anxiety severity predicts poorer treatment response (Compton et al., 2014; Ginsburg et al., 2011; Southam-Gerow et al., 2001), although a recent review found that baseline severity was not a significant predictor of treatment response in four of six studies reviewed (Nilsen at al., 2013). There is some evidence to suggest that youth with certain diagnostic profiles may be less likely to be treatment responders. For example, some studies have suggested that youth with SocAD may be less likely to achieve remission following treatment than youth with GAD or SAD (Compton et al., 2014; Ginsburg et al., 2011) or to maintain treatment gains at longer-term follow-ups (Kerns, Read, Klugman, & Kendall, 2013). However, poorer treatment response in youth with SocAD may in part be due to higher rates of depressive comorbidity among socially anxious youth (Crawley, Beidas, Benjamin, Martin, & Kendall, 2008). Depressive comorbidity in general has been associated with poorer treatment response in several studies (Berman, Weems, Silverman, & Kurtines, 2000; Southam-Gerow et al., 2001), and a recent investigation of the impact of comorbidity on treatment outcome in over 800 youth revealed that youth with externalizing or internalizing comorbidity are less likely to achieve remission of the principal anxiety diagnosis but are not less likely to be classified as treatment responders (Rapee et al., 2013). However, several reviews of the literature have indicated that comorbidity, by and large, does not appear to predict outcome in most studies (Nilsen et al., 2013; Ollendick et al., 2008).

In comparison with research on predictors and moderators of treatment outcome, research on mediators is scant. As Kazdin (2007) and Weersing and Weisz (2002) have pointed out, this is because very few studies have been designed to enable robust tests of meditational hypotheses, which require that hypothesized mediator variables be measured at multiple time points during treatment and prior to change in the outcome variable(s) of interest. In brief, all of the following conditions are necessary to establish mediation:

1. Treatment must result in improvements in symptoms and functioning
2. Treatment must result in changes in the candidate mediator.
3. The candidate mediator must affect symptoms and functioning.
4. The original relationship between treatment and outcome must be attenuated when controlling for the relationship between treatment and the mediator and the mediator and outcome (Weersing & Weisz, 2002).

Few studies have fulfilled all of these conditions, but a number of candidate mediators have been identified on the basis of the impact of treatment on these potential mediators. A meta-analysis conducted by Chu and Harrison (2007) revealed that across 14 intervention studies representing 22 conditions, CBT produced a large mean effect size for behavioral processes (ES = 1.02) and moderate mean effect sizes for physiological (ES = 0.49), cognitive (ES = 0.50) and coping (ES = 0.73) processes. Only a handful of studies, however, have examined whether such processes actually mediate treatment outcome. With respect to cognitive processes, Kendall and Treadwell (2007) found that anxious self-statements and the ratio of positive to negative self-statements partially mediated outcome for child-reported fear and anxiety, and Hogendoorn and colleagues (2014) found that an increase in positive thoughts and use of several coping strategies preceded and contributed to a decrease in anxiety symptoms. In an examination of mediators of outcome for cognitive-behavioral treatment for socially anxious youth, Alfano and colleagues (2009) found that decreased loneliness and increased social effectiveness mediated the relationship pre- and posttreatment anxiety and global functioning.

The preceding sections of this chapter have summarized evidence-based interventions for anxiety disorders in children and adolescents; promising new interventions; and current evidence regarding predictors, moderators, and mediators of such treatments. CBT-based treatments are currently the only interventions for youth anxiety disorders to be regarded as well-established treatments. There is now substantial evidence regarding the positive impact of CBT on diagnostic remission, symptom reduction, and decrease in functional impairment, both immediately following treatment and at longer-term follow-up. Pharmacological interventions have also been shown to be efficacious for anxiety disorders in youth, and the combination of SSRIs and CBT appears to maximize treatment outcomes for youth with SAD, SocAD, and GAD. Few consistent predictors or moderators of outcome have been identified, although emerging evidence is suggests that youth with SocAD may evidence poorer treatment outcomes that youth with SAD or GAD. With regard to mediation, CBT appears to have a moderate to large effect on cognitive and behavioral outcomes, but few controlled studies have measured putative cognitive and behavioral mediators frequently enough over the course of treatment to establish clear evidence of mediation. In short, although there is now compelling evidence to support the efficacy of CBT, relatively little is known about for whom CBT works, under what conditions, or why, and large-scale RCTs are needed to examine the efficacy of alternative treatments such as ABM and CBM alone or in combination with CBT.

EVIDENCE-BASED ASSESSMENT
OF ANXIETY DISORDERS IN CHILDREN AND ADOLESCENTS

Numerous structured and semistructured interviews, self-report measures, and parent-report measures have been used over the years to assess anxiety in children and adolescents. We focus in this section on those diagnostic interviews and measures most commonly used in clinical and research contexts, beginning with semistructured interviews, then moving to broadband anxiety measures and measures of particular anxiety disorder symptoms. Finally, we discuss several broadband measures that assess anxiety symptoms, as well as symptoms of related disorders and childhood conditions.

Assessment of anxious youth, particularly younger children, requires information from multiple sources (Beesdo et al., 2009). Parent reports of anxiety provide added information and value to research as well as to the diagnostic process itself (Kendall et al., 2007; Villabø, Gere, Torgersen, March, & Kendall, 2012). Parent-report interviews and measures also help prevent any biases in anxious children and adolescents who have a difficult time admitting to being socially undesirable (Kendall & Flannery-Schroeder, 1998). In fact, it has been noted that the validity of certain groups of anxious children's self-reports should be questioned due to social desirability concerns (Silverman & Ollendick, 2005). Although teacher ratings can add information to the assessment process, teacher reports are generally considered more helpful when assessing externalizing rather than internalizing behaviors (Loeber, Green & Lahey, 1990). Additionally, factors such as the child having multiple teachers or the timing of the assessment may influence teacher reports, posing challenges in terms of appropriately reconciling or interpreting teacher reports in traditional internalizing disorder assessment contexts. Thus, in the following sections we focus on self- and parent reports only.

When using the assessment tools described in the following sections, it is important to consider that SAD, SocAD, and GAD must be distinguished from developmentally appropriate fears and worries. For example, anxious or oppositional behaviors upon separation from caregivers are normative in children under the age of 5, while fears of rejection and negative evaluation by peers are not uncommon during late childhood and throughout adolescence (Beesdo et al., 2009). Anxiety disorders, in contrast to developmentally appropriate fears and worries, are characterized by fears and worries that are not only distressing but also persistent, extensive, and impairing (Beesdo et al., 2009). A number of the semistructured interviews and measures discussed in subsequent sections contain clinical cutoffs or thresholds that facilitate distinguishing between normative and elevated or clinically significant anxiety.

Cognitive and behavioral characteristics may also be similar across anxiety disorders, as well as between certain anxiety and depressive disorders. For example, youth with both GAD and SocAD may display worries about their competence or performance; however, for youth with SocAD, this worry is limited to evaluative situations, whereas youth with GAD evidence worry about their performance regardless of social context (Whitmore, Kim-Spoon, & Ollendick, 2014). The behavioral presentation of anxiety may also be similar across disorders, so differential diagnosis often requires a careful functional analysis of the antecedents of any given behavior. For example, fear of the dark, fear of being negatively evaluated in social situations, and fears about separation from loved ones may each result in clinging and visible distress when children must separate from parents. In addition to similarities among anxiety disorders, GAD and major depressive disorder (MDD) have high lifetime comorbidity, strong symptom overlap (e.g., fatigue, difficulty concentrating, sleep disturbances), and are both characterized by perseverative cognitive processes (e.g., worry/rumination), all of which may complicate differential diagnosis of GAD and MDD (Moffitt et al., 2007). These similarities across anxiety disorders, as well as between certain anxiety and depressive disorders, reinforce the importance of assessing anxiety disorders using multiple methods and informants, and of choosing measures that demonstrate good discriminant validity.

Structured and Semistructured Diagnostic Interviews

The publication of DSM-5 in 2013 poses challenges to diagnostic interviewing. Some of the structured and semistructured instruments were developed to be consistent with the DSM-IV and have not yet been updated (Leffler, Riebel, & Hughes, 2015). However, the psychometric properties of the instruments we discuss below remain robust. Therefore, until these instruments are updated to reflect the DSM-5 diagnostic changes, they should continue to be administered, as they have shown clinical and research utility.

The *Anxiety Disorders Interview Schedule for the DSM-IV—Child Version, Child and Parent Reports* (ADIS-IV-C/P; Silverman & Albano, 1996) is a semistructured clinical interview that permits the diagnosis of DSM-IV anxiety disorders, mood disorders, and externalizing disorders in youth ages 6–17. The interview is typically administered separately to children and parents and, based on child and parent reports of disorder symptoms and impairment, clinicians assign a *clinical severity rating* (CSR) for each disorder. CSRs range from 0 to 8, with 0 reflecting "no symptoms/impairment" and 8 reflecting "marked symptoms/impairment." A CSR rating of 4 or higher indicates symptoms and impairment at a clinically interfering level. Interrater reliability for ADIS-IV-C/P anxiety diagnoses has been found to be excellent, with kappas ranging from .80–1.00 (Lyneham, Abbott, & Rapee, 2007; Silverman, Saavedra, & Pina, 2001). The ADIS-IV-C/P also has excellent test–retest reliability for anxiety diagnoses, with intraclass correlation coefficients (ICCs) ranging from .81 to .99 for child-reported impairment and from .86 to .99 for parent-rated impairment (Silverman et al., 2001). Convergent validity for the ADIS-IV-C/P has also been established; children with an ADIS diagnosis of SocAD and SAD both scored significantly higher on the Social Anxiety and Separation Anxiety subscales, respectively, of the *Multidimensional Anxiety Scale for Children, Second Edition* (MASC-2; March, 2012). A DSM-5 version of the ADIS-C/P is currently on track for publication using a similar format and structure as the DSM-IV version.

The *Kiddie Schedule for Affective Disorders and Schizophrenia for School-Age Children—Present and Lifetime Versions* (K-SADS-PL; Kaufmann et al., 1997), a semistructured diagnostic interview for youth ages 6–18, is used to assess current and past episodes of psychopathology in children and adolescents according to DSM-III-R and DSM-IV criteria. The K-SADS-PL consists of an initial screen interview that provides an overview of lifetime symptoms of psychopathology, as well as five diagnostic supplement sections (including a supplement for anxiety disorders). Based on information about the presence and quality of symptoms reported by parents and children, symptoms are scored by the clinician on a 0- to 3-point scale (0 = "not available"; 1 = "symptoms not present"; 2 = "subthreshold symptoms"; 3 = "threshold symptoms"). The K-SADS-PL has excellent interrater reliability for assigning current and lifetime diagnoses, and test–retest reliability coefficients range from .80 to .90 for anxiety and depressive disorders (Kaufman et al., 1997). However, relatively few studies have assessed convergence of the K-SADS-PL with other measures of anxiety disorders.

Self- and Parent-Report Measures

Broadband Anxiety

The *Revised Children's Manifest Anxiety Scale, Second Edition* (RCMAS-2) has been widely used since its first edition to identify anxiety symptoms among youth (Reynolds & Richmond, 2008). It is a self-report instrument for children and adolescents ages 6 to 19 years and is composed of a total of 49 items. In addition to a Total Anxiety scale, it yields scores for three anxiety-related scales: Physiological Anxiety, Worry, and Social Anxiety. The RCMAS-2 also yields scores for two Validity scales, an Inconsistent Responding (INC) index, and a Defensiveness (DEF) scale (previously Lie scale), which reveal when respondents have given random responses or have presented themselves in an overly positive manner. Reliability estimates have been improved from the RCMAS to .92 for the Total score (TOT) and .75 to .86 for the scale scores (Reynolds & Richmond, 2008). Although further research is needed to determine RCMAS-2's discriminant validity, because of its substantial overlap with the RCMAS, it is expected to have similar psychometric properties as the RCMAS. Therefore, it appears to be a useful instrument in the assessment and monitoring of treatment in anxious children and adolescents.

The MASC-2 (March, 2012) is a revision of the MASC, a child- and parent-report measure assessing anxiety symptoms (March, Parker, Sullivan, Stallings, & Conners, 1997). It contains 50 items and identifies anxiety symptoms in youth ages 8–19 years. The MASC-2 assesses a broad range of emotional, physical, cognitive, and behavioral symptoms in its six scales: Separation Anxiety/Phobias, GAD, Social Anxiety, Obsessions and Compulsions, Physical Symptoms, and Harm Avoidance. It also has a Validity scale called the Inconsistency Index (response style). The MASC-2 is able to differentiate between anxiety disorders and other disorders, as well as between the various childhood anxiety disorders (March, 2012). It has excellent internal reliability (Parent = .89; Self = .92) and test–retest reliability (Parent = .93; Self = .89) (March, 2013). In addition, it has strong discriminative validity for the three anxiety disorders assessed by its subscales (March, 2012).

The *Screen for Child Anxiety-Related Emotional Disorders* (SCARED; Birmaher et al., 1997), another measure proven to have good discriminative validity, is able to differentiate among varying anxiety disorders and to differentiate anxiety disorders from other disorders, such as depressive disorders (Birmaher et al., 1997, 1999). Both parent and child self-report versions of SCARED contain 38 items that assess the following factors in youth ages 9–18: general anxiety, separation anxiety, social phobia, and physical symptoms of anxiety. It also measures symptoms related to school phobias. Both self-reports have moderate parent–child agreement and good internal consistency, test–retest reliability, and discriminant validity (Birmaher et al., 1999). SCARED is also noted to be sensitive to treatment response (Birmaher et al., 1999). It has been found to have strong sensitivity and specificity to the ADIS-IV-C/P (Muris, Merckelbach, Mayer, & Prins, 2000).

The *Pediatric Anxiety Rating Scale* (PARS; Research Units on Pediatric Psychopharmacology Anxiety Study Group, 2002) is a semistructured interview used by parents and by youth ages 6–17, as well as clinicians, to rate the frequency, severity and impairment of anxiety. It measures anxiety in six areas: Separation, Social Interactions or Performance Situations, Generalized, Specific Phobia, Physical Signs and Symptoms, and Other. It has been particularly useful in treatment studies for clinically anxious children (Research Units on Pediatric Psychopharmacology (RUPP) Anxiety Study Group, 2002). The PARS has two sections that include a 50-item symptom checklist in which items are rated as present or absent during the past week. The second section consists of seven items that measure severity and impairment (rated on a 5-point Likert scale). The Anxiety Severity scale specifically focuses on SAD, SocAD, and GAD. Psychometric properties such as internal consistency are adequate (Research Units on Pediatric Psychopharmacology Anxiety Study Group, 2002). However, convergent and divergent validity may need further investigation (Silverman & Ollendick, 2008). Nevertheless, PARS' utility relative to treatment sensitivity appears promising, as it has paralleled change in other measures of anxiety symptoms and global improvement (Silverman & Ollendick, 2008).

Narrowband Anxiety

The *Penn State Worry Questionnaire for Children* (PSWQ-C; Chorpita, Tracey, Brown, Collica, & Barlow, 1997), a 14-item, self-report measure for youth ages 6–18 years, assesses the ability to control worry and the frequency of worry. Youth rate their agreement with worry items on a 4-point Likert scale, with higher scores representing a tendency to worry more. The psychometric properties of the PSWQ-C for two large community samples demonstrated good internal consistency and test–retest reliability (Chorpita et al., 1997; Muris, Meesters, & Gobel, 2001). Furthermore, recent data suggest that it has favorable discriminate validity for anxiety disorders and excellent internal consistency and convergent validity in a large clinical sample of children and adolescents (Pestle, Chorpita, & Schiffman, 2008). However, among subjects in the clinical sample, the PSWQ-C was not able to differentiate between GAD and MDD/dysthymia, although it did discriminate between individuals with GAD and other anxiety disorders (Pestle et al., 2008). This seeming lack of specificity in the clinical sample could be due to the high comorbidity between GAD and depressive disorders.

A scale that has been specifically designed to discriminate between anxiety and depression is the *Revised Child Anxiety and Depression Scale* (RCADS; Chorpita, Yim, Moffitt, Umemoto, & Francis, 2000), developed for youth ages 6–19 years; it consists of 47 self-report items. Respondents use a 4-point Likert scale to rate how true each item is to them. The RCADS includes the following subscales: Separation Anxiety Disorder (SAD), Social Phobia (SP), Generalized Anxiety Disorder (GAD), Panic Disorder (PD), Obsessive–Compulsive Disorder (OCD), and Major Depressive Disorder (MDD). It also yields a Total Anxiety Scale and a Total Internalizing Scale. Also available is a parent form is also available (*RCADS-P*) that assesses similar youth symptoms of anxiety and depression using the six subscales. The RCADS has been shown to have favorable internal consistency in a community sample of schoolchildren and adolescents (Chorpita et al., 2000), as well as convergent, discriminant, and factorial validity in a clinical sample of youth (Chorpita, Moffitt, & Gray, 2005). Furthermore, it has been shown to assess anxiety and depression symptoms accurately in both clinical and school-based populations (Ebesutani, Bernstein, Nakamura, Chorpita, & Weisz, 2010; Ebesutani et al., 2011). The RCADS-P shows high internal consistency and convergent validity (Ebesutani et al., 2011). Overall, the RCADS appears to have strong utility for both clinical and research settings because it clearly helps to discriminate between anxiety and depression (Chorpita et al. 2000, 2005).

The *Social Anxiety Scale for Children—Revised* (SASC-R; La Greca & Stone, 1993) and the *Social Anxiety Scale for Adolescents* (SAS-A; La Greca & Lopez, 1998) are 22-item scales assessing social anxiety symptoms in children and adolescents, respectively. Respondents rate each item on a 5-point scale according to how much they feel the item is true of them. Both the SASC-R and the SAS-A measure anxiety as it relates to three factors: Fear of Negative Evaluation; Generalized Social Avoidance and Distress; and Social Avoidance Specific to New Situations or Unfamiliar Peers. Each of the three subscales has acceptable internal consistency, with all r's greater than .65, and the measures demonstrate good convergent and discriminant validity (La Greca & Lopez, 1998; La Greca & Stone, 1993). Both measures accurately discriminate between socially anxious individuals and those with no anxiety, and both are sensitive to treatment changes

(Ingles et al., 2010; Tulbure, Szentagotai, Dobrean, & David, 2012). The SASC-R has been used in a number of settings, including community samples, medical samples, and inpatient and outpatient populations (La Greca & Lopez, 1998). Additionally, the SAS-A has been translated into numerous languages, including Spanish, Dutch, German, and Chinese with good test–retest reliability and internal consistency (Ingles et al., 2010; La Greca & Lopez, 1998). Both the SASC-R and the SAS-A facilitate the assessment of adolescent social functioning and friendships.

Another widely used scale for social anxiety, the *Social Phobia and Anxiety Inventory for Children* (SPAIC; Beidel, Turner & Morris, 1995), is a 26-item rating scale that measures children and adolescents' anxiety (ages 8–18 years) in a variety of social situations. The social situations are reflected in its three subscales: Assertiveness/General Conversation, Traditional Social Encounters, and Public Performance. The SPAIC has strong internal consistency and test–retest reliability (Silverman & Ollendick, 2005). Data support the use of this rating scale as a sensitive measure when assessing treatment outcome. It is also a sensitive screening measure with children from diverse backgrounds (Tulbure et al., 2012). Recently, the Social Phobia and Anxiety Inventory for Children–11 (SPAIC-11) and the Social Phobia and Anxiety Inventory for Children's Parents (SPAICP-11) were developed using item response theory (IRT), with reports of social anxiety by children and parents (Bunnell, Beidel, Liu, Joseph, & Higa-McMillan, 2015). Both assessments were developed as brief versions of the child and parent versions of the SPAIC. Although the SPAIC-11 and the SPAICP-11 appear to be psychometrically sound measures, future research is needed to determine additional validation. Preliminary results, however, hold promise for their use as brief assessments of social anxiety for children in research and clinical settings.

Broadband Measures

As noted earlier, pediatric anxiety disorders are highly comorbid with one another, as well as with other psychiatric disorders, including ADHD, depression, and ODD. Therefore, using broadband measures that assess anxiety, in addition to other emotional and behavioral disorders, adds value to the assessment and ultimately the treatment of children with anxiety.

One of the most widely used parent-report measures for assessment and treatment outcome, the *Child Behavior Checklist* (CBCL; Achenbach, 1991; Achenbach, Dumenci, & Rescorla, 2003; Silverman & Ollendick, 2005), assesses not only anxiety but also internalizing and externalizing problems. Additionally, it has eight subscales: Aggressive Behavior, Delinquent Behavior, Withdrawn, Anxious/Depressed, Somatic Complaints, Attention Problems, Social Problems, and Thought Problems. The 118-item parent form was developed for use with school-age children ranging in age from 6 to 18 years. A preschool version has been developed as well for preschoolers ranging in age from 1½ to 5 years (Achenbach & Rescorla, 2000). Parents rate their child on a 0- to 2-point scale (0 = "not true" to 2 = "very true or often true"). Forms also obtain parents' descriptions of problems, disabilities, most important concerns, and child's strengths. The CBCL has been widely used in treatment studies and demonstrates significant correlations with other measures of anxiety and sensitivity to change (Silverman & Ollendick, 2005). Furthermore, the utility of the anxiety scales has been examined using mothers of children with and without anxiety disorders (Kendall et al., 2007). Results indicated that the Anxiety scales significantly discriminated between children with anxiety and those without (Kendall et al., 2007). The CBCL can be used with a wide population. It has been translated into over 90 languages, and multicultural norms have been added. Most recently, there have been scales added to the CBCL that are consistent with DSM-5. For preschoolers, the Autism Spectrum Problems scale contains items consistent with DSM-5 criteria for autism spectrum disorder, and the Anxiety Problems scale has been revised to ensure consistency with DSM-5 criteria for GAD, SAD, and SocAD. The Somatic Problems scale has also been revised for school-age children in order to be consistent with the newly developed DSM-5 category, somatic symptom disorder, which often is related to anxiety.

The *Behavior Assessment System, Third Edition* (BASC-3; Reynolds & Kamphaus, 2015), another multidimensional measure that assesses anxiety, as well as other emotional and behavioral disorders, is a self-report measure for youth and adults ages 2–25 years. There are self-report (SRP; ages 6–25), parent-report (PRS), and teacher-report (TRS) forms. The SRP, TRS, and the PRS contain 100–189 items depending on age (preschool, ages 2–5; child, ages 6–11; adolescent, ages 12–21; or college, ages 18–25). Respondents use a 4-point Likert scale to record whether they agree with each item (0 = "never" to 3 = "almost always"). The BASC-3 PRS and TRS yield five composite scales, each of which includes primary scales: for the PRS, Internalizing Problems (Anxiety, Depression, and Somatization), Externalizing Problems (Hyperactivity, Aggression, and Conduct Problems), Adaptive Skills (Adaptability, Social Skills, Leadership, Study Skills, Functional Communication), Behavioral Symptoms Index (Hyperactivity, Aggression, Depression, Attention Problems, Atypicality, and Withdrawal); and for the TRS, School Problems (Learning Problems and Attention Problems). It also yields seven content scales, which include Anger Control, Bullying, Developmental Social Disorders, Emotional Self-Control, Executive Functioning, Negative Emotionality, and Resiliency. In addition to the content scales, there are three clinical index scales, which include ADHD Probability Index, Autism Probability Index, and Clinical Probability Index. These indices are composed of items from other scales and are empirically derived. The PRS and TRS may be scored online or on paper. Psychometric properties for the BASC-3 are well-established (Reynolds & Kamphaus, 2002, 2015). A Spanish version of the BASC-3 is available for preschool, child, and adolescent PRS forms.

TREATMENT STRUCTURE, KEY COMPONENTS, AND TECHNIQUES ACROSS CBT PROTOCOLS

Numerous variants of CBT and CBT-based treatment manuals exist, but such treatments also contain unifying treatment components. The primary treatment components across CBT protocols include psychoeducation, somatic management skills, cognitive restructuring, gradual exposure to feared situations, and relapse prevention. The *Coping Cat* program (discussed in greater detail below) is one of the best supported versions of CBT for youth with SAD, SocAD, and GAD (Kendall, 1994; Kendall, Furr, & Podell, 2010). The Coping Cat and similar CBT-based protocols for anxious children and adolescents aim to improve functioning by introducing youth to techniques for building reliable coping skills to deal with life's challenges and facing fears. This and similar CBT-based protocols integrate two major components. The first component involves skills training, and the second involves employing learned skills in behavioral practice.

Although many versions of CBT exist, most CBT variants follow a similar treatment structure. In individual CBT, a therapist works primarily with the anxious child or adolescent, usually meeting once per week for approximately 1 hour for an average of 16 weeks (Chorpita et al., 2011; Ishikawa et al., 2007; James et al., 2013; Rapp et al., 2013; Silverman et al., 2008). Often, the therapist also meets with the youth's parent or legal guardian about twice throughout treatment to address parental response to anxious behaviors and to discuss upcoming treatment components with parents. This is especially important prior to behavioral exposure sessions, which can often be distressing for children and adolescents and may require more specific responses from parents (Kendall et al., 2010). When implementing CBT, the therapist plays not only a collaborative and supportive role but also helps to promote independence, responsibility, and self-sufficiency in children and adolescents. Although most CBT-based treatment protocols for pediatric anxiety are distributed to therapists and clients in the format of treatment manuals and workbooks outlining treatment components, experts suggest that therapists should be flexible in their use of manuals, adapting manuals to needs of specific youth, while also making sure to cover important treatment goals.

In addition to encouraging flexibility within a single CBT protocol, intervention researchers have developed variants of CBT for anxious youth in order to adapt treatment to the needs of specific children and adolescents. For example, individual CBT programs (Melfsen et al., 2011; Nauta, Scholing, Emmelkamp, & Minderaa, 2003; Wood, McLeod, Piacentini, & Sigman, 2009) have been modified to incorporate basic CBT skills while increasing parent involvement. Such programs still require approximately 12–20 individual therapy sessions, each lasting 50–90 minutes (specified by the treatment regimen), but also incorporate between four and 16 parent sessions to enhance parent involvement in treatment. Such modifications to the structure of CBT can be especially useful for children who might have less insight into their anxiety symptoms, such as children with autism spectrum disorders and very young children (Waters, Ford, Wharton, & Cobham, 2009; Wood, Drahota, et al., 2009). Group CBT paradigms also increase parental involvement in therapy by incorporating parallel parent sessions, often conducted simultaneously with youth-focused sessions. Programs such as *Cool Kids* and *Take ACTION* (Rapee, 2000; Waters et al., 2009) involve teaching children the core CBT techniques in a group format. Such treatments still involve 10–16 (60- to 120-minute) sessions weekly. However, during sessions, child and parent groups learn similar material. Parent-oriented sessions often include psychoeducation about child anxiety, parenting strategies for managing child anxiety and improving relationships, parental coping techniques including communication and problem-solving techniques, and general therapeutic techniques taught in child sessions.

CBT treatment structure has also been modified in order to target groups of children and adolescents with specific symptom clusters or disorder presentations. For example, Schneider and colleagues (2011) conducted an RCT of a 16-session protocol specifically targeting SAD through a combination of child and parent individualized therapy sessions. Within this protocol, the first 4 weeks of therapy consist of SAD-specific psychoeducation (50-minute sessions) with children and parents separately. Then, the next 8 weeks of treatment consist of weekly sessions split into parent–child portions and parent-only portions. These modifications allow clinicians to target cognitions more specifically and implement situational exposures relevant to children with SAD. Other protocols have employed social skills and/or assertiveness training in combination with CBT skills to target more directly the deficits often experienced by youth with SOC (Alfano et al., 2009; Beidel, Turner, & Morris, 2000; Beidel, Turner, & Young, 2006; White et al., 2013). Similarly to SAD-focused treatments, SocAD-focused interventions incorporate more dis-order-specific psychoeducation and behavioral exposures targeting anxiety in social situations. Most of these treatments involve individual sessions (approximately 2–13 meetings ranging from 15-minute to hourlong sessions) and at least some group therapy component (approximately 7–12, 60- to 90-minute sessions), in which social skills and cognitive techniques can be practiced with other youth in a controlled environment.

The incorporation of manual-based CBT techniques with clinical expertise allows therapists to flexibly adapt treatments. Modern age, population, and disorder-based versions of CBT also allow therapists to better target specific problems exhibited by children and adolescents with varying symptom presentations. Although psychosocial interventions such as CBT and exposure-focused therapies currently have the greatest amount of empirical support, novel behavioral therapies that have recently emerged show promise as alternative or adjunctive treatment options.

EVIDENCE-BASED TREATMENT IN PRACTICE

In the final sections of this chapter we focus on the implementation of CBT in anxious youth using the Coping Cat program (Kendall, 1994; Kendall & Hedtke, 2006), an individual CBT protocol for children ages 7–13 that has been extensively researched and adapted for group, school, and Internet-based treatment (Kendall et al., 1997, 2008, 2010). In its individual format, Coping Cat is a child-focused, skills-based treatment that incorporates parents through several parent sessions (Sessions 4 and 9). Skills delivered in the Coping Cat program are similar to those delivered by other CBT-based manuals and include psychoeducation about anxiety, somatic awareness and relaxation, cognitive restructuring, problem solving, gradual exposures, and relapse prevention. Skills are delivered in a child-friendly format and introduced using the "FEAR" plan (i.e., Feeling frightened?; Expecting bad things to happen?; Attitudes and actions that can help; Rewards and results). Once the exposure-based portion of treatment is introduced, children or adolescents can recall steps from the "FEAR" acronym when they cope with *in vivo* situations that might elicit anxiety (e.g., talking to peers, test-taking, being away from a parent). Each step of the FEAR plan and its corresponding skills is summarized in the sections that follow and may be found in Table 6.2.

The general therapeutic approach of the Coping Cat protocol is similar to that of other CBT-based programs in that it is time-limited, present-focused, and skills-based. The Coping Cat program is 16 weeks in length, which is typically adequate to cover all essential skills and techniques for most children, although treatment may be extended to accommodate additional exposures sessions. The program focuses on identifying and using skills to target current problem or fear areas rather than focus on distal causes of the child's current anxiety. Sessions are organized around the introduction and practice

TABLE 6.2. Common Treatment Components of Coping Cat and other CBT Protocols

Skills training (primarily cognitive)

Psychoeducation
- Corrective education about anxiety is provided (i.e., normalizing experience of anxiety)
- Youth are taught to identify their somatic reactions to anxiety (e.g., sensations such as increased heart rate, sweating, stomachaches)

Affective awareness
- Youth are taught to identify the signs of anxiety, often by breaking down the experience of anxiety into antecedents, thoughts, body sensations, and emotion-related behaviors (i.e., avoidance)

Somatic management skills
- Relaxations skills (e.g., deep breathing, progressive muscle relaxation, visual imagery) are introduced to target somatic reactions to anxiety

Cognitive restructuring
- Youth are taught to identify and challenge inaccurate or negative thoughts using self-talk
- Youth are taught to shift thinking in a more coping-focused direction and to develop coping thoughts

Skills practice (primarily behavioral)

Graduated, controlled behavioral exposures
- Youth develop a hierarchy of feared situations in conjunction with their therapist and, possibly, their parents
- Exposures to feared situations and stimuli are implemented to apply learned skills to situations that are feared and/or avoided

Relapse prevention
- Skills are reviewed
- Consolidation and generalization of treatment gains is emphasized
- Therapist and youth may make plans for overcoming difficult or anxiety-provoking situations in the future

Note. Some versions of CBT focus more or less on different aspects of the treatment, but versions of CBT and exposure-based therapy for social anxiety disorder, generalized anxiety disorder, and separation anxiety disorder include most if not all of these components.

of a set of skills, and these skills are reinforced through weekly STIC ("Show That I Can") tasks to be completed outside of session. Each session is highly structured and includes brief rapport building, review of STIC tasks and previously learned skills, introduction and practice of new skills, and the assignment of a new STIC task to be completed between sessions. Parents may be integrated into the end of sessions by having the child explain new skills and assigned STIC tasks to them. Throughout treatment, the therapist assumes a number of roles (Kendall & Hedtke, 2006), including that of a consultant or collaborator (i.e., someone who does not have all the answers), a diagnostician (integrating data from the verbal reports of child and parent), and a coach (observing the child's performance and providing feedback about strengths and weaknesses). Session 1, which focuses primarily on establishing rapport and providing an overview of treatment, helps to set the tone of the therapeutic relationship and establish the overall structure of treatment.

The "F" step of the FEAR plan (Feeling frightened?) is introduced in Session 2 and elaborated in Sessions 3–5. The primary goals of the "F" step are identifying somatic responses to anxiety, distinguishing somatic responses to anxiety from those elicited by other emotional experiences, and learning to reduce the intensity of these somatic responses through relaxation and other strategies. Session 2 focuses on developing the child's awareness of somatic responses to anxiety through various interactive activities, such as "Feelings Charades" and the creation of a "Feelings Dictionary." The therapist normalizes the experience of anxiety for the child by introducing the idea of the "fight-or-flight response." Children are also asked to begin to develop a hierarchy of anxiety-provoking situations during this session using a "fear ladder" and are introduced to the "F" step of the FEAR plan. During Session 3, the therapist continues to develop the child's somatic awareness of anxiety and encourages him or her to begin to identify his or her own somatic responses of anxiety. In an effort to reinforce the idea that each person may experience anxiety differently, the therapist may provide his or her own examples of somatic responses to anxiety and elicit examples from the child. It may be useful for the therapist to assist the child in making a "body drawing," in which the therapist traces the child's body on a large sheet of paper and encourages the child to identify areas of the body where he or she typically experiences sensations of anxiety. During Session 5, children begin to intervene in the cycle of anxiety by learning relaxation skills, which they continue to practice outside of session. The therapist introduced several relaxations skills using metaphors and imagery (deep breathing, progressive muscle relaxation), and the therapist and child role-play the step-by-step use of these relaxation strategies in situations generated by the therapist and child. Children are encouraged to teach these relaxation skills to their parents at the end of session, and the therapist assists the child in identifying a specific time and place for daily relaxation practice.

The "E" step of the FEAR plan (Expecting bad things to happen?) is introduced in Session 6 and reviewed in Session 7. The primary goals of the "E" step are recognizing anxious self-talk and understanding its contribution to the experience of anxiety. The therapist introduces the idea of self-talk to the child by presenting cartoons with empty thought bubbles and asking the child to generate content for these thought bubbles. The child is then shown cartoons depicting more ambiguous situations and asked to generate two different thoughts that might belong in the bubbles, and to identify different emotions that would be associated with each thought. Variations on this exercise are repeated, progressing to more anxiety-provoking situations and using the child's own thoughts. In this way, the child begins to make the link between thoughts and feelings. Thinking traps may also be introduced in this session (e.g., catastrophizing, all-or-nothing thinking, walking with blinders on, ignoring the positive). Modeling and role plays are used to practice identifying and challenging negative self-talk, and to replace negative self-talk with coping self-talk. These skills are reviewed and reinforced in Session 7.

The "A" step of the FEAR plan (Attitudes and actions that can help) is introduced in Session 7. The primary goal of the "A" step is to improve the child's ability and sense of self-efficacy in coping with anxiety-provoking situations. This goal is achieved primarily through problem solving, which is introduced as a series of steps for coping with both non-anxiety-provoking and anxiety-provoking situations (identify the problem, brainstorm solutions, identify the pros and cons of each solution, pick a solution and try it out, evaluate the outcome). Problem solving is first practiced using neutral situations and applied to more anxiety-provoking situations thereafter. To increase the child's cognitive flexibility, the importance of brainstorming a *variety* of solutions, even if they may seem silly at first, is emphasized and modeled by the therapist.

The "R" step of the FEAR plan (Results and rewards) is introduced in Session 8 and reinforced in the subsequent parent session (Session 9). The primary goal of the "R" step is to introduce the idea of self-monitoring and contingent reinforcement to the child. The child is introduced to the idea of rating and rewarding his or her performance, and the emphasis is placed on effort and successive approximations of a goal rather than on perfectionism or goal attainment. The appropriateness of reward effort and partial successes is discussed with the child, and therapist and child work together to generate a list of possible rewards, both material and nonmaterial, and the idea that rewards can come either from others or from ourselves is explored. Role plays are used throughout this session to reinforce the concepts of self-monitoring and reinforcement. As a way of reviewing the FEAR plan now that all steps have been introduced, the child may create a small FEAR plan card at the end of session for use during upcoming exposures.

The latter part of treatment (Sessions 10–15) focuses on putting the FEAR plan into action during imaginal and *in vivo* exposures conducted with the child in session and assigned for homework outside of session. During Session 9, the therapist should prepare parents for exposures by discussing the rationale for the use, preparing parents for a possible increase in distress upon commencement of exposure sessions, and reinforcing the importance of rewards introduced in to the child in Session 8. It may also be helpful to solicit feedback from parents regarding the child's fear ladder begun in previous sessions. Exposures in the Coping Cat program proceed according to a gradual exposure model, beginning with imaginal exposures or low-anxiety-provoking situations at the bottom of the child's fear ladder and gradually moving up to more feared situations. During each exposure, therapists periodically assess children's distress level using subjective units of distress (SUD) ratings and encourage them to coping strategies in the moment. Children should be encouraged to remain in the situation until their SUD ratings decrease, and postexposure processing with the therapist should call attention to decreases in the child's SUD ratings over time, successful use of coping strategies, and disconfirmation of feared outcomes. Sessions might include one longer or several brief exposures, and additional exposures should be assigned as STIC tasks outside of session in order to facilitate generalization. During the final session, the therapist should review skills with the child and parent and make plans to achieve any remaining goals through continued practice. Children may also be given the option of taping a "commercial" (planned during the previous sessions) in which they celebrate their successes and provide advice to other children about the program. Other means of celebrating treatment completion (e.g., party, award certificate) are also appropriate.

Case Example

In the fictionalized case example to follow, we illustrate anxiety and related psychopathology in a young female and detail the application of evidence-based treatment principles to aid in the amelioration of her symptoms. Relevant background information about the case is provided first, followed by a step-by-step review of the Coping Cat model of treatment, as tailored for use with this child and her family. The case presented is a typical one in terms of age and symptom presentation; however, points of flexibility in the application of this treatment are also highlighted with regard to variations from typical presentations and as appropriate for the particularities of this case.

Background and History

Mila H, a 9-year-old Hispanic female of Cuban American descent, living in the southeastern United States, resides in a single-family home with her mother (Mrs. H), father (Mr. H), younger sister (Victoria, 6), and maternal grandmother (Mrs. A). Mrs. H is employed as a kindergarten teacher, and Mr. H owns and operates a small business. Mrs. A works part-time as a nanny but primarily supports the family as a caregiver who assists with child care and household upkeep. Family income was reported to be approximately $90,000 per year. Of note, Mila's parents indicated that they primarily spoke Spanish at home, both to reinforce dual-language learning and in deference to Mrs. H's mother's limited use of English. They reported that all family members, other than Mrs. A, are fluent English speakers, and Mila indicated that she personally prefers to converse in English with others at home and elsewhere. Mila is in the fourth grade at a parochial school, where she reportedly receives mostly A's and B's in her schoolwork, although there were sporadic indications of poorer academic performance and increased isolation from peers in the most recent academic quarter. During an initial phone screen, Mrs. H described Mila as someone who was "born anxious" and reported current challenges in managing Mila's anxiety at bedtime, at mealtimes, at school, and, particularly, in test-taking situations. Mrs. H indicated that although such concerns were present before, Mila has increasingly evidenced worry and separation distress in the past 3 months as she prepared for state-administered, school-based exams, and she specifically cited an "anxiety attack" that Mila had 2 days before the first school testing day, which resulted in Mila missing school that day, as a motivator for her to contact the clinic at this time. Mrs. H indicated that Mila's increased separation distress and academic worries of late have also been particularly challenging to manage because she works in the same school that Mila attends, and that Mila often made attempts or requested to see her throughout the day as a method to cope with her anxiety. Finally, Mrs. H also reported that Mila was a picky eater who sometimes complained about fears related to choking and vomiting when pressured to eat less-preferred foods.

Mila appeared for an initial assessment with her mother and father at a university-based specialty anxiety research program, where, after providing relevant informed consent and assent to services, she and her parents were administered the ADIS-IV-C/P by an independent evaluator and completed relevant screening questionnaires assessing anxiety, depression, and related cognitive, family, and emotion-related factors of interest. Mila presented as a bright and articulate, but somewhat reserved child who evidenced age-appropriate insight into her anxiety-related concerns. Her mood and affect were generally appropriate to the evaluation context, although she became teary eyed and visibly distressed when asked to separate from her parents for the ADIS interview. She agreed to separate from Mrs. and Mr. H, with an agreement that she could check in with her parents every 15 minutes by text message on her cell phone, while they remained in the waiting room. Mrs. H reported that this checking technique was "sometimes effective" in allowing Mila to separate from them but indicated that they were generally surprised that she was willing to stay with the examiner throughout the testing interval and complete the ADIS-C.

Following the ADIS interviews, the independent evaluator assigned Mila the following diagnoses: GAD (CSR = 5), SAD (CSR = 4) and a subclinical specific phobia, other type (vomiting/choking; CSR = 3). The independent evaluator also noted that some perfectionism-related behaviors and food-related avoidance might be indicative of emergent obsessive–compulsive or eating-disorder-related pathologies, but no additional diagnoses were assigned.

During the interview, Mila and her parents both reported that Mila struggled with chronic worry, particularly related to school performance (starting school, doing homework and in-school work correctly, etc.) and test taking, but also in related domains of performance (in dance class and during gym class at school). Previously, Mr. and Mrs. H had reported that Mila was able to cope with these worries and still perform well academically. However, in recent months, Mila's teacher indicated that Mila appeared to struggle with written assignments, timed work, and preparation for exams, and she shared with Mrs. H her fears Mila was about to experience increasingly poor grades if she did not improve her efforts. Prior to the current intake, Mila completed a psychoeducational evaluation with a school psychologist that indicated no learning disorders and high-average cognitive ability, with some minor deficits in working memory and processing speed that the examiner felt might be due to Mila's visible anxiety during the testing. Mila also reported a number of interpersonal worry situations, including concerns about her hair and appearance, as well as maintaining friendships. Mr. and Mrs. H reported that Mila typically required that her hair be braided a certain way each day, and that her uniform be laid out the night before each school day for her to examine before bedtime. It was unclear to her parents why Mila preferred this "routine," but they indicated that Mila would in fact ruminate or become distressed if she felt her uniform was damaged or her hair was braided incorrectly. Mila and her parents also reported other worries related to natural disasters (hurricanes, thunderstorms), and worries about her parents' health. Mila reportedly had trouble falling asleep on most nights and asked that a parent remain in her bedroom with her until she fell asleep. If they did not follow this dictate, Mila was reported to tantrum and cry until they relented. They also reported increased problems with concentration, restlessness, and fatigue in the past 6 months and a moderate degree of impairment related to these worries and concomitant physiological responses.

In terms of separation distress and related avoidance, Mila indicated that she was specifically worried about harm befalling herself (e.g., being taken by a "kidnap van") or her parents and felt reluctance to separate from her mother, particularly at school, at bedtime, and at other activities, including her dance class (where Mila required that her mom "stay visible" to her at all times). Similar to the behavior observed in session, Mrs. H reported that Mila often texted her during the day, including lunchtime at school, and would become distressed if she did not receive an immediate response by text or in person. To lessen Mila's distress, Mrs. H reported that she often checked in on Mila, as she was able to, throughout the day both to ease initial separations in the mornings (via promises to check in at intervals later) and personally reassure Mila of her safety. That being said, Mila was able to separate from her mother and stay overnight at her cousins' home and attend dropoff playdates with two longtime friends at present, if she was allowed to keep her phone with her throughout. All parties indicated that separation distress and related avoidance caused a moderate amount of interference in Mila's life at present, but they also felt it was slightly less severe than her current problems with more general and academic worries.

Mila reported significant fear of choking and, more specifically, vomiting as a result of choking on food. As a result of this fear, Mila occasionally refused to eat foods that she felt were difficult to swallow easily (e.g., large pieces of beef or pork) or were lengthy in size (e.g., long strings of pasta). Mila's parents could not recall a specific incident that sparked this concern, but they did indicate that she had "waxed and waned" in fear intensity with regard to this domain over the last 2 to 3 years. For example, Mr. H reported that Mila would sometimes eat large pieces of meat if she were in a particularly good mood or distracted. However, Mila reported that she was more consistently fearful of vomiting, in particular, and sometimes even checked labels of foods in the refrigerator to make sure she was not eating "rotten" or expired foods that she believed were likely to make her vomit. Mila also reported that she preferred to avoid long car trips or "spinning rides" at carnivals to limit the likelihood of vomiting. Nonetheless, Mila and her parents concurred that this fear was mild at present and more transient in nature than her generalized worry and separation distress.

Overall, Mila's parents expressed a high degree of motivation for treatment and expressed strong interest in seeing Mila's anxiety and related avoidance behaviors reduced. They also acknowledged that their own behaviors might be reinforcing some of Mila's fears and potentially strengthening them, and wished to learn new skills to cope better and appropriately manage Mila's distress. Mila indicated some interest in reducing her fear and anxiety, but limited, albeit age-appropriate insight, about how to address these concerns or change her avoidant behaviors.

Course of Treatment

Mila received 16 sessions of the *Coping Cat* program (Kendall, 1994; Kendall & Hedtke, 2006) for youth anxiety disorders, delivered via an individual therapy context. In Session 1, the therapist focused primarily on developing rapport with Mila and orienting Mila and Mrs. H to the process and techniques of CBT. Time was devoted to developing rapport with both parties (Mr. H was unable to attend the majority of treatment sessions due to his work schedule) in session and answering pertinent questions about expectations for treatment. Mrs. H acknowledged some level of initial reluctance regarding the exposure components of treatment, noting that she was unsure that all members of her family and her mother, in particular, would be good at tolerating their own distress if they noticed Mila feeling uncomfortable or upset. The therapist acknowledged that these were natural reactions to the notion of exposure and that a graduated or stepped approach, with increasing parental and (if desired) grandparental responsibility for guiding such work could be implemented down the road. Despite this hesitance, the therapist and Mrs. H were heartened by Mila's willingness to separate from Mrs. H during sessions and agreement to follow a visual schedule of the session that the therapist created, with one designated parent check-in only allowed during child-alone components of the initial session. Good rapport was noted, and Mila seemed eager to share her understanding of anxiety and fear with the therapist, and generally seemed engaged in learning new skills provided. Toward the end of session, the clinician introduced both the initial STIC homework task (providing a brief example of a time in the following week when the child felt really great—not upset or worried) and the use of reward points for completion of the STIC task. The purpose of STIC tasks and the use of a reward "bank" were also reviewed with Mila's parents to confirm this as a weekly format for homework and subsequent reinforcement. Finally, the session concluded with the therapist and Mila participating in a fun activity together (watching a humorous video online) that was selected at the beginning of the session to further facilitate positive engagement.

Sessions 2 and 3 consisted of child-directed content aimed at improving Mila's identification of anxious feelings and somatic responses to anxiety, more particularly. At the start of Session 2, the therapist reviewed Mila's STIC task homework, which indicated that Mila "felt great" the prior week when playing with her parents at a local park, and reward points for completion were noted. The therapist used a number of activities in this session to assess and encourage emotion education, including reviewing photos of people expressing varying emotions in magazines and creating a "Feelings Dictionary" by cutting out and mounting such photos on a piece of butcher paper. Mila seemed to enjoy this activity, as well as role-play of various emotion states. The therapist noted that Mila had a good grasp of a variety of emotions but had trouble distinguishing cognitive and physiological aspects of emotions when prompted. As they conducted these emotion education tasks, the therapist worked to normalize Mila's experience of fear and anxiety and discussed how a fantasy role model (Sofia the First) and the therapist worked to overcome prior fears or threats. The therapist noted that they were running short on time and therefore assigned the child and parents to work independently on developing fear ladders that would be expanded in the next two sessions as their STIC tasks for the week. The therapist explained the usage of SUD ratings and how they could be utilized in constructing the hierarchy.

At the start of Session 3, Mrs. H reported that the weeklong interval between Sessions 2 and 3 was a difficult one for Mila because she had two tests at school and was feeling overwhelmed and reluctant to study. Mila noted that she was feeling sick during the week and did not necessarily connect the tests, which she considered to be "easy," to her reluctance to attend school on one of the test days. The therapist praised Mila and Mrs. H for sharing this situation, for attending school despite the distress, and for completing initial fear ladder ratings despite the stress of the prior week. The therapist noted the discrepancy in how Mrs. H attributed Mila's ill feelings to anxiety, whereas Mila felt she was truly unwell on the test day described and indicated that this would in fact be a central focus of Session 3 content. With Mila alone, the therapist spent time discussing a variety of somatic responses to anxiety and, rather than dwell on the recent disputed incident, encouraged Mila to identify body feelings in a safe, neutral situation and contrast these with a more anxiety-provoking one. This tack seemed to work well with Mila, who independently noted to the therapist that the feelings she experienced when she wanted to stay home the past week (stomach distress, feverish feelings) were similar to those many experience in the course of anxiety. Some additional role play was also utilized to further encourage somatic awareness. Then the therapist introduced the "F" step in the four-step FEAR plan or coping model central to the Coping Cat intervention—Feeling frightened? Mila was reminded that in identifying the "F" step she was working to identify anxious feelings more broadly and monitoring somatic responses associated with such anxious feelings. As a final STIC task for Session 3, Mila was asked to record two times in the coming week when she felt anxious and rate her anxiety in each situation based on feelings in her body.

Session 4 was a parent-directed session attended by Mrs. H and her mother, Mrs. A. Since Mrs. A was present, the session was conducted primarily in Spanish. Mr. H's work schedule continued to be a barrier to session attendance. They problem-solved ways to share therapy-related information with him, given that it seemed unlikely that he would be able to attend sessions in the near future. Both Mrs. A and Mrs. H concurred that the prior 2 weeks had been marked by a seeming spike in Mila's anxiety after what seemed like an initial drop in symptoms of worry after Session 1. The therapist gave Mila's mother and grandmother an opportunity to discuss these concerns and normalized the waxing and waning pattern of worry and anxiety endorsed. The therapist also endeavored to understand better the antecedents and consequences of Mila's reported "worry attacks," as Mrs. H called them, since these appeared to be on the rise. Mila's mother and grandmother reported that such worry was often most salient in the morning before school, on the way to school, at the time of separation from Mrs. H at school, and on Sunday night before the start of the school week. Mila's grandmother also indicated that she felt the family members were quite variable in their current responses to Mila's stated worry about school and separation, with some encouraging Mila to cope with it independently and others providing what sounded like excessive verbal reassurance about Mila's safety and academic abilities. The problems with excessive reassurance in the context of generalized anxiety were discussed, as illustrated in the following dialogue:

THERAPIST: Based on what you've been saying, it sounds as though attending school is a big trigger for Mila's anxiety, and she is experiencing a lot of distress in the mornings. What have you tried to help her manage her distress so that she can attend school?

MRS. H: Honestly, I feel like I've tried everything. I try to help her calm down on the way to school by promising her that I'm going to stay safe. She worries that I'll open the door for strangers, that I'll get into a car accident on the way to the store, or pretty much anything else you can imagine. I just try to stay calm and tell her over and over again that mommy is going to be careful and nothing bad is going to happen.

THERAPIST: So it sounds like you provide her a lot of reassurance—is that right?

MRS. A: We all do, all the time! We want to make sure she knows that we are all going to be okay when we're away from each other.

THERAPIST: And do you feel like the reassurance is helpful? In other words, after you reassure her that everyone will be safe, does she appear less anxious and stop asking for your reassurance?

MRS. H: Well . . . no. No matter what I say, usually she keeps asking. Sometimes she'll stop for a few minutes, but then she'll need me to reassure her again about something else.

THERAPIST: Right. Often that happens when we provide reassurance. Providing your child with reassurance may seem to help a little in the short-term. It's also very natural to want to do everything you can to help reduce your child's distress, including reassuring them that everything will be OK. However, providing reassurance may be preventing Mila from developing ways to manage her own worries. As a result, she looks to you and other family members to help her feel better. Mila also may begin to feel as though she needs your reassurance to be sure the situation turns out OK. She never learns that you will be safe, even if she doesn't ask over and over again. Does that make sense?

MRS. A: Yes . . . but what do we do instead? I think Mila will probably become even more upset if we don't reassure her!

THERAPIST: It's true that she might experience more distress for a short while, and you may also feel upset or guilty. But you won't be doing nothing. Mila is learning some helpful skills in this treatment to manage her own anxiety, and it's much more effective to suggest that she use the skills and guide her in doing so. It may take some time, but eventually Mila will become confident that she has the tools to manage her worry on her own, without your reassurance.

Mrs. H and Mrs. A role-played alternative response to Mila's worry statements and requests for reassurance. Both family members seemed encouraged by this alternative plan at the end of session and noted that Mila had established seemingly good rapport with the therapist, indicating that she was happy to continue attending sessions with her.

Session 5 began with a review of Mila's STIC task from Session 3 and discussion of some moderate improvements in Mila's worry the past week, which Mila attributed to the shorter than normal school week and her mother attributed to better management of Mila's school-related worries. The majority of Session 5 was spent introducing the concept of muscle tension and its association with anxiety, and both deep breathing and progressive muscle relaxation techniques. At the end of session, Mila demonstrated some relaxation techniques for Mrs. H and they established a plan to practice a brief version of the progressive muscle relaxation exercise reviewed in session before going to bed on Sundays and weeknights, with a briefer version to be utilized as needed before school. Practice of this relaxation plan was Mila's STIC task for the week.

Session 6 featured the introduction of the second step in the FEAR plan—the "E" step, Expecting bad things to happen?—and the role of cognition in youth anxiety. Mila and her mother continued to report improvements in general worry at this session and Mrs. H attributed much of the improvement to familial changes in responding to Mila's reassurance-seeking and safety-seeking behavior at home and at school. For example, Mrs. H reported that she and Mila agreed to start leaving their cell phones in the car during the school day and to relay any vital messages through Mila's teacher rather than via text message. Although Mila indicated that she did not appreciate all of these changes, she did acknowledge that she has started to manage her worry more independently or with the help of peers or teachers. Mrs. H reported some return of Mila's picky eating and avoidance of meats at mealtimes but agreed to keep presenting such foods for now and observe any changes in the behavior over the next week given Mila's history of variability in such behavior. In session, the therapist introduced cognitive aspects of anxiety to Mila using a series of cartoons, in which Mila indicated the self-talk of characters in "thought bubbles," eventually segueing from discussion of self-talk in low stress situations to self-talk in anxiety-provoking situations, using the cartoon characters to frame this concept throughout. A distinction was made to Mila between anxious self-talk and coping self-talk (thoughts that lead to more distress vs. those leading to less distress), as illustrated in the following dialogue:

THERAPIST: Mila, we've been saying that when we're feeling anxious, a lot of time we're thinking that something bad is going to happen, right?

MILA: Right.

THERAPIST: Sometimes, we call that anxious self-talk. All that means is that when we're telling ourselves that something bad might happen or is going to happen in a situation, that thought often makes us feel anxious. Sometimes we get so stuck on the bad thing we think might happen that we don't consider other things that could happen. These other things may not be bad at all, or they may even be good. Does that ever happen to you?

MILA: Do you mean like when I'm eating meat and all I can think about is the meat getting stuck in my throat and choking?

THERAPIST: That's a really good example. It sounds like your anxious self-talk about choking on the meat gets so strong that it drowns out other self-talk, and it's hard to think about what else could happen. And that probably makes you want to stay away from the meat, right?

MILA: Right.

THERAPIST: Today, we're going to practice coming up with what we call "coping self-talk" or "coping thoughts." Coping self-talk means telling yourself what other things could happen in the situation so that you feel better. Coping self-talk helps you cope and get through the anxiety. Let's look at this magazine picture for a few minutes to practice. Tell me what's happening in the picture, Mila.

MILA: Well, there's a girl standing outside on the playground. She's looking up at the sky. The sky looks really dark, like a storm might be coming.

THERAPIST: Yes, that's what I see, too. Can you think of a thought this girl might have that would make her feel nervous? What would her self-talk sound like?

MILA: Her brain might be telling her, "You might get hit by lightning if you don't run inside right now, or the wind may knock you down and you might get hurt."

THERAPIST: And if that was what her self-talk sounded like, how do you think she would feel?

MILA: Really, really scared.

THERAPIST: How would her body tell her that it was feeling scared?

MILA: Well, she might start to feel really sweaty and shaky, and her heart might start beating really fast. And she would want to run inside right away.

THERAPIST: Good! So it sounds like her self-talk is making her feel scared and making her want to run away. Now, let's think of a coping thought that this girl could use to help her feel better. What else do you think could happen to her?

MILA: Well, she might just end up getting a little wet. And she might even be able to have fun playing in the rain puddles after the storm is over.

THERAPIST: Good! And if that was her self-talk, how do you think she would feel?

MILA: Maybe still a little nervous, but also maybe excited.

THERAPIST: And what do you think she would do?

MILA: She would probably still want to go inside because nobody likes to get really wet. But she would probably just walk instead really calmly.

The "E" step in Mila's FEAR plan was presented formally. Finally, Mila was encouraged to practice coping self-talk in increasingly anxiety-provoking situations by first asking questions from the "F" step ("What's happening in my body?") and then the "E" step. As part of the "E" step, Mila was encouraged to first identify her self-talk, then gather evidence for her thoughts ("Be a detective") by asking herself questions about the likelihood of her anxious thought being true. Mila was provided with a list of common thinking traps to help her to identify common anxious thoughts and help prompt the use of detective-like questions. As usual, the session ended with assignment of Mila's STIC task for the week and a preselected enjoyable activity to share between therapist and client.

Session 7 was largely a review of material covered in the prior section, followed by a brief introduction to the "A" step in the FEAR plan—Attitudes and actions that might help. New content in this session included the introduction of problem-solving steps (e.g., defining the problem; identifying potential solutions; evaluating the pros and cons of selected solutions; selecting a preferred alternative to try out). Mila found these problem-solving steps to be useful and concrete in establishing plans for managing test-related procrastination and worry in particular. Although not explicitly discussed in the treatment manual, the therapist created a laminated card with the problem-solving steps identified by letter and using a humorous acronym selected by Mila in session (PIES; "P" for problem; "I" for ideas about possible solutions; "E" for evaluating solutions; and "S" for selecting a solution). It was later indicated to the therapist by phone that Mila enjoyed using the problem-solving steps so much that her mother purchased a beaded bracelet with the PIES acronym, so that she could wear it at school as a reminder to use her problem-solving steps as needed.

Session 8 of the Coping Cat program typically focuses more explicitly on the delivery of the "R" step in the FEAR plan—Results and rewards. The concept of self-reward for brave behavior was discussed following review of Mila's STIC task at the beginning of this session. A sample dialogue of this conversation follows:

THERAPIST: Mila, today we will be talking about the final step in the FEAR plan— the "R" step. "R" stands for results and rewards. Do you know what a reward is?

MILA: A prize for doing something good?

THERAPIST: That's a really good way to put it! A reward is something that is given when you are happy with the work you've done. Can you think of any rewards you have gotten before? It could be a reward your parent gave you, your teacher gave you, or even one that you gave yourself?

MILA: Well, in school we have a "student of the month." A new kid gets to be student of the month each month, and they get a certificate. Last month I got it!

THERAPIST: Congratulations, Mila—that's great! What an honor! How did you feel when you got rewarded?

MILA: Really happy! I had been trying really hard to go to school every day and walk into the classroom on time. And I tried to be really nice to one of the new kids in my class. It made me feel really good that my teacher noticed all of that.

THERAPIST: Sometimes other people reward us when they're happy with what we've accomplished, like your teacher did. But we can also reward ourselves too when we're happy with how we've performed. Imagine you were at your dance class and you finally were able to successfully perform a dance move you had been trying to do for weeks. How do you think you would feel about it?

MILA: I'd feel amazing! And I would be really proud of myself.

THERAPIST: Sure! And that's an example of a time when you might reward yourself for achieving or being successful at something. What about all those times you practiced though and didn't get the dance move? How do you think you would have felt then?

MILA: Probably pretty frustrated. But determined too!

THERAPIST: Sometimes it can be really helpful to reward ourselves for trying or practicing at something, even if we don't get it right away. Rewarding ourselves in these situations can help us to stay motivated to keep practicing, especially when we're feeling frustrated.

MILA: How would I reward myself though?

THERAPIST: Well, let's talk about some different rewards you would like to earn for being brave and trying new things. We can use this "reward menu" to plan some things you might want to earn.

The remainder of the session was ultimately spent in taking the fear ladders developed earlier in treatment by Mila and her parents, rerating and reevaluating them, then condensing them into a singular hierarchy for use in subsequent exposure-focused sessions. The therapist noted that Mila and her mother were in greater agreement about Mila's hierarchy than earlier in treatment, and that separation and test-related fears, as well as avoidance, had generally been reduced since the onset of treatment. Mila and her mother concurred that rewards for brave actions that might be taken along the lines of this fear ladder were appropriate, and the therapist further encouraged role play between Mila and her mother in session regarding use of Mila's FEAR steps in regard to a couple of low-level sample items from her fear ladder.

Session 9, a parent session, was attended by Mr. and Mrs. H. The concept of situational exposure was introduced more concretely to the parents in this session, and barriers to potential exposures were discussed. Mr. H expressed concern about remaining inconsistencies in the household with regard to management of Mila's fears. For example, he noted that although he and Mrs. H remained firm about continuing to produce foods about which Mila had choking or vomiting fears and preventing checks of food labels by removing these from trigger foods in the refrigerator, Mrs. A, Mila's grandmother, was sneaking preferred, less-feared foods to Mila at between mealtimes because she was "afraid Mila would go hungry." Mrs. H said that because Mrs. A grew up in poverty and often went hungry as a child, she had difficulty conceptualizing the rationale for allowing Mila to go hungry if she refused the feared food. Ways of sensitively approaching this topic with Mrs. A, and compromise solutions that would allow Mrs. A to feel more involved in supporting other exposures to reinforce their rationale and benefit to her were discussed, as well as the possibility of including Mrs. A in future exposure-based sessions, if appropriate. A plan was also clarified for when and how to provide larger side dishes or other foods, along with feared meats or other, similar foods that elicited fears of vomiting or choking to avoid any weight loss or excessive hunger during such exposure meals. The concept of potentially introducing feared foods on a more planful schedule and encouraging everyone to eat them in differing portion sizes, from smaller to larger amounts as an "adventure," was also discussed.

Sessions 10–15 were all exposure-based treatments and involved moving from relatively low-level items on Mila's fear ladder to higher intensity items in subsequent sessions, with between-session exposure opportunities emphasized, and explicit discussion of the role of parents and the grandmother as "coaches" in encouraging and planning such exposures. Before beginning exposures in Session 10, Mila was reminded of the rationale for conducting exposures, and the therapist worked with her to develop a FEAR plan for her first exposure. A sample dialogue for this session follows:

THERAPIST: So far, we've mostly been spending our time in this room learning some different tools to help you when you're feeling scared or worried. The last time we met, I told you that we are going to start to practice using all the tools in your toolbox in some real-life kinds of situations. Although we may stay in this room some of the time, a lot of the time we will be going to other parts of this building or outside to practice some things.

MILA: What kinds of things are we going to practice?

THERAPIST: The last time we met, we made this fear ladder with some different situations that make you feel scared or worried. On the bottom step of the ladder we put some situations that make you a little worried, but not too much. We are going to start by practicing one of those today in session. Do you remember why we want to start with things that make you only a little worried?

MILA: Because if we start with things that make me really scared or worried, I would probably be really upset and not want to do them.

THERAPIST: Right. And if we started with something too hard, how would you rate your performance?

MILA: I'd probably think I did pretty badly. And I probably wouldn't want to try it again.

THERAPIST: Exactly! We want to start with something that's a little tough but not too tough so that you can practice using your FEAR plan and get through it. Some of the things we try might still be difficult because we don't want to go too slowly, but we don't want to go too quickly either. We'll start today with the situation that's on the very bottom of your ladder. Can you read that for me, please?

MILA: Taking a pop quiz. And I gave that one a "3."

THERAPIST: Yes. So Mila, today, I am going to give you a short pop quiz right here in the clinic. The pop quiz has some math problems on it. Let's make a FEAR plan to help you cope with the quiz. What does "F" stand for again?

MILA: "Feeling frightening." I'm feeling a little bit nervous right now. My throat feels a little tight and my legs feel like they want to move around.

THERAPIST: It sounds like your body is definitely telling you that it's feeling nervous. "E" stands for "Expecting bad things to happen." What do you worry might happen during the quiz? Tell me about your self-talk.

MILA: Well, I'm worried that it's going to be too tough and I won't be able to do a lot of the questions. I might feel stupid, and you might think I'm really bad at math.

THERAPIST: It sounds like you're having a lot of worry thoughts right now Mila. Let's come up with some attitudes and actions that could help—the "A" step.

MILA: I could tell myself that nobody always knows the answer to everything. I'm still learning.

THERAPIST: That's a great coping thought Mila! What's our last step in the FEAR plan?

MILA: "Results and rewards."

THERAPIST: Right! So even if you don't know all the answers, do you think you should still reward yourself.

MILA: I think maybe? I'm practicing something that's really hard for me and trying to get better at facing my fears.

THERAPIST: I agree, Mila! Let's come up with a reward you could earn for facing your fears today.

Additional exposures involved classroom-like settings at the university-based research clinic where treatment took place and included replicating fears about performing poorly on written or oral assignments that were too difficult or hard to comprehend and receiving ambiguous feedback from a "teacher." Mila was coached to use SUDS ratings throughout such exposures to indicate points of distress and any habituation that occurred. An emphasis was placed on managing anticipatory anxiety before such exposures through parent-directed and self-prompting to use FEAR and PIES plans as needed. Further sessions included separation-related exposures, such as Mila's mother dropping her off in the school dropoff line rather than walking her to class and purposely being late to pick her up from sessions at the clinic. One session was also dedicated to Mila eating a larger piece of meat with the therapist that had purposely been placed in the family's refrigerator for several days prior to the exposure. This latter exposure proved most difficult for Mila, who indicated that she would continue to worry about the possibility of vomiting for several days after. However, at the next session, Mila reported that she was able to use her FEAR plan steps to effectively manage these worries and that they were reduced sooner than she had anticipated in session.

Although Session 16 was also dedicated to a higher-level exposure involving separation from her mother, Mila and the therapist were also able to spend time reviewing progress and noting the significant improvements she made in sessions. A final evaluation meeting was held with Mila and her mother both to "film a commercial" noting aspects of the Coping Cat program that worked best for her and might benefit other children, and to fill out posttreatment measures. Information from these dimensional rating scales, as well as a brief check on diagnostic status, confirmed that Mila appeared to be in the subclinical range across all primary disorders targeted at pretreatment. Mila and her family members expressed confidence that they had adopted an "exposure lifestyle" and management plan for fear that they believed would continue to help them over the longer term.

CONCLUSION

In this chapter, we have summarized current knowledge about the prevalence and course of anxiety disorders in youth, risk factors for their development, and research-based methods of assessment and treatment. Anxiety disorders appear to be more common than any other mental disorder in childhood and adolescence, and onset may occur as early as preschool. Anxiety disorders are moderately heritable, and temperamental factors such as BI, factors in the familial environment such as insecure attachment and parental overcontrol, and other cognitive and social factors, all play a role in conferring risk for anxiety. The long-term negative consequences associated with early onset of anxiety disorders include impairment during childhood and adolescence in social and academic functioning, as well as occupational impairment and increased risk for additional anxiety, depressive, and substance use disorders in adulthood. Appropriate treatment of anxiety during childhood and adolescence is imperative in forestalling these negative consequences and, fortunately, efficacious treatments for anxiety disorders do exist. CBT, a time-limited treatment that typically includes components such as psychoeducation, somatic management skills, cognitive restructuring, exposures, and relapse prevention, is currently considered a well-established treatment for anxiety disorders and may be effective in upwards of 60–70% of children and adolescents (e.g., Higa-McMillan, Francis, Rith-Najarian, & Chorpita, 2016; Walkup et al., 2008). CBT treatment manuals for anxiety, such as Kendall's Coping Cat program, are now easily accessible to many mental health practitioners and available in a number of formats, including manual-based and Internet-delivered formats.

Despite the growing availability of CBT for anxiety disorders in a variety of modalities, estimates indicate that only 1 youth in 5 with a diagnosable anxiety disorder ever receives treatment for that disorder (Merikangas et al., 2011). Anxiety disorders, clearly, are therefore undertreated in youth, and narrowing the gap between youth in need of CBT and those who actually receive CBT will involve tackling this problem on many fronts: making screening for anxiety disorders in childhood and adolescence a more widespread practice; increasing public knowledge about signs and symptoms of anxiety disorders; making evidence-based treatment more affordable and accessible to low-income families; and continuing to develop novel, technologically enhanced paradigms for training clinicians in the provision of and providing evidence-based therapies to children and adolescents. Clinician attitudes toward evidence-based therapies, or toward certain components of them, may also present a barrier to their dissemination. For example, even among clinicians who have been trained to conduct exposure therapy for anxiety, one-third or fewer clinicans may actually implement exposures with clients due to misconceptions about associated risk of harm or dropout (Harned et al., 2014), despite evidence that use of exposure in children and adolescents is not associated with alliance ruptures or increased dropout (e.g., Chu, Skriner, & Zandberg, 2014).

Finally, despite evidence supporting the efficacy of CBT for youth anxiety disorders, as this chapter has reviewed, relatively little is known about *why* CBT works. It may be the case that certain components of CBT, such as exposure or cognitive restructuring, make a greater contribution to treatment gains than other components. However, the lack of dismantling studies for youth CBT or formal, well-powered tests of mediation make it difficult to isolate certain components of CBT as being more effective than others. Additionally, certain youth characteristics (e.g., demographic, diagnostic, or familial characteristics) may make some youth more responsive to certain evidence-based therapies, but the relative lack of tests of moderation have limited the ability to draw conclusions in this area. Advancements in dismantling studies and tests of both mediation and moderation will make it increasingly possible to streamline and personalize CBT for youth with anxiety, thus facilitating its dissemination.

REFERENCES

Achenbach, T. M. (1991). *Child Behavior Checklist/4–18*. Burlington: University of Vermont.

Achenbach, T. M., Dumenci, L., & Rescorla, L. A. (2003). Are American children's problems still getting worse?: A 23-year comparison. *Journal of Abnormal Child Psychology, 31*(1), 1–11.

Achenbach, T. M., & Rescorla, L. (2000). *ASEBA preschool forms and profiles: An integrated system of multi-informant assessment*. Burlington, VT: ASEBA.

Alfano, C. A., Pina, A. A., Villalta, I. K., Beidel, D. C., Ammerman, R. T., & Crosby, L. E. (2009). Mediators and moderators of outcome in the behavioral treatment of childhood social phobia. *Journal of the American Academy of Child and Adolescent Psychiatry, 48*(9), 945–953.

Altman, C., Sommer, J. L., & McGoey, K. E. (2009). Anxiety in early childhood: What do we know? *Journal of Early Childhood and Infant Psychology, 5*, 157–175.

American Psychiatric Association. (2013). *Diagnostic and statistical manual of mental disorders* (5th ed.). Arlington, VA: Author.

Amin, N., Foa, E. B., & Coles, M. E. (1998). Negative interpretation bias in social phobia. *Behaviour Research and Therapy, 36*(10), 945–957.

Angold, A., Costello, E. J., & Erkanli, A. (1999). Comorbidity. *Journal of Child Psychology and Psychiatry, 40*(1), 57–87.

Axelson, D. A., & Birmaher, B. (2001). Relation between anxiety and depressive disorders in childhood and adolescence. *Depression and Anxiety, 14*(2), 67–78.

Bacow, T. L., May, J. E., Brody, L. R., & Pincus, D. B. (2010). Are there specific metacognitive processes associated with anxiety disorders in youth? *Psychology Research and Behavior Management, 3*, 81–90.

Bar-Haim, Y. (2010). Research review: Attention bias modification (ABM): A novel treatment for anxiety disorders. *Journal of Child Psychology and Psychiatry, 51*(8), 859–870.

Bar-Haim, Y., Lamy, D., Pergamin, L., Bakermans-Kranenburg, M. J., & van IJzendoorn, M. H. (2007). Threat-related attentional bias in anxious and nonanxious individuals: A meta-analytic study. *Psychological Bulletin, 133*(1), 1–24.

Bar-Haim, Y., Morag, I., & Glickman, S. (2011). Training anxious children to disengage attention from threat: A randomized controlled trial. *Journal of Child Psychology and Psychiatry, 52*(8), 861–869.

Barker, E. D., Oliver, B. R., & Maughan, B. (2010). Co-occurring problems of early onset persistent, childhood limited, and adolescent onset conduct problem youth. *Journal of Child Psychology and Psychiatry, 51*(11), 1217–1226.

Barlow, D. H. (2000). Unraveling the mysteries of anxiety and its disorders from the perspective of emotion theory. *American Psychologist, 55*(11), 1247–1263.

Barlow, D. H. (2002). *Anxiety and its disorders: The nature and treatment of anxiety and panic* (2nd ed.). New York: Guilford Press.

Barrett, P. M., Rapee, R. M., Dadds, M. M., & Ryan, S. M. (1996). Family enhancement of cognitive style in anxious and aggressive children. *Journal of Abnormal Child Psychology, 24*(2), 187–203.

Battaglia, M., Pesenti-Gritti, P., Medland, S. E., Ogliari, A., Tambs, K., & Spatola, C. A. (2009). A genetically informed study of the association between childhood separation anxiety, sensitivity to CO_2, panic disorder, and the effect of childhood parental loss. *Archives of General Psychiatry, 66*(1), 64–71.

Beard, C. (2011). Cognitive bias modification for anxiety: Current evidence and future directions. *Expert Review of Neurotherapeutics, 11*(2), 299–311.

Beard, C., & Amir, N. (2009). Interpretation in social anxiety: When meaning precedes ambiguity. *Cognitive Therapy Research, 33*(4), 406–415.

Beesdo, K., Bittner, A., Pine, D. S., Stein, M. B., Höfler, M., Lieb, R., et al. (2007). Incidence of social anxiety disorder and the consistent risk for secondary depression in the first three decades of life. *Archives of General Psychiatry, 64*(8), 903–912.

Beesdo, K., Knappe, S., & Pine, D. S. (2009). Anxiety and anxiety disorders in children and adolescents: Developmental issues and implications for DSM-V. *Psychiatric Clinics of North America, 32*(3), 483–524.

Beidel, D. C., & Turner, S. M. (1997). At risk for anxiety: I. Psychopathology in the offspring of anxious parents. *Journal of the American Academy of Child and Adolescent Psychiatry, 36*(7), 918–924.

Beidel, D. C., Turner, S. M., & Morris, T. L. (1995). A new inventory to assess childhood social anxiety and phobia: The Social Phobia and Anxiety Inventory for Children. *Psychological Assessment, 7*(1), 73–79.

Beidel, D. C., Turner, S. M., & Morris, T. L. (2000). Behavioral treatment of childhood social phobia. *Journal of Consulting and Clinical Psychology, 68*(6), 1072–1080.

Beidel, D. C., Turner, S. M., & Young, B. J. (2006). Social effectiveness therapy for children: Five years later. *Behavior Therapy, 37*(4), 416–425.

Berman, S. L., Weems, C. F., Silverman, W. K., & Kurtines, W. M. (2000). Predictors of outcome in exposure-based cognitive and behavioral treatments for phobic and anxiety disorders in children. *Behavior Therapy, 31*(4), 713–731.

Birmaher, B., Brent, D. A., Chiappetta, L., Bridge, J., Monga, S., & Baugher, M. (1999). Psychometric properties of the Screen for Child Anxiety Related Emotional Disorders (SCARED): A replication study. *Journal of the American Academy of Child and Adolescent Psychiatry, 38*(10), 1230–1236.

Birmaher, B., Khetarpal, S., Brent, D., Cully, M., Balach, L., Kaufman, J., et al. (1997). The Screen for Child Anxiety Related Emotional Disorders (SCARED): Scale construction and psychometric characteristics. *Journal of the American Academy of Child and Adolescent Psychiatry, 36*(4), 545–553.

Bittner, A., Egger, H. L., Erkanli, A., Costello, E. J., Foley, D. L., & Angold, A. (2007). What do childhood anxiety disorders predict? *Journal of Child Psychology and Psychiatry, 48*(12), 1174–1183.

Boden, J. M., Fergusson, D. M., & Horwood, L. J. (2007). Anxiety disorders and suicidal behaviours in adolescence and young adulthood: Findings from a longitudinal study. *Psychological Medicine, 37*(3), 431–440.

Bongers, I. L., Koot, H. M., Van der Ende, J., & Verhulst, F. C. (2003). The normative development of child and adolescent problem behavior. *Journal of Abnormal Psychology, 112*(2), 179–192.

Brady, E. U., & Kendall, P. C. (1992). Comorbidity of anxiety and depression in children and adolescents. *Psychological Bulletin, 111*(2), 244–255.

Britton, J. C., Bar-Haim, Y., Clementi, M. A., Sankin, L. S., Chen, G., Shechner, T., et al. (2013). Training-associated changes and stability of attention bias in youth: Implications for Attention Bias Modification Treatment for pediatric anxiety. *Developmental Cognitivie Neuroscience, 4*, 52–64.

Bunnell, B. E., Beidel, D. C., Liu, L., Joseph, D. L., & Higa-McMillan, C. (2015). The SPAIC-11 and SPAICP-11: Two brief child-and parent-rated measures of social anxiety. *Journal of Anxiety Disorders, 36*, 103–109.

Burckhardt, R., Manicavasagar, V., Batterham, P. J., & Hadzi-Pavlovic, D. (2016). A randomized controlled trial of strong minds: A school-based mental health program combining acceptance and commitment therapy and positive psychology. *Journal of School Psychology, 57*, 41–52.

Chambless, D. L., & Hollon, S. D. (1998). Defining empirically supported therapies. *Journal of Consulting and Clinical Psychology, 66*(1), 7–18.

Chambless, D. L., & Ollendick, T. H. (2001). Empirically supported psychological interventions: Controversies and evidence. *Annual Review of Psychology, 52*, 685–716.

Chorpita, B. F., Daleiden, E. L., Ebesutani, C., Young, J., Becker, K. D., Nakamura, B. J., et al. (2011). Evidence-based treatments for children and adolescents: An updated review of indicators of efficacy and effectiveness. *Clinical Psychology: Science and Practice, 18*(2), 154–172.

Chorpita, B. F., Moffitt, C. E., & Gray, J. (2005). Psychometric properties of the Revised Child Anxiety and Depression Scale in a clinical sample. *Behaviour Research and Therapy, 43*(3), 309–322.

Chorpita, B. F., Tracey, S. A., Brown, T. A., Collica, T. J., & Barlow, D. H. (1997). Assessment of worry in children and adolescents: An adaptation of the Penn State Worry Questionnaire. *Behaviour Research and Therapy, 35*(6), 569–581.

Chorpita, B. F., Yim, L., Moffitt, C., Umemoto, L. A., & Francis, S. E. (2000). Assessment of symptoms of DSM-IV anxiety and depression in children: A revised child anxiety and depression scale. *Behaviour Research and Therapy, 38*(8), 835–855.

Chu, B. C., & Harrison, T. L. (2007). Disorder-specific effects of CBT for anxious and depressed youth: A meta-analysis of candidate mediators of change. *Clinical Child and Family Psychology Review, 10*(4), 352–372.

Chu, B. C., Skriner, L. C., & Zandberg, L. J. (2014). Trajectory and predictors of alliance in cognitive behavioral therapy for youth anxiety. *Journal of Clinical Child and Adolescent Psychology, 43*(5), 721–734.

Compton, S. N., Kratochvil, C. J., & March, J. S. (2007). Pharmacotherapy for anxiety disorders in children and adolescents: An evidence-based medicine review. *Pediatric Annals, 36*(9), 586–590, 592, 594–598.

Compton, S. N., Peris, T. S., Almirall, D., Birmaher, B., Sherrill, J., Kendall, P. C., et al. (2014). Predictors and moderators of treatment response in childhood anxiety disorders: Results from the CAMS trial. *Journal of Consulting and Clinical Psychology, 82*, 212–224.

Costantino, G., & Malgady, R. G. (1994). Storytelling through pictures: Culturally sensitive psychotherapy for Hispanic children and adolescents. *Journal of Clinical Child Psychology, 23*(1), 13–20.

Costello, E. J., Copeland, W., & Angold, A. (2011). Trends in psychopathology across the adolescent years: What changes when children become adolescents, and when adolescents become adults? *Journal of Child Psychology and Psychiatry, 52*(10), 1015–1025.

Costello, E. J., Egger, H. L., & Angold, A. (2004). developmental epidemiology of anxiety disorders. In T. H. Ollendick & J. S. March (Eds.), *Phobic and anxiety disorders in children and adolescents* (pp. 334–380). New York: Oxford University Press.

Costello, E., Mustillo, S., Erkanli, A., Keeler, G., & Angold, A. (2003). Prevalence and development of psychiatric disorders in childhood and adolescence. *Archives of General Psychiatry, 60*(8), 837–844.

Crawley, S. A., Beidas, R. S., Benjamin, C. L., Martin, E., & Kendall, P. C. (2008). Treating socially phobic youth with CBT: Differential outcomes and treatment considerations. *Behavioural and Cognitive Psychotherapy, 36*, 379–389.

Creswell, C., & O'Connor, T. G. (2011). Interpretation bias and anxiety in childhood: Stability, specificity and longitudinal associations. *Behavioural and Cognitive Psychotherapy, 39*(2), 191–204.

Cronk, N. J., Slutske, W. S., Madden, P. A., Bucholz, K. K., & Heath, A. C. (2004). Risk for separation anxiety disorder among girls: Paternal absence, socioeconomic disadvantage, and genetic vulnerability. *Journal of Abnormal Psychology, 113*(2), 237–247.

Cummings, C. M., Caporino, N. E., & Kendall, P. C. (2014). Comorbidity of anxiety and depression in children and adolescents: 20 years after. *Psychological Bulletin, 140*, 816–845.

Degnan, K. A., Almas, A. N., & Fox, N. A. (2010). Temperament and the environment in the etiology of childhood anxiety. *Journal of Child Psychology and Psychiatry, 51*(4), 497–517.

Drake, K. L., & Ginsburg, G. S. (2012). Family factors in the development, treatment, and prevention of childhood anxiety disorders. *Clinical Child and Family Psychology Review, 15*(2), 144–162.

Ebesutani, C., Bernstein, A., Nakamura, B. J., Chorpita, B. F., & Weisz, J. R. (2010). A psychometric analysis of the Revised Child Anxiety and Depression Scale—Parent Version in a clinical sample. *Journal of Abnormal Child Psychology, 38*(2), 249–260.

Ebestuani, C., Chorpita, B. F., Higa-McMillan, C. K., Nakamura, B. J., Regan, J., & Lynch, R. E. (2011). A psychometric analysis of the Revised Child Anxiety and Depression Scales—Parent version in a school sample. *Journal of Abnormal Child Psychology, 39*, 173–185.

Egger, H. L., & Angold, A. (2006). Common emotional and behavioral disorders in preschool children: Presentation, nosology, and epidemiology. *Journal of Child Psychology and Psychiatry, 47*(3–4), 313–337.

Eldar, S., Apter, A., Lotan, D., Edgar, K. P., Naim, R., Fox, N. A., et al. (2012). Attention bias modification treatment for pediatric anxiety disorders: A randomized controlled trial. *American Journal of Psychiatry, 169*(2), 213–220.

Eley, T. C., Bolton, D., O'Connor, T. G., Perrin, S., Smith, P., & Plomin, R. (2003). A twin study of anxiety-related behaviours in pre-school children. *Journal of Child Psychology and Psychiatry, 44*(7), 945–960.

Festa, C. C., & Ginsburg, G. S. (2011). Parental and peer predictors of social anxiety in youth. *Child Psychiatry and Human Development, 42*(3), 291–306.

Field, Z. C., & Field, A. P. (2013). How trait anxiety, interpretation bias and memory affect acquired fear in children learning about new animals. *Emotion, 13*(3), 409–423.

Fox, N. A., Henderson, H. A., Marshall, P. J., Nichols, K. E., & Ghera, M. M. (2005). Behavioral inhibition: Linking biology and behavior within a developmental framework. *Annual Review of Psychology, 56*, 235–262.

Friedman, M. J., Resick, P. A., Bryant, R. A., Strain, J., Horowitz, M., & Spiegel, D. (2011). Classification of trauma and stressor-related disorders in DSM-5. *Depression and Anxiety, 28*(9), 737–749.

Garber, J., & Weersing, V. R. (2010). Comorbidity of anxiety and depression in youth: Implications for treatment and prevention. *Clinical Psychology: Science and Practice, 17*(4), 293–306.

Ginsburg, G. S., Becker, E. M., Keeton, C. P., Sakolsky, D., Piacentini, J., Albano, A. M., et al. (2014). Naturalistic follow-up of youths treated for pediatric anxiety disorders. *JAMA Psychiatry, 71*(3), 310–318.

Ginsburg, G. S., Drake, K. L., Winegrad, H., Fothergill, K., & Wissow, L. S. (2016). An open trial of the Anxiety Action Plan (AxAP): A brief pediatrician-delivered intervention for anxious youth. *Child and Youth Care Forum, 45,* 19–32.

Ginsburg, G. S., Kendall, P. C., Sakolsky, D., Compton, S. N., Piacentini, J., Albano, A. M., et al. (2011). Remission after acute treatment in children and adolescents with anxiety disorders: Findings from the CAMS. *Journal of Consulting and Clinical Psychology, 79*(6), 806–813.

Ginsburg, G. S., Siqueland, L., Masia-Warner, C., & Hedtke, K. A. (2005). Anxiety disorders in children: Family matters. *Cognitive and Behavioral Practice, 11*(1), 28–43.

Gonzalez, A., Peris, T. S., Vreeland, A., Kiff, C. J., Kendall, P. C., Compton, S. N., et al. (2015). Parental anxiety as a predictor of medication and CBT response for anxious youth. *Child Psychiatry and Human Development, 46*(1), 84–93.

Gottesman, I. I., & Gould, T. D. (2003). The endophenotype concept in psychiatry: Etymology and strategic intentions. *American Journal of Psychiatry, 160*(4), 636–645.

Gregory, A., Caspi, A., Moffitt, T., Koenen, K., Eley, T., & Poulton, R. (2007). Juvenile mental health histories of adults with anxiety disorders. *American Journal of Psychiatry, 164*(2), 301–308.

Halldorsdottir, T., & Ollendick, T. H. (2014). Comorbid ADHD: Implications for the treatment of anxiety disorders in children and adolescents. *Cognitive and Behavioral Practice, 21*(3), 310–322.

Hancock, K. M., Swain, J., Hainsworth, C. J., Dixon, A. L., Koo, S., & Munro, K. (2016). Acceptance and commitment therapy versus cognitive behavior therapy for children with anxiety: Outcomes of a randomized controlled trial. *Journal of Clinical Child and Adolescent Psychology.* [Epub ahead of print]

Harned, M. S., Dimeff, L. A., Woodcock, E. A., Kelly, T., Zavertnik, J., Contreras, I., et al. (2014). Exposing clinicians to exposure: A randomized controlled dissemination trial of exposure therapy for anxiety disorders. *Behavior Therapy, 45*(6), 731–744.

Higa-McMillan, C. K., Francis, S. E., Rith-Najarian, L., & Chorpita, B. F. (2016). Evidence base update: 50 years of research on treatment for child and adolescent anxiety. *Journal of Clinical Child and Adolescent Psychology, 45*(2), 91–113.

Hofmann, S. G., Wu, J. Q., & Boettcher, H. (2014). Effect of cognitive-behavioral therapy for anxiety disorders on quality of life: A meta-analysis. *Journal of Consulting and Clinical Psychology, 82*(3), 375–391.

Hogendoorn, S. M., Prins, P. J., Boer, F., Vervoort, L., Wolters, L. H., Moorlag, H., et al. (2014). Mediators of cognitive behavioral therapy for anxiety-disordered children and adolescents: Cognition, perceived control, and coping. *Journal of Clinical Child and Adolescent Psychology, 43*(3), 486–500.

Hudson, J. L., Dodd, H. F., Lyneham, H. J., & Bovopoulous, N. (2011). Temperament and family environment in the development of anxiety disorder: Two-year follow-up. *Journal of the American Academy of Child and Adolescent Psychiatry, 50*(12), 1255–1264.

Hudson, J. L., Rapee, R. M., Deveney, C., Schniering, C. A., Lyneham, H. J., & Bovopoulos, N. (2009). Cognitive-behavioral treatment versus an active control for children and adolescents with anxiety disorders: A randomized trial. *Journal of the American Academy of Child and Adolescent Psychiatry, 48*(5), 533–544.

Ingles, C. J., La Greca, A. M., Marzo, J. C., Garcia-Lopez, L. J., & Garcia-Fernandez, J. M. (2010). Social Anxiety Scale for Adolescents: Factorial invariance and latent mean differences across gender and age in Spanish adolescents. *Journal of Anxiety Disorders, 24*(8), 847–855.

Ishikawa, S., Okajima, I., Matsuoka, H., & Sakano, Y. (2007). Cognitive behavioural therapy for anxiety disorders in children and adolescents: A meta-analysis. *Child and Adolescent Mental Health, 12*(4), 164–172.

James, A. C., James, G., Cowdrey, F. A., Soler, A., & Choke, A. (2013). Cognitive behavioural therapy for anxiety disorders in children and adolescents. *Cochrane Database of Systematic Reviews, 6,* CD004690.

Kaufman, J., Birmaher, B., Brent, D., Rao, U. M. A., Flynn, C., Moreci, P., et al. (1997). Schedule for Affective Disorders and Schizophrenia for School-Age Children—Present and Lifetime version (K-SADS-PL): Initial reliability and validity data. *Journal of the American Academy of Child and Adolescent Psychiatry, 36*(7), 980–988.

Kazdin, A. E. (2007). Mediators and mechanisms of change in psychotherapy research. *Annual Review of Clinical Psychology, 3,* 1–27.

Keenan, K., & Hipwell, A. E. (2005). Preadolescent clues to understanding depression in girls. *Clinical Child and Family Psychology Review, 8*(2), 89–105.

Keeton, C. P., & Ginsburg, G. S. (2008). Combining and sequencing medication and cognitive-behaviour therapy for childhood anxiety disorders. *International Review of Psychiatry, 20*(2), 159–164.

Kendall, P. C. (1994). Treating anxiety disorders in children: Results of a randomized clinical trial. *Journal of Consulting and Clinical Psychology, 62*(1), 100–110.

Kendall, P. C., & Flannery-Schroeder, E. C. (1998). Methodological issues in treatment research for anxiety disorders in youth. *Journal of Abnormal Child Psychology, 26*(1), 27–38.

Kendall, P. C., Flannery-Schroeder, E., Panichelli-Mindel, S. M., Southam-Gerow, M., Henin, A., & Warman, M. (1997). Therapy for youths with anxiety disorders: A second randomized clinical trial. *Journal of Consulting and Clinical Psychology, 65*(3), 366.

Kendall, P. C., Furr, J. M., & Podell, J. L. (2010). Child-focused treatment of anxiety. In J. R. Weisz & A. E. Kazdin (Eds.), *Evidence-based psychotherapies for children and adolescents* (2nd ed., pp. 45–59). New York: Guilford Press.

Kendall, P. C., & Hedtke, K. (2006). *Cognitive-behavioral therapy for anxious children: Therapist manual* (3rd ed.). Ardmore, PA: Workbook.

Kendall, P. C., Hudson, J. L., Gosch, E., Flannery-Schroeder, E., & Suveg, C. (2008). Cognitive-behavioral therapy for anxiety disordered youth: A randomized clinical trial evaluating child and family modalities. *Journal of Consulting and Clinical Psychology, 76*(2), 282–297.

Kendall, P. C., Puliafico, A. C., Barmish, A. J., Choudhury, M. S., Henin, A., & Treadwell, K. S. (2007). Assessing anxiety with the Child Behavior Checklist and the Teacher Report Form. *Journal of Anxiety Disorders, 21*(8), 1004–1015.

Kendall, P. C., Settipani, C. A., & Cummings, C. M. (2012). No need to worry: The promising future of child anxiety research. *Journal of Clinical Child and Adolescent Psychology, 41*(1), 103–115.

Kendall, P. C., & Treadwell, K. R. (2007). The role of self-statements as a mediator in treatment for youth with anxiety disorders. *Journal of Consulting and Clinical Psychology, 75*(3), 380–389.

Kerns, C. M., Read, K. L., Klugman, J., & Kendall, P. C. (2013). Cognitive behavioral therapy for youth with social anxiety: Differential short and long-term treatment outcomes. *Journal of Anxiety Disorders, 27*(2), 210–215.

Kertz, S. J., & Woodruff-Borden, J. (2011). The developmental psychopathology of worry. *Clinical Child and Family Psychology Review, 14*(2), 174–197.

Kessler, R. C., Petukhova, M., Sampson, N. A., Zaslavsky, A. M., & Wittchen, H. U. (2012). Twelve-month and lifetime prevalence and lifetime morbid risk of anxiety and mood disorders in the United States. *International Journal of Methods in Psychiatric Research, 21*(3), 169–184.

Khanna, M. S., & Kendall, P. C. (2010). Computer-assisted cognitive behavioral therapy for child anxiety: Results of a randomized clinical trial. *Journal of Consulting and Clinical Psychology, 78*(5), 737–745.

Kley, H., Heinrichs, N., Bender, C., & Tuschen-Caffier, B. (2012). Predictors of outcome in a cognitive-behavioral group program for children and adolescents with social anxiety disorder. *Journal of Anxiety Disorders, 26*(1), 79–87.

Kraemer, H. C., Wilson, G. T., Fairburn, C. G., & Agras, W. S. (2002). Mediators and moderators of treatment effects in randomized clinical trials. *Archives of General Psychiatry, 59*(10), 877–883.

La Greca, A. M., & Lopez, N. (1998). Social anxiety among adolescents: Linkages with peer relations and friendships. *Journal of Abnormal Child Psychology, 26*(2), 83–94.

La Greca, A. M., & Stone, W. L. (1993). Social Anxiety Scale for Children—Revised: Factor structure and concurrent validity. *Journal of Clinical Child Psychology, 22*(1), 17–27.

Larson, K., Russ, S. A., Kahn, R. S., & Halfon, N. (2011). Patterns of comorbidity, functioning, and service use for US children with ADHD, 2007. *Pediatrics, 127*(3), 462–470.

Lau, J. Y., Molyneaux, E., Telman, M. D., & Belli, S. (2011). The plasticity of adolescent cognitions: Data from a novel cognitive bias modification training task. *Child Psychiatry and Human Development, 42*(6), 679–693.

Lau, J. Y., Pettit, E., & Creswell, C. (2013). Reducing children's social anxiety symptoms: Exploring a novel parent-administered cognitive bias modification training intervention. *Behaviour Research and Therapy, 51*(7), 333–337.

Leffler, J. M., Riebel, J., & Hughes, H. M. (2015). A review of child and adolescent diagnostic interviews for clinical practitioners. *Assessment, 22*(6), 690–703.

Leyfer, O., Gallo, K. P., Cooper-Vince, C., & Pincus, D. B. (2013). Patterns and predictors of comorbidity of DSM-IV anxiety disorders in a clinical sample of children and adolescents. *Journal of Anxiety Disorders, 27*(3), 306–311.

Loeber, R., Green, S. M., & Lahey, B. B. (1990). Mental health professionals' perception of the utility of children, mothers, and teachers as informants on childhood psychopathology. *Journal of Clinical Child Psychology, 19*(2), 136–143.

Luby, J. L. (2013). Treatment of anxiety and depression in the preschool period. *Journal of the American Academy of Child and Adolescent Psychiatry, 52*(4), 346–358.

Lyneham, H. J., Abbott, M. J., & Rapee, R. M. (2007). Interrater reliability of the Anxiety Disorders Interview Schedule for DSM-IV: Child and Parent version. *Journal of the American Academy of Child and Adolescent Psychiatry, 46*(6), 731–736.

Manassis, K., Fung, D., Tannock, R., Sloman, L., Fiksenbaum, L., & McInnes, A. (2003). Characterizing selective mutism: Is it more than social anxiety? *Depression and Anxiety, 18*(3), 153–161.

Manassis, K., Wilansky-Traynor, P., Farzan, N., Kleiman, V., Parker, K., & Sanford, M. (2010). The feelings club: Randomized controlled evaluation of school-based CBT for anxious or depressive symptoms. *Depression and Anxiety, 27*(10), 945–952.

March, J. S. (2012). *Multidimensional Anxiety Scale for Children, Second Edition (MASC-2)*. North Tonawanda, NY: Multi-Health Systems.

March, J. S., Parker, J. D., Sullivan, K., Stallings, P., & Conners, C. K. (1997). The Multidimensional Anxiety Scale for Children (MASC): Factor structure, reliability, and validity. *Journal of the American Academy of Child and Adolescent Psychiatry, 36*(4), 554–565.

Melfsen, S., Kühnemund, M., Schwieger, J., Warnke, A., Stadler, C., Poustka, F., et al. (2011). Cognitive behavioral therapy of socially phobic children focusing on cognition: A randomised wait-list control study. *Child and Adolescent Psychiatry and Mental Health, 5*(1), 1–12.

Merikangas, K. R., He, J. P., Burstein, M., Swanson, S. A., Avenevoli, S., Cui, L., et al. (2010). Lifetime prevalence of mental disorders in US adolescents: Results from the National Comorbidity Survey Replication–Adolescent Supplement (NCS-A). *Journal of the American Academy of Child and Adolescent Psychiatry, 49*(10), 980–989.

Merikangas, K. R., He, J., Burstein, M., Swendsen, J., Avenevoli, S., Case, B., et al. (2011). Service utilization for lifetime mental disorders in U.S. adolescents: Results of the National

Comorbidity Survey—Adolescent Supplement. *Journal of the American Academy of Child and Adolescent Psychiatry, 50,* 32–45.

Moffitt, T. E., Harrington, H., Caspi, A., Kim-Cohen, J., Goldberg, D., Gregory, A. M., et al. (2007). Depression and generalized anxiety disorder: Cumulative and sequential comorbidity in a birth cohort followed prospectively to age 32 years. *Archives of General Psychiatry, 64*(6), 651–660.

Mohatt, J., Bennett, S. M., & Walkup, J. T. (2014). Treatment of separation, generalized, and social anxiety disorders in youths. *American Journal of Psychiatry, 171,* 741–748.

Muris, P., Meesters, C., & Gobel, M. (2001). Reliability, validity, and normative data of the Penn State Worry Questionnaire in 8–12-yr-old children. *Journal of Behavior Therapy and Experimental Psychiatry, 32*(2), 63–72.

Muris, P., Merckelbach, H., Mayer, B., & Prins, E. (2000). How serious are common childhood fears? *Behaviour Research and Therapy, 38*(3), 217–228.

Muris, P., van Brakel, A. M., Arntz, A., & Schouten, E. (2011). Behavioral inhibition as a risk factor for the development of childhood anxiety disorders: A longitudinal study. *Journal of Child and Family Studies, 20*(2), 157–170.

Nauta, M. H., Scholing, A., Emmelkamp, P. M. G., & Minderaa, R. B. (2003). Cognitive-behavioral therapy for children with anxiety disorders in a clinical setting: No additional effect of a cognitive parent training. *Journal of the American Academy of Child and Adolescent Psychiatry, 42*(11), 1270–1278.

Nilsen, T. S., Eisemann, M., & Kvernmo, S. (2013). Predictors and moderators of outcome in child and adolescent anxiety and depression: A systematic review of psychological treatment studies. *European Child and Adolescent Psychiatry, 22*(2), 69–87.

Nolte, T., Guiney, J., Fonagy, P., Mayes, L. C., & Luyten, P. (2011). Interpersonal stress regulation and the development of anxiety disorders: An attachment-based developmental framework. *Frontiers in Behavioral Neuroscience, 5,* 55.

Ollendick, T. H., Jarrett, M. A., Grills-Taquechel, A. E., Hovey, L. D., & Wolff, J. C. (2008). Comorbidity as a predictor and moderator of treatment outcome in youth with anxiety, affective, attention deficit/hyperactivity disorder, and oppositional/conduct disorders. *Clinical Psychology Review, 28*(8), 1447–1471.

Pahl, K. M., Barrett, P. M., & Gullo, M. J. (2012). Examining potential risk factors for anxiety in early childhood. *Journal of Anxiety Disorders, 26*(2), 311–320.

Perez-Edgar, K., Bar-Haim, Y., McDermott, J. M., Gorodetsky, E., Hodgkinson, C. A., Goldman, D., et al. (2010). Variations in the serotonin-transporter gene are associated with attention bias patterns to positive and negative emotion faces. *Biological Psychology, 83*(3), 269–271.

Pestle, S. L., Chorpita, B. F., & Schiffman, J. (2008). Psychometric properties of the Penn State Worry Questionnaire for children in a large clinical sample. *Journal of Clinical Child and Adolescent Psychology, 37*(2), 465–471.

Piacentini, J., Bennett, S., Compton, S. N., Kendall, P. C., Birmaher, B., Albano, A. M., et al. (2014). 24- and 36-week outcomes for the Child/Adolescent Anxiety Multimodal Study (CAMS). *Journal of the American Academy of Child and Adolescent Psychiatry, 53*(3), 297–310.

Pine, D. S. (2007). Research review: A neuroscience framework for pediatric anxiety disorders. *Journal of Child Psychology and Psychiatry, 48*(7), 631–648.

Pine, D. S., Cohen, P., Gurley, D., Brook, J., & Ma, Y. (1998). The risk for early-adulthood anxiety and depressive disorders in adolescents with anxiety and depressive disorders. *Archives of General Psychiatry, 55*(1), 56–64.

Rapee, R. M. (2000). Group treatment of children with anxiety disorders: Outcome and predictors of treatment response. *Australian Journal of Psychology, 52*(3), 125–129.

Rapee, R. M. (2014). Preschool environment and temperament as predictors of social and nonsocial anxiety disorders in middle adolescence. *Journal of the American Academy of Child and Adolescent Psychiatry, 53*(3), 320–328.

Rapee, R. M., Lyneham, H. J., Hudson, J. L., Kangas, M., Wuthrich, V. M., & Schniering, C. A. (2013). Effect of comorbidity on treatment of anxious children and adolescents: Results from a large, combined sample. *Journal of the American Academy of Child and Adolescent Psychiatry, 52*(1), 47–56.

Rapp, A., Dodds, A., Walkup, J. T., & Rynn, M. (2013). Treatment of pediatric anxiety disorders. *Annals of the New York Academy of Sciences, 1304,* 52–61.

Read, K. L., Comer, J. S., & Kendall, P. C. (2013). The Intolerance of Uncertainty Scale for Children (IUSC): Discriminating principal anxiety diagnoses and severity. *Psychological Assessment, 25*(3), 722–729.

Research Units on Pediatric Psychopharmacology (RUPP) Anxiety Study Group. (2002). The Pediatric Anxiety Rating Scale (PARS): Development and psychometric properties. *Journal of the American Academy of Child and Adolescent Psychiatry, 41*(9), 1061–1069.

Reynolds, C. R., & Kamphaus, R. W. (2002). *The clinician's guide to the Behavior Assessment System for Children (BASC).* New York: Guilford Press.

Reynolds, C. R., & Kamphaus, R. W. (2015). *Behavior Assessment System for Children, Third Edition (BASC-3).* New York: Pearson Assessments.

Reynolds, C. R., & Richmond, B. O. (2008). *Revised Children's Manifest Anxiety Scale, Second Edition (RCMAS-2).* New York: Pearson.

Roberson-Nay, R., Klein, D. F., Klein, R. G., Mannuzza, S., Moulton, J. L., III, Guardino, M., et al. (2010). Carbon dioxide hypersensitivity in separation-anxious offspring of parents with panic disorder. *Biological Psychiatry, 67*(12), 1171–1177.

Rooksby, M., Elouafkaoui, P., Humphris, G., Clarkson, J., & Freeman, R. (2015). Internet-assisted delivery of cognitive behavioural therapy (CBT) for childhood anxiety: Systematic review and meta-analysis. *Journal of Anxiety Disorders, 29,* 83–92.

Rozenman, M., Amir, N., & Weersing, V. R. (2014). Performance-based interpretation bias in clinically anxious youths: Relationships with attention, anxiety, and negative cognition. *Behavior Therapy, 45*(5), 606–618.

Schneider, S., Blatter-Meunier, J., Herren, C., Adornetto, C., In-Albon, T., & Lavallee, K. (2011). Disorder-specific cognitive-behavioral therapy for separation anxiety disorder in young children: A randomized waiting-list-controlled trial. *Psychotherapy and Psychosomatics, 80*(4), 206–215.

Segool, N. K., & Carlson, J. S. (2008). Efficacy of cognitive-behavioral and pharmacological treatments for children with social anxiety. *Depression and Anxiety, 25*(7), 620–631.

Seidel, L., & Walkup, J. T. (2006). Selective serotonin reuptake inhibitor use in the treatment of the pediatric non-obsessive–compulsive disorder anxiety disorders. *Journal of Child and Adolescent Psychopharmacology, 16*(1–2), 171–179.

Shechner, T., Rimon-Chakir, A., Britton, J. C., Lotan, D., Apter, A., Bliese, P. D., et al. (2014). Attention bias modification treatment augmenting effects on cognitive behavioral therapy in children with anxiety: Randomized controlled trial. *Journal of the American Academy of Child and Adolescent Psychiatry, 53*(1), 61–71.

Silverman, W. K., & Albano, A. M. (1996). *The Anxiety Disorders Interview Schedule for DSM-IV, Child version: Clinician manual.* New York: Oxford University Press.

Silverman, W. K., & Ollendick, T. H. (2005). Evidence-based assessment of anxiety and its disorders in children and adolescents. *Journal of Clinical Child and Adolescent Psychology, 34*(3), 380–411.

Silverman, W. K., & Ollendick, T. H. (2008). *Child and adolescent anxiety disorders: A guide to assessments that work.* New York: Oxford University Press.

Silverman, W. K., Pina, A. A., & Viswesvaran, C. (2008). Evidence-based psychosocial treatments for phobic and anxiety disorders in children and adolescents. *Journal of Clinical Child and Adolescent Psychology, 37*(1), 105–130.

Silverman, W. K., Saavedra, L. M., & Pina, A. A. (2001). Test–retest reliability of anxiety symptoms and diagnoses with the Anxiety Disorders Interview Schedule for DSM-IV: Child and Parent versions. *Journal of the American Academy of Child and Adolescent Psychiatry, 40*(8), 937–944.

Southam-Gerow, M. A., Kendall, P. C., & Weersing, V. R. (2001). Examining outcome variability: Correlates of treatment response in a child and adolescent anxiety clinic. *Journal of Clinical Child Psychology, 30*(3), 422–436.

Sportel, B. E., de Hullu, E., de Jong, P. J., & Nauta, M. H. (2013). Cognitive bias modification versus CBT in reducing adolescent social anxiety: A randomized controlled trial. *PLoS ONE, 8*(5), e64355.

Stanton, H. E. (1994). Self-hypnosis: One path to reduced test anxiety. *Contemporary Hypnosis, 11*, 14–18.

Storch, E. A., Abramowitz, J., & Goodman, W. K. (2008). Where does obsessive–compulsive disorder belong in DSM-V? *Depression and Anxiety, 25*(4), 336–347.

Thomas, A., & Chess, S. (1977). *Temperament and development.* Oxford, UK: Brunner/Mazel.

Tulbure, B. T., Szentagotai, A., Dobrean, A., & David, D. (2012). Evidence based clinical assessment of child and adolescent social phobia: A critical review of rating scales. *Child Psychiatry and Human Development, 43*(5), 795–820.

Van Ameringen, M., Mancini, C., & Farvolden, P. (2003). The impact of anxiety disorders on educational achievement. *Journal of Anxiety Disorders, 17*(5), 561–571.

Vassilopoulos, S. P., Banerjee, R., & Prantzalou, C. (2009). Experimental modification of interpretation bias in socially anxious children: Changes in interpretation, anticipated interpersonal anxiety, and social anxiety symptoms. *Behaviour Research and Therapy, 47*(12), 1085–1089.

Vassilopoulos, S. P., Blackwell, S. E., Misailidi, P., Kyritsi, A., & Ayfanti, M. (2014). The differential effects of written and spoken presentation for the modification of interpretation and judgmental bias in children. *Behavioral and Cognitive Psychotherapy, 42*, 535–554.

Verduin, T. L., & Kendall, P. C. (2003). Differential occurrence of comorbidity within childhood anxiety disorders. *Journal of Clinical Child and Adolescent Psychology, 32*(2), 290–295.

Villabø, M., Gere, M., Torgersen, S., March, J. S., & Kendall, P. C. (2012). Diagnostic efficiency of the child and parent versions of the Multidimensional Anxiety Scale for Children. *Journal of Clinical Child and Adolescent Psychology, 41*(1), 75–85.

Walkup, J. T., Albano, A. M., Piacentini, J., Birmaher, B., Compton, S. N., Sherrill, J. T., et al. (2008). Cognitive behavioral therapy, sertraline, or a combination in childhood anxiety. *New England Journal of Medicine, 359*(26), 2753–2766.

Warren, S. L., Huston, L., Egeland, B., & Sroufe, L. (1997). Child and adolescent anxiety disorders and early attachment. *Journal of the American Academy of Child and Adolescent Psychiatry, 36*(5), 637–644.

Waters, A. M., Ford, L. A., Wharton, T. A., & Cobham, V. E. (2009). Cognitive-behavioural therapy for young children with anxiety disorders: Comparison of a child + parent condition versus a parent only condition. *Behaviour Research and Therapy, 47*(8), 654–662.

Waters, A. M., Pittaway, M., Mogg, K., Bradley, B. P., & Pine, D. S. (2013). Attention training towards positive stimuli in clinically anxious children. *Developmental and Cognitive Neuroscience, 4*, 77–84.

Weersing, V. R., Gonzalez, A., Campo, J. V., & Lucas, A. N. (2008). Brief behavioral therapy for pediatric anxiety and depression: Piloting an integrated treatment approach. *Cognitive and Behavioral Practice, 15*(2), 126–139.

Weersing, V. R., & Weisz, J. R. (2002). Mechanisms of action in youth psychotherapy. *Journal of Child Psychology and Psychiatry, 43*(1), 3–29.

White, S. W., Ollendick, T., Albano, A. M., Oswald, D., Johnson, C., Southam-Gerow, M. A., et al. (2013). Randomized controlled trial: Multimodal anxiety and social skill intervention for adolescents with autism spectrum disorder. *Journal of Autism and Developmental Disorders, 43*(2), 382–394.

Whitmore, M. J., Kim-Spoon, J., & Ollendick, T. H. (2014). Generalized anxiety disorder and social anxiety disorder in youth: Are they distinguishable? *Child Psychiatry and Human Development, 45*(4), 456–463.

Wood, J. J., Drahota, A., Sze, K., Har, K., Chiu, A., & Langer, D. A. (2009). Cognitive behavioral therapy for anxiety in children with autism spectrum disorders: A randomized, controlled trial. *Journal of Child Psychology and Psychiatry, 50*(3), 224–234.

Wood, J. J., McLeod, B. D., Piacentini, J. C., & Sigman, M. (2009). One-year follow-up of family versus child CBT for anxiety disorders: Exploring the roles of child age and parental intrusiveness. *Child Psychiatry and Human Development, 40*(2), 301–316.

Wittchen, H. U., Nocon, A., Beesdo, K., Pine, D. S., Höfler, M., Lieb, R., et al. (2008). Agoraphobia and panic. *Psychotherapy and Psychosomatics, 77*(3), 147–157.

Yeganeh, R., Beidel, D. C., Turner, S. M., Pina, A. A., & Silverman, W. K. (2003). Clinical distinctions between selective mutism and social phobia: An investigation of childhood psychopathology. *Journal of the American Academy of Child and Adolescent Psychiatry, 42*(9), 1069–1075.

Zahn-Waxler, C., Shirtcliff, E. A., & Marceau, K. (2008). Disorders of childhood and adolescence: Gender and psychopathology. *Annual Review of Clinical Psychology, 4*, 275–303.

CHAPTER 7

Specific Phobias

Ella L. Oar, Lara J. Farrell, Simon P. Byrne,
and Thomas H. Ollendick

THE DSM-5 DEFINITION OF SPECIFIC PHOBIAS

Although it is common for children to have a variety of fears during their development, a significant proportion of them experience more intense, frequent, and intransigent fears that meet diagnostic criteria for a specific phobia. In specific phobias, which are characterized by a persistent fear of an object or situation, the level of fear is disproportionate to the level of danger associated with the feared stimulus (American Psychiatric Association, 2013). In order to be considered clinically significant, the fear must cause not only distress but also cause interference in the child's life. Furthermore, while subclinical fears may be transient and not require treatment, diagnosable phobias must be present for at least 6 months and frequently require treatment (American Psychiatric Association, 2013).

In order to meet diagnostic criteria of specific phobia, the fear stimulus must almost always provoke an anxiety response. In children, this anxiety may be characterized by a fight-or-flight response: it can also be expressed by crying, tantrums, freezing, or clinging (American Psychiatric Association, 2013). Furthermore, while adults typically have insight that their fears are unrealistic, children often have less awareness (Ollendick & Muris, 2015).

The fifth edition of the *Diagnostic and Statistical Manual of Mental Disorders* (DSM-5; American Psychiatric Association, 2013) classifies phobias into common subtypes: fear of animals (e.g., dogs or spiders), fear of environmental stimuli (e.g., heights or the dark), fear of blood–injection–injury (BII; e.g., needles or injections), situational fears (e.g., enclosed spaces) and other fears (e.g., loud noises or costumed characters). Due to their more focused nature and often favorable treatment response, phobias have often been regarded as a less serious mental disorder, once being referred to as "simple" phobias. However, current research suggests that childhood phobias are not only prevalent but also may be highly complex and disruptive to a child and family's life.

PREVALENCE AND COURSE

Specific phobias are the most common of the anxiety disorders experienced by children and adolescents (Essau, Conradt, & Petermann, 2000). At any one time they are estimated to affect 5–10% of young people in the community and up to 15% in mental health settings (Bener, Ghuloum, & Dafeeah, 2011; Kessler, Chiu, Demler, & Walters, 2005; Ollendick, Hagopian, & King, 1997). The lifetime prevalence rate is approximately 12.5% (Kessler, Berglund, et al., 2005). The most common types of phobias among children are animal fears and environmental fears (Last, Perrin, Hersen, & Kazdin, 1992; Milne et al., 1995; Stinson et al., 2007).

Phobias typically start young, with a median age of onset of approximately 7–9 years (Kessler, Chiu, et al., 2005; Stinson et al., 2007), then decrease in prevalence from the age of 10 on (Muris, Merckelbach, Gadet, & Moulaert, 2000). Different phobia presentations throughout development reflect increasing levels of cognitive ability: During infancy, fears are typically more concrete in nature (e.g., animals or strangers), becoming more abstract during childhood (e.g., ghosts) and adolescence (e.g., agoraphobia or social fears; Ollendick, Davis, & Muris, 2004). Animal phobias tend to occur around age 7, BII phobias around age 9, situational phobias around age 13, and claustrophobia around 20 years of age (Öst, 1987). Although some childhood phobias spontaneously remit without the need for intervention, most children continue to exhibit symptoms into adolescence and adulthood unless treated (Ollendick, Davis, et al., 2004).

Specific phobias may be associated with significant interference and disruption in the life of a child and his or her family. Phobias have the potential to disrupt a young person academically (Dweck & Wortman, 1982; Ialongo, Edelsohn, Werthamer-Larsson, Crockett, & Kellam, 1995), cause social and personal distress (Ollendick & King, 1994; Ollendick, King, & Muris, 2002), and affect daily functioning (Essau et al., 2000). Because phobias often occur during a critical period in development, the effects of the disruption can be far-reaching. For example, a child who is fearful of dogs may be unable to play outdoors or visit dog-owning friends, potentially affecting his or her physical and social development as he or she enters adolescence (Ollendick, King, & Muris, 2004). Furthermore, it has also been suggested that untreated childhood phobias may lead to the development of other psychiatric disorders in adulthood, including the development of anxiety disorders, mood disturbance, and substance use (Kendall, Safford, Flannery-Schroeder, & Webb, 2004).

COMMON COMORBID CONDITIONS

A further reason for considering the seriousness of specific phobias in childhood is that they often present with comorbid psychiatric disorders. Indeed, comorbidity appears to be the rule, rather than the exception with 25–72% of phobic youth across community and clinical studies meeting criteria for at least one other disorder (Costello,

Egger, & Angold, 2004; Last et al., 1992; Ollendick, King, & Muris, 2002; Ollendick, Öst, Reuterskiöld, & Costa, 2010). Most commonly, phobias are comorbid with another anxiety disorder, especially other phobias, with 50% of phobic youth meeting criteria for another specific phobia (Costello et al., 2004). Comorbidity with mood disorders and externalizing disorders in children has also been observed (Last et al., 1992).

ETIOLOGICAL/CONCEPTUAL MODELS OF SPECIFIC PHOBIAS

The etiology of specific phobias is not fully understood; however, a multifactorial model provides the best account (Merckelbach, de Jong, Muris, & van Den Hout, 1996). A variety of factors, including genetics, evolutionary preparedness, learning, and parenting styles, are implicated in the etiology of a specific phobia. In addition, information-processing biases and parental accommodation are believed to be implicated in the maintenance of a phobia.

There appears to be a modest, yet significant genetic contribution toward the development of specific phobias (Distel et al., 2008). There is also research to suggest that phobias are highly familial; that is, children more often exhibit the same type of phobia as their parents (LeBeau et al., 2010). For example, Fyer, Mannuzza, Chapman, Martin, and Klein (1995) found that first-degree relatives of individuals with a specific phobic disorder were two- to fourfold more likely to develop the same type of phobia. Moreover, a biological predisposition is consistent with phobias typically focusing on objects or situations that appear to be adaptive (Menzies & Clarke, 1995). For example, childhood phobias typically focus on stimuli that are advantageous to avoid for survival, such as spiders, the dark, and heights. The evolutionary preparedness model of phobic stimuli is also consistent with children reporting they are unable to recall a direct or indirect encounter with the stimulus that triggered such fears (Poulton & Menzies, 2002).

The role of learning in the development of phobias has been extensively researched. Rachman (1977) proposed that the acquisition of a phobia may occur through three different learning pathways: direct conditioning with the feared stimulus, vicarious conditioning through a model, or by transmission of negative information. A traumatic "conditioning" experience has frequently been used to explain the development of a phobia: A neutral stimulus comes to be associated with an aversive outcome (an unconditioned stimulus), such that the neutral stimulus takes on its aversive properties (becoming a conditioned stimulus). For example, a child who is bitten by a dog may go on to develop dog phobia. While this account is intuitive and grounded in learning theory, it has a number of shortcomings, including the fact phobias can occur without an obvious conditioning episode, and furthermore, that conditioning does not always result in a phobia (Davey, 1992; Menzies & Clarke, 1995). Hence, other research suggests phobias may be acquired without direct contact with the feared stimulus, either through modeling from other people or through information from the environment (see Askew & Field, 2008). For example, a dog phobia may be transmitted to a child either through watching a parent react fearfully to a dog or by hearing about a dog attack through popular media.

More recent research suggests parenting factors may also increase vulnerability to the development of a phobia, as well as help to maintain the phobia. For example, anxious children are more likely to experience an overprotective or intrusive style of parenting (Barrett, Rapee, Dadds, & Ryan, 1996; Rapee, Schniering, & Hudson, 2009). Overprotective parents are more likely to intervene to prevent their child from experiencing perceived harm, to accommodate avoidance of the feared stimulus, and to model fearful behavior toward the feared stimulus (Milliner, Farrell, & Ollendick, 2013). This parenting style communicates the potential threat associated with the stimulus to the child, while preventing the child from experiencing disconfirming evidence through contact with the stimulus.

In addition to these etiological factors, avoidance and information-processing biases are believed to be implicated in the maintenance of a phobia. Early on, Mowrer (1960) proposed that behavioral avoidance of the feared stimulus maintains a phobia through operant conditioning; that is, avoidance is negatively reinforced by reducing anxiety triggered by the presence of the stimulus and thereby preventing the individual from learning it is nonharmful. More recent research from adults suggests that individuals experiencing phobias have biases toward interpreting and attending to threats related to their feared stimulus. Hyperattention toward threat-related cues may be advantageous in certain circumstances; however, this preferential encoding can also lead to a maladaptive preservation of the fear response (see Bar-Haim, Lamy, Pergamin, Bakermans-Kranenburg, & van IJzendoorn, 2007, for a review). For example, participants with spider phobia took longer to process the color of words related to their fear (e.g., "web") than neutral words (e.g., "car"), suggesting that they have automatic attention toward threat-relevant stimuli (Watts, McKenna, Sharrock, & Trezise, 1986). Individuals with phobias also often have inflated perceptions of harm or risk associated with their feared stimulus, which maintains their fear (Merckelbach et al., 1996). For example, individuals with dog and spider phobias are reported to have unrealistic expectations of harm from their feared stimulus (Arntz, Lavy, Van den Berg, & Van Rijsoort, 1993; Di Nardo et al., 1988).

Although less is known about the role of cognition in children with specific phobias, Byrne, Rapee, Malhi, Sweller, and Hudson (2014) recently examined how harm beliefs in 27 children with dog phobia predict avoidance and distress before and after exposure therapy. Children were shown a live dog and asked to rate the extent to which they believed the dog would harm them (e.g., the dog would bite or attack). Harm beliefs predicted distress during a pretreatment behavioral approach task (BAT) and avoidance during a posttreatment BAT. These results are consistent with theory in adults, suggesting that harm beliefs have a maintaining role in a child's phobic response as well.

EVIDENCE-BASED TREATMENTS FOR SPECIFIC PHOBIAS IN CHILDREN

Cognitive-behavioral treatments that incorporate techniques such as *in vivo* exposure, cognitive restructuring, participant modeling, contingency management, and psychoeducation and skills training have the strongest evidence base for phobic youth (Davis, Jenkins, & Rudy, 2012; Davis & Ollendick, 2005). To date, empirical support for cognitive-behavioral therapy (CBT) has been demonstrated in 11 studies, including four large, randomized controlled trials (RCTs) (Ollendick et al., 2015; Ollendick, Öst, et al., 2009; Öst, Svensson, Hellstrom, & Lindwall, 2001; Silverman et al., 1999) and seven smaller clinical trials (Flatt & King, 2010; Leutgeb, Schäfer, Köchel, & Schienle, 2012; Leutgeb & Schienle, 2012; Muris, Merckelbach, Holdrinet, & Sijsenaar, 1998; Muris, Merckelbach, Van

Haaften, & Mayer, 1997; Oar, Farrell, Waters, Conlon, & Ollendick, 2015; Waters et al., 2014; see Table 7.1 for a summary of these studies). The majority of these studies have evaluated the effectiveness of an intensive CBT approach, known as one-session treatment (OST; Öst et al., 2001) with only one of the large RCTs examining a standard weekly format (Silverman et al., 1999).

The first large RCT for phobic youth, conducted by Silverman and colleagues (1999), examined the efficacy of an exposure-based cognitive self-control (SC) and exposure-based contingency management (CM) treatment relative to an education support (ES) condition. Children and adolescents ($N = 81$; ages 6–16 years) with a diverse range of specific phobias participated in the study. Treatments involved 10 sessions, each 80 minutes in duration, with parents and children seen separately at the beginning of sessions, then together at the end of each session. Findings were mixed. The SC condition (88%) was found to have the greatest proportion of youth who no longer meet criteria for a phobia diagnosis. Moreover, children in the SC (80%) and CM (80%) conditions reported either little or no fear on ratings of subjective distress toward their phobic stimuli in comparison to the ES (25%) condition. However, no differences were observed between the conditions on self-report measures. Thus, Silverman and colleagues (1999) found considerable support for exposure-based procedures, particularly SC for phobic youth.

Following this, Öst and colleagues (2001) conducted the first RCT of an intensive single CBT session (e.g., OST) for phobic youth. Sixty children and adolescents (ages 7–17 years) from Sweden, with various specific phobias, participated in the study. Youth were randomly assigned to either OST alone, OST with a parent present (i.e., parents observed their child's session and at times acted as a model for their child), or to a wait-list control condition. Youth in the OST conditions had significantly improved outcomes on measures of subjective distress, behavioral avoidance, and ratings of phobia severity at posttreatment, in comparison to those in the wait-list control condition (Öst et al., 2001). Moreover, treatment gains were maintained at 1-year follow-up. The authors had hypothesized that the presence of the parents during treatment would facilitate change. Unexpectedly, differences were not observed between the two OST conditions. While speculative, this finding may be due to the fact that most of the parents were not actively involved in the treatment process; rather, for most of the session, they were passive observers.

In a subsequent trial, the largest trial for phobic youth to date, Ollendick, Öst, and colleagues (2009) randomly assigned 196 children and adolescents to OST alone, an education support treatment (EST; a non-exposure-based treatment), or a wait-list control. Children were recruited from two sites across Sweden and the United States. OST and EST were found to be superior to the wait-list control. Moreover, OST was superior to EST on clinician ratings of phobia severity, percentage of participants diagnosis free (55% OST vs. 23% EST) at posttreatment, child ratings of anxiety during the behavioral avoidance test, and treatment satisfaction (Ollendick, Öst, et al., 2009). Treatment gains were maintained at 6-month follow-up.

Developments in Psychosocial Treatments

Although CBT is effective for most children and adolescents with phobias (25–90% diagnosis free), there still remains a significant proportion of youth who only partially

TABLE 7.1. Summary of Psychosocial Phobia Treatment Studies in Children and Adolescents

Study	Sample	Conditions	Treatment outcome (primary assessment measures)
		Intensive CBT—OST	
Muris et al. (1997)	N = 22	OST	OST > EMDR
	Spider phobias (9–14 years)	EMDR	(Subjective anxiety and behavioral avoidance)
Muris et al. (1998)	N = 26	OST	OST > EMDR > Computer exposure
	Spider phobias (8–17 years)	EMDR Computer Exposure	(Subjective anxiety, spider fear, and behavioral avoidance)
Öst et al. (2001)	N = 60	OST child alone	OST child alone = OST parent present > WL
	Diverse range phobia (7–17 years)	OST parent present WL	(Clinician-rated phobia severity, subjective anxiety, and behavioral avoidance)
Ollendick, Öst, et al. (2009)	N = 196 Diverse range phobia (7–16 years)	OST EST WL	OST > EST > WL (Clinician-rated phobia severity, % of participants diagnosis free, subjective anxiety, and treatment satisfaction)
Flatt & King (2010)	N = 43 Diverse range phobia (7–17 years)	OST Psychoeducation WL	OST = psychoeducation > WL (Behavioral avoidance and self-efficacy ratings)
Leutgeb et al. (2012)	N = 32	OST	OST > WL
	Spider phobias (8–13 years)	WL	(Behavioral avoidance, subjective fear and disgust, and physiological measures)
Leutgeb & Schienle (2012)	N = 30	OST	OST > WL
	Spider phobias (8–14 years)	WL	(Behavioral avoidance, subjective fear and disgust, and physiological measures)
Waters et al. (2014)	N = 37	OST + ATP	OST + ATP = OST + ATC
	Diverse range phobia (6–17 years)	OST + ATC	(Clinician-rated phobia severity and global functioning)
			OST+ ATP > OST + ATC on phobic beliefs
Ollendick et al. (2015)	N = 97	OST	OST = PA-OST
	Diverse range phobia (6–15 years)	PA-OST	(Clinician-rated phobia severity and % of participants diagnosis free) *(continued)*

TABLE 7.1. (*continued*)

Oar, Farrell, Waters, et al. (2015)	N = 24 Blood–injection–injury phobia (7–17 years)	1-week baseline 2-week baseline 3-week baseline	BII symptoms and phobia severity remained relatively stable during the baseline periods, then significantly improved following OST
		Nonintensive CBT	
Silverman et al. (1999)	N = 81 Diverse range phobia (7–16 years)	CM SC ES	SC > CM = ES; SC = CM > ES % of participants diagnosis free, subjective anxiety
Vigerland et al. (2013)	N = 30 Diverse range phobia (8–12 years)	6 session Internet-delivered CBT	Significant reductions in phobia severity posttreatment

Note. ATC, attention training control; ATP, attention training toward positive stimuli; CM, contingency management; EMDR, eye movement desensitization and reprocessing; ES, education support; EST, education support treatment; OST, one-session treatment; PA, parent augmented; PBO, placebo; SC, cognitive self-control; WL, wait-list control condition.

respond or do not respond at all to this treatment (Ollendick et al., 2015; Ollendick, Öst, et al., 2009; Öst et al., 2001; Silverman et al., 1999). Novel approaches to augmenting CBT offer great promise in terms of further improving outcomes for these youth. Ollendick and colleagues (2015) recently conducted a study evaluating the relative efficacy of parent-augmented OST relative to child-alone OST in a sample of 97 phobic youth (ages 6–15 years). Parent-augmented OST involved parent components targeting psychoeducation (e.g., contingency management and developing and conducting exposure tasks), observation of their child during treatment, guidance setting up exposure tasks for their child at home, and once weekly telephone calls for 4 weeks to encourage ongoing exposure practice at home. Surprisingly, parent involvement did not enhance OST treatment outcome, with no significant differences observed between the groups at posttreatment or 6-month follow-up. Following treatment, approximately 50% of youth in both groups were diagnosis free. The authors speculated that the findings may have been due to two reasons: (1) After seeing the significant progress their child made in the OST, parents developed unrealistically high expectations regarding their child's progress with child–parent guided exposure following treatment and may have become more frustrated and less tolerant of children avoidance behavior; and (2) many of the parents in the study may not have benefited from the augmented OST, as many did not present with risk factors (e.g., high anxiety and overprotective parenting style) that the enhanced treatment was targeting (Ollendick et al., 2015).

In an innovative study, Waters and colleagues (2014) examined the augmenting effects of attention training toward positive stimuli in combination with OST. Attention training is purported to work through the modification of attentional biases toward threat stimuli, which are believed to be involved in the development and maintenance of anxiety disorders (Cowart & Ollendick, 2011; Waters et al., 2014). Thirty-seven children and adolescents (ages 6–17 years), with a diverse range of specific phobias, participated in the study. Youth were randomly assigned to either attention training to positive stimuli (ATP+OST) prior to their OST or control attention training before OST (ATC+OST). Children in the ATP+OST condition were found to have significantly greater reductions in phobic belief ratings during their OST and at 3-month follow-up. Moreover, at post-treatment, youth in the ATP+OST condition had an improved attention bias toward positive stimuli, which predicted a greater reduction in the diagnostic severity of their phobia at 3-month follow-up. Surprisingly, however, no differences were observed between the conditions on clinician-, parent-, or child-rated outcomes of phobia diagnostic severity, symptom reduction, or global functioning at posttreatment or follow-up. While encouraging, Waters and colleagues suggested that a larger sample size and a stronger dose of attention training, matched specifically to the children's phobia type, may be necessary to achieve improved clinical outcomes.

Recently, advances have also been made in relation to the treatment of particular phobia subtypes in youth. To date in the child and adolescent literature, BII phobia subtype has been largely neglected. Across the existing trials Öst and colleagues (2001) included the greatest number of youth with BII phobia subtype ($n = 14$). These youth were found to respond significantly less favorably to treatment on a postassessment BAT. Subsequently, Ollendick, Öst, and colleagues (2009) and Ollendick and colleagues (2015) excluded children and adolescents with BII from their large RCTs for a number of reasons, including their poorer treatment response, unique physiological response (e.g., fainting) and barriers to delivery of the OST (e.g., the need for health professionals). In a recent multiple-baseline controlled trial, Oar, Farrell, Waters, and colleagues (2015) examined the effectiveness of an adapted OST for pediatric BII phobia. Twenty-four children were randomly assigned to a 1-, 2-, or 3-week monitoring period of their BII symptoms; following this they completed an education session, an intensive exposure session maximized to 3 hours (e.g., OST) and a 4-week e-therapy maintenance program (Oar, Farrell, & Ollendick, 2015). During the baseline periods, BII symptoms remained relatively stable; however, they improved significantly following the OST. At 1-month follow-up, 58% of youth were diagnosis free, and this increased to 62% by 3-month follow-up.

The development of Internet-based psychological therapies may also lead to inexpensive, accessible, and effective treatment of specific phobias in children. In a recent open trial, Vigerland and colleagues (2013) evaluated the effectiveness of a 6-week Internet-delivered CBT treatment program. Thirty children (ages 8–12 years) with primary diagnosis of specific phobia participated in the study. The treatment consisted of both parent and child modules that included education relating to specific phobia, exposure hierarchies, and reward systems. At posttreatment, significant reductions were observed in children's symptom severity, with large effect sizes and 35% of the sample no longer meeting criteria for a phobia after treatment. Treatment gains were maintained at 3-month follow-up.

Current Status of Psychosocial Treatments

The aforementioned studies provide strong empirical support for OST for the treatment of youth with phobias. In summary, OST has been found to be superior to a wait-list control (Flatt & King, 2010; Ollendick, Öst, et al., 2009; Öst et al., 2001), psychological placebo (Ollendick, Öst, et al., 2009) and other psychological therapies (Muris et al., 1997, 1998). OST's efficacy has been demonstrated by multiple research groups, with children who have a diverse range of specific phobias, from around the world (e.g., Sweden, United States, Netherlands, Austria, and Australia). According to criteria for evidence-based treatments developed by Chambless and colleagues (1998) and Chambless and Ollendick (2001), OST meets criteria for designation as a *well-established* treatment for children and adolescents with specific phobia (Davis, Jenkins, et al., 2012; Davis, May, & Whiting, 2011; Davis & Ollendick, 2005; Ollendick & Davis, 2013).

The relative efficacy of parent-augmented OST has now been evaluated in two large RCTs (Ollendick et al., 2015; Öst et al., 2001) across two countries and independent research groups. Both studies found that parent-augmented OST produced comparable effects to child-alone OST, which is an already *well-established* treatment. Hence, according to the criteria of Chambless and colleagues (1998) and Chambless and Ollendick (2001), parent-augmented OST should similarly be considered a *well-established* treatment for youth with phobias.

As previously discussed, only one large RCT (Silverman et al., 1999) has examined less intensive CBT approaches (ten 80-minute sessions) for youth with specific phobia. This trial compared two variations of exposure-based treatments to an education support condition. In line with Chambless and colleagues (1998) and Chambless and Ollendick (2001), weekly spaced CBT for phobic youth should be considered *probably efficacious*.

Children and adolescents with specific phobias have also been included in trials with other anxious youth (generalized anxiety disorder, social anxiety disorder, and separation anxiety disorder) evaluating the effectiveness of broad-based CBT approaches (Davis et al., 2011). These treatments similarly tend to involve less intensive exposure programs and are delivered in a standard weekly format over a period of time (e.g., 10–16 sessions), as is typical in most outpatient settings (Spence, Holmes, March, & Lipp, 2006). A complete review of broad-based approaches for child anxiety is beyond the scope of this chapter. Davis and colleagues (2011) noted that while broad-based treatments are useful in order to increase power, generalizability, and external validity, the relative efficacy of these treatment approaches for specific disorders, such as specific phobias, remains unclear.

Finally, OST augmented with attention training toward positive stimuli, Internet-delivered CBT, and adapted OST for BII have been examined in only one study each (Oar, Farrell, Waters, et al., 2015; Vigerland et al., 2013; Waters et al., 2014) with promising results, and should be considered *experimental treatments* in terms of efficacy for youth with phobias.

Pharmacological Treatments

There is limited evidence for the use of pharmacological agents as stand-alone treatments for specific phobia in children and adults. To date, only a few case reports (Abene & Hamilton, 1998; Balon, 1999) and small controlled trials (Alamy, Wei, Varia, Davidson, & Connor, 2008; Benjamin, Ben-Zion, Karbofsky, & Dannon, 2000) have been published.

Fairbanks and colleagues (1997) conducted a small, 9-week open trial of fluoxetine (40 mg children and 80 mg adolescents) in 16 youth with a range of anxiety disorders. Four of the six participants with a specific phobia responded to treatment. Selective serotonin reuptake inhibitors (SSRIs) such as fluoxetine have also been found to be effective for pediatric generalized anxiety disorder, social anxiety disorder, separation anxiety disorder, and obsessive–compulsive disorder (Pediatric OCD Treatment Study (POTS) Team, 2004; Walkup et al., 2008). Hence, medications are often used as an adjunct to behavioral therapy for youth with phobias and comorbid anxiety disorders (Reinblatt & Walkup, 2005). More recently, Ollendick, Davis, and Sirbu (2009) recommended the use of SSRI medications as an alternative approach for youth with treatment-refractory specific phobia who have been unresponsive to first-line psychological therapies.

A promising new development in the treatment of specific phobia has been the use of D-cycloserine (DCS), a cognitive enhancer, to augment exposure therapy. DCS is a partial N-methyl-D-aspartate (NMDA) agonist, that has been found in animal and human clinical studies to accelerate fear reduction during exposure (Norberg, Krystal, & Tolin, 2008). The drug has no anxiolytic properties; rather, it is thought to work through its effect on the formation and consolidation of fear-extinction learning. DCS is purported to strengthen extinction memories, thus assisting in the recall of these memories when confronted with the phobic stimuli (Ressler et al., 2004). DCS has been found to be effective with adults with specific phobia of heights (Ressler et al., 2004) and has also been trialed in adults with spider phobias (Guastella, Dadds, Lovibond, Mitchell, & Richardson, 2007). Recently researchers have begun to examine the effectiveness of DCS-augmented exposure therapy in pediatric samples. For example, Byrne and colleagues (2015) examined whether DCS could augment OST for children experiencing dog or spider phobias. The researchers were particularly interested in whether DCS enhanced fear extinction, such that the new learning would generalize to different feared stimuli and contexts. In a double-blind RCT, children received either 50 mg of DCS ($n = 18$) or a placebo ($n = 17$) prior to receiving a single 1-hour session of exposure therapy for their phobia. Return of fear was measured with BATs 1 week after treatment to a different example of their feared stimulus (a different dog or spider), presented in both the original treatment context and an alternative context. Most notably, when the new stimulus was presented in an alternative context, the DCS group showed less avoidance and fear. This suggests that DCS may augment OST by enabling the fear extinction learning to better generalize and extend beyond the treatment setting.

Predictors and Moderators of Treatment Response

Four large RCTs and one small clinical trial (Flatt & King, 2010; Ollendick et al., 2015; Ollendick, Öst, et al., 2009; Öst et al., 2001; Silverman et al., 1999) have examined predictors of treatment success in phobic youth (see Farrell, Waters, Milliner, & Ollendick, 2013). Collapsed across these trials conducted in Australia, Sweden, and the United States, these studies found that gender, socioeconomic status, ethnicity, severity of the diagnosis, type of phobia, and parent overprotectiveness were not related to treatment outcome. However, in regard to age, comorbidity and parent psychopathology findings have been mixed. In a recent study, Ollendick and colleagues (2015) found that age predicted treatment outcome, with older children rated by clinicians as having greater reductions in the clinical severity of their phobias, and rated by their parents as having greater improvements in managing their phobias, than those in younger children. In contrast, other trials (Flatt & King, 2010; Ollendick, Öst, et al., 2009; Öst et al., 2001; Silverman et al., 1999) have not found effects associated with age. Furthermore, although Silverman and colleagues (1999) found that poorer treatment response was associated with self-reported depression (Berman, Weems, Silverman, & Kurtines, 2000), these findings have not been replicated. In fact, Öst and colleagues (2001) and Ollendick and colleagues (Ollendick, Öst, et al., 2010; Ollendick et al., 2015) found no evidence that comorbid disorders or heightened internalizing or externalizing problems were related to treatment outcome. Finally, in regard to parent factors, Silverman and colleagues found that parental psychopathology, characterized by anxiety, depression, and hostility, were associated with child treatment failure. In comparison, parental anxiety was not found to be associated with child treatment in the Ollendick and colleagues (2015) study.

There is limited research examining moderators of treatment response for phobic youth, with only one published study to date. In an effort to examine the utility of parent involvement in the treatment of phobic youth, Ollendick and colleagues (2015) investigated whether gender, age, internalizing or externalizing problems, parent overprotectiveness, and parent anxiety moderated treatment response to either child-alone OST or parent-augmented OST. Surprisingly, support was not found for any of the potential moderators. Further research is needed in this area to help clinicians to develop individualized treatment approaches that successfully target more difficult-to-treat phobic presentations in youth.

EVIDENCE-BASED ASSESSMENT AND TREATMENT IN PRACTICE

Assessment

A thorough evidence-based assessment is necessary not only for the purposes of diagnostic classification of a specific phobia but also to inform treatment planning and to adequately evaluate treatment outcome. Assessments for specific phobias in children and adolescents should be multimethod (e.g., clinical/diagnostic interview, behavioral observation, self- and parent-report questionnaires) and multi-informant (e.g., child, parent and teacher) to ensure a complete diagnostic picture of youth across contexts and settings (Silverman & Ollendick, 2005). Moreover, all aspects of the child's phobic response (e.g., cognitions, physiology and behavior) should be investigated. Given that specific phobias commonly occur alongside other psychological problems, a broad assessment of psychopathology is recommended to assist with differential diagnosis, as well as the identification of comorbid conditions.

Diagnostic Classification and Differential Diagnosis

Inasmuch as fear and avoidance of circumscribed objects or situations characterize a number of anxiety and obsessive–compulsive spectrum disorders, differential diagnosis between these disorders and a specific phobia can be difficult. Another source of diagnostic inaccuracy involves the challenge of determining whether a child's fear exceeds the clinical threshold for a diagnosis. Moreover, when working with children, clinicians must consider whether a child's fear is developmentally inappropriate.

To establish an accurate diagnosis, the clinician needs to consider the focus of the child's apprehension and associated symptoms. According to DSM-5, for a child to meet diagnostic criteria for a specific phobia, their fear must not be associated with separation from a primary caregiver (e.g., separation anxiety disorder), fears relating to negative evaluation (e.g., social phobia), or a persistent fear of having a panic attack (losing control or going crazy; e.g., panic disorder; American Psychiatric Association, 2013). If a child or adolescent presents with phobic symptoms following a traumatic event (e.g., car accident, dog attack, or traumatic hospital admission), it is necessary to consider a differential diagnosis of a trauma- or stressor-related disorder such as posttraumatic stress disorder (PTSD). To assist in distinguishing between a phobia and PTSD, the clinician needs to assess whether the child is currently experiencing any other symptoms of PTSD, such as recurrent intrusive and involuntary memories of the event or dissociative reactions (American Psychiatric Association, 2013). Obsessive–compulsive disorder (OCD) also needs to be ruled out when assessing for a specific phobia. If the focus of the child's fear is the result of an obsession (e.g., a child who fears vomit due to obsessive thoughts related to contamination) and if a child presents with other symptoms of OCD (e.g., checking his or her school bag or counting the steps as he or she walks, or experiencing intrusive unwanted thoughts about harming others), a diagnosis of OCD should be given.

An additional source of diagnostic error in childhood specific phobia is difficulty in determining whether a fear exceeds the clinical threshold. As noted earlier, experiencing transitory fears is a normal part of child development, with the content of fears following a predictable course, from infancy and toddlerhood to childhood and adolescence. Many children experience mild fears of particular objects or situations (e.g., the dark; Ollendick & Muris, 2015); however, these fears do not necessarily interfere with their day-to-day functioning and tend not to persist. According to DSM-5, diagnosis of a phobia is warranted if the child's fear causes substantial distress and is associated with significant impairment in functioning for at least 6 months (American Psychiatric Association, 2013).

Clinical Interview and Diagnostic Interviews

Clinical interviews are an essential component of any specific phobia assessment; they not only assist with establishing a diagnosis, but they also allow the clinician to gather further information about the idiographic phobic response of the individual (Hood & Antony, 2012). Several structured and semistructured diagnostic interviews have been developed to assess child psychiatric disorders (Kaufman et al., 1997; Shaffer, Fisher, Lucas, Dulcan, & Schwab-Stone, 2000). For phobic and anxiety disorders, the Anxiety Disorders Interview Schedule for DSM-IV—Child and Parent versions (ADIS-IV C/P; Silverman & Albano, 1996), is the "gold standard" (Ollendick & Davis, 2012). The ADIS-IV C/P consists of specific modules designed to assess for childhood anxiety disorders, mood disorders, and externalizing disorders. The interview can be delivered wholly, or if completing a brief assessment, in individual modules (e.g., specific phobia). At the conclusion of the interview, clinicians rate the severity of each disorder on a 9-point scale, ranging from 0 ("not present") to 8 ("very severe"). Ratings of 4 or above indicate a clinically significant diagnosis (Silverman & Albano, 1996).

It is recommended that when administering the Specific Phobia module of the ADIS-IV-C/P, clinicians ask a number of supplementary questions relating to phobic objects or situations given a fear rating of 4 or above by the parent or child. Example supplementary questions may include asking parents about their child's physical and emotional reaction (e.g., crying, running away, fainting) when confronted with the phobic object or situation. Furthermore, children and parents can be questioned about avoidance behaviors and impairment associated with the child's phobia (e.g., "Are there places your child will not go because he or she is afraid of dogs?" and "Has your child's fear impacted socializing with friends in anyway?"). The information gathered through additional questioning provides greater understanding of the nature and diagnostic severity of the child's phobia, which is crucial for treatment planning. See Table 7.2 for example supplementary questions for dog and dark phobias.

TABLE 7.2. Supplementary Questions for the ADIS-IV-C/P Specific Phobia Module

Dogs

- Are there places you cannot go because you are afraid of dogs?
  - Parks
  - Friends' houses
  - Beach
- Does the size/color/breed/age of the dog make a difference?
- Does it make a difference if the dog is on a lead or loose?
- Are there particular parts of dogs' bodies (e.g., teeth, claws, head) that you are more afraid of?
- Is there anything a dog does that particularly bothers you (e.g., jump or bark)?
- Are you able to watch dogs on television or in movies?
- What do you do if you see a dog (e.g., cry, freeze, run away)?
- If you went to the house of a friend who owns a dog, would you be able to go in if you knew the dog was restrained (e.g., closed in the backyard)? What if it was not?

Dark

- Do you keep lights on in your bedroom, closet, hall, or bathroom at night? How many? Which ones?
- Do you sleep alone? Share a room with a sibling? Sleep with your parents either in their bedroom or yours?
- Do you fight with your mom or dad about sleeping in your own bedroom at night?
- Have you ever slept alone? How many times a week do you sleep with your parents?
- Are there places in the house that you won't go after dusk (e.g., upstairs, basement, attic, rooms with no lights on, garage, outside)?
- Are you able to play games at night (i.e., flashlight tag or ghost in the graveyard?) or go trick or treating?
- How do you feel when going to the movies and being in a darkened cinema? (Does the child cling more to parents or stay close to their friends or avoid going?)
- Do you avoid being outdoors after dark? Do you refuse to put the rubbish out at night for your parents or take your brother and sister with you?
- If you left a schoolbook you needed in the car in the driveway, would you be able to go out at night and collect it?

Note. Adapted from Ollendick (2001) with permission from the author.

Questionnaires

In addition to diagnostic interviews, it is recommended that questionnaires be administered as part of a comprehensive assessment of phobic youth. Questionnaires should examine not only specific phobia symptoms but also broad psychopathology. The Child Behavior Checklist (CBCL; Achenbach, 2001) and the Behavior Assessment System for Children (BASC; Reynolds & Kamphaus, 2004) are ideal measures because they screen for a wide range of psychopathology and have multiple versions for children, parents, and teachers. Broad measures should also be accompanied by more specific measures of child anxiety and fear. Overall anxiety can be assessed using measures such as the Multidimensional Anxiety Scale for Children (MASC; March, 1997) and the Spence Children's Anxiety Scale—Child and Parent Versions (SCAS; Spence, 1998).

The most widely used and well-validated self-report measure for specific phobia in youth is the Fear Survey Schedule for Children—Revised (FSSC-R; Ollendick, 1983). This measure is designed to assess fearfulness in children and adolescents, ages 7–16 years, and provides information about a range of specific and social phobias. The measure requires youth to rate their fearfulness of 80 specific objects and situations on a 3-point scale (0 = "none," 1 = "some," 2 = "a lot"). A parent version of the FSSC-R is also available. It asks parents to rate their children's fearfulness of the same 80 specific objects and situations and uses an identical rating scale and scoring system (Silverman & Nelles, 1989; Weems, Silverman, Saavedra, Pina, & Lumpkin, 1999). The FSSC-R yields a total score and five factor scores, including Fear of the Unknown, Fear of Failure and Criticism, Fear of Minor Injury and Small Animals, Fear of Danger and Death, and Medical Fears. Inspection of phobia specific items can assist in identifying the presence and severity of different types of phobia. It has well-established reliability and validity, and has been normed for youth of various ages and nationalities (Ollendick, 1983; Ollendick, King, & Frary, 1989). Additionally, the FSSC-R has been shown to discriminate among phobia types (Weems et al., 1999). Recently, a shortened 25-item version was published (Muris, Ollendick, Roelofs, & Austin, 2014).

In the adult literature, a number of questionnaires are available to assess the different specific phobia subtypes (Hood & Antony, 2012). A smaller number of questionnaires have been developed for children; however, their psychometric properties are not well established at this time (Silverman & Ollendick, 2008). One measure that does have sound psychometric properties is the 29-item Spider Phobia Questionnaire for Children (SPQ-C; Kindt, Brosschot, & Muris, 1996), which provides the clinician with an overall spider fear score.

Behavioral Approach Tasks

BATs are an integral part of any phobia assessment, as they allow for a direct observation of the child's phobic response (Ollendick & Davis, 2012). A BAT is a standardized and controlled test that involves asking the child to approach the feared object or stimulus. For example, a child who is fearful of dogs may be brought to a closed door and informed that inside the room is a dog on a leash. The child is then instructed to enter the room, walk over to the dog, and pet the dog on the head for 20 seconds. Children are informed that the task is voluntary, and they can stop at any time. For example, for child with a a costume character phobia:

> "Now I want to see how being around a costumed character is for you. Sitting in this room, there is a costumed character. I want to see if you can go into the room and shake hands with the character for 20 seconds. Remember, you don't have to do this if you don't want to. Just try your best."

The degree to which the child approaches the feared object or situation provides an objective measure of phobic avoidance (e.g., does not enter the room vs. pets dog for 10 seconds). At various time points (beginning, during and after) in the task the clinician may ask the child to rate his or her fear from 0 ("not at all scared") to 8 ("very, very scared"). BAT performance is scored by measuring the percentage of steps completed by the child and his or her fear rating (see Table 7.3; Ollendick, King, & Muris, 2004). Clinicians may also obtain information about the child's phobic beliefs (e.g., "What do you worry will happen if you enter the room?") prior to the task. Moreover, physiological data (e.g., heart rate) may also be collected to allow for assessment across all components (e.g., cognitive, physiological, and behavioral) of the phobic response (Ollendick & Davis, 2012).

Although they may be challenging to organize (e.g., having a dog come into the office, obtaining costumes), BATs provide a wealth of knowledge beyond what may be obtained by clinical interviews and questionnaires. They give a foundation on which to establish an exposure hierarchy for treatment (Cowart & Ollendick, 2013). The child's behavior during the BAT provides insight into the ideal starting point for treatment and how the child will cope with interacting with the phobic object or situation. Moreover, they provide information regarding the child's motivation to overcome the fear and the

TABLE 7.3. Example of BAT Steps for a Phobia of Costume Characters

1. Does not open door.
2. Opens door, but does not go in.
3. Steps inside the room.
4. Stays 6 feet away from costume character.
5. Stands at arm's length from costume character for < 10 seconds and does not attempt to shake hands.
6. Stands at arm's length from costume character for 10 seconds, no attempt to shake hands.
7. Stands at arm's length from costume character for < 20 seconds and does not attempt to shake hands.
8. Stands at arm's length away from costume character for ≥ 20 seconds but does not attempt to shake hands.
9. Stands within arm's reach of costume character, reaches out to character but does not make contact.
10. Stands within arm's reach of costume character and shakes hands for < 20 seconds.
11. Stands within arm's reach to costume character and shakes hands ≥ 20 seconds.

Note. Adapted from Ollendick (2001) with permission from the author.

willingness to engage in therapy. BAT assessment protocols can be developed and adjusted for a range of phobia types (Milliner et al., 2013).

Treatment—Key Treatment Components

OST incorporates a combination of cognitive-behavioral techniques, including exposure, cognitive challenges, participant modeling, contingency management, and psychoeducation into a single intensive session (Davis & Ollendick, 2005; Zlomke & Davis, 2008). It is considered a *well-established* treatment for childhood specific phobia (Davis et al., 2011; Davis & Ollendick, 2005; Davis, Ollendick, & Öst, 2012). The following is a description of the key treatment components of OST and tips for maximizing treatment success.

Functional Analysis

Prior to OST, a functional assessment session (45–60 minutes) is carried out with the child and his or her parents (Öst & Ollendick, 2001). The aim of the session is to (1) determine the catastrophic beliefs involved in the maintenance of the child's phobia; (2) create an exposure hierarchy to guide the OST; and (3) explain to the family the rationale for treatment.

ELICITING PHOBIC BELIEFS

The functional assessment session assists in transitioning families from assessment to treatment and gives the clinician an opportunity to build further rapport with the child and increase his or her motivation for treatment (Davis, Ollendick, Reuther, & Muson, 2012). The beginning of this session is an opportune time to provide the child and his or her parents with feedback regarding the child's phobia diagnosis and any other comorbid problems. Following this, the clinician uses a conversational approach, asking open-ended questions in order to elicit the child's catastrophic beliefs and expectations regarding the feared stimuli (see Figure 7.1; Öst et al., 2001). Because metacognition is not fully developed until early adolescence, obtaining catastrophic cognitions from young children may be challenging (Holmbeck, Greenley, & Franks, 2004). It is recommended that the clinician discuss with the child concrete examples of times when he or she has encountered the phobic object or situation and ask the child to recall his or her thoughts at the time (e.g., "What did you worry would happen when you saw the dog in the park?"). It may also be helpful to have the child recollect the first time he or she encountered the phobic object, the most recent confrontation, and the worst encounter with the phobic object (Davis, Ollendick, Reuther, et al., 2012). Moreover, if the child has completed a BAT as part of the assessment, the clinician can have the child draw on this experience by him or her to recall the thought that went through his or her mind during the task, and what he or she feared would happen if he or she approached the feared object or situation. An objective measure of a child's phobic beliefs can be obtained by having the youth rate (using a Likert scale) how likely it is that this belief will occur (likelihood; e.g., "What is the chance a dog will bite you?"), how bad it would be if the belief occurred (danger), and how sure he or she is that he or she could could cope if the belief occurred (self- efficacy; Ollendick, 2001; Ollendick, Raishevich, Davis, Sirbu, & Öst, 2010; Waters et al., 2014).

Ratings can be obtained before, during, and after treatment, for the child's top three phobic beliefs, to assist with tracking changes associated with treatment and to ensure that exposure tasks address the child's catastrophic cognitions.

DEVELOPING AN EXPOSURE HIERARCHY

Developing an exposure hierarchy is another important part of the functional assessment session. This involves working with the child and parent to identify the different aspects

---

The following handout is designed to assist in eliciting and rating children's phobic beliefs. The aim is to identify two phobic beliefs and to rate these in terms of likelihood, severity, and coping. Ensure that the beliefs are as specific as possible (e.g., "The dog will jump on me and I will be badly scratched" or "I will get hurt"). It is intended to be used a guide rather than as a structured interview. Start the session by chatting with the child and spending time building rapport. Provide the following rationale for the functional analysis:

"We are going to work together to try and figure out exactly what it is about dogs that is scary for you, so that I will know the best way to help you. We will try to discover the thoughts you have that make you feel so scared. I will be asking you a lot of questions, and you will need to help me understand all about this fear so that we can tackle it together during our next session.

What is it about dogs that causes you to feel so afraid?
- *Is it the size?*
- *The way it moves?*
- *The noises it makes?*
- *It might bite?*

What do you think will happen if you see a dog?
- *In the yard?*
- *In your home?*
- *In the woods?*
- *Would you run away?*
- *Feel sick?*

What is this worst thing that could happen when you are near a dog?

Phobic Beliefs—Record the child's two strongest beliefs.

1. _____

2. _____

	Phobic Belief 1	Phobic Belief 2
*How likely is it that (**PHOBIC BELIEF**) will happen?*	/8	/8
*If (**PHOBIC BELIEF**) did happen, how bad would that be for you?*	/8	/8
*How confident are you that you could cope (**PHOBIC BELIEF**)?*	/8	/8

FIGURE 7.1. Functional analysis guide: Dog phobia. Adapted from Ollendick (2001) with permission from the author.

of the phobic stimulus, and different situations involving the phobic stimulus that evoke the child's fear or avoidance (Davis, Ollendick, Reuther, et al., 2012; Young, Ollendick, & Whiteside, 2014). Initially, the clinician needs to gather information regarding the characteristics of the feared object the child finds most distressing—for example, for a child with a spider phobia: "Does the size of the spider make a difference?"; "Does the type of spider make a difference (e.g., daddy long legs vs. huntsman vs. red back)?"; "Are hairy spiders harder to be around?" The clinician also needs to obtain information about the different situations that trigger the child's fear. For a child with a spider phobia, the clinician could ask: "How scared would you feel watching a movie (e.g., a Harry Potter film) with spiders?"; "Would it be scarier if you saw a spider sitting in a web or walking up a wall?"; "Would it make a difference if you saw a spider in the bush versus in the house?" Following this, the child can provide a fear rating for each aspect or situation using a fear thermometer (Likert scale) to rank them from "least distressing" to "most distressing." It may be helpful to write or draw the different aspects and situations onto cards that the child can order from easiest to hardest (Young et al., 2014). This will also help the child to compare the situations. The hierarchy should initially consist of some steps that are easy enough for the child to complete immediately (e.g., look at pictures of a spider), then, at the higher levels, steps that are more challenging than day-to-day experiences with the feared object (e.g., holding a spider in his or her hand, letting it crawl on his or her arm). Early steps, which are achievable, are used in order to engage the child in the OST, and to build confidence and trust (Davis, Ollendick, Reuther, et al., 2012). The latter steps in the exposure hierarchy may include more challenging tasks that directly target the child's catastrophic beliefs and involve overlearning to enhance symptom improvement and maintain treatment gains.

Rationale for Treatment

At the end of the functional assessment session, the rationale for OST should be explained to the family. Ensuring that family members have a good understanding of the reasoning behind exposure and the nature of intensive treatments (e.g., to kick-start overcoming the fear) is essential for keeping them engaged and motivated to continue exposure practice following OST. The family is informed that during OST, the child and clinician work as team to face the child's fear gradually and test out the phobic beliefs through a serious of exposure tasks (Davis, Ollendick, Reuther, et al., 2012; Öst & Ollendick, 2001)—for example:

> "We are going to work together as a team to help you overcome your fear of dogs. We will do this in slow, small steps. Throughout the session we will do a number of experiments to test out whether the things you fear will actually happen when you are with a dog."

The child is informed that his or her permission will always be sought before carrying out an exposure task and that he or she is in control of the pacing of the session, and that it is necessary to experience some anxiety during the OST in order to overcome his or her fear; however, this will only be a moderate level of fear (e.g., fear rating 6/10) and will not repeat or beat the worst level of fear he or she has experienced (Öst & Ollendick, 2001)—for example:

"When you first start facing your fear of dogs, you are likely feel a bit uncomfortable, around a 6 on the thermometer. During the session we will never repeat or beat the highest level of fear you have ever felt. However, we know that you do need to experience some anxiety if you are to overcome your fear."

Integral to the success of OST is explaining to families that a fear the child has had for months, or even years, will not remit after one session. OST should be viewed as a "kick-start" and the first step in overcoming the child's fear—for example:

"An important thing to remember is that a fear you have had for a long time, say, since you were 5 years old, won't go away after one session; however, if you keep practicing what you learned after our session you will become less and less afraid over the next few months."

It is important for children and parents to understand that following their OST practice is essential, and that if they engage in regular exposure activities, over the weeks or months after the treatment, the child's fear will diminish (Davis, Ollendick, Reuther, et al., 2012). The clinician should also take time to address any questions the child or parents may have and to normalize any anticipatory anxiety the child may experience prior to attending the session—for example:

"Most children and teenagers tell me they are worried about attending the session. I want to assure you that during our time together I won't do anything to surprise you. You are in charge. When you come and see me it is not like school. I am not a teacher, and you won't get into trouble if you do not wish to do something."

Preparing for OST

Considerable preparation is required before undertaking OST with a child or adolescent. Prior to OST clinicians need to ensure that they (1) have appropriate materials and stimuli for exposure; (2) find appropriate people to be involved in the session (e.g., dog handler, nurse, beekeeper, or meteorologist); (3) consider any safety or ethical issues that may arise when conducting exposure; and (4) prepare themselves for OST by seeking supervision if necessary, researching the child's phobic stimuli (e.g., why does it storm?) and practice interacting with the child's phobic stimulus (e.g., handling a spider; Reuterskiold & Öst, 2012). For more detailed information regarding preparing for OST for different phobia subtypes, refer to Reuterskiold and Öst (2012).

Information gathered during the initial assessment, BAT, and functional analysis will guide the type of materials and stimuli needed for the OST. Additionally, it is important to have enough stimuli to be able to graduate exposure steps effectively. For example, if a child reports being more fearful of active dogs, the clinician would want to start the OST with a calm dog, and finish the final hour of treatment with an active dog. When working with animals, it is necessary to plan for their housing and to determine who will care for the animal prior to or during the session. Moreover, the clinician needs to consider whether any materials need to be purchased to ensure that the animal is healthy and well looked after, and to keep the office clean (e.g., water bowl, old blanket, cleaning products, poo bags). In relation to natural environment phobias such as a storm phobia, the clinician needs to consider the time of year and possibly delay treatment until the spring or summer months when storms are more common, and to be on call to schedule the treatment session on short notice. Alternatively, it may be possible to collaborate with personnel at science museums or universities who may have storm or rain simulation equipment. In relation to a darkness phobia, treatments are ideally completed at the child's home in the late afternoon or early evening. The therapist may need to provide glow sticks and torches. When working with a BII phobic, the therapist might have to purchase ingredients to make fake blood or acquire medical equipment (e.g., finger pricks or blood test tubes) for the child to look at. Furthermore, he or she may need to ensure that a pathology nurse is involved in the session. For children with a situational phobia, such as an elevator phobia, it is essential for clinician to go outside of the office to seek out and identify stimuli that might be used to evoke differing levels of anxiety (e.g., glass elevators, steel-enclosed elevators). If a child has previously been stuck in a particular elevator (e.g., at a local shopping center) arranging to use this elevator (if possible) would be ideal during the final hour of OST. For a flying phobia, the clinician can organize with an airline to go into the cockpit of a plane and even potentially to take short flights. Finally, for other phobia types such as vomit phobia, therapists can download smartphone applications that produce sounds of someone vomiting. Therapists can also visit websites such as "rate my vomit" to find images of people vomiting and search for vomit recipes online. For costume characters, a therapist can arrange to visit a theme park (e.g., Disneyland or Dreamworld) or find a local sports team mascot who will assist with exposure. Also purchasing or hiring a range of different costumes may be necessary.

Orchestrating coordination among oneself, the child, his or her family, and any other people who need to be involved in the delivery of OST (e.g., dog owner, nurse, beekeeper) can be challenging. It is helpful to be up front with the family and explain this challenge from the outset. This will ensure that the family is aware of and understands the need to be flexible with the timing of the appointment. Furthermore, it may be necessary for the child to miss some school to attend the appointment. Families are generally comfortable with this given that OST involves only a single session and assessment appointments can be scheduled outside of school hours. It is recommended to families that OST appointments be scheduled in the morning, if at all possible, because children can be quite anxious prior to the session and a morning appointment prevents them from worrying throughout the day. Additionally, in the morning, children are often well rested, as opposed to exhausted, following a long day at school. Families are also encouraged to take their child for a special lunch (e.g., child's choice) after the session to celebrate their achievements.

Prior to conducting the OST session, ethical or safety issues need to be considered, in relation to not only the patient but also the therapist and others who are assisting with the exposure (Wolitzky-Taylor, Viar-Paxton, & Olatunji, 2012). When working with animals, it is important to contemplate and to mitigate any potential risks. For example, if you are completing a spider phobia treatment and have collected spiders from your home, it is essential to consult with an expert to determine whether any are poisonous. Also, when working with dogs, it is necessary to screen the dogs to ensure they have no history of biting or jumping on people and are able to follow basic commands. If conducting exposure outside of the clinic, it is important to visit the area before the session and assess for risks (e.g., if you are completing a height phobia treatment). If the child is being treated for an injection phobia consent needs to be obtained from the parent before completing any medical procedure, which is the usual process in health settings.

Maintaining the child's and family's confidentiality also needs to be considered (Wolitzky-Taylor et al., 2012). When conducting exposure outside of the clinic, you may be approached by inquisitive onlookers and asked about what you are doing. It is helpful to discuss with the child and parent about how you will respond if this occurs. Furthermore, while in public situations, the clinician should refrain from doing things that draw attention to the nature of the relationship between him- or herself and the child (e.g., do not record fear ratings while in public or loudly discuss issues associated with therapy; Wolitzky-Taylor et al., 2012). As previously discussed, at times, another person may need to assist with exposure therapy. These people also need to be briefed regarding confidentiality. It is recommended that volunteers or others involved in the session sign a confidentiality agreement.

OST Itself

EXPOSURE

Prolonged and massed exposure is the key element of OST (Öst, 1989). During the session, the child is assisted to repeatedly confront the feared object or situation repeatedly in a graduated and controlled manner (Öst & Ollendick, 2001). Hypothetically, this process leads to habituation of the child's fear and extinguishes avoidance. During OST, exposure is conducted through a number of behavioral experiments designed to test the child's phobic beliefs associated with interacting with the feared object or situation. Davis, Ollendick, Reuther, and colleagues (2012) outline a four-step process when conducting a behavioral experiment: (1) suggesting and negotiating a possible exposure task with the child, (2) having the clinician demonstrate the proposed task, (3) encouraging and assisting the child to perform the task, and (4) reinforcing the child for attempting or successfully completing the task. These steps can also be supplemented with cognitive challenges (see below). See Figure 7.2 for a handout that can be used to guide behavioral experiments.

At times during the OST session, a child may be reluctant or unwilling to engage in exposure. To continue to progress with the session, Davis, Ollendick, and Öst (2009) recommend use of "foot in the door" and "door in the face" techniques. The "foot in the door" technique involves initially suggesting very easy and achievable exposure tasks to build rapport with the child and to increase their confidence and sense of self-efficacy. Following this, as the session progresses the clinician uses the "door in the face" technique to suggest a highly challenging exposure task that is well advanced beyond the task that the child is currently completing, in the hope that negotiation following this will result in the child agreeing to complete an intermediate exposure step, so that the session continues to move forward (Davis, Ollendick, Reuther, et al., 2012).

To assist in the generalization of learning over the course of OST, exposure tasks should ideally be repeated, carried out using multiple stimuli (e.g., small, medium and large dog) and across different contexts (e.g., interact with a dog in a therapy room, a

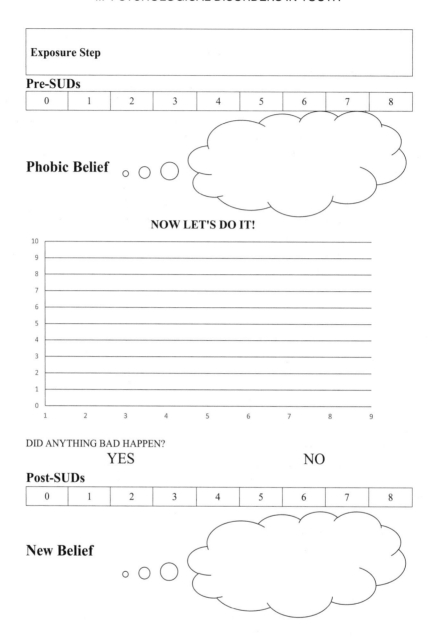

FIGURE 7.2. Behavioral Experiment Handout

fenced yard, and an open park), and toward the end of the session, assuming the child has progressed sufficiently—to involve overlearning (e.g., place your hand in a dog's mouth, only if the dog has been trained to do so safely). To keep children motivated, and to maximize success, exposure tasks should be as fun and engaging as possible (e.g., hiding glow sticks in the dark or making different types of fake vomit). It is recommended that throughout the session, and with the parent's permission, the therapist take photos of the child smiling and engaged in exposure tasks (e.g., patting a dog). Following the session, these pictures can be e-mailed to families, with parents encouraged to print them and place them around the house, and to show others (e.g., siblings and grandparents) how their child was able to successfully face his or her fear. We have found that the photos help to keep a child motivated and can be used to encourage the child to practice. Furthermore, the photos serve to increase a child's sense of self-efficacy. Additionally, following treatment, families can be asked to e-mail or text-message photos of the child practicing exposure to therapist. To manage fatigue over the course of the OST, especially for a young child, it is recommended that the therapist give the child a 10-minute break at the end of each hour. During this time the child can have a snack, chat with his or her parents, or use the bathroom.

When conducting exposure with children and animals, therapists need to be aware that that the unexpected will likely happen and the session is unlikely to go 100% according to plan. During OST, for example, a dog may jump up on a child or a spider might get caught in the child's hair, or when playing hide and seek in the dark, the child might get caught up in curtains or trip over something, or the pathology nurse might not be able to find the child's vein when performing a blood draw. It is important when these unexpected events occur for you, as therapist, to model remaining calm and being empathetic to the child (e.g., "You got a fright when the dog jumped up on you!") and help the child to calm down (e.g., "Let's just sit here and calm down for a minute"). Once the child is calm, spend time reviewing the situation and help the child to use the incident as a learning experience (e.g., "Yes, the dog did jump on you, but let's think this through. Are you OK now? What happened when the dog jumped on you? Yes, you got a fright, but you were able to cope with it. So your biggest fear came true but you were able to handle it. Good for you!"). Following this, recommence the exposure.

COGNITIVE CHALLENGES

During OST, catastrophic cognitions and expectancies are challenged through the exposure tasks (e.g., behavioral experiments) that either confirm or disconfirm these cognitions. This is in contrast to a traditional cognitive restructuring approach using Socratic questioning (Davis, Ollendick, Reuther, et al., 2012). Hence, during OST, the therapist does not generate with the child alternative cognitions or counter automatic thoughts (Davis, Ollendick, Reuther, et al., 2012; Öst & Ollendick, 2001; Zlomke & Davis, 2008). Exposure tasks need to be set up in a manner that challenges the child's catastrophic beliefs, rather than focus broadly on what the child avoids. Broad, nontargeted exposure may not address the child's underlying phobic beliefs, whereas very specific exposure tasks (e.g., behavioral experiments) in a briefer time period are more likely to achieve the goal of correcting the catastrophic belief (Öst, 2012). Behavioral experiments typically proceed with the clinician questioning the child about what he or she thinks or predicts will happen during the exposure task (e.g., "What do you think will happen if we release the spider from the container?"). The exposure task is then carried out. Following this, the clinician discusses with the child what actually happened and whether his or her catastrophic cognition or expectancies came true (e.g., "We let the spider out of its container, and what happened? Did it run toward you and climb up your arm?"). This process helps the child to obtain new learning about the phobic stimuli. Moreover, he or she learns that he or she is able to cope in the presence of the feared stimuli, and the experience corrects the phobic beliefs maintaining his or her fear and avoidance.

PARTICIPANT MODELING

Another fundamental element of OST, participant modeling, assists with breaking down more complex or difficult exposure steps into more manageable tasks (Davis et al., 2009; Zlomke & Davis, 2008). It involves a model (most often the clinician) demonstrating a behavior, then including the observer in the modeled action. For example, the clinician may demonstrate to the child how to catch a spider using a container. Following this, the clinician might ask the child to place his or her hand on top of the clinician's own, so that they catch the spider together. This would be repeated until the child's fear habituates and the clinician is able to gradually phase out the physical contact and verbal instructions. The goal in participant modeling is for the child eventually to be able to independently engage in the exposure step. Modeling during OST serves two important purposes: (1) helping to build skills (e.g., how to safely pat a dog), and (2) reducing fear through observational learning (e.g., watching someone have a blood test). It can be used for a range of phobia types (Davis, Ollendick, Reuther, et al., 2012).

REINFORCEMENT

Reinforcement is also an important component of OST that is used to shape and encourage children's approach behavior. Throughout the OST session, the clinician provides the child with positive attention, praise, and social support for completing behavioral experiments and interacting with the feared object or situation. Typically tangible reinforcers (e.g., food, toys, stickers) are not used during OST, with social reinforcers favored (Davis, Ollendick, Reuther, et al., 2012). Moreover, during the session, selective attention can be used not only to encourage approach behavior but also to discourage avoidance. For example, the clinician may decrease the amount of attention he or she gives the child who pats the dog on the back (as opposed to the head); however, as the child moves back to patting the dog on the head, the clinician reinitiates attending to the child and provides praise (e.g., "I really like the way you are patting the dog's head"). Additionally, during the OST session, the clinician needs to be careful not to inadvertently reinforce the child's avoidance behavior by allowing the child to avoid the situation, by praising a failed attempt at approaching stimuli, or by providing unnecessary reassurance or excessively comforting an upset child (Davis, Ollendick, Reuther, et al., 2012).

PSYCHOEDUCATION AND SKILLS TRAINING

Another essential OST element is the provision of psychoeducation and skills training. Psychoeducation is used to (1) keep the child engaged and interested during the session, (2) keep the child focused on the feared stimuli (e.g., "How many legs does a spider have? Spiders are members of the Arachnid family, all of which have eight legs"), (3) correct any false assumptions or myths the child may have in relation to the feared object, and (4) address deficits in the child's skills set (e.g., how to safely catch a spider; Davis, Ollendick, Reuther, et al., 2012).

Following OST

At the conclusion of the OST, the clinician invites the child's parents into the session and has the child review, and demonstrate what was achieved during the session (Davis et al., 2009). A behavioral experiment can also be shown to parents, with instructions provided so they can carry out potential future exposures on their own. Families should again be reminded of the rationale for treatment (e.g., OST is a kick-start) and encouraged to keep practicing self-guided exposure for the next few months to consolidate gains. Parents are encouraged to schedule regular opportunities for exposure practice (see Figure 7.3). At this stage, or a week later at a postassessment appointment, the clinician should discuss with family members that while trying to overcome fear, the child will at times experience setbacks. It is important for the clinician to explain to the family the difference between a "setback" (e.g., a brief return of fear) and a "relapse" (e.g., the child is experiencing same levels of fear and in as many places as in pretreatment; Davis, Ollendick, Reuther, et al., 2012). If the child experiences a setback, the family members are encouraged to draw on the skills they learned during OST and to try to approach the situation again and increase frequency of exposure practice. If they are still having difficulty, family members can contact their therapist for a phone consult or, if necessary, have a booster session.

Descriptions of OST for Dog Phobia

We describe in this section the use of OST with the most common specific phobia in children and youth: fear of dogs. It should be noted that when conducting an OST, the exposure tasks completed, as well as the pace of the session, vary considerably from one child to the next. Thus, the clinician has to adjust his or her approach according to how the child responds (e.g., fear and behavior) to each task.

As noted, dog phobia is the most common childhood specific phobia. It is important to have a number of dogs (ideally, three different dogs) involved in the session to allow for generalization of the child's skills and to sufficiently test the child's phobic beliefs (e.g., "The dog will bite me"). Ideally, the dogs should vary in size (e.g., small, medium or large) and activity level (e.g., calm or active). The order in which the dogs are presented to the child depends on information obtained during the initial assessment, BAT, and functional analysis. It is important to commence the session with each dog in a controlled setting, such as a large-group meeting room; however, as the child feels more confident, the dog can be taken to an outside grass area or walked to a nearby park. The following is a description of a 1-hour component of OST for dog phobia, describing the nature of the exposure tasks. The same progression (e.g., patting, walking on a lead, being off a lead, feeding the dog) of exposure tasks can be used for each new dog that is introduced to the child. For a summary of an entire 3-hour dog phobia OST, see Table 7.4.

The session begins with the dog on one side of the room, held on a lead by an assistant. The therapist and child sit on chairs in front of the dog (a couple of meters away, depending on how fearful the child is), and the assistant describes the dog (e.g., shape, size, color). The child or therapist may want to ask the assistant some questions about the dog, such as its name and age. Following this, the therapist can set up a behavioral experiment whereby the child is asked to predict what will happen if the therapist approaches

Exposure Ideas
- Visit a local dog park.
- Go to an off-the-lead dog beach.
- Go to a dog breeding show.
- Watch a sheep dog or dog agility competition.
- Visit a pet shop.
- Visit a volunteer dog therapy group.
- Watch a dog-training session.
- Dog-sit for a friend who goes away.
- Visit friends who own dogs.

Make a list of friends who own dogs (e.g., Lucy and Max [border collie]).

_____
_____
_____
_____

Week	Exposure tasks	Reward
1		
2		
3		
4		

FIGURE 7.3. Home practice for exposure: Dog phobia.

the dog. The therapist can then model for the child how to approach an unfamiliar dog (e.g., ask the assistant if it is OK to pat the dog and allow the dog to sniff his or her hand before patting it) and ask whether the child's prediction came true. The therapist can then sit near the dog and continue to pat it, while inviting the child to gradually approach the dog. The child may initially stand behind the therapist. It may be easier for the child to start by patting the dog's back (as opposed to its head). Participant modeling can be used, in which the child places his or her hand on top of the therapist's and initially they pat the dog together. Following this, the therapist can gradually remove his or her hand so that the child is patting the dog alone. The therapist should work toward leading the child to pat the dog's head. While patting the dog, and throughout the session, the therapist can educate the child about the benefits of owning a dog, the role of dogs in our society, and safe dog handling behavior. The dialogue below is an example of education provided to a child during exposure:

THERAPIST: Why do you think people own dogs?

CHILD: I'm not sure. We don't have a dog.

THERAPIST: Well maybe we could try and work it out by asking Maggie's handler, Geoff.

TABLE 7.4. OST for Dog Phobia

Hour 1: Psychology clinic and park
- Pat a small dog on a lead held by an assistant.
- Walk the small dog on a lead around the clinic room.
- Walk the small dog on a lead outside of the clinic, to the park.
- Have the small dog off the lead in the clinic room.
- Call the small dog to come to you in the clinic room.
- Throw a ball for the small dog to chase.
- Feed the small dog a treat.

Hour 2: Psychology clinic and park
- Pat a medium-size dog on a lead held by an assistant.
- Walk the medium-size dog on a lead around the clinic room.
- Walk the medium-size dog on a lead outside of the clinic.
- Have the medium-size dog off the lead in the clinic room.
- Call the medium-size dog to come to you in the clinic room.
- Throw a ball for the medium-size dog to chase.
- Feed the medium-size dog a treat.

Hour 3: Psychology clinic and park
- Pat a large-size dog on a lead held by an assistant.
- Walk the large-size dog on a lead around the clinic room.
- Walk the large-size dog on a lead outside of the clinic.
- Have the large-size dog off the lead in the clinic room.
- Call the large-size dog to come to you in the clinic room.
- Throw a ball for the large-size dog to chase.
- Feed the large-size dog a treat.

ASSISTANT: I own a dog because she keeps me company and helps me to stay active. I have to walk Maggie two times every day for 40 minutes. She also is good at protecting my family and barks if someone comes to our door.

THERAPIST: Wow! So just like Geoff, lots of people own dogs because they make good friends and keep you company. . . . Some dogs even have jobs! Do you know some jobs that a dog may have?

CHILD: Well, guide dogs help people who are blind and also sniffer dogs at the airport.

THERAPIST: Great! Yes, dogs help humans in many ways. Those are great examples. Also, some dogs visit nursing homes to make old people happy or may come into schools so children can read to them, or there are also police dogs that help police officers find drugs or missing people.

Once the child feels comfortable patting the dog (e.g., fear rating of 2 on a 0- to 8-point scale), the therapist moves on to the next step. Typically, children are more fearful when the dog is moving around. The therapist and the child together can walk the dog around the room on the lead. The therapist holds the part of the lead that is closest to the dog, and the child holds the end. When the child feels comfortable, the therapist can let go of the lead and continue to walk beside the child and dog. The child eventually walks the dog around the room alone, and the therapist and child can then walk the dog to a park or outside. The child can be encouraged to go for small walks with the dog alone— still within the therapist's eyesight, however (e.g., "I want you to walk Maggie to the big tree over there and then back to me"). Following this, the therapist and the child return to the clinic. The next task involves letting the dog off the lead. This is often a difficult step for children when they perceive the dog is no longer under the assistant's control. For children who become stuck or are reluctant to proceed with an exposure task, "foot-in-the-door" techniques (Davis, Ollendick, Reuther, et al., 2012) may be used to help the child progress, as suggested earlier. For example:

> THERAPIST: You did such a wonderful job walking Maggie. For our next step, I will give you a choice—we can feed Maggie or ask Geoff to let her off her lead. What would you like to do?
>
> CHILD: Let her off the lead.

It is suggested that prior to commencing this exposure task, the child and therapist sit on the side of the room opposite the dog and the dog's handler. Before letting the dog off the lead, the child should be asked to predict how the dog will behave, for example:

> THERAPIST: In a minute I will ask Geoff to let Maggie off her lead. What do you think will happen?
>
> CHILD: I think she is going to go crazy! She will run toward us and jump on me!
>
> THERAPIST: OK, Geoff, please let Maggie off the lead . . . (laughing) So what happened when Geoff let Maggie off the lead?
>
> CHILD: She did not move—she just sat there.
>
> THERAPIST: What a lazy dog! OK, we will just sit here and watch Maggie for a bit longer . . . She still has not moved. So was your prediction correct?
>
> CHILD: No.
>
> THERAPIST: What did you learn from this?
>
> CHILD: That what I thought would happen did not. I guess I was wrong.

To continue the progress of the session, the therapist and child can watch what happens if the handler encourages the dog to move around. They can eventually practice calling the dog toward them and throwing a ball for the dog. The final exposure step involves the child feeding the dog. It is important for the therapist to model to the child how to feed a dog by placing dog biscuits on his or her hand, keeping the fingers and palm flat. Again, participant modeling can be used, with the child placing his or her hand under the therapist's hand, then swapping, with the therapist's hand under the child's, and finally the child feeding the dog alone, for example:

> THERAPIST: What do you think will happen if you feed Maggie?
>
> CHILD: She will bite my hand.

THERAPIST: OK, you have seen me feed Maggie. So let's try it out together. You put your hand under my hand. Well done! You helped me feed Maggie a biscuit. So what happened? Do we still have all our fingers?

CHILD: Yes! It felt kind of slobbery and wet but it was OK. She did not bite me.

The task was repeated again, with the therapist's hand on top, and following this, three more times, with the child's hand on top, until the child reported a fear rating of 1 on a scale of 0–8.

THERAPIST: OK, you have done so well. Let's now have a go of you doing it alone. Is there anything you worry will happen?

CHILD: I am still a bit worried she will bite me.

THERAPIST: OK, well, let's try it out to see what happens. You did it! You fed Maggie a couple of biscuits. Good on you. So what happened?

CHILD: She didn't bite me, she just licked my hand a lot.

This progression of steps can be completed with all the dogs of different sizes and activity levels (see Table 7.4). Finish the OST by having the family observe the child interacting with a dog. Discuss with the family the progression of the child's OST and generate ideas for exposure tasks at home for the next month.

CONCLUSION

While it is common for young people to experience a variety of fears during development, a significant proportion of them go on to experience more serious and interfering specific phobias. Specific phobias are characterized by a marked and persistent fear of an object or situation that causes significant disruption in a child's daily life. A variety of factors are implicated in the development of a phobia, including genetics, an evolutionary "preparedness," learning/conditioning experiences with the feared stimulus, and an overprotective parenting style. In addition, behavioral avoidance and cognitive biases toward the feared stimulus are believed to maintain this disorder. Evidence-based assessment for a specific phobia should ideally be multimodal (e.g., using an interview, a measurement of behavioral avoidance, and questionnaires) and involve multiple informants (e.g., the child, parents, and teachers). It should assess all aspects of the phobia, including its effects on behavior, physiology, and cognition. CBT and, more specifically, OST is considered to be the first-line treatment of choice for childhood specific phobias and has a well-established evidence base. Researchers have recently attempted to augment exposure for childhood phobias with increased parent involvement, attention retraining, and use of a pharmacological adjunct, D-cycloserine. Moreover, researchers are now also aiming to address difficulties in accessing treatment for phobic youth through trials of Internet-delivered CBT. Much progress has been made in treating specific phobias in youth (Ollendick & Muris, 2015); however, we must do more to enhance their effectiveness and to determine for whom these treatments work best.

REFERENCES

Abene, M. V., & Hamilton, J. D. (1998). Resolution of fear of flying with fluoxetine treatment. *Journal of Anxiety Disorders, 12*(6), 599–603.

Achenbach, T. M. (2001). *Manual for the Child Behavior Checklist 4–18 and 2001 profile*. Burlington: University of Vermont.

Alamy, S., Wei, Z., Varia, I., Davidson, J. R. T., & Connor, K. M. (2008). Escitalopram in specific phobia: Results of a placebo-controlled pilot trial. *Journal of Psychopharmacology, 22*(2), 157–161.

American Psychiatric Association. (2013). *Diagnostic and statistical manual of mental disorders* (5th ed.). Arlington, VA: Author.

Arntz, A., Lavy, E., Van den Berg, G., & Van Rijsoort, S. (1993). Negative beliefs of spider phobics: A psychometric evaluation of the spider phobia beliefs questionnaire. *Advances in Behaviour Research and Therapy, 15*(4), 257–277.

Askew, C., & Field, A. P. (2008). The vicarious learning pathway to fear 40 years on. *Clinical Psychology Review, 28*(7), 1249–1265.

Balon, R. (1999). Fluvoxamine for phobia of storms. *Acta Psychiatrica Scandinavica, 100*(3), 244–246.

Bar-Haim, Y., Lamy, D., Pergamin, L., Bakermans-Kranenburg, M. J., & van IJzendoorn, M. H. (2007). Threat-related attentional bias in anxious and nonanxious individuals: A meta-analytic study. *Psychological Bulletin, 133*(1), 1–24.

Barrett, P. M., Rapee, R. M., Dadds, M. M., & Ryan, S. M. (1996). Family enhancement of cognitive style in anxious and aggressive children. *Journal of Abnormal Child Psychology, 24*(2), 187–203.

Bener, A., Ghuloum, S., & Dafeeah, E. E. (2011). Prevalence of common phobias and their sociodemographic correlates in children and adolescents in a traditional developing society. *African Journal of Psychiatry, 14*(2), 140–145.

Benjamin, J., Ben-Zion, I. Z., Karbofsky, E., & Dannon, P. (2000). Double-blind placebo-controlled pilot study of paroxetine for specific phobia. *Psychopharmacology, 149*(2), 194–196.

Berman, S. L., Weems, C. F., Silverman, W. K., & Kurtines, W. M. (2000). Predictors of outcome in exposure-based cognitive and behavioral treatments for phobic and anxiety disorders in children. *Behavior Therapy, 31*(4), 713–731.

Byrne, S. P., Rapee, R. M., Malhi, G., Sweller, N., & Hudson, J. (2014). *An examination of harm beliefs in children with dog phobia*. Doctoral thesis, Macquarie University, Sydney, Australia.

Byrne, S. P., Rapee, R. M., Richardson, R., Malhi, G. S., Jones, M., & Hudson, J. L. (2015). D-Cycloserine enhances generalization of fear extinction in children. *Depression and Anxiety, 32*(6), 408–414.

Chambless, D. L., Baker, M. J., Baucom, D. H., Beutler, L. E., Calhoun, K. S., Crits-Christoph, P., et al. (1998). Update on empirically validated therapies: II. *Clinical Psychologist, 51*(1), 3–16.

Chambless, D. L., & Ollendick, T. H. (2001). Empirically supported psychological interventions: Controversies and evidence. *Annual Review of Psychology, 52*(1), 685–716.

Costello, E. J., Egger, H. L., & Angold, A. (2004). Developmental epidemiology of anxiety disorders. In T. H. Ollendick & J. S. March (Eds.), *Phobic and anxiety disorders in children and adolescents: A clinician's guide to effective psychosocial and pharmacological interventions* (pp. 61–91). New York: Oxford University Press.

Cowart, M. J. W., & Ollendick, T. H. (2011). Attention training in socially anxious children: A multiple baseline design analysis. *Journal of Anxiety Disorders, 25*(7), 972–977.

Cowart, M. J. W., & Ollendick, T. H. (2013). Specific phobias. In C. A. Essau & T. H. Ollendick (Eds.), *The Wiley-Blackwell handbook of the treatment of childhood and adolescent anxiety* (pp. 353–368). Chichester, UK: Wiley.

Davey, G. C. L. (1992). Classical conditioning and the acquisition of human fears and phobias: A review and synthesis of the literature. *Advances in Behaviour Research and Therapy, 14*(1), 29–66.

Davis, T. E., III, Jenkins, W. S., & Rudy, B. M. (2012). Empirical status of one-session treatment. In T. E. Davis III, T. H. Ollendick, & L. G. Öst (Eds.), *Intensive one-session treatment of specific phobias* (pp. 19–42). New York: Springer.

Davis, T. E., III, May, A., & Whiting, S. E. (2011). Evidence-based treatment of anxiety and phobia in children and adolescents: Current status and effects on the emotional response. *Clinical Psychology Review, 31*(4), 592–602.

Davis, T. E., III, & Ollendick, T. H. (2005). Empirically supported treatments for specific phobia in children: Do efficacious treatments address the components of a phobic response? *Clinical Psychology: Science and Practice, 12*(2), 144–160.

Davis, T. E., III, Ollendick, T. H., & Öst, L. G. (2009). Intensive treatment of specific phobias in children and adolescents. *Cognitive and Behavioral Practice, 16*(3), 294–303.

Davis, T. E., III, Ollendick, T. H., & Öst, L. G. (Eds.). (2012). *Intensive one-session treatment of specific phobias.* New York: Springer.

Davis, T. E., III, Ollendick, T. H., Reuther, E. T., & Muson, M. S. (2012). One-session treatment: Principles and procedures with children and adolescents. In T. E. Davis III, T. H. Ollendick, & L. G. Öst (Eds.), *Intensive one-session treatment of specific phobias* (pp. 19–42). New York: Springer.

Di Nardo, P. A., Guzy, L. T., Jenkins, J. A., Bak, R. M., Tomasi, S. F., & Copland, M. (1988). Etiology and maintenance of dog fears. *Behaviour Research and Therapy, 26*(3), 241–244.

Distel, M. A., Vink, J. M., Willemsen, G., Middeldorp, C. M., Merckelbach, H., & Boomsma, D. I. (2008). Heritability of self-reported phobic fear. *Behavior Genetics, 38*(1), 24–33.

Dweck, C. S., & Wortman, C. B. (1982). Learned helplessness, anxiety, and achievement motivation: Neglected parallels in cognitive, affective, and coping responses. In H. Krohne & L. Laux (Eds.), *Achievement, stress, and anxiety* (pp. 93–125). Washington, DC: Hemisphere.

Essau, C. A., Conradt, J., & Petermann, F. (2000). Frequency, comorbidity, and psychosocial impairment of specific phobia in adolescents. *Journal of Clinical Child Psychology, 29*(2), 221–231.

Fairbanks, J. M., Pine, D. S., Tancer, N. K., Dummit, E. S., III, Kentgen, L. M., Martin, J., et al. (1997). Open fluoxetine treatment of mixed anxiety disorders in children and adolescents. *Journal of Child and Adolescent Psychopharmacology, 7*(1), 17–29.

Farrell, L. J., Waters, A. M., Milliner, E. L., & Ollendick, T. H. (2013). Prognostic indicators of treatment response for children with anxiety disorders. In D. McKay & E. A. Storch (Eds.), *Handbook of treating variants and complications in anxiety disorders* (pp. 37–55). New York: Springer.

Flatt, N., & King, N. J. (2010). Brief psycho-social interventions in the treatment of specific childhood phobias: A controlled trial and a 1-year follow-up. *Behaviour Change, 27*(3), 130–153.

Fyer, A. J., Mannuzza, S., Chapman, T. F., Martin, L. Y., & Klein, D. F. (1995). Specificity in familial aggregation of phobic disorders. *Archives of General Psychiatry, 52*(7), 564–573.

Guastella, A. J., Dadds, M. R., Lovibond, P. F., Mitchell, P., & Richardson, R. (2007). A randomized controlled trial of the effect of D-cycloserine on exposure therapy for spider fear. *Journal of Psychiatric Research, 41*(6), 466–471.

Holmbeck, G. N., Greenley, R. N., & Franks, E. A. (2004). Developmental issues in evidence-based practice. In P. M. Barrett & T. H. Ollendick (Eds.), *The handbook of interventions that work with children and adolescents—from prevention to treatment* (pp. 27–48). West Sussex, UK: Wiley.

Hood, H. K., & Antony, M. M. (2012). Evidence-based assessment and treatment of specific phobias in adults. In T. E. Davis III, T. H. Ollendick, & L. G. Öst (Eds.), *Intensive one-session treatment of specific phobias* (pp. 19–42). New York: Springer.

Ialongo, N., Edelsohn, G., Werthamer-Larsson, L., Crockett, L., & Kellam, S. (1995). The significance of self-reported anxious symptoms in first grade children: Prediction to anxious symptoms and adaptive functioning in fifth grade. *Journal of Child Psychology and Psychiatry, 36*(3), 427–437.

Kaufman, J., Birmaher, B., Brent, D. A., Rao, U. M. A., Flynn, C., Moreci, P., et al. (1997). Schedule for Affective Disorders and Schizophrenia for School-Age Children—Present and Lifetime Version (K-SADS-PL): Initial reliability and validity data. *Journal of the American Academy of Child and Adolescent Psychiatry, 36*(7), 980–988.

Kendall, P. C., Safford, S., Flannery-Schroeder, E., & Webb, A. (2004). Child anxiety treatment: Outcomes in adolescence and impact on substance use and depression at 7.4-year follow-up. *Journal of Consulting and Clinical Psychology, 72*(2), 276–287.

Kessler, R. C., Berglund, P., Demler, O., Jin, R., Merikangas, K. R., & Walters, E. E. (2005). Lifetime prevalence and age-of-onset distributions of DSM-IV disorders in the National Comorbidity Survey Replication. *Archives of General Psychiatry, 62*(6), 593–602.

Kessler, R. C., Chiu, W., Demler, O., & Walters, E. E. (2005). Prevalence, severity, and comorbidity of 12-month DSM-IV disorders in the National Comorbidity Survey Replication. *Archives of General Psychiatry, 62*(6), 617–627.

Kindt, M., Brosschot, J. F., & Muris, P. (1996). Spider Phobia Questionnaire for Children (SPQ-C): A psychometric study and normative data. *Behaviour Research and Therapy, 34*(3), 277–282.

Last, C. G., Perrin, S., Hersen, M., & Kazdin, A. E. (1992). DSM-III-R anxiety disorders in children: Sociodemographic and clinical characteristics. *Journal of the American Academy of Child and Adolescent Psychiatry, 31*(6), 1070–1076.

LeBeau, R. T., Glenn, D., Liao, B., Wittchen, H.-U., Beesdo-Baum, K., Ollendick, T. H., et al. (2010). Specific phobia: A review of DSM-IV specific phobia and preliminary recommendations for DSM-V. *Depression and Anxiety, 27*(2), 148–167.

Leutgeb, V., Schäfer, A., Köchel, A., & Schienle, A. (2012). Exposure therapy leads to enhanced late frontal positivity in 8- to 13-year-old spider phobic girls. *Biological Psychology, 90*(1), 97–104.

Leutgeb, V., & Schienle, A. (2012). Changes in facial electromyographic activity in spider-phobic girls after psychotherapy. *Journal of Psychiatric Research, 46*(6), 805–810.

March, J. S. (1997). *Multidimensional Anxiety Scale for Children.* North Tonawanda, NY: Multi-Health Systems.

Menzies, R. G., & Clarke, J. C. (1995). The etiology of phobias: A nonassociative account. *Clinical Psychology Review, 15*(1), 23–48.

Merckelbach, H., de Jong, P. J., Muris, P., & van Den Hout, M. A. (1996). The etiology of specific phobias: A review. *Clinical Psychology Review, 16*(4), 337–361.

Milliner, E. L., Farrell, L. J., & Ollendick, T. H. (2013). Phobic anxiety. In P. Graham & S. Reynolds (Eds.), *Cognitive behaviour therapy for children and families* (3rd ed., pp. 255–274). Cambridge, UK: Cambridge University Press.

Milne, J. M., Garrison, C. Z., Addy, C. L., McKeown, R. E., Jackson, K. L., Cuffe, S. P., et al. (1995). Frequency of phobic disorder in a community sample of young adolescents. *Journal of the American Academy of Child and Adolescent Psychiatry, 34*(9), 1202–1211.

Mowrer, O. H. (1960). *Learning theory and behavior.* New York: Wiley.

Muris, P., Merckelbach, H., Gadet, B., & Moulaert, V. (2000). Fears, worries, and scary dreams in 4- to 12-year-old children: Their content, developmental pattern, and origins. *Journal of Clinical Child Psychology, 29*(1), 43–52.

Muris, P., Merckelbach, H., Holdrinet, I., & Sijsenaar, M. (1998). Treating phobic children: Effects of EMDR versus exposure. *Journal of Consulting and Clinical Psychology, 66*(1), 193–198.

Muris, P., Merckelbach, H., Van Haaften, H., & Mayer, B. (1997). Eye movement desensitisation and reprocessing versus exposure *in vivo*: A single-session crossover study of spider-phobic children. *British Journal of Psychiatry, 171*(1), 82–86.

Muris, P., Ollendick, T. H., Roelofs, J., & Austin, K. E. (2014). The Short Form of the Fear Survey Schedule for Children—Revised (FSSC-R-SF): An efficient, reliable, and valid scale for measuring fear in children and adolescents. *Journal of Anxiety Disorders, 28*(8), 957–965.

Norberg, M. M., Krystal, J. H., & Tolin, D. F. (2008). A meta-analysis of D-cycloserine and the facilitation of fear extinction and exposure therapy. *Biological Psychiatry, 63*(12), 1118–1126.

Oar, E. L., Farrell, L. J., & Ollendick, T. H. (2015). One session treatment for specific phobias: An adaptation for pediatric blood–injection–injury phobia in youth. *Clinical Child and Family Psychology Review, 18*(4), 370–394.

Oar, E. L., Farrell, L. J., Waters, A. M., Conlon, E. G., & Ollendick, T. H. (2015). One-session treatment for pediatric blood–injection–injury phobia: A controlled multiple baseline trial. *Behaviour Research and Therapy, 73*, 131–142.

Ollendick, T. H. (1983). Reliability and validity of the Revised Fear Survey Schedule for Children (FSSC-R). *Behaviour Research and Therapy, 21*(6), 685–692.

Ollendick, T. H. (2001). *Phobia Project resources.* Blacksburg: Child Study Center, Virginia Polytechnic University.

Ollendick, T. H., & Davis, T. E., III. (2012). Evidence based assessment and treatment of specific phobia in children and adolescents. In T. E. Davis III, T. H. Ollendick, & L. G. Öst (Eds.), *Intensive one-session treatment of specific phobias* (pp. 19–42). New York: Springer.

Ollendick, T. H., & Davis, T. E., III. (2013). One-session treatment for specific phobias: A review of Öst's single-session exposure with children and adolescents. *Cognitive Behaviour Therapy, 42*(4), 275–283.

Ollendick, T. H., Davis, T. E., III, & Muris, P. (2004). Treatment of specific phobia in children and adolescents. In P. M. Barrett & T. H. Ollendick (Eds.), *Handbook of interventions that work with children and adolescents* (pp. 273–299). New York: Wiley.

Ollendick, T. H., Davis, T. E., III, & Sirbu, C. (2009). Specific phobias. In D. McKay & E. A. Storch (Eds.), *Cognitive behavior therapy for children: Treating complex and refractory cases* (pp. 171–199). New York: Springer.

Ollendick, T. H., Hagopian, L. P., & King, N. J. (1997). Specific phobias in children. In G. C. L. Davey (Ed.), *Phobias: A handbook of theory, research and treatment* (pp. 201–223). Chichester, UK: Wiley.

Ollendick, T. H., Halldorsdottir, T., Fraire, M. G., Austin, K. E., Noguchi, R. J. P., Lewis, K. M., et al. (2015). Specific phobias in youth: A randomized controlled trial comparing one-session treatment to a parent-augmented one-session treatment. *Behavior Therapy, 46*, 141–155.

Ollendick, T. H., & King, N. J. (1994). Fears and their level of interference in adolescents. *Behaviour Research and Therapy, 32*(6), 635–638.

Ollendick, T. H., King, N. J., & Frary, R. B. (1989). Fears in children and adolescents: Reliability and generalizability across gender, age and nationality. *Behaviour Research and Therapy, 27*(1), 19–26.

Ollendick, T. H., King, N. J., & Muris, P. (2002). Fears and phobias in children: Phenomenology, epidemiology, and aetiology. *Child and Adolescent Mental Health, 7*(3), 98–106.

Ollendick, T. H., King, N. J., & Muris, P. (2004). Phobias in children and adolescents. In M. Maj, H. S. Akiskal, J. J. Lopez-Ibor, & A. Okasha (Eds.), *Phobias* (pp. 245–279). Chichester, UK: Wiley.

Ollendick, T. H., & Muris, P. (2015). The scientific legacy of Little Hans and Little Albert: Future direction for research on specific phobias in youth. *Journal of Clinical Child and Adolescent Psychology, 44*(4), 689–706.

Ollendick, T. H., Öst, L. G., Reuterskiöld, L., & Costa, N. (2010). Comorbidity in youth with specific phobias: Impact of comorbidity on treatment outcome and the impact of treatment on comorbid disorders. *Behaviour Research and Therapy, 48*(9), 827–831.

Ollendick, T. H., Öst, L. G., Reuterskiold, L., Costa, N., Cederlund, R., Sirbu, C., et al. (2009). One-session treatment of specific phobias in youth: A randomized clinical trial in the United States and Sweden. *Journal of Consulting and Clinical Psychology, 77*(3), 504–516.

Ollendick, T. H., Raishevich, N., Davis, T. E., III, Sirbu, C., & Öst, L. G. (2010). Specific phobia in youth: Phenomenology and psychological characteristics. *Behavior Therapy, 41*(1), 133–141.

Öst, L. G. (1987). Age of onset in different phobias. *Journal of Abnormal Psychology, 96*(3), 223–229.

Öst, L. G. (1989). One-session treatment for specific phobias. *Behaviour Research and Therapy, 27*(1), 1–7.

Öst, L. G. (2012). One-session treatment: Principles and procedures with adults. In T. E. Davis III, T. H. Ollendick, & L. G. Öst (Eds.), *Intensive one-session treatment of specific phobias* (pp. 19–42). New York: Springer.

Öst, L. G., & Ollendick, T. H. (2001). *Manual for one-session treatment of specific phobias.* Unpublished manuscript, Department of Psychology, Stockholm University and Child Study Centre, Department of Psychology, Virginia Polytechnic Institute and State University, Blacksburg, VA.

Öst, L. G., Svensson, L., Hellstrom, K., & Lindwall, R. (2001). One-session treatment of specific phobias in youths: A randomized clinical trial. *Journal of Consulting and Clinical Psychology, 69*(5), 814–824.

Pediatric OCD Treatment Study (POTS) Team. (2004). Cognitive-behavior therapy, sertraline, and their combination for children and adolescents with obsessive–compulsive disorder. *Journal of the American Medical Association, 292*(16), 1969–1976.

Poulton, R., & Menzies, R. G. (2002). Non-associative fear acquisition: A review of the evidence from retrospective and longitudinal research. *Behaviour Research and Therapy, 40*(2), 127–149.

Rachman, S. (1977). The conditioning theory of fearacquisition: A critical examination. *Behaviour Research and Therapy, 15*(5), 375–387.

Rapee, R. M., Schniering, C. A., & Hudson, J. L. (2009). Anxiety disorders during childhood and adolescence: Origins and treatment. *Annual Review of Clinical Psychology, 5*(1), 311–341.

Reinblatt, S. P., & Walkup, J. T. (2005). Psychopharmacologic treatment of pediatric anxiety disorders. *Child and Adolescent Psychiatric Clinics of North America, 14*(4), 877–908.

Ressler, K. J., Rothbaum, B. O., Tannenbaum, L., Anderson, P., Graap, K., Zimand, E., et al. (2004). Cognitive enhancers as adjuncts to psychotherapy: Use of D-cycloserine in phobic individuals to facilitate extinction of fear. *Archives of General Psychiatry, 61*(11), 1136–1144.

Reuterskiold, L., & Öst, L. G. (2012). Real world applications of one-session treatment. In T. E. Davis III, T. H. Ollendick, & L. G. Öst (Eds.), *Intensive one-session treatment of specific phobias* (pp. 127–141). New York: Springer.

Reynolds, C. R., & Kamphaus, R. W. (2004). *BASC-2: Behavior Assessment System for Children, second edition manual.* Circle Pines, MN: American Guidance Service.

Shaffer, D., Fisher, P., Lucas, C. P., Dulcan, M. K., & Schwab-Stone, M. E. (2000). NIMH Diagnostic Interview Schedule for Children Version IV (NIMH DISC-IV): Description, differences from previous versions, and reliability of some common diagnoses. *Journal of the American Academy of Child and Adolescent Psychiatry, 39*(1), 28–38.

Silverman, W. K., & Albano, A. M. (1996). *The Anxiety Disorders Interview Schedule for DSM-IV—Child and Parent Versions.* London: Oxford University Press.

Silverman, W. K., Kurtines, W. M., Ginsburg, G. S., Weems, C. F., Rabian, B., & Serafini, L. T. (1999). Contingency management, self-control, and education support in the treatment of childhood phobic disorders: A randomized clinical trial. *Journal of Consulting and Clinical Psychology, 67*(5), 675–687.

Silverman, W. K., & Nelles, W. B. (1989). An examination of the stability of mothers' ratings of child fearfulness. *Journal of Anxiety Disorders, 3*(1), 1–5.

Silverman, W. K., & Ollendick, T. H. (2005). Evidence-based assessment of anxiety and its disorders in children and adolescents. *Journal of Clinical Child and Adolescent Psychology, 34*(3), 380–411.

Silverman, W. K., & Ollendick, T. H. (2008). Assessment of child and adolescent anxiety disorders. In J. Hunsley & E. Mash (Eds.), *A guide to assessments that work* (pp. 181–206). New York: Oxford University Press.

Spence, S. H. (1998). A measure of anxiety symptoms among children. *Behaviour Research and Therapy, 36*(5), 545–566.

Spence, S. H., Holmes, J. M., March, S., & Lipp, O. V. (2006). The feasibility and outcome of clinic plus Internet delivery of cognitive-behavior therapy for childhood anxiety. *Journal of Consulting and Clinical Psychology, 74*(3), 614–621.

Stinson, F. S., Dawson, D. A., Chou, S. P., Smith, S., Goldstein, R. B., Ruan, W. J., et al. (2007). The epidemiology of DSM-IV specific phobia in the USA: Results from the National Epidemiologic Survey on Alcohol and Related Conditions. *Psychological Medicine, 37*(7), 1047–1059.

Vigerland, S., Thulin, U., Ljótsson, B., Svirsky, L., Öst, L. G., Lindefors, N., et al. (2013). Internet-delivered CBT for children with specific phobia: A pilot study. *Cognitive Behaviour Therapy, 42*(4), 303–314.

Walkup, J. T., Albano, A. M., Piacentini, J., Birmaher, B., Compton, S. N., Sherrill, J. T., et al. (2008). Cognitive behavioral therapy, sertraline, or a combination in childhood anxiety. *New England Journal of Medicine, 359*(26), 2753–2766.

Waters, A. M., Farrell, L. J., Zimmer-Gembeck, M., Milliner, E. L., Tiralongo, E., Donovan, C. L., et al. (2014). Augmenting one session treatment of children's specific phobias with attention training towards positive stimuli. *Behaviour Research and Therapy, 62*, 107–119.

Watts, F. N., McKenna, F. P., Sharrock, R., & Trezise, L. (1986). Colour naming of phobia-related words. *British Journal of Psychology, 77*(1), 97–108.

Weems, C. F., Silverman, W. K., Saavedra, L. M., Pina, A. A., & Lumpkin, P. W. (1999). The discrimination of children's phobias using the Revised Fear Survey Schedule for children. *Journal of Child Psychology and Psychiatry, 40*(6), 941–952.

Wolitzky-Taylor, K. B., Viar-Paxton, M. A., & Olatunji, B. O. (2012). Ethical issues when considering exposure. In T. E. Davis III, T. H. Ollendick, & L. G. Öst (Eds.), *Intensive one-session treatment of specific phobias* (pp. 195–208). New York: Springer.

Young, B. J., Ollendick, T. H., & Whiteside, S. P. (2014). Changing maladaptive behaviors, Part 1: Exposure and response prevention. In E. S. Sburlati, H. J. Lyneham, C. A. Schniering, & R. M. Rapee (Eds.), *Evidence-based CBT for anxiety and depression in children and adolescents: A competencies based approach* (pp. 194–207). West Sussex, UK: Wiley.

Zlomke, K., & Davis, T. E., III. (2008). One-session treatment of specific phobias: A detailed description and review of treatment efficacy. *Behavior Therapy, 39*(3), 207–223.

CHAPTER 8

Panic Disorder

Donna B. Pincus, Ashley Korn,
and Maria DiFonte

Panic disorder has been long viewed as one of the most severe and impairing anxiety disorders to affect youth. Distressing physiological sensations such as heart racing, shortness of breath, nausea, dizziness, feelings of "unreality," trembling, palpitations, and sweating appear to arise "out of the blue" and often lead to catastrophic cognitions and avoidance of any situations that might bring on panic-like sensations (Diler et al., 2004; Ollendick & Pincus, 2008). Thus, it is common for youth with panic disorder to avoid activities that are a normal part of everyday life such as school, classrooms, public transportation, crowds, movies, restaurants, school functions, and other developmentally appropriate activities because they are frightened that they might experience distressing physical sensations during these situations (Kearney, Albano, Eisen, Allan, & Barlow, 1997; Mattis & Pincus, 2004).

With developmentally appropriate activities curtailed, it is not surprising that youth with panic disorder also frequently experience interference and distress in many domains of their lives, including their academic, social, and family functioning. If not effectively treated, panic disorder and agoraphobia may place teens at increased risk for increased medical and emergency room use, for future psychopathology, and for poor medical and emotional health (Colman, Wadsworth, Croudace, & Jones, 2007). We provide in this chapter a detailed review of the literature on panic disorder in youth, including its definition, nature of the disorder, etiological models of panic, and a review of evidence-based assessment methods and treatment approaches. We conclude with a case illustration demonstrating the use of state-of-the-art cognitive-behavioral components for treating panic disorder in youth.

THE DSM-5 DEFINITION OF PANIC DISORDER

There are two primary symptoms in the diagnostic criteria for panic disorder. First, the child or adolescent must experience recurrent, unexpected panic attacks. As described in the fifth edition of the *Diagnostic and Statistical Manual of Mental Disorders* (DSM-5; American Psychiatric Association, 2013) a *panic attack* is defined as sudden intense fear or discomfort, which can peak within minutes. Symptoms of a panic attack include, but are not limited to, shortness of breath, heart palpitations, sweating, and trembling. To be diagnosed with panic disorder, these symptoms cannot be explained by another medical condition or mental disorder, or be the side effects of a drug or medication. Second, a minimum of one panic attack must be followed by at least 1 month of incessant worry about future panic attacks or consequences of the attack, such as death or losing control of one's body. Also, during the time following an attack, the child or adolescent may begin to display maladaptive behaviors in order to avoid triggering another panic attack. Additionally, the panic attacks must be unexpected; that is, they do not occur solely in response to a specific trigger. In the previous version of the DSM (DSM-IV), a diagnosis of panic disorder had to be accompanied by a specification regarding whether the individual also presented with symptoms of agoraphobia. However, with the development of the DSM-5, panic disorder and agoraphobia are now separate diagnoses. Youth with panic disorder are likely to experience impairments in many dimensions of functioning, including interpersonal relationships, academics, and psychosocial functioning (Essau, Conradt, & Petermann, 2000).

PREVALENCE AND COURSE

Studies have found that nearly 10% of children and adolescents experience at least one type of anxiety disorder (Merikangas et al., 2010). Children and adolescents between ages 13 and 18 have a lifetime prevalence rate of 2.3% for developing panic disorder specifically, with females having a higher prevalence rate (2.7%) than males (2.0%) (Merikangas et al., 2010). Another report of panic disorder in children and adolescents suggests that prevalence rates can be as high as 5% (Vallance & Garralda, 2008). In a relatively large sample (n = 472) of youth who are repeatedly referred for clinical treatment, the prevalence rate of panic disorder has been reported to be as high as 6% (Biederman et al., 1997). If symptoms of panic persist into adulthood, the 1-year prevalence rate for adults with panic disorder in the United States is between 2 and 3% (American Psychiatric Association, 2013). The gender difference for developing panic disorder is also found in adults; in self-reports of individuals with panic disorder, female respondents report experiencing more panic-related symptoms, such as shortness of breath, faintness, or choking, than do male respondents (Sheikh, Leskin, & Klein, 2002).

According to DSM-5 (American Psychiatric Association, 2013), panic disorder is rarely found in children younger than age 14 years old; it occurs in about 0.4% of this age group. This prevalence rate may be low because it is often difficult to distinguish whether their anxiety derives from a specific situation or object, separation from their primary caregivers, or the fear of having future panic attacks. According to the National Comorbidity Survey Replication Study, roughly one-fourth of individuals who develop panic disorder do so before age 16 (Kessler et al., 2005). Typically, the onset of panic disorder occurs when an individual is between 15 and 19 years of age (Silverman & Field, 2011).

When panic disorder symptoms emerge in childhood, several reasons have been proposed as to why the severity and chronicity of symptoms increase. First, mild symptoms early on may be dismissed as a "fearful phase," and parents may not seek out help in these early stages. Second, parents may not know how to help their distressed child, or they may feel anxious about being unable to soothe their child, then reinforce their child's symptoms by helping the child avoid panic-evoking situations. Sometimes parents intervene immediately in situations that they believe might bring about a panic attack, without giving their child the opportunity to face anxiety-inducing situations and learn coping strategies. Parents may accompany children to everyday activities in order to be "easily accessible" in the event that the child has a panic attack, or they may inadvertently reinforce the youth's avoidance of activities by providing differential attention to the child's avoidant behaviors in comparison to his or her approach behaviors. Not surprisingly, children struggling with anxiety disorders, including panic disorder, are more likely to have impairments in school, within their family, and in social relationships (Hughes, Loureau-Waddell, & Kendall, 2008). Many children with panic disorder fear being on school buses, in their classrooms, or in restaurants, as they worry that it will be difficult for them to be able to get out of these locations if they experience a panic attack (Kearney et al., 1997).

When panic disorder is left untreated, symptoms tend to vacillate between periods of recurrent panic attacks, along with anticipatory fear of future attacks, and periods when the individual does not have persistent symptoms. However, due to the high comorbidity of panic disorder and many other mental health disorders, such as depression, bipolar disorders, and other anxiety disorders (Kessler et al., 2006), the course of untreated panic disorder is very complicated. Adolescents and adults tend to have similar a course for untreated symptoms; however, with increasing age, concern for future panic attacks intensifies (American Psychiatric Association, 2013). Additionally, panic disorder has been found to have extreme homotypic continuity, suggesting that children with panic disorder are likely to be diagnosed continuously with panic disorder throughout adolescence and into early adulthood (Costello, Mustillo, Erkanli, Keeler, & Angold, 2003). Similarly, even when panic disorder is treated in children, it has been reported that the 3-year remission rate is around 70%, which is the lowest rate compared to other anxiety disorders, including separation anxiety disorder, which has a recovery rate of 82% (Bernstein, Borchardt, & Perwien, 1996).

COMMON COMORBID CONDITIONS

Youth diagnosed with panic disorder have a high likelihood of developing comorbid disorders; comorbidity rates up to 90% have been reported (Essau et al., 2000). One of the most common comorbid diagnoses to occur with panic disorder is depression; in fact, one study reported that approximately 63% of patients being treated for panic disorder experienced at least one major depressive episode during their lives (Stein, Tancer, & Uhde, 1990). Among children who have chronic or untreated panic disorder, some may later develop a form of bipolar disorder that is highly comorbid with panic disorder in both childhood and adulthood (Sala et al., 2010; Sugaya et al., 2013). Panic disorder has also been found to be comorbid with other anxiety disorders in children (Doerfler, Toscanojr, & Connor, 2008; Gallo, Chan, Buzzella, Whitton, & Pincus, 2012). In a recent study of panic disorder in youth between ages 8 and 17, about 51% of youth also had comorbid social anxiety disorder, roughly 48% also had generalized anxiety disorder, around 45% met criteria for a specific phobia, and approximately 25% also met criteria for major depressive disorder (Achiam-Montal, Tibi, & Lipsitz, 2013). When children and adolescents have comorbid anxiety disorders or major depression, their anxiety symptoms have been found to be much more severe than those of youth who meet criteria for only one of the comorbid disorders (Doerfler et al., 2008).

Future comorbidity problems for children with panic disorder may also include substance-related disorders, which have also been found to be highly comorbid with panic disorder and may possibly serve as the adolescent or adult's coping mechanism for his or her anxious thoughts and symptoms (Otto, Pollack, Sachs, O'Neil, & Rosenbaum, 1992; Robinson, Sareen, Cox, & Bolton, 2009). Children who have experienced sexual abuse have an increased likelihood of developing comorbid panic disorder and posttraumatic stress disorder (Leskin and Sheikh, 2002). Panic disorder has also been linked to several co-occurring medical conditions both in childhood and adulthood, including asthma (Friedman & Morris, 2006; Goodwin, Pine, & Hoven, 2003; Perna, Bertani, Politi, Colombo, & Bellodi, 1997), chronic obstructive pulmonary disease (COPD; Smoller et al., 2003), dizziness, and cardiac arrhythmias (Peacock & Whang, 2013); however, the exact relationship between these physiological symptoms and panic disorder is unknown. Moreover, several studies that have found a significant association between the presence of panic disorder and allergies in children (e.g., Friedman & Morris, 2006; Kovalenko et al., 2001).

ETIOLOGICAL/CONCEPTUAL MODEL(S) OF PANIC DISORDER

There are several possible reasons that individuals, particularly children, develop panic disorder, and these different pathways are quite complex. Several key theories of the development of panic disorder posit that panic is the consequence of multiple, contributing factors. For example, Clark (1986) posits that in panic disorder, an internal or external stimulus increases one's perceived threat, which amplifies one's bodily sensations, leads to cataclysmic misinterpretations, and in turn, heightens perceived threat. Barlow (2002) and Barlow, Raffa, and Cohen (2002) propose a "triple vulnerability" model of the etiological components of panic disorder, such that an individual's biological vulnerabilities (e.g., genetic risk factors), general psychological vulnerabilities (e.g., the child's temperament and experiences of lack of control with stressful events), and specific psychological vulnerabilities (e.g., anxieties acquired through parent modeling) synergistically combine to make an individual more susceptible to developing panic symptoms. Children who have an inherited vulnerability to experience negative emotion, and who have been exposed to negative, stressful events in their environment, have a higher probability of developing symptoms such as increased physical sensations, intensified physiological arousal, and overwhelming fear (Barlow et al., 2002; Mattis & Ollendick, 1997). We now expand on each of these etiological factors—genetic/biological vulnerabilities, general psychological vulnerabilities, and specific psychological vulnerabilities—in turn.

Genetic/Biological Vulnerabilities

The development of panic disorder has been found, in many studies, to have a genetic component. Heritability rates of panic disorder are among the highest of any type of anxiety disorder and were found to be as great as 44% (Kendler et al., 1995). One way to measure heritability of panic disorder is to look at the likelihood that children of parents with panic disorder will eventually develop panic disorder symptoms themselves. It has been found that there is a direct association between parental panic disorder and off-spring panic disorder, whether or not the parent has comorbid major depressive disorder (Biederman et al., 2001). Genetic heritability has been shown through various pathways, including direct parent-to-child symptoms of panic disorder, or through different forms of temperament, including both behavioral inhibition and anxiety sensitivity in the child (Smoller et al., 2005; Van Beek & Griez, 2003).

Another empirically based theory for the etiology of panic disorder involves an individual's biological systems. The neuroanatomical hypothesis of Gorman, Kent, Sullivan, and Coplan (2000) suggests that panic attacks have behavioral responses similar to a conditioned fear response, such as autonomic arousal and avoidance of fear-evoking stimuli. The fear response pathway in the brain, which includes the amygdala, hippocampus, thalamus, and brainstem, is highly over-activated and is extremely sensitive to physical sensations and external situations. Dysregulation of normal amygdala activation then leads individuals to misinterpret their bodily sensations and continually have panic attacks (Gorman et al., 2000). In addition to this hypothesis, Bourin, Baker, and Bradwejn (1998) found that several neurotransmitter and neuromodulator systems are associated with panic disorder. These include serotonin, gamma-aminobutyric acid (GABA), norepinephrine, and dopamine, which have been shown to have a strong impact on an individual's conditioned responses.

General Psychological Vulnerabilities

Research has shown that the temperamental construct of behavioral inhibition may be a potential mediator through which panic disorder is passed down genetically. Rosenbaum and colleagues (2000) found that children of parents with comorbid panic disorder and major depression had an increased likelihood of displaying signs of behavioral inhibition in their youth. Other researchers have also established an association among childhood behavioral inhibition, social anxiety, and panic disorder in late adolescence and early adulthood (Rosenbaum, Biederman, Bolduc, & Chaloff, 1991; Sportel, Nauta, de Hullu, de Jong, & Hartman, 2011). Smoller and colleagues (2005) discovered that the cortiotropin-releasing hormone (CRH) gene is strongly associated with symptoms of behavioral inhibition, and this gene is frequently found concurrently in parents with panic disorder and their children.

The generational aggregation of panic disorder may also occur through several alternative pathways, one of which may be an individual's level of anxiety sensitivity, which has been shown to be quite heritable (Van Beek & Griez, 2003). Anxiety sensitivity plays an important role in the emergence of panic disorder. If a child or adolescent is particularly sensitive to physical sensations and fearful of external events, in a threatening situation, he or she may overreact and experience an overwhelming sense of fear, which can eventually lead to a panic attack. A vicious cycle may ensue as the individual becomes aware of his or her anxiety and worries about the threat of future panic attacks. As Pilecki, Arentoft, and McKay (2011) discussed in their etiological model of panic disorder, individuals who have had early experiences of lack of control over their environments or an anxious temperament may have a predisposition toward panicky tendencies. A child who is highly sensitive to anxiety-provoking situations and has aversive reactions to his or her resulting bodily sensations may develop catastrophic cognitions about these physiological sensations, which result in panic attacks and fear in regards to future attacks (Pileki et al., 2011).

Hayward, Killen, Karemer, and Taylor (2000) explored which specific risk factors were predictors of panic disorder symptoms in adolescents. They found that both anxiety sensitivity and negative affect predicted the likelihood that adolescents would have four-symptom panic attacks. While the constructs of anxiety sensitivity and neuroticism have empirical evidence for heritability, both are clearly major components of cognitive theories for the development of panic disorder. These theories, focusing on the individual's maladaptive cognitions as the main predictor or causal factor for panic disorder, have been long-standing in research on panic disorder.

A child's experiences may even contribute to the emergence of panic disorder in late adolescence or early adulthood. Craske, Poulton, Tsao, and Plotkin (2001) examined the possible pathways for developing panic disorder specifically in children, through their sample of 992 children who were 3 years old. Over the course of this longitudinal study, researchers sought to predict the development of a variety of anxiety disorders at ages 18 and 21 by measuring children's anxious temperament at age 3, and tracking their or their families' experiences with illness, along with their level of anxiety symptoms. Higher incidence of respiratory problems, including asthma and COPD, was more common in children who developed panic disorder (Craske et al., 2001). Also, it has been shown that children who are exposed to physical or sexual abuse are at increased risk of either developing panic disorder or having panic attacks in late adolescence or early adulthood (Goodwin, Fergusson, & Horwood, 2005). Similarly, a proportion of adults with panic disorder also report having been sexually molested in their youth; about 24% of females and 5% of males with panic disorder who participated in the National Comorbidity Survey reported having experienced early sexual abuse (Leskin & Sheikh, 2002).

Specific Psychological Vulnerabilities

Parents may also pass down panic disorder to their children through modeling or priming. Many researchers have examined how parents with a variety of anxiety disorders serve as models for how young children interpret and react to their surroundings. Not surprisingly, when parents are fearful of either their environment or social settings, or of more specific objects, they are likely to display symptoms in their interactions with their child, especially in how they reinforce and punish their child's behaviors, which has a major impact on shaping how the child behaves and interacts with others. Mothers with panic disorder have been shown to be more likely to express significantly high levels of expressed emotion and to be less likely to promote autonomy in their children (Challacombe & Salkovskis, 2009; Moore, Whaley, & Sigman, 2004). Moore and colleagues (2004) found that anxious mothers were less warm toward their children and also more likely to catastrophize their situations, which significantly predicted children's level of anxiety. Also, children who are not given the opportunity to be autonomous due to their parent's anxiety have an increased probability of developing anxiety symptoms themselves (Whaley, Pinto, & Sigman, 1999).

The effects of anxious parenting on children have been explored in a study by Schneider, Unnewehr, Florin, and Margraf (2002). These authors found that children of parents with panic disorder showed a significant increase in their anxious interpretations when they were primed for panic situations. Although the children in this study were not diagnosed with panic disorder, they may be at a higher risk of developing panic disorder, since they are more inclined to interpret situations through a panic "lens." Children are likely to model their parents' anxious behaviors, as their experiences with their parents make up the largest proportion of their total learning experiences, especially prior to the start of school. These children, starting from a very young age, may be developing an anxious schema on how to react to threatening or even ambiguous situations. McNally (2002) suggests that parental modeling of anxious behaviors also may have an impact on children's anxiety sensitivity, which is a clear risk factor in developing a variety of anxiety disorders, including panic disorder.

EVIDENCE-BASED TREATMENTS FOR PANIC DISORDER

Review of the Existing Evidence Base: Psychosocial Treatments

Cognitive-behavioral therapy (CBT) is currently the state-of-the-art psychological treatment for youth with anxiety disorders generally, and for panic disorder in particular. The current leading CBT method specific to panic disorder in youth is the Panic Control Treatment for Adolescents (PCT-A; Hoffman & Mattis, 2000; Mattis & Ollendick, 1997; Pincus, May, Whitton, Mattis, & Barlow, 2010). Prior to the development of PCT-A, Ollendick (1995) was the first to examine the treatment of panic disorder in children and adolescents using a multiple baseline design study. Ollendick's treatment method included cognitive-behavioral components taken from effective treatments of panic disorder in adults (Barlow, Craske, Cerny, & Klosko, 1989). Ollendick (1995) included four adolescent participants who were diagnosed with panic disorder with agoraphobia. Following treatment, all participants showed a significant drop in panic attack frequency and agoraphobic avoidance, as well as enhanced mood and greater self-efficacy in coping with anxiety. This early study was a catalyst for studying ways to tailor cognitive-behavioral methods to treat panic disorder in children and adolescents.

Following the promising results from Ollendick (1995), Hoffman and Mattis (2000) adapted and piloted PCT-A, an 11-session CBT-based protocol originally developed for adults, which addresses three main aspects of panic: cognitive misinterpretations, the hyperventilatory response, and conditioned reactions to physical sensations (Barlow et al., 1989). The developmentally adapted PCT-A protocol retained the main treatment components of adult panic control treatment but simplified the language and used age-appropriate examples to foster understanding and engagement. Hoffman and Mattis noted that agoraphobic avoidance behaviors, such as skipping school, had been observed in the majority of adolescents with panic, and that this aspect is particularly detrimental to adolescents, who may be missing out on important developmental activities. Therefore, an exposure component was added in order to help adolescents overcome feared situations. A parental treatment component was also developed to guide parents in understanding panic disorder. Pincus and colleagues (2010) conducted a randomized controlled trial (RCT) to evaluate this 11-session PCT-A. This study included 26 participants ages 14–17, diagnosed with panic disorder, with or without agoraphobia. Participants were randomly assigned to immediate PCT-A or to a self-monitoring control group. The PCT-A group, in comparison to the control group, showed significant reductions from pre- to posttreatment in the severity and frequency of panic symptoms. PCT-A participants' average panic severity was reduced to subclinical levels at posttreatment, and these reductions were maintained over 6 months following treatment. Participants also showed improvements in anxiety sensitivity, general anxiety, and depressive symptoms, which point to the possibility that the skills learned in PCT-A, such as identifying and correcting cognitive distortions, can generalize to other issues. Adolescents' avoidance of developmentally appropriate activities, a key target of the treatment, also was significantly reduced. The acceptability and satisfaction with the treatment was rated highly by the participants and their families. Parental involvement was seen as an important component based on parent reports. Overall, this randomized clinical trial showed strong initial support for the efficacy of PCT-A to treat adolescents diagnosed with panic disorder.

New Promising Intensive Format of PCT-A

During the first RCT of PCT-A (Pincus et al., 2010), the primary reason that participants declined to participate in the study was the lengthy treatment (12 weeks). Many parents inquired about whether there were any other, more expedient forms of treatment available, so that their children could return more rapidly to participating in developmentally important activities. Patients in the first RCT of PCT-A also indicated that they would have benefited from having therapists accompany them during *in vivo* exposures. Thus, a larger RCT was conducted to pilot-test the efficacy of an intensive, 8-day treatment program for youth with panic disorder and agoraphobia (Gallo et al., 2012; 2014; Hardway, Pincus, Gallo, & Comer, 2015; Pincus et al., 2015; Pincus, Leyfer, Hardway, Elkins, & Comer, 2014). The 8-day, intensive protocol incorporated similar treatment components to those in the 11-session PCT-A, but delivered the same "dose" of treatment over a shorter time period (8 days). The study design of this intensive format of PCT-A allowed for the investigation of the relative benefit of parent involvement in treatment. Unlike the 11-session version of PCT-A, the 8-day intensive format of treatment was modified to include therapist-assisted *in vivo* exposures.

Angelosante, Pincus, Whitton, Cheron, and Pian (2009) outlined the structure and key features, and described the implementation of this intensive panic intervention for adolescents. The first session is spent building rapport, presenting psychoeducation about panic to the patient and their family, and gaining a better understanding of the patient's anxiety and panic symptoms. Patients learn about the fight-or-flight system and the reasons that it is adaptive to survival. The second session focuses on helping the patient understand the relationship between the physiological, cognitive and behavioral aspects of panic disorder. In the third session, patients learn that the physical sensations of panic are not harmful by conducting a series of symptom induction exercises called *interoceptive exposure exercises*. The fourth and fifth sessions consist of therapist-assisted *in vivo* exposures; patients work with therapists to enter previously avoided situations. Adolescents continue working on exposures independently during the sixth and seventh sessions. In the final session, the therapist reviews the skills learned, talks about relapse prevention strategies, and establishes a plan and schedule for future exposure practice. Throughout treatment, there are homework assignments that require patients to monitor and record their anxiety and panic experiences, challenge their automatic thoughts and beliefs, and continue practicing interoceptive and *in vivo* exposures. During the 4 weeks following treatment, therapists check in via telephone to monitor patients' progress. The goal of the check-in is to transfer control from the therapist to the patient, so that the patient gradually begins to work independently toward attaining his or her therapy goals.

There are some important considerations that therapists should be aware of when using this treatment in youth with panic disorder. Angelosante and colleagues (2009) noted that although rapport may be difficult to establish over such a short period of time, it is essential that trust between therapist and patient be established to set the stage for successful exposures. It is suggested that the therapist take on the role of a coach who will help guide youth as they adopt and practice new skills. This idea of a "coach" is likely to be very familiar and easily grasped by adolescents and should help to facilitate trust. Also of importance is making sure the patient is actively participating by creating his or her own goals throughout treatment, which allows the therapist to actively support those goals and enhance rapport. The authors acknowledge that the full-day sessions of *in vivo* exposures is likely new and challenging for therapists who typically are accustomed to conducting briefer, 50- to 60-minute office-based sessions. They state that these sessions take planning and preparation, and the ability to maintain adolescents' motivation and positivity throughout the day. It is also important to allow patients to take over the responsibility of directing themselves through exposures, so that they have the skills to conduct exposures independently posttreatment. During the 11-session PCT-A, the transfer of control from therapist to patient can take place gradually, but in the 8-day intensive program, it is important to get the patient actively involved on the first day of exposures. Therapists can facilitate this involvement by allowing patients to choose their next exposure, and helping them to brainstorm ways to increase the level of challenge with each exposure practice (e.g., by removing safety behaviors such as holding a "good luck charm," which only further escalates anxiety in the long term). By using these skills, therapists are helping patients to develop skills for continued improvement even once treatment ends.

Preliminary studies of this intensive, 8-day format of PCT-A show promise. In an RCT (Pincus et al., 2015) 52 adolescent patients, ages 11–17, were randomly assigned to one of three treatment conditions: (1) intensive adolescent panic treatment without parent involvement, (2) intensive adolescent panic treatment with parent involvement, or (3) a wait-list condition. Participants in both of the intensive treatment conditions showed significantly greater reductions in panic attack frequency and the severity of their panic symptomatology after the program compared to participants in the wait-list condition. Panic attack severity was measured by the 7-item Panic Disorder Severity Scale (PDSS;

Elkins, Pincus, & Comer, 2014; Pincus et al., 2015). Adolescents who received intensive treatment also reported significant improvement in their fear and avoidance ratings over the course of treatment, as measured by the Anxiety Disorders Interview Schedule for DSM-IV for Children/Parents (Silverman & Albano, 1996). Adolescents who were randomly assigned to the individual treatment and the treatment that included parents showed comparable improvement on all measures of panic. Adolescents who received the intensive panic treatment showed significant reductions in comorbid clinical diagnoses, including specific phobias, generalized anxiety disorder, and social phobia (Gallo et al., 2012). These findings suggest that the skills learned in the intensive program, like those in the weekly program, can generalize to other issues not specifically targeted by the treatment. Hardway and colleagues (2015) investigated whether this intensive treatment for panic disorder also conferred a corollary benefit of ameliorating symptoms of patients' depression; results of this study showed that younger patients benefited more from treatment without parent involvement than did older patients with regard to depression symptoms. A study of the rate and shape of change over the course of the intensive panic treatment showed that panic severity showed linear change, decreasing steadily throughout the intensive treatment, while fear and avoidance ratings showed cubic change, peaking slightly at the first session of treatment, decreasing at the second session of treatment, then improving steadily through the fourth session (Gallo, Cooper-Vince, Hardway, Pincus, & Comer, 2014).

Chase, Whitton, and Pincus (2012) conducted a nonrandomized controlled trial comparing weekly versus intensive PCT-A. Both treatments showed very large treatment effects, and symptom improvements were maintained at a 6-month follow-up. Potentially, there are many additional benefits of the 8-day intensive treatment, such as greater treatment accessibility and more rapid reduction in symptoms, so that patients can return more quickly to healthy functioning. Overall, results of the studies evaluating both the weekly and intensive formats of PCT-A are quite promising. Further studies on intensive PCT-A are currently under way, to better understand potential mechanisms underlying changes in treatment.

Pharmacological Interventions

Very few studies have focused specifically on the use of psychopharmacological treatments for children and adolescents with panic disorder. Most of the larger studies to date have focused on the use of psychopharmacological treatments for more prevalent anxiety disorders (e.g., social phobia, generalized anxiety disorder, or separation anxiety disorder), and have excluded youth with panic disorder. (For a detailed review of pharmacological interventions for anxiety disorders in youth, see Wolff et al., Chapter 4, this volume.) To date, only two small, open-label studies and one retrospective chart analysis have specifically focused on the use of selective serotonin reuptake inhibitors (SSRIs) to treat children and adolescents with panic disorder. Masi and colleagues (2001) examined charts of 18 patients, between ages 7 and 16, diagnosed with panic disorder and treated with SSRIs. The majority (83.3%) showed significant improvements in their panic symptomatology, with more than half reporting full remission. There were frequent side effects of the medication reported, but they were mild and transient, and did not result in the reduction of dose. The mean dose at initial response was 22 mg and the mean dose at follow-up was 23.9 mg, suggesting that doses did not have to be significantly increased over time and they were much smaller than the amount needed to treat adults (typically 40 mg). The patients also showed rapid improvement after an average period of only 3 weeks. Two open-label pilot studies conducted by Renaud, Birmaher, Wassick, and Bridge (1999) and Fairbanks and colleagues (1997) pointed out the efficacy and safety of SSRIs in the treatment of children and adolescents with panic disorder. Fairbanks and colleagues' study had a total sample of 16 children, ages 9–17, five of whom were diagnosed with panic disorder. Overall, the majority of patients in this study showed clinical improvement and minimal side effects, with improvements on average beginning at 5 weeks. Renaud and colleagues' study included 12 subjects, ages 8–18, all diagnosed with panic disorder. In this study, benzodiazepines were used in conjunction with SSRIs for those presenting with severe symptoms. The use of SSRIs alone and in combination with short-term use of benzodiazepines was shown to be safe and effective.

A review of the pharmacological management of panic disorder in adults conducted by Marchesi (2008) summarized studies that have shown tricyclic antidepressants, monoamine oxidase inhibitors (MAOIs), benzodiazepines, and SSRIs to be more effective than placebo in the treatment of panic disorder in adults. Although there were no comparable treatment effect differences among the four classes of drugs, their less aversive side effect profile compared to the others makes SSRIs the drug class of choice. However, the noted disadvantages of SSRIs may be especially problematic for those with panic disorder. SSRI side effects include anxiety, agitation, insomnia, tremors, and nausea; these symptoms may be triggers for panic attacks in patients with panic disorder. Tricyclic antidepressants were the first and most studied drug class, but their side effects in comparison to the newer class of SSRIs made them less advantageous. MAOIs are only considered a second-line treatment due to their side effects. Benzodiazepines are very commonly prescribed because they act quickly and are very tolerable, but they come with many disadvantages, such as side effects, reduced effect on often comorbid depression, and the risk of tolerance, withdrawal, and abuse. For these reasons, benzodiazepines are not the first choice in treating panic disorder. However, benzodiazepines have been used in combination with SSRIs to help patients get through the initial negative response to SSRIs activation side effects, which typically last 4 to 6 weeks. Giving benzodiazepines in these first few weeks has been shown to reduce severity and frequency of panic attacks when starting SSRI treatment (Marchesi, 2008).

In summary, the existing preliminary studies that have examined the efficacy of SSRIs and benzodiazepines in youth with panic disorder have shown initial positive effects on reducing symptoms of panic, with minimal side effects. SSRIs have been shown to be beneficial in the treatment of adults with panic disorder, and in children and adolescents with other anxiety disorders. Benzodiazepines may also function over the short term to reduce severe symptoms at presentation and when beginning the use of SSRIs in order to combat negative side effects. However, there is little evidence of the efficacy of benzodiazepines for treatment of children and adolescents with anxiety; thus, this drug is not currently recommended. SSRIs remain the most promising pharmacological treatment, and the evidence base for the use of SSRIs in treating children and adolescents with panic disorder is growing. RCTs are still needed to confirm the safety and efficacy of using SSRIs with children and adolescents with panic disorder.

Predictors and Moderators of Treatment Response

Examining predictors and moderators of treatment response in youth with panic may allow for better understanding of prognosis following treatment and for more personalized adjustments to interventions in order to suit individual patients best. A number of factors may be both predictors of treatment response in youth with panic and moderators of treatment response, which can change the magnitude or direction of the effects of treatment. For example, predictors and moderators of panic treatment outcome might include child and adolescent characteristics such as age, gender, or level of motivation, parent and family characteristics such as family functioning and parenting stress, or therapist and intervention characteristics such as therapeutic alliance or treatment duration. Presence of comorbid disorders may be another factor that is important to consider due to the high rate of comorbid anxiety, mood, or other disorders and panic disorder in youth.

Although numerous studies in the child literature have examined predictors and moderators of treatment for child anxiety disorders generally (e.g., Rapee et al., 2013), very few studies have specifically examined predictors and moderators in samples of youth with panic disorder specifically. Thus, relatively little is known about the conditions under which panic treatment for adolescents is most effective. One recent study (Elkins, Gallo, Pincus & Comer, 2016) examined the moderating roles of baseline fear and avoidance in the intensive treatment of 52 adolescents with panic disorder, with or without agoraphobia (PDA), randomized to either an intensive CBT panic treatment ($n = 37$) or a wait-list condition ($n = 17$). In this study, PDA diagnosis, symptom severity, and number of feared and avoided situations were assessed at baseline and 6-week, posttreatment/post wait list. Hierarchical regression analyses examined the relative contributions of treatment condition, number of baseline feared or avoided situations, and their interactions in the prediction of posttreatment/wait-list PDA symptoms. The results of this study showed that the main effect of intensive CBT treatment on posttreatment PDA symptoms was not uniform across participants, with larger treatment effects found among participants with lower, relative to higher, baseline levels of fear and avoidance. These findings help to clarify which adolescents may benefit most from an intensive treatment format.

Other predictors of treatment outcome that may be particularly relevant to examine in youth with panic disorder are level of motivation, readiness to change, therapeutic alliance between the patient and therapist, and patient and family involvement and engagement with treatment. These constructs have yet to be examined in samples of youth with panic disorder, but they have been shown to influence treatment outcomes in youth with other anxiety disorders (e.g., La Greca, Silverman, & Lochman, 2009; Shirk & Karver, 2003). Factors such as engagement and therapeutic alliance are likely to be particularly relevant for youth with panic disorder given that CBT requires the motivation to engage in exposures that might cause temporary but heightened anxiety. Having a strong therapeutic alliance with one's therapist might help adolescents with panic to engage in exposures more readily. Furthermore, factors such as family involvement and engagement in the treatment process may impact the success of treatment for panic disorder in youth given that the interoceptive and *in vivo* exposures that youth must conduct outside of therapy sessions often require parental support and encouragement.

In studies particular to CBT interventions for panic disorder in adults, several predictors of treatment have emerged that may well be relevant for treatment of panic in youth. Dow and colleagues (2007) found younger age at first experienced panic attack, comorbid social anxiety, and higher severity of agoraphobic avoidance when unaccompanied by another person were all predictors of worse outcomes. Panic attacks experienced at a young age were also associated with stronger dysfunctional beliefs and fears regarding panic, further stressing the importance of early intervention. Further studies on the predictors and moderators of treatment outcomes following CBT for adolescents with panic are under way and will help clinicians better adapt these treatments to their individual patients and their families.

EVIDENCE-BASED ASSESSMENT AND TREATMENT IN PRACTICE

Assessment

Differential Diagnosis

Differential diagnoses are important to consider when assessing children and adolescents with panic disorder because it is quite common for these youth to have other primary diagnoses. Children may only be assigned a diagnosis of panic disorder when they experience panic attacks that do not occur solely in the context of other forms of anxiety or mood disorders. If their panic attacks occur only in the context of separation situations, for example, but children do not experience worry about a future panic attack, then they cannot be given a diagnosis of panic disorder. Similarly, children who have certain medical conditions, such as asthma, diabetes, cardiopulmonary conditions, and hyperthyroidism, cannot be diagnosed with panic disorder if they experience panic attacks as a direct response to physiological symptoms associated with their condition (American Psychiatric Association, 2013). For clinicians, it is very important to be cognizant of whether the patient has any other medical conditions, and to make a good judgment regarding whether that medical problem is a trigger for the panic attacks (Ollendick, Mattis, & Birmaher, 2004). Finally, when assessing adolescents for panic disorder, it is important to determine whether substances, including over-the-counter medications, prescription drugs, alcohol, or any other substances, are eliciting the panic attacks. This also applies to stimulants of the central nervous system, such as caffeine or amphetamines. Panic disorder may only be diagnosed if panic attacks occur prior to the initiation of substance use (American Psychiatric Association, 2013).

Structured and Semistructured Clinical Interviews

One of the field's "gold-standard" methods for assessing panic in youth is using a comprehensive diagnostic clinical interview. One of the most well-established clinical interviews for diagnosing youth with panic is the semistructured Anxiety Disorders Interview Schedule for the DSM-IV—Child version (ADIS-IV-C; Silverman & Albano, 1996), which has been found to be very reliable in assessing a variety of childhood anxiety disorders. The ADIS interview comprises sections that comprehensively assess all anxiety disorders occurring in youth, along with sections assessing commonly comorbid disorders (e.g., depression, attention problems, substance use disorders, and posttraumatic stress disorder) and sections assessing school-related and peer-related functioning. In assessing the presence of panic disorder, clinicians gather pertinent information regarding the presence, frequency, and severity of unexpected panic attacks, as well as the degree to which worry about panic attacks is causing impairment in the child and family's functioning. The parent ADIS interview allows parents or caregivers to provide their perspective on the severity and interference caused by the child's symptoms. Each category of anxiety is assigned a clinical severity rating on a scale of 0 to 8, ranging from "mild" to "severe" levels of interference and distress, respectively (Silverman, Saavedra, & Pina, 2001). Generally a clinical severity rating score above a 4 is determined to be clinically significant. Wood, Piacentini, Bergman, McCracken, and Barrios (2002) compared the panic disorder scores of both the Child and Parent versions of the ADIS to those of the validated Multidimensional Anxiety Scale for Children (March, Parker, Sullivan, Stallings, & Conners, 1997) and found that the scores from both measures were significantly correlated. The ADIS-C/P remains the "gold-standard" semistructured interview tool used to assess and diagnose children's panic disorder symptoms.

Self-Report and Parent-Report Measures

In addition to the ADIS, self-report measures should be included in a diagnostic assessment of youth with panic disorder. The PDSS was designed to assess panic symptoms and impairment in persons over age 18 with current or lifetime panic disorder diagnoses. Cronbach's alpha for the PDSS has been found to be between .88 and .92 (Houck, Spiegel, Shear, & Rucci, 2002; Shear et al., 2001). Building on this work, researchers recently developed a child/adolescent version of the PDSS, called the *Panic Disorder Severity Scale for Children* (PDSS-C; Elkins et al., 2014). This seven-item measure was tailored for children and adolescents in several ways, including the replacement of questions about work interference with questions about school interference. This measure has been reported to have strong reliability and other psychometric properties (Elkins et al., 2014), and to date is the only known panic-specific child self-report measure.

Other youth self-report measures that can be particularly useful in assessing panic disorder symptoms include the *Childhood Anxiety Sensitivity Index* (CASI; Silverman et al., 1991), the MASC (March et al., 1997), and the *Screen for Child Anxiety and Related Emotional Disorders* (SCARED; Birmaher et al., 1997; Muris, et al., 1998). Spence (1997) developed a child-report scale, the *Spence Children's Anxiety Scale* (SCAS-C), which is used to measure a variety of anxiety and related disorders, including panic disorder, social phobia, and obsessive–compulsive disorder in children between ages 8 and 12.

To supplement these child self-report measures, parent reports are very beneficial to conceptualize fully the child or adolescents' distress levels and impairment due to panic. Some commonly used parental reports include the *Parent Anxiety Rating Scale* (PAR; Doris et al., 1971) and the *Child Behavior Checklist* (CBCL; Achenbach & Edelbrock, 1983; Achenbach & Rescorla, 1991). Another psychometrically sound parent-report measure for child anxiety levels is the *Spence Children's Anxiety Scale—Parent version* (SCAS-P; Spence, 1998). One final parent-report measure for assessing child anxiety levels is the *Screen for Child Anxiety Related Emotional Disorders—Revised* (SCARED-R; Birmaher et al., 1997), which has moderate-to-high agreement between the child and parent versions. A list of some of the key child and parent self-report measures used in the assessment of panic is also provided in Table 8.1.

TABLE 8.1. Commonly Used Self-Report and Parent-Report Measures for Assessing Panic Disorder and Related Disorders In Youth

Measure	Researchers	Disorders assessed	Population assessed	Reliability
		Self-report measures		
Panic-focused measures				
Panic Disorder Severity Scale— Children (PDSS-C)	Elkins & colleagues (2014)	Panic disorder with or without agoraphobia	11- to 17-year-olds	0.82 (Elkins et al., 2014)
Child Anxiety Sensitivity Index (CASI)	Silverman & colleagues (1991)	Panic disorder and GAD	7- to 17-year-olds	0.76 (Chorpita & Daleiden, 2000)
Broader child anxiety-focused measures				
Multidimensional Anxiety Scale for Children (MASC)	March & colleagues (1997)	Physical symptoms, harm avoidance, social anxiety, and separation/panic disorders	8- to 13-year-olds	0.74 (Baldwin & Dadds, 2007)
Spence Children's Anxiety Scale (SCAS)	Spence (1997)	Social phobia, panic disorder, SAD, OCD, GAD, physical injury	6- to 18-year-olds	0.92 (Spence, 1998)
Screen for Child Anxiety Related Emotional Disorders—Revised (SCARED-R)	Birmaher & colleagues (1997)	Separation anxiety, GAD, panic disorder, OCD, PTSD, social, specific, and school anxiety	7- to 17-year-olds	0.74–0.93 (Birmaher et al., 1999; Muris et al., 2004)
		Parent-report measures		
Parent Anxiety Rating Scale	Doris & colleagues (1971)	General fears and anxieties of childhood		0.82 (Doris et al., 1971)
Child Behavior Checklist	Achenbach & Edelbrock (1983)	Behavior and emotional problems		0.8–0.94 (Achenback & Rescorla, 2001)
Spence Children's Anxiety Scale—Parent (SCAS-P)	Spence (1998)	Separation anxiety, GAD, panic disorder, OCD, PTSD, social, specific, and school anxiety		0.8–0.91 (Nauta et al., 2004)
Screen for Child Anxiety-Related Emotional Disorders—Revised (SCARED-R)	Birmaher & colleagues (1997)	Separation anxiety, GAD, panic disorder, OCD, PTSD, social, specific, and school anxiety		0.64–0.87 (Muris et al., 2004)

Note. GAD, generalized anxiety disorder; OCD, obsessive–compulsive disorder; PTSD, posttraumatic stress disorder; SAD, social anxiety disorder.

Objective Measures

A final way to assess panic symptoms of youth is through objective measures, which can be conducted in sessions or in a laboratory setting. Some of these assessment tools include skin conductance and heart rate variability measures. Scarpa, Raine, Venables, and Mednick (1997) studied both of these physiological features in young children. Three-year-olds who were behaviorally inhibited displayed significantly increased heart rate variability and skin conductance, along with longer skin conductance latency, than same-age children who were not inhibited (Scarpa et al., 1997). Although these children were not necessarily anxious and did not have panic disorder, behaviorally inhibited children are at risk of developing panic disorder later in their lives. Additionally, children of parents with panic disorder have displayed a slight decrease in cardiac vagal function compared to children of parents without panic disorder, which may suggest a possible heritable trait in abnormal heart rate variability for individuals with panic disorder (Srinivasan, Ashok, Vaz, & Yeragani, 2002).

One study that examined heart rate and other physiological markers in children of parents with panic disorder found that, compared to children with parents who do not have any mental health problems, these children experienced a higher heart rate and increased behavioral inhibition during mildly stressful scenes (Battaglia et al., 1997). However, other physiological measures, including respiratory rates and cortisol secretion, did not appear to be significantly different between groups. Battaglia and his colleagues suggest that the differences in heart rate may be signs of a vulnerability to panic disorder. Similar findings of increased heart rate variability have been found in adults with panic disorder (Friedman & Thayer, 1998; Stein & Asmundson, 1994). Since there is a lack of these types of studies with young patient samples, it would be helpful if future studies could include measures of physiological responses in their assessment of panic disorder in children to deepen our understanding of children and adolescents' experience of panic and to better understand whether therapy has the potential to change these physiological responses in some way. Although physiological equipment is still costly, relatively cumbersome, and prone to error, and may be impractical for therapists to utilize in community and clinical settings, future research studies might examine the potential clinical utility of using physiological data to enhance treatment. For example, if youth with panic disorder could visually observe their heightened heart rate during an exposure, while also noticing that no catstrophic outcomes occurred (e.g., having a heart attack or going crazy), this might potentially be clinically helpful. Furthermore, physiological data could be used to provide real-time feedback to youth in session, for example, if they could watch how their heart rate decreases after using cognitive restructuring exercises effectively. Thus, future research that incorporates physiological assessment could shed light on new ways to potentially enhance our current treatment methods.

Additional Measures

Several other areas of functioning are important to assess in patients with panic disorder, including sleep problems and overall family functioning. One of the more common sleep measures for children is the *Children's Sleep Habits Questionnaire* (CSHQ; Owens, Spirito, & McGuinn, 2000), which is a parent report measure that assesses children's sleep patterns, including sleep-onset delay, sleep latency, sleep-disordered breathing, bed-time resistance, and parasomnias. An assessment tool that is used to determine the level of functioning of the child's entire family is the *McMaster Family Assessment Device* (FAD; Epstein, Baldwin, & Bishop, 1983). This scale measures the family's level of communication, affective responsiveness, problem-solving skills, behavior control, roles, general functioning, and affective involvement with other members. The FAD has been shown to be effective in identifying families at risk for a variety of negative outcomes, including child psychopathology, and helps determine whether the family should seek out preventive interventions before problems arise within the family (Akister & Stevenson-Hinde, 1991).

Future Improvements in Assessment

Although existing child and parent reports, clinician observations, and other objective measures of anxiety symptoms in children may be helpful in assessing anxiety disorders in youth, further work is needed to determine how panic disorder, specifically, is assessed. The many limitations to self-report and parent-report measures include inaccurate reporting, either over- or underreporting the number of panic symptoms the child has, or the severity of these symptoms. For example, if a child is referred to seek treatment, parents may be in denial about their child having a disorder, and may therefore underreport symptoms the child is experiencing. Also, the child may not be attuned to what is triggering his or her panic attacks or what the physiological sensations mean. Many studies have found inconsistencies between child and parent reports for youth anxiety in both community and clinical sample populations (Barbosa, Tannock, & Manassis, 2002; Birmaher et al., 1997; Bögels & van Melick, 2004). However, despite the limitations of self-report measures, Bögels and van Melick (2004) suggest that when multiple reporters contribute information about a child's anxiety symptoms, the conclusions about the child's current situation and severity level of symptoms are much more accurate than when the child or the parent is the sole reporter. Future research should investigate how self-report responses of children and adolescents with panic disorder compare to their physiological symptoms because this also has not yet been examined.

Treatment

Key Treatment Components and Important Considerations

PCT-A, a cognitive-behavioral treatment, shares many treatment components with general CBT for anxiety in youth. However, the unique symptomatology of panic disorder requires some specific adaptations, some unique treatment techniques to address the fear of physical sensations, and some special considerations. The key treatment components of PCT-A are psychoeducation, cognitive restructuring, *in vivo* exposure to feared stimuli/situations, and interoceptive exposure. PCT-A is typically offered in 11 sessions over the course of 12 weeks, but it can also be delivered in a more intensive format by massing treatment sessions and delivering the same "dose" of treatment over a shorter time period. It is critical even before delivering PCT-A to ensure that the patient is motivated to change/get better, and this can be the first challenging task even prior to implementing the treatment. Given that PCT-A requires the patient to learn, implement, and practice new skills, it can be helpful to start therapy by assessing ways that the patient's life could be happier if panic were not interfering. The therapist can describe the overall goals of treatment as teaching the patient how to better understand, manage, and ultimately reduce and take the "fear" out of panic attacks. The therapist might work with the patient to generate a list of goals the patient has prior to treatment (e.g., "I want to be able to go to movies again"; "I want to hang out with my friends again without panic interfering") as one way of increasing the patient's motivation to get involved with treatment. The therapist might also help the patient to generate several lists, "benefits and costs of change" and "benefits or costs of no change." Another important consideration prior to implementing PCT-A is the developmental age of the child or adolescent. It is important for the therapist to tailor the treatment to the patient's developmental level by using examples and illustrations that are relevant and understandable. To assist in this process, the patient may be provided an accompanying panic treatment workbook (e.g., *Riding the Wave Workbook*; Pincus, Ehrenreich, & Spiegel, 2008) that contains information about panic disorder, handouts, and homework to complete each week, and instructions on how to conduct therapeutic exercises such as interoceptive exposure and *in vivo* situational exposures. Therapists can also assess parents' motivation to learn new skills that support their child's progress. Therapists can provide parents with reading (e.g., a guide to understanding their child's panic disorder) that reviews the skills youth will learn throughout treatment so that the parents feel included in the process and learn the same "tools" or therapeutic techniques as their child. Parents may also be encouraged to attend parts of some sessions.

PSYCHOEDUCATION

The first few sessions of panic treatment for youth are dedicated to rapport building and psychoeducation. The psychoeducation component is used to explain to youth and their parents the structure and purpose of treatment, and to teach them about the nature of panic attacks and panic disorder. It is important in these early sessions to establish a common language for discussing feelings (e.g., What exactly do adolescents mean when they say, "I'm freaking out"?) and to make sure patients are actively engaged in treatment. Engaging younger children in treatment may mean incorporating concrete, interactive activities to illustrate therapy concepts (e.g., using a large outline of the child's body to illustrate the parts of the body involved in the fight-or-flight system) and using positive reinforcement such as praise or stickers to reward children for completing components of treatment. Including youth in the discussion of panic (e.g., by garnering children's input when talking about the places panic attacks frequently occur) can help to increase engagement and motivation of youth. Most importantly in these early psychoeducation sessions, youth are taught about the nature of panic and introduced to the "three-component model of anxiety," which includes cognitions, physical feelings, and behaviors. Youth are taught to identify their own "triggers" of panic attacks by becoming more aware of the specific thoughts, feelings, and behaviors that ignite panic attacks. As homework, youth are asked to monitor their thoughts, feelings, and behaviors in the context of panic attacks. This helps them to begin to recognize the factors that trigger and maintain the maladaptive cycle of panic. (See the Thoughts–Feelings–Behavior Monitoring Sheet in the next section.)

Relaxation training is another component that may be used and is usually taught during the psychoeducation phase. Relaxation training includes techniques such a breathing retraining (diaphragmatic breathing) to teach patients not to "overbreathe," which may cause hyperventilation. However, it is important to make sure that relaxation techniques are not used during later exposure sessions. Exposures are supposed to induce anxiety, and the anxiety should be experienced fully until it diminishes; using relaxation techniques or safety behaviors disrupts this process. Riding out panic feelings teaches patients that these feelings will not last forever, that they are not dangerous, and that patients can cope with panic when it occurs. Relaxation skills are also used to help youth with panic become more aware of what their bodies feel like when tense, and how this tension can trigger panic attacks as part of the three-component model of panic.

COGNITIVE SKILLS

The next major component of panic treatment is teaching cognitive skills to youth. The goal of this cognitive work is to first teach youth to identify panic thoughts and other maladaptive cognitions, and to recognize common cognitive distortions or "thinking traps" in panic (e.g., overestimation of negative outcomes and catastrophic thinking). Youth are taught to identify inaccurate and maladaptive thoughts, which often trigger panic attacks (e.g., "My heart pounding will go on forever") and the perceived catastrophic consequences of having a panic attack (e.g., "My heart racing means I'm actually about to have a heart attack; my body can't handle this"). Youth are also asked to produce evidence and facts to support or refute these thoughts, then to evaluate the evidence in order to determine how realistic these thoughts are. They are also taught how to come up with more accurate, coping thoughts to replace the maladaptive thoughts. This cognitive restructuring skill can be practiced by using a Cognitive Restructuring or "Detective Thinking" Worksheet (included in the next section). Youth are also taught to compare the perceived probability of the occurrence of a negative event with the real probability of this event occurring. When the imagined or feared situation is perceived as "likely to happen," then the next step is to discuss all of the possible consequences (e.g., that the child or adolescent would be able to cope with the feared situation, and that the situation would not be a catastrophe). Engaging in this process allows youth to develop more realistic thoughts about physical symptoms and concerns about having a panic attack, and gives them skills to overcome maladaptive thought patterns that may induce a panic attack or lead to avoidance or agoraphobic behaviors.

INTEROCEPTIVE EXPOSURE

Importantly, the fear of physical sensations that leads to panic attacks and the subsequent development of panic disorder requires the incorporation of a unique intervention component to treat panic disorder that is not typically used for other anxiety disorders. Interoceptive exposure is used to target this fear of physical sensations just as *in vivo* exposure targets feared situations. During an interoceptive exposure, the physical sensations experienced during panic are induced in a variety of ways, such as running in place to increase heart rate, breathing through a straw to simulate hyperventilation, or spinning around to induce dizziness. Patients are often asked what they "predict" will happen if they bring on physical feelings, and these predictions are often that catastrophic events will occur (e.g., "I will most certainly have a heart attack or won't be able to handle the feelings"). Instead of feeling like a "victim" of panic, the patient is taught to think like a "scientist" and to notice the physical symptoms at their peak during each exercise. Each exercise lasts anywhere from about 30 seconds to 2 minutes. After each exercise is conducted, the patient is asked whether the symptoms generated were similar or different from naturally occurring panic attacks. The therapist encourages patients to compare their predictions of what would occur to what actually happened after conducting the exercises. Typically, patients are surprised that their catastrophic predictions did not occur. Typically, patients are led to conduct three trials of each exercise, and most notice that with each trial, they have lower levels of anxiety. Patients are taught the concept of exposure and habituation, and are encouraged to continue to practice the exercises that were most similar to their naturally occurring panic (see the homework sheet, Practicing Symptom Exposures Record, in the next section). When interoceptive exposures are practiced, patients begins to learn that the physical sensations are not going to be catastrophic, and that when they occur "in real life," they can ride out the wave of anxiety without avoiding situations that induce physical feelings. Patients can also challenge overestimating or catastrophizing thoughts associated with the physical sensations and learn to ride out these sensations with lessened anxiety. Interoceptive exposures can also be paired with *in vivo* exposures in order to increase the intensity or to better recreate the feared situation.

IN VIVO SITUATIONAL EXPOSURE

One of the most important components of panic treatment for adolescents is conducting an *in vivo* exposure, as this targets avoidance of feared situations. There are a number of commonly feared situations for youth with panic disorder, including crowded places, being separated from parents, being in a mall or movie theater, sitting in a classroom, or riding in a car. The first step in conducting *in vivo* exposures is to work with patients and their parents to create a fear hierarchy or "bravery ladder" that lists feared situations from least to most anxiety provoking (see the Fear Avoidance Hierarchy Worksheet in the next section). Patients and therapists then collaboratively discuss a plan for entering each of these situations in turn. For patients who are resistant to implementing exposures, therapists can enhance motivation by reminding patients of the reasons why they wanted to get better. Therapists and parents should praise youth accordingly as they gradually reenter situations they previously avoided, and small rewards can be implemented for youth to reinforce approach behaviors and keep motivation high. After each situation is practiced successfully, patients are encouraged to move onto the next higher step on the fear hierarchy. Some *in vivo* exposures can be completed in session, whereas others can be assigned as "homework," then discussed in the next session. It is important to make sure patients are not using safety behaviors during exposures, such as carrying a water bottle or playing with their cellphone, because safety behaviors support the maintenance of maladaptive thoughts about the situation, such as thinking that if they do not drink water, they will have a panic attack. During exposures, patients are encouraged to challenge maladaptive thoughts and behaviors using the skills they learned in the cognitive restructuring component. Although completing *in vivo* exposures may seem daunting to patients and are initially very anxiety provoking, overcoming their fear of the situation and enhancing their ability to cope on their own, without safety behaviors, is vital to overcoming panic and maintaining improvements posttreatment.

SKILLS CONSOLIDATION AND RELAPSE PREVENTION

In the final session of treatment, the skills learned are reviewed, and plans for continued practice are formulated. Further practice allows patients to strengthen their skills and become comfortable approaching more situations or stimuli that they have previously avoided. Future planning also facilitates continued treatment gains and maintenance of improvements past the end of treatment. It is often helpful during this last session of treatment to describe that it is normal for panic to re-occur during stressful periods in one's life. Patients should be encouraged to review the skills learned in treatment, and not to worry that an occasional reoccurrence of a panic attack means that they are having a "setback." Furthermore, it may be helpful to discuss with the family the ways that the child's relationships with friends and family members might change now that panic has subsided. Parents commonly express conflicting feelings: joy, when they see their child return to normal activities, and sadness at not feeling relied upon in the same way as when their child was panicking. Therapists can encourage a discussion of ways to keep parent–child relationships strong (e.g., scheduling pleasant activities together) now that panic is not interfering.

When developing a treatment, it is important to determine the relative contribution of each component to treatments gains in order to make sure that each is necessary, or to determine whether some other combination of treatment components would be sufficient. Micco, Choate-Summers, Ehrenreich, Pincus, and Mattis (2007) examined session-by-session treatment gains in adolescent panic treatment to better elucidate the effects of individual PCT-A components. The study showed that two components led to sudden "significant treatment gains" (defined as an improvement above two standard deviations from the mean on the outcome measure of interest). Following the administration of the psychoeducation component, there was a significant reduction in panic attack frequency. After the cognitive restructuring segment, there was a decrease in overall anxiety symptoms. However, this study was limited in its power to closely examine the effect of each component because of overlap in the presentation of components, small sample size, and because the sudden gains criteria may have missed some smaller but clinically significant changes in symptoms. The authors suggest that future studies dismantle the treatment in order to better study each component, such as examining the effect of PCT-A administered without situational exposures or only looking at one component at a time, such as psychoeducation. Research investigating the relative importance of each PCT-A component and other treatment factors, such as the optimal levels of parental involvement, is under way.

Table 8.2 is a session-by-session outline of the PCT-A and intensive PCT-A treatment protocols.

TABLE 8.2. Outline of Sessions for PCT-A and Intensive PCT-A

PCT-A[a]

Session no.	Focus	Treatment components
1 and 2	Psychoeducation	Teaching patients and their families about the nature of anxiety, model of panic attacks, fight-or-flight system, and physiology of hyperventilation
3 and 4	Cognitive skills	Identifying cognitive errors such as catastrophic thinking and overestimation, monitoring thoughts, and cognitive restructuring
5	Interoceptive exposure	Engaging in a series of symptom induction exercises to learn that physical sensations are not harmful
6–10	Situational exposure	*In vivo* situational exposures, including use of the fear hierarchy, elimination of safety behaviors, and home–work exposures
11	Skills consolidation and relapse prevention	Reviewing skills learned and creating a plan for future practice

Intensive PCT-A[b]

Corresponding 11-week PCT-A session no.	Intensive treatment session no.	Focus
1–5	1–3	Psychoeducation, cognitive skills, interoceptive exposure
6 and 7	4 and 5	Intensive *in vivo* exposure with therapist accompaniment
8–10	6 and 7	Continued exposures, independently or with family
11	8	Skills consolidation and relapse prevention

Note. Adapted from Pincus, Ehrenreich, and Spiegel (2008). Copyright © 2008 Oxford University Press. Adapted by permission.
[a]Pincus, Ehrenreich, Mattis, Whitton, and Barlow (2010); Pincus, Ehrenreich, and Mattis (2008).
[b]Pincus, Ehrenreich, and Mattis (2008); Pincus, Ehrenreich, and Spiegel (2008); Angelosante et al. (2009).

Key Measures, Tools, and Recording Sheets to Be Used during Treatment

There are a number of important measures to be used during an initial assessment and some that continue to be useful throughout treatment. An initial assessment battery typically comprises a semistructured interview such as the ADIS-C/P or a comparable semistructured interview or unstructured clinical interview that assesses key diagnostic criteria for panic disorder. The ADIS interview is often complemented with child self-report measures that assess symptoms of panic such as the PDSS-C, general anxiety symptoms such as the MASC-C, and related constructs such as anxiety sensitivity using the CASI (all of these measures were described earlier). The PDSS-C can be used either daily or weekly throughout treatment to track changes in panic symptomatology over time. It may also be helpful to have youth track their mood (anxiety and depression) and panic attacks on a daily basis using a calendar or daily mood monitoring sheet. A rating scale of 0–8 is typically used, with 0 being "no anxiety/depression," 4 being "moderate," and 8 being "as much as I can imagine." Patients can also keep a log of their panic attacks that includes a description of the situation, the likely triggers of the panic attack, a rating of the highest level of anxiety (0–8 scale), and how the patient coped with it.

Parents or caregivers should also complete self-report measures to complement the youth's self-report. These measures could include parent reports of the child's panic symptomatology, or related symptomatology (e.g., sleep), as well as reports of family functioning and parenting stress. The compilation of the interview measures, parent and child self-report measures, and daily mood and panic logs can help provide a means of tracking changes in patients' panic symptoms, as well as concomitant changes, over the course of treatment.

Tools and Recording Sheets

THOUGHTS–FEELINGS–BEHAVIORS MONITORING SHEET

The Thoughts–Feelings–Behaviors Monitoring Sheet can be created to help patients begin to recognize triggers of panic attacks. It is also used to teach patients how to "break down" anxiety and panic into three components: thoughts, feelings, and behaviors. The sheet provides space for patients to write in the context of the anxiety-provoking situation that occurred (e.g., including the date/time, who they were with, and what occurred). One helpful design for the monitoring sheet is to include a visual depiction of three blank circles; each one is separately labeled, "What I Think," "What I Feel," and "What I Do." Patients practice breaking down anxiety by writing in each circle the thoughts, physical feelings, and behaviors they experienced or exhibited during the anxiety-provoking situation. Samples of such sheets are included in the *Riding the Wave Workbook* (Pincus, Ehrenreich, & Spiegel, 2008).

COGNITIVE RESTRUCTURING OR "DETECTIVE THINKING" WORKSHEET

The Cognitive Restructuring Worksheet can also be called the "Detective Thinking" worksheet for younger youth who might enjoy the idea that searching for "facts" about one's thoughts is similar to being a detective. The purpose of this worksheet is to help youth practice identifying maladaptive thoughts and their associated "thinking traps" or cognitive errors (e.g., overestimation, catastrophic thinking). There are several columns on this chart. The first column includes space for the patient to write down the situation that occurred. Next, the patient has a column to record his or her automatic thoughts. The next column includes space for the patient to record any cognitive errors or "thinking traps" that might have occurred. In the following three columns, the patient records the evidence or facts that the thought is true, the evidence that the thought is not true, and an alternative coping thought that is more consistent with the facts or evidence. Youth utilize this worksheet specifically during the cognitive component of treatment, but the final column of "alternative coping thoughts" can be referred to throughout treatment, especially to motivate patients prior to conducting exposures. An example of this type of cognitive worksheet is included in the *Riding the Wave Workbook* (Pincus, Ehrenreich, & Spiegel, 2008). Instructions for how to use this worksheet in a step-by-step fashion is included in the *Mastery of Anxiety and Panic for Adolescents: Therapist Guide* (Pincus, Ehrenreich, & Mattis, 2008).

PRACTICING SYMPTOM EXPOSURES RECORD

The Practicing Symptom Exposures record allows the patient to record his or her interoceptive exposure practice. The patient is asked to list the exercise in which he or she engaged (e.g., running in place, breathing through a straw), the date and time, the physical sensations he or she experienced, the intensity of the sensations on a 0- 8-point scale, their similarity to actual panic, and any anxious thoughts he or she had during the exercise. The practice of "bringing on" physical sensations can facilitate exposure to fear and, ultimately, fear extinction. Using this worksheet can help therapists track how often patients are practicing and whether their anxiety levels are gradually reducing. Patients can be reminded that although they may continue to experience intense physical sensations after completing each exercise, they will likely notice that their anxiety levels are gradually decreasing.

FEAR AVOIDANCE HIERARCHY OR "BRAVERY LADDER" WORKSHEET

The patient and therapist use the Fear and Avoidance Hierarchy or "Bravery Ladder" Worksheet collaboratively (and often with parent input) prior to conducting *in vivo* exposures. The Fear Avoidance Hierarchy Worksheet contains a grid that allows patients to describe 10 different situations that they have avoided due to panic, ranging from the easiest or least anxiety provoking (ranked situation "10") to the hardest, or most anxiety provoking (ranked situation "1"). Next to the description of each situation, patients can rate how much they fear the situation and avoid the situation, on a 0- to 8-point scale. The last column next to each situation indicates whether the child completed the exposure. There is space in this column for a check mark or sticker that the child can give him- or herself or that the therapist or parent can provide after exposures are completed. After treatment is completed, the therapist can make a revised version of the Fear Avoidance Hierarchy to include even more difficult exposures as part of a plan for continued practice.

Case Example

Laura,* a 17-year-old white female, was referred to treatment after her mother called our anxiety clinic complaining that her daughter had been withdrawing from most of her activities over the past 6 months. She described how her daughter was one of the "stars" of the track team in her high school, but she began skipping track practice and making excuses for why she could not attend track meets. Laura's teachers also noted on her most

---

*This is a fictionalized case based on the integration of information from multiple cases. The name and disorder characteristics do not identify a particular patient.

recent report card that she was not attending gym class regularly, and she frequently asked for passes to use the restroom throughout the school day. When Laura's mother questioned her about these behaviors, Laura reported that she thought she might have something wrong with her heart, or that she might have asthma, because she frequently felt like she could not get enough air and felt her heart racing. Laura's mother reported that she had taken Laura to several different doctors, including the emergency room on several occasions, due to Laura reporting a sudden, severe onset of breathlessness, chest pain, and dizziness. After several medical workups, which all found Laura to be functioning normally, it was suggested that the family consult with a psychologist to assess the possibility of Laura having panic disorder.

During the initial interview, Laura reported that she was having sudden rushes of physical symptoms, and she constantly was worried that another rush of these symptoms would occur. Although these distressing symptoms first started during track practice, they also started occurring when Laura was in school, prompting her to ask for passes to use the restroom, where she would "splash her face with water" and wait for the feelings to subside. Laura's mother reported that she was worried about her daughter and had asked Laura to call her when these feelings occurred. Laura began calling her mother on her cellphone throughout the day and frequently asked her mother to pick her up early from school. Laura's mother reported that she decided to quit her job because she felt her daughter needed her full attention. Laura also reported during the initial assessment session that had been drinking moderately with her friends in order to "numb out" her frightening physical feelings. She also said she was avoiding all the things she used to enjoy, such as running, going to movies, going to concerts, going shopping with friends, and traveling. She had even faked being sick to avoid school field trips due to fear of having a panic attack on the bus. Laura stated that she feared her peers would see her "freaking out." Laura reported that she was very motivated to get better, as her world had been "shrinking" since she stopped attending most activities that she used to enjoy. Laura's mother stated that, more than anything, she wanted "her adventurous daughter back." After the assessment, Laura was scheduled for an intensive, 8-day treatment for panic disorder. What follows is an overview of Laura's treatment sessions, along with sample excerpts of dialogue between Laura and the therapist.

INTENSIVE SESSION 1

In Session 1, the therapist spoke with Laura about her motivation to get better and helped her generate a "pros and cons" list for completing the intensive treatment. Laura wrote that on the top of her "pros" list was "getting my life back again" and "being a regular teenager" and "feeling in control of my body." The only "con" she could think of was that she knew that getting better would mean that she would have to be willing to experience anxiety. In this session, the therapist introduced the concept of breaking down anxiety (the three-component model) in the following way:

THERAPIST: One of the most important ways to start helping you feel better is to break down this feeling of panic you're describing that feels so overwhelming.

LAURA: Yes, it is incredibly overwhelming.

THERAPIST: One way to better deal with overwhelming feelings is to break them down into smaller parts. The smaller parts can feel much easier to work with. For example, take these panicky waves you are experiencing. Could you describe the last situation you were in where you had one of these waves of panic?

LAURA: I was eating breakfast by the window in the kitchen on a Sunday morning in my pajamas. It was the most relaxing place in the house, my favorite meal of the day, on my favorite day of the week, and I couldn't imagine why these nervous feelings came on for no reason.

THERAPIST: What types of thoughts do you recall having on that Sunday morning?

LAURA: I recall that I wasn't thinking of anything scary at all. I was just eating waffles and drinking water.

THERAPIST: Can you recall any physical feelings you were having?

LAURA: Well, I recall that I was feeling very warm, due to the sun streaming in the window. It was a very hot day, and we don't have air conditioning in the house.

THERAPIST: Do you recall anything else you were doing or thinking?

LAURA: Well, besides eating breakfast, I think I was probably shaking my leg, which is often a nervous habit. Oh, and I actually was remembering that the last time I had felt similarly warm was the last time I was riding in the car with my friends. That was also the last time I had those panicky feelings. And I was remembering how I couldn't handle the scary feelings of my heart racing fast and dizziness, and I had to get out of the car. And then while I was eating breakfast, I started worrying that those panicky feelings might come back, so I took several big gulps of water and huge deep breaths to try to "push down" the feelings and to cool myself down. That's when I noticed the panicky wave of feelings coming over me.

THERAPIST: So it sounds like you had a number of things that could have triggered panicky feelings that Sunday morning. Let's break them down and write them on this worksheet. (*Takes out the Thoughts–Feelings–Behaviors Monitoring Sheet.*) You were feeling warm—let's write this in the "physical feelings" circle. You said you were thinking about a situation where you didn't feel you could cope with your feelings, let's write this in the "thoughts" circle. And you said that your leg was shaking and you started taking big gulps of water and taking deep breaths. Let's write these in the "behaviors" circle. Take a look at how a physical feeling of being extra warm triggered some anxious thoughts, and these anxious thoughts triggered some behaviors. Each of these "circles"—your thoughts, feelings, and behaviors—can trigger panic. Each of these parts can feed the next part, so it becomes a cycle. But we can break the cycle. The first step, though, is learning how to break down panicky feelings into thoughts, feelings, and behaviors.

LAURA: Wow, all this time, I thought my panicky feelings came from "out of the blue."

THERAPIST: During our work together, you will learn about how to become more aware of your own triggers for panic. And you will get really good at breaking down your panic attacks into these three parts. Together, we will learn how to "break" this cycle of panic. I will teach you skills that address each of these parts—your thoughts, feelings and behaviors. I will teach you ways to become more aware of your thoughts, and to change the thoughts that aren't true. We will learn why the physical feelings of anxiety are not actually harmful or dangerous at all, in fact, they are protective. And we will learn how to become more aware of the types of behaviors you might be doing that could inadvertently bring on more panic. As you learn each of these skills, you might notice that you are becoming less afraid of having a panic attack. And as you become less afraid of having a panic attack, the panic attacks come on less frequently. Together, we will "retrain" your brain not to react with fear when there is no real danger.

INTENSIVE SESSION 2

During Session 2, Laura was taught how to become more aware of her panic-related maladaptive cognitions that might lead to panic. She was also taught ways to recognize "thinking traps" or cognitive errors that can contribute to the cycle of panic. She enjoyed learning how to restructure her maladaptive thoughts by examining the evidence that the thought was true or not true. The therapist used the "Detective Thinking" Worksheet with Laura to teach her a concrete way to practice restructuring her thoughts. What follows is an excerpt of sample dialogue from Session 2.

THERAPIST: Can you identify one thought that you frequently have when you panic?

LAURA: I can think of many thoughts that race through my mind. One thought I often have is "My heart racing will never stop. My body can't handle this, I'm going to have a heart attack."

THERAPIST: Let's take the first thought you mentioned, "My heart racing will never stop." What evidence do you have that this thought is true? In previous panic situations, has your heart racing gone on forever and never stopped?

LAURA: Well, I guess in all previous situations, my heart racing eventually stopped and slowed down. I guess this is one of those "thinking traps"—I am overestimating the probability that something bad will happen, but I guess this really never does happen.

THERAPIST: Let's take the next thought you mentioned, "My body can't handle this, I am going to have a heart attack." How many panic attacks would you say you had in the past month?

LAURA: At least five per week, so I would say about 20 per month, for the past 6–8 months.

THERAPIST: How many of these resulted in a heart attack?

LAURA: (*laughing*) None.

THERAPIST: Did your body "handle" the heart racing?

LAURA: Yes. I guess it handled it just fine.

THERAPIST: What else could heart racing mean, besides that you are having a heart attack?

LAURA: Well, I remember from the last session, we learned that heart racing is a normal part of the fight-or-flight system. It means that my body is trying to protect me from either real or imagined danger by pumping the blood quickly to my legs so that I can leave the situation. So, actually, heart racing doesn't seem so scary when I think that it is just my body's protective system that is working well. Maybe I am "catastrophizing" when I say that I am sure I will have a heart attack. And maybe I'm also completely overestimating the likelihood of this happening.

THERAPIST: That is great that you remembered all of that information! Remembering what panic really is can be quite helpful. It helps you remember that all of these physical sensations are actually not an "attack" at all. It is simply the fight-or-flight system, doing its job at a time when there is no real danger around. You are doing a great job of becoming more aware of your panic thoughts. The next thing we will learn is how to come up with some more accurate coping thoughts you might think that are more consistent with the real facts.

INTENSIVE SESSION 3

During Session 3, the therapist reviewed with Laura every physical symptom that she experiences during a panic attack, then explained in detail how every one of these physical symptoms is evolutionarily protective. The therapist also explained the concepts of habituation and exposure. The therapist introduced these concepts in the following way:

THERAPIST: Have you ever watched a scary movie that made you startle at points and almost jump out of your seat at the movie theater?

LAURA: Yes, I have. I actually love scary movies.

THERAPIST: Have you ever watched the same scary movie multiple times?

LAURA: Yes, I have. My friends and I used to like to watch them before sleepover parties.

THERAPIST: After watching the same movie, say, three or four times, do you still find that you are startled quite as intensely as the first time you watched the movie?

LAURA: No. It's funny, but the scary parts don't seem scary anymore. It is almost like my body just got used to the movie.

THERAPIST: That is also similar to what happens when you enter a situation that you are scared of because you've been avoiding it due to panic. The first time you enter the situation, your anxiety level might reach a high point. If I could have you stay in the situation for a long while, do you think your anxiety would stay at that high point?

LAURA: Well, I guess eventually it would go down.

THERAPIST: That's right! As you give your brain a chance to learn that nothing bad or catastrophic is going to happening to you, even when you're nervous, then your anxiety level comes down. Every time you practice entering that feared situation, and you are experiencing anxiety, you are giving your brain a chance to develop new learning about that situation. And quite naturally, your anxiety starts to come down. This concept of how your anxiety starts to come down after repeated exposures is called *habituation*. It applies to lots of different fears and situations. When you practice entering situations that you were previously avoiding due to fear, we call this conducing "exposure" practices.

LAURA: Oh, I think I understand—so as I conduct exposures, the process of habituation happens and new learning happens and I gradually get less afraid?

THERAPIST: Exactly. And we can also conduct exposures that help you become less afraid of the physical symptoms of anxiety—we call these "interoceptive exposure exercises." Interoceptive exposure is a special type of exposure practice where you learn not to let what you feel scare you.

The majority of the session was devoted to symptom induction exercises, or interoceptive exposure exercises. The therapist first modeled how to conduct each exercise (e.g., spinning in a chair, breathing through a cocktail straw, running in place, tensing all muscles, shaking head from side to side). Then the patient conducts each exercise, one at a time. After each exercise, the therapist asked Laura to describe the sensations she felt, the strength of the sensations, how much anxiety she felt, and how similar the sensations were to real panic. Although Laura initially wanted to stop her chair spinning after only 15 seconds, the therapist encouraged her to really bring on the physical sensations so that she could learn to "ride the wave" of panic. Laura was very responsive to praise and encouragement. At one point, Laura admitted to the therapist that she was thinking about pleasant things, such as her upcoming birthday, to distract herself during the interoceptive exposures. The therapist reviewed the concept of exposure and the importance of letting herself really experience these sensations to allow the processes of habituation and extinction to occur. Laura was reminded to see herself as a "scientist" who observes what happens when the anxiety and symptoms get to their peak, rather than as a "victim" of panic. Laura reported that she was shocked to see that after only three trials of each interoceptive exercise, her fear of the sensation decreased. She particularly liked the running-in-place exercise because it helped her to see that feelings of heart racing dissipated naturally. At the end of Session 3, Laura reported that she was already feeling happier, as she could imagine herself going to her track practices again. Laura's parents joined for the last part of this session, and Laura had her parents conduct the symptom induction exercises together. Her parents reported that they could not believe how "intense" the physical feelings were when they conducted each exercise. Laura stated to her parents, "See, now you both can understand me. This is how I've been feeling every day. But now I know why I've been feeling this way." Laura was instructed to practice the three exercises that were most similar to her naturally occurring panic (running in place, spinning in a chair, and breathing through a straw) and to record her practice on the Practicing Symptom Exposures Record Form.

INTENSIVE SESSIONS 4 AND 5

Sessions 4 and 5 were devoted to conducting *in vivo* situational exposures. Prior to beginning exposures, therapist and patient completed the Fear and Avoidance Hierarchy or "Bravery Ladder" Worksheet. Laura described how she has been avoiding all of the situations on the worksheet, but that she was ready to begin facing her fears in order to "get her life back." Prior to setting out on exposures, the therapist also discussed with Laura the concept of "safety behaviors" (e.g., bringing along a cellphone, a water bottle, distracting herself) as being subtle forms of avoidance. Although, in the short term, these techniques may temporarily reduce anxiety, they ultimately cause fears to grow and "feed" the cycle of panic. Laura was willing to remove all safety objects and agreed to be aware of any safety behaviors she was exhibiting (e.g., distracting herself or trying to relax) that could make the exposures less effective. The therapist helped Laura to write down a list of these safety behaviors so that Laura could be aware of them. Throughout the remainder of Sessions 4 and 5, Laura conducted the following *in vivo* exposures: watching a movie, sitting in the middle of the theater, running on a track, going to a crowded restaurant, going on the subway, going to the mall, and taking a dance class. She conducted exposures for approximately 5 hours per day. She was able to stay in each of these situations successfully, without leaving once her anxious feelings arose. Laura reported being surprised at how quickly her symptoms were reduced and how she enjoyed watching and tracking her anxiety levels as they came down. For some of the more difficult exposures, the therapist accompanied Laura for a few minutes, then allowed Laura to complete the exposure on her own. Some situations were practiced repeatedly—once with the therapist, and several times without the therapist. Laura reported feeling much more energized and accomplished by the time she completed Session 5 of treatment. The therapist met with Laura at the end of session to create a plan for continued independent practice over the next few days.

INTENSIVE SESSIONS 6 AND 7

These two sessions were devoted to further *in vivo* exposure practice. Laura conducted some exposures on her own, and others with her parents. The patient was scheduled to return for Session 8, the final session of treatment.

INTENSIVE SESSION 8

In the final session of treatment, the therapist helped Laura to reflect on how much she had accomplished in a short period of time. The therapist had Laura answer the following questions: What do you remember about the first time you came to treatment? What were the most important things you learned in therapy? What will you never forget? What coping thoughts do you find have been most useful to you? What differences do you notice in how you react to stressful situations? What are your hopes for the future? After discussing Laura's answers to these questions, Laura and the therapist created a plan for continued exposure practice. Laura liked the idea of combining interoceptive exposures with *in vivo* exposures to make the exposures "harder." Together, the therapist and Laura completed a new Fear and Avoidance Hierarchy Form, listing new situations that she could practice and a tentative plan for when she would practice these exposures. Laura was reminded that practicing the skills she learned in real-life situations is the most important and essential part of treatment. The therapist also discussed with Laura the differences between normal anxiety, a lapse, or a full-blown relapse. Laura invited her parents to join at the end of session. Her parents expressed how proud they were of her accomplishments and said they would do "whatever it took" to give her opportunities to continue to practice her exposures. The therapist encouraged the family to celebrate Laura's hard work. Laura expressed that, to celebrate, she wanted to combine an exposure with a reward—she wanted the whole family to try a short "fun run/race" that was being held in their town later that month to support a good cause. Her parents expressed how thrilled they were to "get their adventurous daughter back."

REFERENCES

Achenbach, T. M., & Edelbrock, C. S. (1983). *Manual for the Child Behavior Checklist and Revised Child Behavior Profile.* Burlington: University of Vermont, Department of Psychiatry.

Achenbach, T. M., & Rescorla, L. (2001). Reliability, internal consistency, cross-informant agreement, and stability. In *Manual for the ASEBA school-age forms & profiles: An integrated system of multi-informant assessment* (pp. 99–135). Burlington, VT: ASEBA.

Achiam-Montal, M., Tibi, L., & Lipsitz, J. D. (2013). Panic disorder in children and adolescents with noncardiac chest pain. *Child Psychiatry and Human Development, 44*(6), 742–750.

Akister, J., & Stevenson-Hinde, J. (1991). Identifying families at risk: Exploring the potential of the McMaster Family Assessment Device. *Journal of Family Therapy, 13*(4), 411–421.

American Psychiatric Association. (2013). *Diagnostic and statistical manual of mental disorders* (5th ed.). Arlington, VA: Author.

Angelosante, A. G., Pincus, D. B., Whitton, S. W., Cheron, D., & Pian, J. (2009). Implementation of an intensive treatment protocol for adolescents with panic disorder and agoraphobia. *Cognitive and Behavioral Practice, 16*(3), 345–357.

Baldwin, J. S., & Dadds, M. R. (2007). Reliability and validity of parent and child versions of the Multidimensional Anxiety Scale for Children in community samples. *Journal of the American Academy of Child and Adolescent Psychiatry, 46*(2), 252–260.

Barbosa, J., Tannock, R., & Manassis, K. (2002). Measuring anxiety: Parent–child reporting differences in clinical samples. *Depression and Anxiety, 15*(2), 61–65.

Barlow, D. H. (2002). *Anxiety and its disorders: The nature and treatment of anxiety and panic* (2nd ed.). New York: Guilford Press.

Barlow, D. H., Craske, M. G., Cerny, J. A., & Klosko, J. S. (1989). Behavioral treatment of panic disorder. *Behavior Therapy, 20*(2), 261–282.

Barlow, D. H., Raffa, S. D., & Cohen, E. M. (2002). Psychosocial treatments for panic disorders, phobias, and generalized anxiety disorder. In P. Nathan & J. Gorman (Eds.), *A guide to treatments that work* (2nd ed., pp. 301–366). New York: Oxford University Press.

Battaglia, M., Bajo, S., Strambi, L. F., Brambilla, F., Castronovo, C., Vanni, G., et al. (1997). Physiological and behavioral responses to minor stressors in offspring of patients with panic disorder. *Journal of Psychiatric Research, 31*(3), 365–376.

Bernstein, G. A., Borchardt, C. M., & Perwien, A. R. (1996). Anxiety disorders in children and adolescents: A review of the past 10 years. *Journal of the American Academy of Child and Adolescent Psychiatry, 35*(9), 1110–1119.

Biederman, J., Faraone, S. V., Hirshfield-Becker, D. R., Friedman, D., Robin, J., & Rosenbaum, J.

F. (2001). Patterns of psychopathology and dysfunction in high-risk children of parents with panic disorder and major depression. *American Journal of Psychiatry, 158*(1), 49–57.

Biederman, J., Faraone, S. V., Marrs, A., Moore, P., Garcia, J., Ablon, S., et al. (1997). Panic disorder and agoraphobia in consecutively referred children and adolescents. *Journal of the American Academy of Child and Adolescent Psychiatry, 36*(2), 214–223.

Birmaher, B., Brent, D. A., Chiapetta, L., Bridge, J., Monga, S., & Baugher, M. (1999). Psychometric properties of the Screen for Child Anxiety Related Emotional Disorders Scale (SCARED): A replication study. *Journal of the American Academy of Child and Adolescent Psychiatry, 38*(10), 1230–1236.

Birmaher, B., Khetarpal, S., Brent, D., Cully, M., Balach, L., Kaufman, J., & Neer, S. M. (1997). The Screen for Child Anxiety Related Emotional Disorders (SCARED): Scale construction and psychometric characteristics. *Journal of the American Academy of Child and Adolescent Psychiatry, 36*(4), 545–553.

Bögels, S. M., & van Melick, M. (2004). The relationship between child-report, parent self-report, and partner report of perceived parental rearing behaviors and anxiety in children and parents. *Personality and Individual Differences, 37*(8), 1583–1596.

Bourin, M., Baker, G. B., & Bradwejn, J. (1998). Neurobiology of panic disorder. *Journal of Psychosomatic Research, 44*(1), 163–180.

Challacombe, F., & Salkovskis, P. (2009). A preliminary investigation of the impact of maternal obsessive–compulsive disorder and panic disorder on parenting and children. *Journal of Anxiety Disorders, 23*(7), 848–857.

Chase, R. M., Whitton, S. W., & Pincus, D. B. (2012). Treatment of adolescent panic disorder: A nonrandomized comparison of intensive versus weekly CBT. *Child and Family Behavior Therapy, 34*(4), 305–323.

Chorpita, B. F., & Daleiden, E. L. (2000). Properties of the Childhood Anxiety Sensitivity Index in children with anxiety disorders: Autonomic and nonautonomic factors. *Behavior Therapy, 31*(2), 327–349.

Clark, D. M. (1986). A cognitive approach to panic. *Behaviour Research and Therapy, 24*(4), 461–470.

Colman, I., Wadsworth, M. E., Croudace, T. J., & Jones, P. B. (2007). Forty-year psychiatric outcomes following assessment for internalizing disorder in adolescence. *American Journal of Psychiatry, 164*(1), 126–133.

Costello, E. J., Mustillo, S., Erkanli, A., Keeler, G., & Angold, A. (2003). Prevalence and development of psychiatric disorders in childhood and adolescence. *Archives of General Psychiatry, 60*(8), 837–844.

Craske, M. G., Poulton, R., Tsao, J. C., & Plotkin, D. (2001). Paths to panic disorder/agoraphobia: An exploratory analysis from age 3 to 21 in an unselected birth cohort. *Journal of the American Academy of Child and Adolescent Psychiatry, 40*(5), 556–563.

Diler, R. S., Birmaher, B., Brent, D. A., Axelson, D. A., Firinciogullari, S., Chiapetta, L., et al. (2004). Phenomenology of panic disorder in youth. *Depression and Anxiety, 20*(1), 39–43.

Doerfler, L. A., Toscanojr, P. F., & Connor, D. F. (2008). Separation anxiety and panic disorder in clinically referred youth. *Journal of Anxiety Disorders, 22*(4), 602–611.

Doris, J., McIntyre, A., Kelsey, C., & Lehman, E. (1971, September). *Separation anxiety in nursery school children.* Paper presented at the 79th annual convention of the American Psychological Association, Washington, DC.

Dow, M. G., Kenardy, J. A., Johnston, D. W., Newman, M. G., Taylor, C. B., & Thomson, A. (2007). Prognostic indices with brief and standard CBT for panic disorder: I. Predictors of outcomes. *Psychological Medicine, 37*(10), 1493–1502.

Elkins, R. M., Gallo, K. P., Pincus, D. B., Comer. J. S. (2016). Moderators of intensive CBT for adolescent panic disorder: The roles of fear and avoidance. *Child and Adolescent Mental Health, 21*(1), 30–36.

Elkins, R. M., Pincus, D. B., & Comer, J. S. (2014). A psychometric evaluation of the Panic

Disorder Severity Scale for children and adolescents. *Psychological Assessment, 26*(2), 609–618.

Epstein, N. B., Baldwin, L. M., & Bishop, D. S. (1983). The McMaster Family Assessment Device. *Journal of Marital and Family Therapy, 9*(2), 171–180.

Essau, C. A., Conradt, J., & Petermann, F. (2000). Frequency, comorbidity, and psychosocial impairment of anxiety disorders in German adolescents. *Journal of Anxiety Disorders, 14*(3), 263–279.

Fairbanks, J. M., Pine, D. S, Tancer, N. K., Dummit, E. S., III, Kentgen, L. M., Martin, J., et al. (1997). Open fluoxetine treatment of mixed anxiety disorders in children and adolescents. *Journal of Child and Adolescent Psychopharmacology, 7*(1), 17–29.

Friedman, A. H., & Morris, T. L. (2006). Allergies and anxiety in children and adolescents: A review of the literature. *Journal of Clinical Psychology in Medical Settings, 13*(3), 318–331.

Friedman, B., & Thayer, J. (1998). Autonomic balance revisited: Panic anxiety and heart rate variability. *Journal of Psychosomatic Research, 44*(1), 133–151.

Gallo, K. P., Chan, P. T., Buzzella, B. A., Whitton, S. W., & Pincus, D. B. (2012). The impact of an 8-day intensive treatment for adolescent panic disorder and agoraphobia on comorbid diagnoses. *Behavior Therapy, 43*(1), 153–159.

Gallo, K. P., Cooper-Vince, C. E., Hardway, C. L., Pincus, D. B., & Comer, J. S. (2014). Trajectories of change across outcomes in intensive treatment for adolescent panic disorder and agoraphobia. *Journal of Clinical Child and Adolescent Psychology, 43*(5), 742–750.

Goodwin, R. D., Fergusson, D. M., & Horwood, L. J. (2005). Childhood abuse and familial violence and the risk of panic attacks and panic disorder in young adulthood. *Psychological Medicine, 35*(6), 881–890.

Goodwin, R. D., Pine, D. S., & Hoven, C. W. (2003). Asthma and panic attacks among youth in the community. *Journal of Asthma, 40*(2), 139–145.

Gorman, J. M., Kent, J. M., Sullivan, G. M., & Coplan, J. D. (2000). Neuroanatomical hypothesis of panic disorder, revised. *American Journal of Psychiatry, 157*(4), 493–505.

Hardway, C. L., Pincus, D. B., Gallo, K. P., & Comer, J. S. (2015). Parental involvement in intensive treatment for adolescent panic disorder and its impact on depression. *Journal of Child and Family Studies, 24*(11), 3306–3317.

Hayward, C., Killen, J. D., Kraemer, H. C., & Taylor, C. B. (2000). Predictors of panic attacks in adolescents. *Journal of the American Academy of Child and Adolescent Psychiatry, 39*(2), 207–214.

Hoffman, E. C., & Mattis, S. G. (2000). A developmental adaptation of panic control treatment for panic disorder in adolescence. *Cognitive and Behavioral Practice, 7*(3), 253–261.

Houck, P. R., Spiegel, D. A., Shear, M. K., & Rucci, P. (2002). Reliability of the self-report version of the panic disorder severity scale. *Depression and Anxiety, 15*(4), 183–185.

Hughes, A. A., Lourea-Waddell, B., & Kendall, P. C. (2008). Somatic complaints in children with anxiety disorders and their unique prediction of poorer academic performance. *Child Psychiatry and Human Development, 39*(2), 211–220.

Kearney, C. A., Albano, A. M., Eisen, A. R., Allan, W. D., & Barlow, D. H. (1997). The phenomenology of panic disorder in youngsters: An empirical study of a clinical sample. *Journal of Anxiety Disorders, 11*(1), 49–62.

Kendler, K. S., Walters, E. E., Neale, M. C., Kessler, R. C., Heath, A. C., & Eaves, L. J. (1995). The structure of the genetic and environmental risk factors for six major psychiatric disorders in women: Phobia, generalized anxiety disorder, panic disorder, bulimia, major depression, and alcoholism. *Archives of General Psychiatry, 52*(5), 374–383.

Kessler, R. C., Berglund, P., Demler, O., Jin, R., Merikangas, K. R., & Walters, E. E. (2005). Lifetime prevalence and age-of-onset distributions of DSM-IV disorders in the National Comorbidity Survey Replication. *Archives of General Psychiatry, 62*(6), 593–602.

Kessler, R. C., Chiu, W., Jin, R., Ruscio, A. M., Shear, K., & Walters, E. E. (2006). The epidemiology of panic attacks, panic disorder, and agoraphobia in the National Comorbidity Survey Replication. *Archives of General Psychiatry, 63*(4), 415–424.

Kovalenko, P. A., Hoven, C. W., Wu, P., Wicks, J., Mandell, D. J., & Tiet, Q. (2001). Association between allergy and anxiety disorders in youth. *Australian and New Zealand Journal of Psychiatry, 35*(6), 815–821.

La Greca, A. M., Silverman, W. K., & Lochman, J. E. (2009). Moving beyond efficacy and effectiveness in child and adolescent intervention research. *Journal of Consulting and Clinical Psychology, 77*(3), 373–382.

Leskin, G. A., & Sheikh, J. I. (2002). Lifetime trauma history and panic disorder: Findings from the National Comorbidity Survey. *Journal of Anxiety Disorders, 16*(6), 599–603.

March, J. S., Parker, J. D., Sullivan, K., Stallings, P., & Conners, C. K. (1997). The Multidimensional Anxiety Scale for Children (MASC): Factor structure, reliability, and validity. *Journal of the American Academy of Child and Adolescent Psychiatry, 36*(4), 554–565.

Marchesi, C. (2008). Pharmacological management of panic disorder. *Neuropsychiatric Disease and Treatment, 4*(1), 93–106.

Masi, G., Toni, C., Mucci, M., Millepiedi, S., Mata, B., & Perugi, G. (2001). Paroxetine in child and adolescent outpatients with panic disorder. *Journal of Child and Adolescent Psychopharmacology, 11*(2), 151–157.

Mattis, S. G., & Ollendick, T. H. (1997). Panic in children and adolescents: A developmental analysis. In T. H. Ollendick & R. J. Prinz (Eds.), *Advances in clinical child psychology* (Vol. 10, pp. 27–74). New York: Plenum Press.

Mattis, S. G., & Pincus, D. B. (2004). Treatment of SAD and panic disorder in children and adolescents. In P. M. Barrett & T. H. Ollendick (Eds.), *Handbook of interventions that work with children and adolescents: Prevention and treatment* (pp. 145–169). West Sussex, UK: Wiley.

McNally, R. J. (2002). Anxiety sensitivity and panic disorder. *Biological Psychiatry, 52*(10), 938–946.

Merikangas, K. R., He, J., Burstein, M., Swanson, S. A., Avenevoli, S., Cui, L., et al. (2010). Lifetime prevalence of mental disorders in U.S. adolescents: Results from the National Comorbidity Survey Replication–Adolescent Supplement (NCS-A). *Journal of the American Academy of Child and Adolescent Psychiatry, 49*(10), 980–989.

Micco, J. A., Choate-Summers, M. L., Ehrenreich, J. T., Pincus, D. B., & Mattis, S. G. (2007). Identifying efficacious treatment components of panic control treatment for adolescents: A preliminary examination. *Child and Family Behavior Therapy, 29*(4), 1–23.

Moore, P. S., Whaley, S. E., & Sigman, M. (2004). Interactions between mothers and children: Impacts of maternal and child anxiety. *Journal of Abnormal Psychology, 113*(3), 471–476.

Muris, P., Dreessen, L., Bögels, S., Weckx, M., & Melick, M. (2004). A questionnaire for screening a broad range of DSM-defined anxiety disorder symptoms in clinically referred children and adolescents. *Journal of Child Psychology and Psychiatry, 45*(4), 813–820.

Muris, P., Merckelbach, H., Mayer, B., van Brakel, A., Thissen, S., Moulaert, V., et al. (1998). The screen for child anxiety related emotional disorders (SCARED) and traditional childhood anxiety measures. *Journal of Behavior Therapy and Experimental Psychiatry, 29*(4), 327–339.

Nauta, M. H., Scholing, A., Rapee, R. M., Abbott, M., Spence, S. H., & Waters, A. (2004). A parent-report measure of children's anxiety: Psychometric properties and comparison with child-report in a clinic and normal sample. *Behaviour Research and Therapy, 42*(7), 813–839.

Ollendick, T. H. (1995). Cognitive behavioral treatment of panic disorder with agoraphobia in adolescents: A multiple baseline design analysis. *Behavior Therapy, 26*(3), 517–531.

Ollendick, T. H., Mattis, S. G., & Birmaher, B. (2004). Panic disorder. In T. L. Morris & J. S. March (Eds.), *Anxiety disorders in children and adolescents* (2nd ed., pp. 189–211). New York: Guilford Press.

Ollendick, T. H., & Pincus, D. (2008). Panic disorder in adolescents. In R. G. Steele, T. D. Elkin, & M. Roberts (Eds.), *Handbook of evidence-based therapies for children and adolescents: Bridging science and practice* (pp. 83–102). New York: Springer.

Otto, M. W., Pollack, M. H., Sachs, G. S., O'Neil, C. A., & Rosenbaum, J. F. (1992). Alcohol dependence in panic disorder patients. *Journal of Psychiatric Research, 26*(1), 29–38.

Owens, J. A., Spirito, A., & McGuinn, M. (2000). The Children's Sleep Habits Questionnaire (CSHQ): Psychometric properties of a survey instrument for school-aged children. *Sleep, 23*(8), 1043–1052.

Peacock, J., & Whang, W. (2013). Psychological distress and arrhythmia: Risk prediction and potential modifiers. *Progress in Cardiovascular Diseases, 55*(6), 582–589.

Perna, G., Bertani, A., Politi, E., Colombo, G., & Bellodi, L. (1997). Asthma and panic attacks. *Biological Psychiatry, 42*(7), 625–630.

Pilecki, B., Arentoft, A., & McKay, D. (2011). An evidence-based causal model of panic disorder. *Journal of Anxiety Disorders, 25*(3), 381–388.

Pincus, D. B., Ehrenreich, J. T., & Mattis, S. G. (2008). *Mastery of anxiety and panic for adolescents: Therapist guide.* New York: Oxford University Press.

Pincus, D. B., Ehrenreich, J. T., & Spiegel, D. A. (2008). *Riding the Wave workbook.* New York: Oxford University Press.

Pincus, D. B., Leyfer, O., Hardway, C., Elkins, R., & Comer, J. (2014, November). Recent advances in the development of psychological treatments for adolescents with panic disorder. In A. Asnaani (Symposium Chair), *Novel and innovative applications of evidence-based treatments for emotional disorders in adolescent patients.* Paper presented at the 48th annual meeting of the Association for Behavioral and Cognitive Therapies, Philadelphia, PA.

Pincus, D. B., May, J. E., Whitton, S. W., Mattis, S. G., & Barlow, D. H. (2010). Cogntive-behavioral treatment of panic disorder in adolescence. *Journal of Clinical Child and Adolescent Psychology, 39*(5), 638–649.

Pincus, D. B., Whitton, S. W., Gallo, K., Weiner, C. L., Chow, C., Hardway, C. L., et al. (2015). *Intensive treatment of adolescent panic disorder: Results of a randomized controlled trial.* Manuscript in preparation.

Rapee, R. M., Lyneham, H. J., Hudson, J. L., Kangas, M., Wuthrich, V. M., & Schniering, C. A. (2013). Effect of comorbidity on treatment of anxious children and adolescents: Results from a large, combined, sample. *Journal of American Academy of Child and Adolescent Psychiatry, 52*(1), 47–55.

Renaud, J., Birmaher, B., Wassick, S. C., & Bridge, J. (1999). Use of selective serotonin reuptake inhibitors for the treatment of childhood panic disorder: A pilot study. *Journal of Child and Adolescent Psychopharmacology, 9*(2), 73–83.

Robinson, J., Sareen, J., Cox, B., & Bolton, J. (2009). Self-medication of anxiety disorders with alcohol and drugs: Results from a nationally representative sample. *Journal of Anxiety Disorders, 23*(1), 38–45.

Rosenbaum, J. F., Biederman, J., Bolduc, D. R., & Chaloff, J. (1991). Behavioral inhibition in children: A possible precursor to panic disorder or social phobia. *Journal of Clinical Psychiatry, 52*(Suppl.), 5–9.

Rosenbaum, J. F., Biederman, J., Hirshfeld-Becker, D., Kagan, J., Snidman, N., Friedman, D., et al. (2000). A controlled study of behavioral inhibition in children of parents with panic disorder and depression. *American Journal of Psychiatry, 157*(12), 2002–2010.

Sala, R., Axelson, D. A., Castro-Fornieles, J., Goldstein, T. R., Ha, W., Liao, F., et al. (2010). Comorbid anxiety in children and adolescents with bipolar spectrum disorders. *Journal of Clinical Psychiatry, 71*(10), 1344–1350.

Scarpa, A., Raine, A., Venables, P. H., & Mednick, S. A. (1997). Heart rate and skin conductance in behaviorally inhibited Mauritian children. *Journal of Abnormal Psychology, 106*(2), 182–190.

Schneider, S., Unnewehr, S., Florin, I., & Margraf, J. (2002). Priming panic interpretations in children of patients with panic disorder. *Journal of Anxiety Disorders, 16*(6), 605–624.

Shear, M. K., Rucci, P., Williams, J., Frank, E., Grochocinski, V., Vander Bilt, J., et al. (2001).

Reliability and validity of the Panic Disorder Severity Scale: Replication and extension. *Journal of Psychiatric Research, 35*(5), 293–296.

Sheikh, J. I., Leskin, G. A., & Klein, D. F. (2002). Gender differences in panic disorder: Findings from the National Comorbidity Survey. *American Journal of Psychiatry, 159*(1), 55–58.

Shirk, S. R., & Karver, M. (2003). Prediction of treatment outcome from relationship variables in child and adolescent therapy: A meta-analytic review. *Journal of Consulting and Clinical Psychology, 71*(3), 452–464.

Silverman, W. K., Albano, A. M. (1996). *Anxiety Disorders Interview Schedule for DSM-IV: Child Version, Child and Parent Interview Schedules.* San Antonio, TX: Psychological Corporation.

Silverman, W. K., & Field, A. P. (Eds.). (2011). *Anxiety disorders in children and adolescents.* Cambridge, UK: Cambridge University Press.

Silverman, W. K., Fleisig, W., Rabian, B., & Peterson, R. A. (1991). Childhood Anxiety Sensitivity Index. *Journal of Clinical Child and Adolescent Psychology, 20*(2), 162–168.

Silverman, W. K., Saavedra, L. M., & Pina, A. A. (2001). Test–retest reliability of anxiety symptoms and diagnoses with the Anxiety Disorders Interview Schedule for DSM-IV: Child and Parent versions. *Journal of the American Academy of Child and Adolescent Psychiatry, 40*(8), 937–944.

Smoller, J. W., Pollack, M. H., Wassertheil-Smoller, S., Barton, B., Hendrix, S. L., Jackson, R. D., et al. (2003). Prevalence and correlates of panic attacks in postmenopausal women: Results from an ancillary study to the women's health initiative. *Archives of Internal Medicine, 163*(17), 2041–2050.

Smoller, J. W., Yamaki, L. H., Fagerness, J. A., Biederman, J., Racette, S., Laird, N. M., et al. (2005). The corticotropin-releasing hormone gene and behavioral inhibition in children at risk for panic disorder. *Biological Psychiatry, 57*(12), 1485–1492.

Spence, S. (1998). A measure of anxiety symptoms among children. *Behaviour Research and Therapy, 36*(5), 545–566.

Spence, S. H. (1997). Structure of anxiety symptoms among children: A confirmatory factor-analytic study. *Journal of Abnormal Psychology, 106*(2), 280–297.

Sportel, B., Nauta, M. H., de Hullu, E., de Jong, P. J., & Hartman, C. A. (2011). Behavioral inhibition and attentional control in adolescents: Robust relationships with anxiety and depression. *Journal of Child and Family Studies, 20*(2), 149–156.

Srinivasan, K., Ashok, M., Vaz, M., & Yeragani, V. K. (2002). Decreased chaos of heart rate time series in children of patients with panic disorder. *Depression and Anxiety, 15*(4), 159–167.

Stein, M., & Asmundson, G. (1994). Autonomic function in panic disorder: Cardiorespiratory and plasma catecholamine responsivity to multiple challenges of the autonomic nervous system. *Biological Psychiatry, 36*(8), 548–558.

Stein, M. B., Tancer, M. E., & Uhde, T. W. (1990). Major depression in patients with panic disorder: Factors associated with course and recurrence. *Journal of Affective Disorders, 19*(4), 287–296.

Sugaya, N., Yoshida, E., Yasuda, S., Tochigi, M., Takei, K., Otani, T., et al. (2013). Prevalence of bipolar disorder in panic disorder patients in the Japanese population. *Journal of Affective Disorders, 147*(1), 411–415.

Vallance, A., & Garralda, E. (2008). Anxiety disorders in children and adolescents. *Psychiatry, 7*(8), 325–330.

Van Beek, N., & Griez, E. (2003). Anxiety sensitivity in first-degree relatives of patients with panic disorder. *Behaviour Research and Therapy, 41*(8), 949–957.

Whaley, S. E., Pinto, A., & Sigman, M. (1999). Characterizing interactions between anxious mothers and their children. *Journal of Consulting and Clinical Psychology, 67*(6), 826–836.

Wood, J. J., Piacentini, J. C., Bergman, R. L., McCracken, J., & Barrios, V. (2002). Concurrent validity of the anxiety disorders section of the Anxiety Disorders Interview Schedule for DSM-IV: Child and Parent versions. *Journal of Clinical Child and Adolescent Psychology, 31*(3), 335–342.

CHAPTER 9

Posttraumatic Stress Disorder

Stephanie M. Keller, Mark Burton,
and Norah C. Feeny

THE DSM-5 DEFINITION OF POSTTRAUMATIC STRESS DISORDER

Posttraumatic stress disorder (PTSD) is characterized by exposure to a traumatic event and the subsequent development of symptoms that fall into four clusters (i.e., intrusions, avoidance, negative alterations in cognition and mood, and alterations in arousal and reactivity). The diagnostic criteria for PTSD are generally similar for both adults and children, though the clinical presentation of PTSD can differ across developmental stages. The current PTSD criteria outlined in the fifth edition of the *Diagnostic and Statistical Manual of Mental Disorders* (DSM-5; American Psychiatric Association, 2013) reflect these developmental considerations by including a preschool subtype for children 6 years of age and younger. This chapter provides a brief introduction of PTSD prevalence and diagnosis in youth, followed by an overview of evidence-based interventions for youth with PTSD. Finally, we provide a clinical guide of evidence-based assessment tools and treatment procedures for youth with PTSD.

In order to meet criteria for PTSD, an individual has to experience a traumatic stressor, defined by the DSM-5 (American Psychiatric Association, 2013) as directly experiencing a traumatic event (e.g., sexual assault, motor vehicle accident), witnessing a traumatic event (e.g., witnessing domestic violence), indirectly learning about a traumatic event that a close family member or friend experienced (e.g., learning about a family member being murdered), or experiencing repeated exposure to extreme details of a traumatic event, not through media or electronic sources (e.g., first responder). In addition to traumatic exposure, the individual must experience persistent and impairing symptoms in four separate clusters, including at least one *intrusion* symptom, which involves repeatedly reexperiencing the trauma in some form (e.g., trauma-related nightmares, emotionally and/or physiologically upset when reminded of the trauma, or flashbacks). Children may express these intrusive symptoms through repetitive play or more generalized frightening dreams (e.g., monsters harming them). The individual must also experience at least one *avoidance* symptom (e.g., trying not to think or talk about the traumatic event, staying away from the location where the trauma occurred). Two *negative alterations in cognition and mood* are also required for a PTSD diagnosis. These negative shifts may be evidenced by persistent negative beliefs about the self (e.g., "I am to blame for the trauma") or the world (e.g., "The world is a scary place"), persistent negative emotions (e.g., fear, guilt), reduced interest in pretrauma hobbies or activities, feeling detached from others, or an inability to feel positive emotions. While adults and children over 6 years of age require one avoidance symptom and two negative alterations in cognition and mood to be diagnosed with PTSD, children under 6 years old must express only one symptom in *either* the avoidance or negative alterations in cognition and mood cluster. Finally, two *alterations in arousal and reactivity* such as increased irritability, reckless or impulsive behavior, sleep difficulties, reduced concentration, hypervigilance, and exaggerated startle are required for a PTSD diagnosis. Overall, in order to be diagnosed with PTSD, an individual must experience a traumatic event, experience symptoms in each of the previously mentioned four clusters, experience these symptoms persistently for at least 1 month, and exhibit impairment in functioning in at least one domain (e.g., relationships, school performance). Historically, the criteria for PTSD in children and adults have been similar.

In an attempt to be more developmentally sensitive, the PTSD diagnostic criteria outlined in DSM-5 (American Psychiatric Association, 2013) include a preschool subtype. As previously mentioned, the primary change was a reduction in the number of avoidance symptoms required for a PTSD diagnosis in young children. The addition of the preschool subtype was guided by empirical findings that suggest young children tend to display symptoms in more behaviorally oriented ways and often failed to meet the symptom threshold for the avoidance cluster of PTSD symptoms (Scheeringa, Peebles, Cook, & Zeanah, 2001). For example, in a study of 62 children aged 0–18 years who were hospitalized with injuries, only 2% of children under age 7 endorsed enough avoidance symptoms to qualify for a diagnosis of PTSD (Scheeringa, Wright, Hunt, & Zeanah, 2006) based on DSM-IV (American Psychiatric Association, 2000) criteria. The level of cognitive ability required for reflection on internal states can make it difficult for young children to endorse symptoms of PTSD such as feeling detached from family members and cognitive avoidance of trauma reminders (e.g., Perrin, Smith & Yule, 2000; Scheeringa, Zeanah, & Cohen, 2011). Although young children may not be able to describe their PTSD symptoms, researchers and clinicians advocate (e.g., Scheeringa, Zeanah, et al., 2011) paying attention to behavioral manifestations of these symptoms, such as social withdrawal, restricted or repetitive play, regressive behavior (e.g., toileting issues), posttrauma-onset separation anxiety, or extreme temper tantrums (Perrin et al., 2000; Scheeringa et al., 2011). Overall, it is important for PTSD criteria to be appropriately developmentally sensitive to ensure a proper assessment, diagnosis, and potential future treatment.

PREVALENCE AND COURSE

A high percentage of youth report exposure to traumatic events, with rates ranging widely from 16 to 86% (e.g., Cuffe et al., 1998; Gwadz, Nish, Leonard, & Strauss, 2007). In a nationally representative survey of over 4,000 youth under the age of 18 years, over 60% reported directly experiencing or witnessing victimization (i.e., witnessing or experiencing intentional harm by another person) at least once in the past year (Finkelhor, Turner, Ormrod, & Hamby, 2009) and over 38% reported exposure to two or more victimizations. While rates of trauma exposure are high, most children and adolescents who experience trauma do not go on to develop PTSD (e.g., Copeland, Keeler, Angold, & Costello, 2007). In a large, nationally representative sample of 10,123 adolescents between ages 13 and 18 years, the lifetime prevalence of a PTSD diagnosis was 5% (Merikangas et al., 2010). Generally, among both adults and children, males are more likely to experience traumatic events, but females are more likely to develop PTSD (e.g., Kilpatrick et al., 2003) with lifetime PTSD prevalence rates among adolescents reported as 8.0% in females and 2.3% in males (Merikangas et al., 2010). Generally, it has been suggested that the likelihood of traumatic exposure increases during adolescence, particularly for interpersonal traumas such as physical and sexual assault (Finkelhor et al., 2009). For example, 9.8% of children between ages 0 and 17 reported experiencing a sexual trauma at some point in their lifetime. However, among adolescents ages 14–17, the lifetime prevalence rate was 16.3% (Finkelhor et al., 2009).

PTSD symptoms among children are often chronic if left untreated (e.g., De Young, Kenardy, Cobham, & Kimble, 2012). For example, among 200 adolescent survivors of a shipping disaster, over 50% developed PTSD, and close to 20% still met criteria for PTSD between 5 and 8 years after the trauma (Yule et al., 2000). Taken together, these data suggest that trauma exposure is common among youth, a minority of traumatized children and adolescents go on to develop PTSD, and that once present, these symptoms are often chronic if untreated.

As with adults, trauma reactions in youth are not restricted to symptoms of PTSD. A nationally representative survey of 4,023 adolescents ages 12–17 (Kilpatrick et al., 2003) found that of those who developed PTSD as a result of trauma, comorbidity was common, with comorbid depression, substance abuse/dependence, or both occurring in 2.5% of boys and 4.7% of girls with PTSD. Overall, PTSD exhibits high comorbidity rates with depression and substance use among adolescents exposed to a wide variety of traumas (e.g., Macdonald, Danielson, Resnick, Saunders & Kilpatrick, 2010).

Of note, most research examining PTSD and comorbid conditions has included school-age and adolescent youth, as opposed to younger children. In light of the addition of the PTSD preschool subtype in DSM-5, which suggests that very young children express symptoms in a distinct way, it will be important to study comorbid symptom presentation in this age group. At least one study has demonstrated high rates of comorbidity in a sample of preschool-age children following Hurricane Katrina (Scheeringa & Zeanah, 2008). Among those children who met criteria for PTSD (50%), 88.6% met criteria for at least one comorbid disorder, including major depressive disorder (MDD; 42.9%), panic disorder (33.3%), attention-deficit/hyperactivity disorder (ADHD; 33.3%), oppositional defiant disorder (ODD; 60.6%), and separation anxiety disorder (21.2%; Scheeringa & Zeanah, 2008). Taken together, these findings highlight the importance of assessing a wide range of symptoms in children of all ages with PTSD.

ETIOLOGICAL/CONCEPTUAL MODELS
OF PTSD IN CHILDHOOD AND ADOLESCENCE

There are a number of empirically supported theoretical models of PTSD development in adults (e.g., Brewin & Holmes, 2003; Dalgleish, 2004; Ehlers & Clark, 2000; Foa, Huppert, & Cahill, 2006). Comparatively few comprehensive conceptual models have been formulated to account for the development of PTSD in youth. However, a number of models may serve as a framework for identifying factors that impact PTSD development in children. Some have modified adult-based PTSD theories to map onto childhood PTSD development, while others have created child-specific models. The following section provides a brief overview of theoretical models to highlight factors that are thought to contribute to PTSD development and maintenance in youth.

Neurobiological and Physiological Models

Generally, trauma appears to impact the systems that regulate fear and stress responses. Among both children and adults, the most widely studied brain regions associated with trauma and PTSD are within the limbic system, including structures such as the amygdala and hippocampus. Research also examines the interaction among brain regions and other physiological systems, such as the endocrine system, autonomic nervous system, and immune system (Charmandari, Tsigo, & Chrousos, 2005; Heim & Nemeroff, 2009; for a review of physiology of PTSD in youth, see Kirsch, Wilhelm, & Goldbeck, 2011). While there is growing evidence to suggest that neurobiological and physiological changes occur following trauma exposure, there are no comprehensive models describing the biological underpinnings of PTSD in youth. Additionally, although PTSD symptoms are thought to arise from the disruption of these systems following trauma exposure, there is also evidence to suggest that certain physiological characteristics may be preexisting risk factors for the development of PTSD rather than consequences of the traumatic event (e.g., Heim & Nemeroff, 2009). The generalization of adult findings to youth is not appropriate given the need to consider both developmental and maturational processes. For example, there is literature to support significantly reduced hippocampal volumes, a brain region involved in processing memories, in adults with PTSD when compared with healthy controls (e.g., Bremner et al., 1995; Teicher, Anderson, & Polcari, 2012). However, neither cross-sectional nor longitudinal studies of maltreated youth have replicated these findings (e.g., Carrion et al., 2001; De Bellis, Hall, Boring, Frustaci, & Moritz, 2001; Tupler & DeBellis, 2006). Findings do, however, suggest that maltreated youth, in comparison to nonmaltreated youth, have higher basal levels of cortisol, a hormone that regulates changes that occur in the body in response to stress, which may lead to damage in brain structures such as the hippocampus in some individuals later in life (De Bellis & Zisk, 2014).

Research into early biological predictors of PTSD symptoms in youth has primarily been conducted in hospital settings and emergency rooms (e.g., Delahanty, Nugent, Christopher, & Walsh, 2005; Kassam-Adams et al., 2005). Among children seen in the hospital following accident or injury, it appears that heart rate while being transported to the emergency room and urinary cortisol levels taken soon after the accident/injury, predict the development of PTSD symptoms (Delahanty et al., 2005; Kassam-Adams, Garcia-Espana, Fein, & Winston, 2005). There is likely an interaction between a child's physiological functioning and ecology following trauma exposure. For example, higher parental PTSD symptoms were particularly deleterious for children who excreted low levels of cortisol soon after their accident, whereas parental PTSD symptoms did not impact children with high levels of initial cortisol (Nugent, Ostrowski, Christopher, & Delahanty, 2007). Similarly, higher parental PTSD symptoms were associated with more symptoms in their children, particularly among children with low in-hospital heart rate. These findings suggest that children who are not at increased risk for the development of PTSD on the basis of their initial biological response may still develop PTSD symptoms, partly due to their parent's response to the trauma (Nugent et al., 2007). Overall, the literature on the neurobiological and physiological pathways of PTSD in youth is still developing, and comprehensive models need to take into account multiple developmental considerations, including child stage of development, maturational processes, as well as factors related to the child's environment.

Five-Factor Model

This model suggests that multiple risk factors (i.e., pretrauma characteristics, trauma features, and posttrauma factors) interact to predict a child's posttrauma reactions (La Greca, Silverman, Vernberg, & Prinstein, 1996). *Exposure to trauma* and trauma-related characteristics comprise the first factor in this model. Variables associated with the trauma itself, such as trauma type, severity, and duration, have been shown to predict PTSD symptoms (Copeland et al., 2007). For example, youth who perceive higher threat to their life during the trauma and experience higher levels of ongoing life disruption due to the trauma exposure are at higher risk for developing PTSD symptoms (Yelland et al., 2010). The second factor accounts for a child's *preexisting characteristics,* or variables that were present prior to trauma exposure (e.g., age, ethnicity). Meta-analytic findings do suggest that pretrauma characteristics play a small role in predicting PTSD development in youth (Trickey, Siddaway, Meiser-Stedman, Serpell, & Field, 2012). The third factor in this model involves the child's *posttrauma environment* and includes contextual factors such as parental functioning and social support. The posttrauma environment may either "magnify or attenuate" a child's reaction to trauma. Indeed, posttrauma variables such as social support have been found to have a moderate-to-large effect on PTSD development in youth (Trickey et al., 2012). Specifically, poor support following trauma exposure, particularly from family members, predicts higher levels of PTSD symptoms among children (e.g., Valentino, Berkowitz, & Stover, 2010). The fourth factor involves the child's *coping skills.* The model suggests that the relationship between PTSD symptoms and coping skills is bidirectional, such that poor coping skills may predict higher PTSD symptoms, but that PTSD symptoms may also subsequently reduce the child's ability to cope. Generally, negative coping strategies such as self-blame and anger are predictive of higher levels of PTSD symptoms (e.g., Vernberg, Silverman, La Greca, & Prinstein, 1996). Finally, the fifth factor, *additional stressful life events,* may differentially impact each of the previous four factors. For example, additional life stressors (e.g., parental divorce) may serve to "magnify" a child's reactions to the original trauma. Overall, there has been empirical support for multiple components of this conceptual model, though no studies to date have examined each component of the model within the same sample. Given that this model was originally conceptualized for survivors of natural disasters, further research is needed to examine its utility among individuals who have experienced other types of traumas (e.g., physical or sexual abuse). The five-factor model is helpful in framing a variety of trauma-related and environmental predictors of PTSD development in youth, but it does not account for cognitive or physiological processes that are also likely to play a role in risk for PTSD.

Developmental Trajectory Model

This model highlights both intrinsic (e.g., within the child) and extrinsic (e.g., outside of the child) factors (Pynoos, Steinberg, & Piacentini, 1999). The developmental trajectory model also accounts for maturational processes, highlighting that PTSD may be expressed differently depending on the age/developmental stage of the child. Finally, the model suggests that separate factors contribute to immediate versus long-term reactions to traumatic stressors. This developmental model also highlights the challenges that trauma introduces into the neurodevelopment of children, particularly in learning to integrate and cope with intense emotional reactions. For example, different facets of emotional development may be interrupted depending on the age of trauma exposure. If the trauma occurs during preschool age, children may have difficulty differentiating between their emotions (e.g., anger vs. sadness). However, trauma exposure during adolescence may negatively impact an adolescent's ability to understand the origins (e.g., "Why am I sad?") and consequences of negative emotions (e.g., "How is my sadness negatively impacting me or others around me?") (Pynoos et al., 1999; Saarni & Harris, 1991). More specifically, factors theorized to contribute to PTSD development within this model include proximal trauma reminders (e.g., situations/places/people that are reminders, media coverage of the traumatic event, physiological reactions), proximal secondary stressors (e.g., disruption of school schedule, loss of property/resources), the child's ecology (e.g., family functioning, parental psychopathology), and intrinsic factors (e.g., temperament, genetics, acquired developmental milestones). Overall, this comprehensive model highlights the role of development and maturation processes in predicting PTSD symptoms in youth.

Cognitive Models

Multiple cognitive models have been proposed to explain the development of PTSD (for a review, see Dalgleish, 2004). Ehlers and Clark's (2000) model suggest that individuals with PTSD develop a sense of ongoing threat within their environment that is maintained by (1) negative appraisals of the trauma itself (e.g., "The world is dangerous") and/or posttrauma events (e.g., "Why can't I get over this?") and (2) poorly elaborated or poorly integrated trauma memories. Maladaptive coping strategies (e.g., avoidance, rumination, thought suppression) interfere with the integration and elaboration of the trauma memory, altering the negative appraisals and reducing the sense of current threat. There is a growing body of empirical support for the applicability of this cognitive model in youth (e.g., Ehlers, Mayou, & Bryant, 2003; Meiser-Stedman, Dalgleish, Glucksman, Yule, & Smith, 2009; Stallard, 2003; Stallard & Smith, 2007). For example, higher levels of maladaptive cognitive coping strategies such as thought suppression (i.e., trying to forget about the trauma), distraction (i.e., doing something to forget about the trauma), and rumination (i.e., wishing that the trauma could have happened differently) were associated with PTSD development (Stallard, 2003) in a study of children ages 5–18 years who experienced a motor vehicle accident. Similarly, in a study of children ages 5–16 who experienced a motor vehicle accident, negative appraisals (e.g., perceived alienation from others after the trauma) were a significant predictor of PTSD 3 and 6 months post-accident (Ehlers et al., 2003). Taken together, there is preliminary support suggesting that cognitive models may be useful for conceptualizing PTSD in children. However, the majority of studies examining cognitive models of PTSD in youth have focused on older children (mean age = 12 years 3 months [Ehlers et al., 2003]; mean age = 14 years 6 months [Stallard, 2003]). Similarly, others have suggested (Salmon & Bryant, 2002) that cognitive theories of youth PTSD need to include more developmentally sensitive components, such as stage of language and memory development.

Parental Model

This model highlights the role of parental functioning, parent–child relationships, and familial functioning in PTSD development, particularly for young children (Scheeringa & Zeanah, 2001). Three types of parenting styles are suggested as negatively impacting a child's posttrauma adjustment: overprotective, reenacting, and withdrawn parenting. Parents who adopt the first negative parenting style, the withdrawn parent, are generally withdrawn, unresponsive, and unavailable to provide support to their child. This parenting style may be most often observed in parents with previous trauma histories (Scheeringa & Zeanah, 2001). Overprotective parents often have a fear that their child will be retraumatized in some way, or they feel guilty because they were unable to protect their child from experiencing a trauma. Therefore, they become overprotective and constrict their child's development. Finally, the reenacting type of parent becomes preoccupied with trauma reminders. A parent exhibiting this style may repeatedly discuss the trauma or question the child about the details of the experience. All three of these parenting styles are suggested to exacerbate the child's PTSD symptoms and hinder natural recovery following a trauma. Clinically, this model suggests that clinicians attend to the caregiver's symptomatology prior to attending to the child's symptoms (Scheeringa & Zeanah, 2001) in order to allow the parent to be better able to respond to the needs of the child.

Generally, this relational model offers a helpful framework for understanding the role of family dynamics in youth PTSD. The primary focus of this model is the way in which the child's PTSD symptoms are influenced by parental distress. However, this model does not account for situations, common among childhood cancer survivors, in which parents display significantly higher PTSD symptoms than their child (e.g., for a review of PTSD in childhood cancer survivors, see Bruce, 2006). Similarly, relational models do not propose potential moderating factors that may impact the strength of the relationship between parenting and PTSD in youth.

Overall then, compared to the literature on adults, conceptual models of PTSD development in children are still in the early stages. Emotional processing (e.g., Foa & Kozak, 1986) and learning (e.g., Lang, Craske, & Bjork, 1999) theories, prominent in the adult literature, have rarely been examined in youth samples. Others have proposed including components of early attachment theories and the role of chronic trauma exposure (van der Kolk, 2005) in theoretical accounts of youth PTSD. While some promising theories have been proposed, further empirical examination within diverse samples and across developmental stages is warranted.

EVIDENCE-BASED TREATMENTS FOR PTSD

There is a growing body of research examining the efficacy of psychotherapy and pharmacotherapy treatment options for PTSD in youth. Compared to the adult treatment literature, there are relatively few randomized controlled trials (RCTs) in youth samples. To date, trauma-focused psychotherapy has received the strongest empirical support (Cohen et al., 2010). Pharmacotherapy trials have been fewer, and there are no current U.S. Food and Drug Administration (FDA)–approved medications for PTSD treatment in youth. In the next section we briefly outline the evidence for current empirically supported treatment options. Following the review of the evidence, we provide guidelines for assessment and descriptions of the treatment protocols.

Psychotherapy

There is a growing number of promising evidence-based psychotherapy options for children and adolescents with PTSD (Cohen et al., 2010; Feeny, Foa, Treadwell, & March, 2004). The American Academy of Child and Adolescent Psychiatry considers trauma-focused psychotherapy to be the first-line treatment for youth with PTSD (Cohen et al., 2010). We review in the next section the evidence for the three treatments with the strongest empirical support to date: trauma-focused cognitive-behavioral therapy (TF-CBT), prolonged exposure for adolescents (PE-A), and cognitive-behavioral intervention for trauma in schools (CBITS). These three treatments are considered "well established" based on the American Psychological Association (1995, 2006), Division 12 (Clinical Psychology) Task Force on Psychological Intervention Guidelines (Chambless & Hollon, 1998). "Well-established" treatments are those with the highest level of support, reflecting converging evidence from multiple well-designed studies.

TF-CBT (Cohen, Manarino, & Deblinger, 2006) has received the strongest empirical support and is the most widely disseminated trauma-focused treatment for youth ages 3–17 years (Saxe, MacDonald, & Ellis, 2007). RCTs suggest that TF-CBT leads to greater reduction in PTSD symptoms than do other forms of psychotherapy, including supportive therapy (Cohen & Manarino, 1996) and client-centered therapy (Cohen, Deblinger, Mannarino, & Steer, 2004). Intent-to-treat analyses suggest that TF-CBT remains effective in the long-term, with treatment gains often maintained 12 months after completing treatment (Cohen, Mannarino, & Knudsen, 2005). In addition to reductions in PTSD symptoms, TF-CBT has also been effective in reducing depressive symptoms and shame (Deblinger, Manarino, Cohen, & Steer, 2006). One RCT (Sheeringa, Weems, Cohen, Amaya-Jackson, & Guthrie, 2011) found that TF-CBT was effective in reducing PTSD symptoms even in very young children (ages 3–6). However, further research is needed to better understand how implementation of and reaction to TF-CBT may differ depending on developmental level.

Prolonged exposure (PE) therapy, an empirically supported treatment for adults with PTSD, has recently been adapted for use in adolescent samples (PE-A; Foa, Chrestman,

& Gilboa-Schechtman, 2008). Recent RCTs have indicated that PE-A is more effective in reducing PTSD symptoms than time-limited dynamic therapy (Gilboa-Schectman et al., 2010) and supportive therapy (Foa, McLean, Capaldi, & Rosenfield, 2013), with large overall effects found in both studies (Cohen's d = 1.71 and 2.72, respectively). PE-A has also been shown to produce long-term gains, with adolescents maintaining their treatment gains 17 months posttreatment (Gilboa-Schechtman et al., 2010). PE-A has shown promising results. However, additional RCTs with larger sample sizes are needed to further support the use of PE for adolescents.

CBITS (Jaycox, 2004) is a brief, 10-session, group-based intervention that is implemented in a school setting. CBITS has been shown to be effective in reducing PTSD symptoms in two RCTs: one showing a medium effect (R^2 = .43) for CBITS with recently immigrated Latino third to eighth graders (Kataoka et al., 2003), and the other showing a large effect (Cohen's d = 1.08) for a largely Latino sample of sixth graders exposed to violence (Stein et al., 2003). This treatment protocol is particularly helpful in settings in which there has been a schoolwide or community-based trauma with a large number of children exposed to a similar trauma (e.g., school shooting, natural disaster).

Although these therapies have shown the strongest empirical support, a few other CBT treatments have also shown promise, including Alternatives for Families: A Cognitive Behavioral Therapy (AF-CBT, formerly known as Abuse-Focused CBT; Kolko & Swenson, 2002), and Child–Parent Psychotherapy (CCP; Lieberman, 2004). These protocols have stronger empirical support than non-CBT approaches such as psychodynamic therapy and medication (Feeny et al., 2004), and they have been shown to be superior to non-trauma-focused psychotherapy approaches such as nondirective supportive therapy (Cohen, Mannarino, Murray, & Igelman, 2006).

Pharmacotherapy

A number of pharmacological agents have been examined for treatment of youth with PTSD, including antipsychotics, beta-blockers, selective serotonin reuptake inhibitors (SSRIs), and antiseizure medications (for a review of pharmacological treatment in youth PTSD, see Strawn, Keeshin, DelBello, Geracioti, & Putnam, 2010). However, results have been mixed, and in many trials, medication has not been superior to placebo in reducing PTSD symptoms (e.g., Cohen, Mannarino, Perel, & Staron, 2007; Robb et al., 2010). SSRIs including paroxetine and sertraline are FDA approved for PTSD treatment in adults. Open trials of SSRIs for youth with PTSD have produced promising results (e.g., Seedat, Lockhat, Kaminer, Zungu-Dirwayi, & Stein, 2001), but in the only controlled trial, failed to demonstrate significant benefit compared to placebo (Robb, Cueva, Sporn, Yang, & Vanderburg, 2010). Recently, Cohen and colleagues (2007) examined the efficacy of using an SSRI as an adjunct to TF-CBT. A small sample of sexually abused youth ages 10–17 years were randomized to either a 12-week course of TF-CBT + sertraline or TF-CBT + placebo. Both groups experienced similar reductions in PTSD symptoms and depression symptoms (Cohen et al., 2007). Notably, the authors indicated that a large portion of parents refused to allow their children to take part in the trial due to medication-related concerns.

Taken together, results from pharmacotherapy trials do not support medication as a first-line intervention for youth with PTSD (Strawn et al., 2010). Recent guidelines set forth by the American Academy of Child and Adolescent Psychiatry (Cohen et al., 2010) suggest that clinicians should consider recommending psychiatric treatment of youth PTSD only for those who do not respond to evidence-based trauma-focused psychotherapy. Similarly, others (e.g., Cohen et al., 2007; Strawn et al., 2010) have suggested that using an SSRI as an add-on to evidence-based psychotherapy may be considered for children who have severe trauma-related symptoms or PTSD in addition to a comorbid psychological disorder that requires treatment (e.g., depression).

Predictors of Treatment Response

There are few well-established predictors of PTSD treatment response among youth. Similarly, little is known regarding which type of treatment is most effective for a particular client. Research is also needed to understand and examine the processes that drive therapeutic improvement in evidence-based treatments for PTSD. In a review of psychological treatment for youth exposed to trauma, treatment type, specifically, receiving CBT, and parental involvement in treatment were predictors of better treatment response (Silverman et al., 2008). Demographic factors, therapeutic alliance, and social support have also been examined as predictors of treatment outcome.

Similar to the pattern in adults, demographic variables such as age, gender, and ethnicity have not emerged as consistent predictors of treatment outcome among youth receiving TF-CBT (Cohen et al., 2004). With regard to ethnicity, it appeared that TF-CBT was equally effective in treating children of European American and African American backgrounds (Cohen et al., 2004). However, in a study examining TF-CBT and client-centered therapy, higher socioeconomic status predicted better treatment outcome (Cohen & Mannarino, 2000).

A strong *therapeutic alliance,* or relationship between client and therapist, is consistently predictive of better therapy outcomes in adult samples (Martin, Garske, & Davis, 2000). Few studies have examined the role of treatment alliance in youth PTSD treatment. In a recent trial comparing TF-CBT to treatment as usual among 156 traumatized adolescents ages 10–18 years, a stronger therapeutic alliance emerged as a significant predictor of better treatment outcome, but only in the TF-CBT group (Ormhaug, Jensen, Wentzel-Larsen, & Shirk, 2014). In a recent report analyzing the same sample of 156 youth, higher therapist and patient ratings of treatment alliance predicted patient treatment satisfaction but only the patient scale was significantly related to change in symptoms (Ormhaug, Shirk, & Wentzel-Larsen, 2015). Similarly, strong therapeutic alliance has been shown to predict better treatment outcome for adult survivors of childhood sexual assault, with this relationship being mediated by emotion regulation capacity during therapy (Cloitre, Stovall-McClough, Miranda, & Chemtob, 2004). The authors suggest that emotion regulation difficulties are common for traumatized youth, emphasizing the importance of this mechanism in understanding the impact of therapeutic alliance during treatment for this population. More studies are needed to understand the role of therapeutic alliance in psychotherapy for children.

Social support, a strong predictor of PTSD development (Brewin, Andrews, & Valentine, 2000), has recently received attention as a potential variable impacting treatment outcome in youth. Social support is a multifaceted construct, and a number of types of support have been found to predict treatment outcome in youth. For example, child perceptions of support have been found to relate to treatment response. Children who perceived that others did not believe them (e.g., when they disclosed the abuse) and perceptions that others blamed them for the trauma had a poorer response to TF-CBT or client-centered therapy than children without such beliefs (Cohen & Mannarino, 2000). On the other hand, higher levels of parent-reported parental support have also been shown to relate to improved treatment outcome for children (Cohen & Mannarino, 1998, 2000).

Finally, there is preliminary evidence that supports neurobiological markers of treatment response (Cisler et al., 2015). In a recent study of 23 adolescent girls with PTSD related to physical or sexual assault who completed TF-CBT, pretreatment amygadala reactivity predicted treatment response. Prior to treatment, participants completed an implicit threat processing task during functional magnetic resonance imaging (fMRI), in which their amygdala response was measured while they viewed faces with fearful or neutral expressions. Adolescents who showed greater amygdala activation to both threatening/fearful faces and neutral faces showed less symptom reduction across TF-CBT. However, adolescents with greater symptom reduction across TF-CBT showed amygdala activation only to threat images. These results are preliminary, but they suggest that pretreatment amygdala reactivity in response to fearful or threatening stimuli positively predicts symptom reduction during TF-CBT (Cisler et al., 2015). Overall, as the treatment efficacy literature grows, it will be important to pinpoint both psychosocial and neurobiological variables that reliably and consistently predict treatment response in order to improve and tailor PTSD treatment for youth. Promising potential predictors, based on the limited research available, include parental involvement in CBTs, a strong therapeutic alliance, and perceived parental/social support.

EVIDENCE-BASED ASSESSMENT AND TREATMENT IN PRACTICE

Assessment

Regardless of treatment modality, there are often barriers to seeking treatment (e.g., lack of resources, transportation difficulties, insurance coverage). In order to increase utilization of services and improve adherence, it is important for clinicians to provide a clear rationale for each component of the treatment and to educate both parents and children on common symptoms of PTSD (Sharma-Patel et al., 2011). Specifically, providing a developmentally appropriate rationale addressing potential differences in posttrauma reactions based on developmental stage can personalize the treatment and increase trust between the therapist and child. As a clinician, it is also important to assess child safety, particularly for children who have chronic trauma histories or may be at risk of current danger. Engaging a nonoffending caregiver in the treatment plan, whether it is just to make a few phone calls or to have the caregiver attend sessions, can help to ensure child safety. In fact, parental involvement in treatment has been found to improve treatment outcome for youth with trauma-related symptoms (Silverman et al., 2008). Similarly, some have suggested that a parent's ability to support his or her child and maintain his or her own support network is a crucial factor in promoting mental health in children exposed to traumatic events (e.g., McGloin & Widom, 2001). Thus, some have suggested that a clinician may want to discuss, early in treatment, with the parent whether he or she feels it would be important to engage in his or her own mental health treatment (Yule,

Smith, Perrin, & Clark, 2013). This may be especially important for cases in which both the parent and child were exposed to the target trauma. Generally, however, the child's treatment should not be contingent on the parent seeking treatment (Yule et al., 2013).

Developmental stage is an important consideration for assessment of PTSD in youth. As we discussed previously, a preschool subtype was added to the DSM-5 PTSD diagnosis (American Psychiatric Association, 2013). However, differences in trauma reactions are also found between school-age (i.e., > 6 years of age) and adolescent children. For example, among a generalized trauma sample of children ages 7–14 years, those in later stages of pubertal development were more likely to meet criteria for multiple PTSD symptom clusters compared to those in earlier stages (Carrion, Weems, Ray, & Reiss, 2002), suggesting that younger children are less likely to report enough symptoms to meet criteria for PTSD. However, the children exhibiting subthreshold PTSD had similar levels of functional impairment compared to children who met full criteria (Carrion et al., 2002). Therefore, it is essential to provide age-appropriate assessment, including reports from others (i.e., teachers and parents), in order to fully understand how trauma relates to symptoms of PTSD in youth.

Differential Diagnosis

Given that PTSD exhibits high comorbidity rates with other psychological disorders and symptoms, including, depression, substance use, internalizing symptoms, and externalizing disorders such as ODD and ADHD (e.g., Ford et al., 2000; Kilpatrick et al., 2003; Macdonald et al., 2010), thorough assessment is required to provide the appropriate diagnostic picture. Considering these high comorbidity rates, it is important for clinicians working with traumatized youth to assess for a wide variety of symptoms, in addition to those specific to PTSD.

Clinicians working with youth should employ the proper assessment measures and techniques to understand whether symptoms should be classified as part of a PTSD diagnosis or a separate psychological disorder. The American Academy of Child and Adolescent Psychiatry (Cohen, et al., 2010) recommends routine screening for trauma exposure in initial assessments with children. Subsequent assessment can identify whether reactions to the trauma have resulted in a pathological response, which may or may not include symptoms of PTSD. For example, a clinician seeing a child with attention difficulties and a history of abuse might be able to rule out ADHD if attention problems occur solely when the child is reexperiencing a trauma.

Clinical Interviews

The unique difficulties regarding the assessment of PTSD in children complicate the development of structured clinical interviews for this population. One approach has been to adapt empirically supported adult assessments for use with children. For example, the *Clinician-Administered PTSD Scale for Children and Adolescents* (CAPS-CA; Nader et al., 1996) is designed for use with children ages 8–15 years and is based on the widely used Clinician-Administered PTSD Scale for adults (CAPS; Blake, Weathers, Nagy & Kaloupek, 1995). Similar to the CAPS for adults, the CAPS-CA assesses frequency and intensity of PTSD symptoms. The CAPS and CAPS-CA assess for additional trauma-related symptoms, such as dissociation, and for global functioning and impairment. The CAPS-CA has a number of features and additional questions to make it more applicable to the assessment of children. The instructions for the CAPS-CA are worded specifically for children and provide more detailed information explaining PTSD symptoms. For example, the instructions include a practice question to make sure the child understands the difference between the frequency and intensity ratings. Some questions are altered as well (e.g., assessing scholastic functioning as opposed to occupational functioning). The CAPS-CA also contains three additional items tailored specifically to children:

Item 23. Impact on developmental functioning: Loss of acquired skill
Item 29. Shame
Item 33. Changes in attachment

The CAPS-CA has demonstrated acceptable internal consistency (Erwin, Newman, McMackin, Morrisey, & Kaloupek, 2000) and construct validity (Carrion et al., 2002).

The Child PTSD Symptom Scale (CPSS; Foa, Johnson, Feeny, & Treadwell, 2001) was also adapted from an adult PTSD assessment tool (PTSD Symptom Scale—Interview version (PSS-I; Foa, Riggs, Dancu, & Rothbaum, 1993) for use with children. Like the adult version, it has both a clinician-administered and a self-report version, and like the CAPS-CA, it measures the DSM-IV PTSD symptoms. However, unlike the CAPS-CA, the CPSS asks about frequency of symptoms in the last 2 weeks specifically, and does not include separate questions for rating intensity. Frequency ratings are made on a Likert-type scale that ranges from 0 ("not at all or only at one time") to 3 ("5 or more times a week/almost always"). In addition to the 17 DSM-IV symptom items, the CPSS also includes seven functional impairment items, designed to assess whether PTSD symptoms have impacted areas of the child's life (e.g., family relationships, academic functioning). The CPSS has demonstrated high internal consistency and convergent validity with other measures of childhood PTSD (e.g., Foa et al., 2001).

While it is preferable to utilize an instrument that assesses symptom frequency and intensity (i.e., the CAPS-CA or the CPSS), simply assessing for the presence of PTSD symptoms in a comprehensive diagnostic interview may be more appropriate in many clinical settings. Comprehensive diagnostic interviews for children include the Kiddie Schedule for Affective Disorders and Schizophrenia for School-Age Children—Present and Lifetime Version (K-SADS-PL; Kaufman, et al., 1997); the Diagnostic Interview for Children and Adolescents (DICA; Reich, 2000); The National Institute of Mental Health (NIMH) Diagnostic Interview Schedule for Children, Version IV (NIMH DISC-IV; Shaffer, Fisher, Lucas, Dulcan, & Schwab-Stone, 2000); and The Anxiety Disorders Interview Schedule for DSM-IV for Children (ADIS-C; Silverman, Saavedra, & Pina, 2001). These measures are structured around diagnostic criteria from the DSM-IV and, when available, revised accordingly for the DSM-5. Each of these measures contains parent and child versions because both reports are beneficial to the diagnosis of childhood psychopathology.

While a description of the psychometrics for each of these measures is beyond the scope of this review, the K-SADS-PL is commonly used in samples of traumatized youth across the developmental spectrum (e.g., Cohen et al., 2004, 2007). The K-SADS-PL has been shown to reliably assess PTSD in young children between ages 2 and 5 years using only parent report (Birmaher et al., 2010). The ability of this measure to assess multiple traumas and age groups makes it particularly clinically useful. The K-SADS-PL is a semi-structured diagnostic interview analogous to the Structured Clinical Interview for DSM-IV-Axis I Disorders (SCID-IV; First, Spitzer, Gibbon, & Williams, 2002) for adults, and like the SCID, the K-SADS contains a specific module to diagnose PTSD. In this module, symptoms of PTSD are assessed and marked present or absent either currently or in the past. A diagnosis of PTSD is determined based on DSM symptom cluster thresholds. Psychometric studies show concurrent validity for diagnoses using the K-SADS-PL, as well as good test–retest reliability for a diagnosis of PTSD (Kaufman et al., 1997).

Self-Report Measures

A number of self-report measures have been developed to assess symptoms of PTSD and other trauma reactions in children. One validated self-report measure of PTSD symptoms is the Self-Report version of the Child PTSD Symptom Scale (CPSS). Like the adult version (the PSSI), the CPSS can be administered as an interview or self-report measure. As with the interview version, the current self-report measure assesses the 17 DSM-IV PTSD symptoms and contains seven social function questions. A validated DSM-5 version is not yet available as of this writing.

The Children's Revised Impact of Events Scale (CRIES; Smith, Perrin, Dyregrov, & Yule, 2003) is also derived from an adult assessment tool, the Impact of Events Scale (IES; Horowitz, Wilner, & Alvarez, 1979). The CRIES is a 13-item PTSD screening tool that assesses four intrusion, four avoidance, and five arousal symptoms. Factor analysis of the 13 items (Smith et al., 2003) showed a clear distinction between intrusion and avoidance symptoms; however, all of the arousal symptoms loaded onto the intrusion factor, suggesting that intrusion and arousal symptoms are closely related in children. Furthermore, a cutoff score of 30 on the CRIES has been shown to accurately predict a PTSD diagnosis for 75–83% of children in samples with high and low PTSD base rates (Perrin, Meiser-Stedman & Smith, 2005), suggesting high specificity and sensitivity for the measure. This study also showed that an eight-item version of the CRIES that excluded arousal symptoms was as accurate as the 13-item CRIES in predicting PTSD diagnosis, suggesting that hyperarousal symptoms may not be necessary for the diagnosis of PTSD in children. However, a factor analysis of the CRIES in a Chinese sample of traumatized youth (Zhang, Zhang, Wu, Zhu, & Dyregrov, 2011) supported a three-factor structure but suggested that these factors were highly correlated.

There are a number of self-report measures designed to assess reactions to trauma beyond the DSM core symptoms. For example, the Children's Impact of Traumatic Event Scale—Revised (CITES-R; Wolfe & Gentile, 1991) comprises 78 items assessing 11 clinical subscales. These subscales include DSM PTSD reactions (Intrusive Thoughts, Avoidance, and Hyperarousal), sexual anxiety, attributions about the abuse (Self-Blame/Guilt, Personal Vulnerability, Believing in a Dangerous World, and A Sense of Empowerment), social reactions (Negative Reactions by Others and Social Support), and eroticism. Items are worded as statements, and the respondent indicates whether the statement is "very true," "somewhat true," or "not true." Internal consistency for the CITES-R subscales has been shown to be highest for the main PTSD scales, with the other scales showing less consistency (Chaffin & Shultz, 2001).

The Trauma Symptom Checklist for Children (TSCC; Briere, 1996) also measures a broad range of trauma reactions. This 54-item measure includes six subscales (Anxiety, Depression, Posttraumatic Stress, Sexual Concerns, Dissociation, and Anger). In addition to the clinical scales, this measure includes two validity scales (Underresponse and Hyperresponse) to determine abnormal response styles that may invalidate the results. The items comprise a list of thoughts, feelings, or behaviors to which the respondent responds from 0 ("Never") to 3 ("Almost all the time"). The clinical scales show moderate to high reliability (.77–.89; Briere, 1996).

In conclusion, while most assessments of PTSD in children are adapted from adult measures, they include some developmentally specific modifications. As the diagnosis of PTSD becomes more developmentally sensitive (i.e., the inclusion of the preschool subtype), childhood assessments will require greater modifications. Proper assessment development and implementation will ensure that as the diagnosis for childhood PTSD evolves, clinicians will be equipped to identify and treat the many reactions that manifest in children after a traumatic experience.

Treatment

As we discussed previously, there are a number of empirically supported treatments for childhood PTSD. The three CBT approaches with the strongest empirical support to date include TF-CBT (Cohen & Mannarino, 1993), CBITS (Stein et al., 2003), and PE-A (Foa et al., 2008), but other CBT treatments have also shown promise. Several primary components have been theorized to be important in CBT for children and adolescents with PTSD, including *exposure, cognitive processing/reframing,* and *parental training* (Cohen, Mannarino, Berlinger, & Deblinger, 2000). Whereas Cohen and colleagues (2000) describe the empirical support for each of these components, we address in this review important clinical considerations for implementing each of these therapeutic strategies in order to help bridge the gap between the empirical base and clinical practice.

Exposure

Exposure techniques are often utilized in the treatment of anxiety disorders in adults and children. For the treatment of PTSD in adults, exposure-based therapies have the strongest empirical evidence for treatment efficacy (Institute of Medicine, 2008). While the research with PTSD in children is less developed, exposure techniques have been shown to be efficacious for adolescents ages 12–18 years (e.g., Gilboa-Schechtman et al., 2010). PE-A involves 12–15 sessions and includes the core exposure elements used in adults, as well as more extensive case management and a stronger emphasis on relapse prevention.

The primary types of exposure include imaginal and *in vivo* techniques. Imaginal exposure involves describing and repeatedly retelling the traumatic memory in session in the presence of the therapist. *In vivo* exposure involves engaging in objectively safe, real-life situations that the adolescent is avoiding because they serve as reminders of the trauma or make him or her feel unsafe (e.g., for a motor vehicle accident [MVA] survivor, being in a car; being around people who remind a child of an abuse perpetrator). PE-A (Foa et al., 2008) devotes eight or nine sessions to both imaginal and *in vivo* exposure work. Much as in prolonged exposure for adults, *in vivo* exposure involves the creation of a fear hierarchy of avoided people, places, and situations that act as triggers for the traumatic memory. The adolescent is encouraged to engage with these trauma reminders between sessions. For example, an MVA survivor may be encouraged to sit in a vehicle in a driveway or be a passenger while a family member drives around the block or to the store. Imaginal exposure involves having the adolescent retell the narrative of the trauma memory, preferably in the present tense and with his or her eyes closed to allow for optimal engagement with the memory. Imaginal exposures are audio-recorded, and clients are instructed to listen to the recordings for homework. Other empirically supported trauma-focused treatments such as TF-CBT and CBITS also include modified imaginal and *in vivo* exposure components (e.g., fear hierarchy in CBITS).

One consideration that is especially important in assigning *in vivo* exposure tasks for adolescents is ensuring that the situation is objectively safe. As with any abuse victim, it is necessary to ensure that exposures will not increase risk of harm. However, for children and adolescents, this risk is increased due to their lack of autonomy and reduced ability to avoid potentially harmful situations. For example, an adult who has moved away from the neighborhood where an assault occurred may be able to drive back there as an *in vivo* exposure. However, an adolescent may lack the means to do this and may not be able to accurately assess the objective safety of such a situation. For adolescents completing *in vivo* exposure, it may be helpful to have an additional person, such as a trusted nonperpetrating relative, collaborate on the fear hierarchy and accompany the adolescent during exposures. Imaginal exposures may be difficult for children and adolescents, depending on developmental stage because of difficulty engaging with the memory either due to problems with attention or understanding the task. Additional strategies can be used if verbal narration is too difficult. For example, the CBITS exposure protocol (Jaycox, 2004) involves imagining the memory, drawing the memory, or writing about the traumatic event. Similarly, TF-CBT involves constructing a trauma narrative. The considerations regarding exposure listed earlier are even more important when working with preschool-age children. For this population, the collaborative development (i.e., between child and parent) of a trauma narrative has been shown to be an effective exposure technique (Cohen & Mannarino, 1997; Lieberman, Van Horn & Ippen, 2005).

Cognitive Processing/Reframing

Cognitive therapy is designed to identify an individual's maladaptive cognitions and alter or reframe them to reduce psychopathology. For the treatment of adults with PTSD, cognitive processing therapy (CPT; Resick & Schnicke, 1992) is one such approach that focuses on addressing distorted cognitions about the trauma. TF-CBT, an adaptation of CPT (Cohen et al., 2000) for the treatment of children and adolescents, includes a cognitive processing component. TF-CBT is a brief (i.e., 12- to 18-session) intervention designed for both children and adolescents. Overall, TF-CBT involves skills described as PRACTICE (Psychoeducation and Parenting skills, Relaxation techniques, Affective expression and modulation, Cognitive coping, Trauma narrative and processing, *In vivo* mastery of trauma reminders, Conjoint parent–child sessions, and Enhancing future safety and development). TF-CBT seeks to correct distorted cognitions about a traumatic event (i.e., self-blame) through first identifying the distorted thoughts, then evaluating the reasons behind them, and finally, discussion, replacing the distorted thought with a more accurate one. There are multiple opportunities for clinicians to receive training in TF-CBT, including initial online workshops (*http://tfcbt.musc.edu*).

Other treatments also incorporate cognitive components. For example, PE-A involves processing of the traumatic event (e.g., discussing the process of talking through the memory) immediately after imaginal exposure, and CBITS dedicates two sessions to discussing the role of negative cognitions in PTSD and how to combat negative thoughts. The CBITS protocol (Jaycox, 2004) includes psychoeducation, relaxation, cognitive skills, exposure-based components, and social problem solving. The treatment is done within the school setting; therefore, a discussion of confidentiality is necessary during the first session to ensure that group members do not share others' experiences outside the group setting. Although parents are not directly involved in the treatment, there are parent and teacher education sessions about the CBITS program, as well as common reactions to trauma exposure.

As with exposure techniques, it is essential to take into account developmental stage when employing cognitive techniques. For adolescents, who are more capable of abstract reasoning than young children, cognitive reframing techniques used with adults may be appropriate. However, for younger children, these strategies need to be modified. For example, a 16 year-old may be able to engage in a discussion about the evidence for and against a negative thought, such as "It is my fault that the trauma occurred." A 7 year-old, however, may not be able to engage directly with his or her thought in the same way. In such cases, therapists can utilize more direct cognitive techniques such as helping young children to replace negative thoughts with positive ones (e.g., generating Helpful Other Thoughts in CBITS; Jaycox, 2004). This allows for cognitive change while bypassing the abstract thinking required in Socratic questioning. In addition, it is important for clinicians to listen closely to any negative cognition mentioned spontaneously during exposure exercises, as children may not be as easily able to identify these cognitions when asked directly. Finally, clinicians treating youth with PTSD should attempt to include trusted others, such as a nonperpetrating parent, to assist with the child's cognitive processing, as they may be a source of comfort for an especially reserved child.

Parent or Caregiver Involvement

It is often beneficial to include parents and other caregivers, especially when treating young children. Caregivers can help the child understand and engage in therapy and help the therapist understand the child's symptoms and functioning. Parents may play an important role in how a child reacts to a traumatic situation and are often the child's primary source of information, comfort, and support following a traumatic event. Therefore, it is crucial that parents not engage in the disconfirming and avoidant behaviors sometimes displayed by loved ones of trauma victims (i.e., placing blame on or not believing the victim). Including parents in treatment can help the parent (1) process the trauma along with the child, (2) reduce the negative emotions (e.g., guilt that they could not protect their child from exposure to trauma) that may be hindering their ability to help their child, and (3) implement changes in parenting practices.

There are a number of treatments for childhood PTSD that include the parent. For example, TF-CBT includes two components involving the parents. The first is a parent skills module that teaches praise, selective attention, time-out, and contingency reinforcement strategies. The second is a series of sessions with the child and parent together that come after the other components of treatment have been implemented. These sessions are designed to encourage open communication about the trauma between the child and parent. In contrast, AF-CBT (Kolko & Swenson, 2002) is a treatment designed for physical abuse victims and their families. AF-CBT is considered a "promising" treatment for child abuse victims by the National Child Traumatic Stress Network (see *www.nctsn.org*). Specifically, this treatment is often used in situations where there is frequent conflict in the home and use of physical discipline (clinicians seeking more information on training are encouraged to visit *www.afcbt.org*). In addition to addressing the child's reaction to parental violence, this treatment also has a number of parent-focused components for both offending and nonoffending parents. These include recognizing and managing abuse triggers and learning appropriate developmental expectations. This approach differs from other child-focused, as well as adult-focused, treatments for abuse victims in that the cause of the abuse, as opposed to the reaction, is directly targeted.

Other treatments designed for older children and adolescents, such as PE-A and CBITS do not require a parent-specific component, likely reflecting the increased autonomy of older children. Parent involvement in the treatment of early childhood trauma however, may be necessary for symptom change, as evidenced by data showing that abuse-specific components of AF-CBT (i.e., parent skills focused on preventing maltreatment) were uniquely related to positive treatment outcomes for abused children (Kolko, Iselin, & Gully, 2011).

Treatment for Preschool-Age Children

Treatment for this age group is enhanced by the inclusion of parents and caregivers because of trusted adults' ability to facilitate a child's engagement, and because of the strong influence of attachment in early childhood. TF-CBT has shown promising efficacy in this age group (Scheeringa et al., 2011). CPP (Lieberman, 2004; Lieberman & Van Horn, 2013) is a treatment for preschool children exposed specifically to parent-related adversity (e.g., parent mental illness) or other traumatic events (e.g., exposure to violence). In this treatment, joint child–parent sessions focus not only on parent training and developing a trauma narrative, as in TF-CBT, but also on supporting developmentally appropriate interactions between the parent and child (Lieberman et al., 2005). In this way, CPP treats the attachment between child and parent as a specific mechanism of change in therapy. CPP was been shown to be effective in reducing traumatic stress symptoms for children ages 3–5 years, all of whom who had witnessed marital violence, and a portion of whom experienced additional traumatic stressors such as physical abuse and sexual abuse, and witnessing community violence (Lieberman et al., 2005). This is a sensible approach when there is reason to believe that the attachment between the parent and child may be a contributing factor. However, some important drawbacks to this approach must be considered. First, a comprehensive knowledge of attachment theory is likely required for implementation of this treatment, which restricts the number of clinicians capable of implementing this therapy. Second, some parents may have had a direct role or been complacent in their child's abuse, which makes involvement of either parent difficult, if not impossible. In these situations, it is necessary to involve other, nonperpetrating caregivers, which is not always a possibility. Third, the focus on the parent–child relationship may ignore other important social influences, such as peers and siblings. Finally, given the high levels of resilience to adverse events displayed by young children (Masten, 2001), caution should be exercised when deciding to implement treatment. This is not to say that treatment would not be necessary in some cases, but time for natural recovery should be allowed.

In conclusion, like assessment for childhood PTSD, treatment has evolved to be developmentally sensitive. The growing number of empirically supported treatments for childhood PTSD is largely modeled on evidence-based adult treatments. These approaches have demonstrated that children as young as preschoolers can benefit from the same techniques used with adults. However, it is essential that these treatments include developmentally sensitive modifications, such as including a caregiver, when necessary.

Case Example

This section provides a case example of implementing an empirically supported, manualized group-based intervention for youth between ages 11 and 15 years. As previously mentioned, CBITS (Jaycox, 2004) is a short-term intervention implemented in a school setting. The case example highlights the course of CBITS treatment for a student named Lily.* We present Lily's course of treatment, including clinical recommendations and session dialogue. The clinician followed the manualized CBITS intervention protocol outlined in the treatment manual (Jaycox, 2004). Clinicians seeking more information on training in CBITS should consult the CBITS website (*https://cbitsprogram.org*).

BACKGROUND AND PRETREATMENT ASSESSMENT

Lily, a 14-year-old African American female freshman in high school, was referred to the CBITS program by her school counselor. She was raised by her mother in a single-parent household and never met her biological father. Lily reported that she had one older brother (age 19) whom she "really never sees." When Lily was 12 years old, she was waiting at a bus stop with her best friend [Jenny] when she witnessed a stabbing of a stranger. When asked to briefly describe what happened, Lily reported that she witnessed a young male jump out of a car, stab a young female, grab her purse, and get back into the car. Lily saw the young woman "bleeding all over" and quickly ran away from the scene. When asked about her current upsetting thoughts about the event, Lily said, "That could have happened to me or Jenny." Lily reported that she had seen a therapist for one session about 2 months earlier, but she never went back because "the lady just sided with my mom the whole time." Lily obtained a score of 23 on the CPSS, indicating PTSD symptoms in the clinical range. She also completed the Child Depression Inventory (CDI; Kovacs, 1981) and scored 18, indicating moderate depressive symptoms. With regard to PTSD symptoms, Lily reported that she had thoughts on a daily basis such as, "This could have happened to me or Jenny." Lily was also upset by trauma reminders, such as seeing buses on the street, young men who looked like the assailant, and being around

---

*This case represents a composite of various clients we have seen in our clinical work. All identifying information has been altered to protect confidentiality. Any resemblance to a specific individual is purely coincidental.

strangers (e.g., going to restaurants or to the mall). She was also experiencing moderate levels of cognitive and behavioral trauma-related avoidance (see Session 2 below for a detailed description of trauma-related avoidance) and detachment from others. Specifically, Lily put it this way: "I don't want to get close to anyone because what if something bad happens to them or something?" Finally, she reported significant difficulty sleeping and nightmares of "people bleeding."

Prior to starting CBITS, the clinician held a group parental informational meeting in order to discuss the primary components of CBITs, highlight the program as one that builds skills to better cope with stressors, educate parents on common reactions to trauma, and answer questions they had about the treatment. Parents were not involved in the group sessions. At the parental meeting, Lily's mother stated that she was worried that Lily "ignores me a lot and just sits in her room. She hardly sees her friends at all anymore."

SESSION 1

Lily and five other group members attended the first group session. First, confidentiality was discussed. Next, an overall rationale for CBITS was provided to the students (see the CBITS manual for the full rationale; Jaycox, 2004). The rationale included defining a trauma, giving examples of potential traumatic events, and asking group members to discuss how a trauma might change the way we *think, feel,* and *act.* At the end of the session, each student was asked to provide a brief statement of why he or she was attending the group and what he or she would like to work on in the group. Lily stated, "I am here because I saw someone get hurt by someone else. I want to get closer to people."

The students, including Lily, were fairly quiet and reserved in the first session. Particularly in high school settings, students may be reluctant to open up about their experiences for fear that other group members will discuss the group material with students outside the group. For this reason, reviewing confidentiality at the beginning of the session is critical.

SESSION 2

At the beginning of Session 2, common reactions to trauma were discussed (for a handout of common reactions to trauma, see the CBITS manual; Jaycox, 2004). Group members disclosed trauma-related difficulties that they were experiencing. Lily reported that she felt "alone" and "didn't want to talk or think about the trauma at all." Finally, she said, "I don't like to be around Jenny [her best friend]" because "the trauma happened to both of us but she's over it and so I feel stupid being upset still." At the end of the session, a breathing exercise was introduced and group members were asked to practice the exercise every day. Lily reported that she often uses "loud music to drown out whatever is going on in my head to get to sleep at night." The clinician suggested that Lily listen instead to relaxing music before bed while doing the deep breathing to help her sleep.

SESSIONS 3 AND 4

The aim of these sessions was to introduce cognitive therapy and provide group members with cognitive strategies they could use to combat negative thoughts. At the beginning of the session, the clinician introduced the idea of a fear thermometer (0- to 10-point scale of distress) as a way to measure how scared or upset the students feel. Lily reported that she felt a 0 ("completely calm") when she went on family vacation when she was 8 years old. She reported that she felt a 10 ("completely upset/afraid") during the trauma. Following the introduction of the fear thermometer, the session shifted to focus on cognitive therapy. Transcript from Session 3 introducing the link between thoughts and feelings follows (see the CBITS manual for Fear Thermometer Handouts and Rationale for Cognitive Therapy; Jaycox, 2004).

> CLINICIAN: Now that we have a way to measure how we are feeling, we are going to talk about how different types of thoughts you have going through your mind can lead you to have different types of feelings. Let's say, for example, that it's Friday night and you are going to a birthday party. Your friend was supposed to pick you up at about 7:00 P.M. and drive you to the party. It's 7:45 P.M. and your friend hasn't arrived yet, and she hasn't called or texted you either. What type of emotions are you feeling?
>
> GROUP MEMBER 1: Really annoyed and irritated.
>
> GROUP MEMBER 2: Worried about her. What if she got hurt?
>
> GROUP MEMBER 3: Like, bad about myself because she probably forgot about me or doesn't care about me.
>
> CLINICIAN: OK, so you all feel differently, even though it's the same situation. Let's see what types of thoughts would lead you to feel this way. Group Member 1, why would you feel irritated?
>
> GROUP MEMBER 1: Because she's late and didn't call. She's being rude.
>
> CLINICIAN: And Group Member 2, the thought you had was, "She could have gotten hurt," so you became worried. And Group Member 3, you were thinking that she didn't really care about you, so you were feeling a little ashamed and left out. When we say things to ourselves in our heads, it can make us feel a certain way. And each of you had different thoughts in that situation which caused you each to feel differently.

Following this dialogue, the clinician introduced various strategies for combatting negative thoughts (see CBITS manual for handouts that can be distributed to students; Jaycox, 2004). A portion of this dialogue follows:

> CLINICIAN: So, let's keep going with this example. There are different ways that we can check out our thoughts to make sure they are right or make sure they are helpful to us. So, let's say you are feeling worried because you think your friend got hurt and that's why she's late. Do you think there could be any other reason she's late?
>
> GROUP MEMBER 1: Well, maybe she forgot her phone at home, or it died or something.
>
> CLINICIAN: Exactly, so there are other ways of thinking about this situation. And, how might you feel if you think that the reason she didn't call you is because she accidentally forgot her phone at home?

GROUP MEMBER 1: Well, better, I guess. Not as worried.

CLINICIAN: Great, so by checking out your thoughts and figuring out if there were other ways to think about the situation, you were able to see that you can feel better about that situation.

In Sessions 3 and 4, the clinician went through multiple situations/examples in a similar fashion and introduced additional strategies to challenge negative thoughts. Group members were asked to practice using these strategies between group sessions. The clinician started off Session 4 by asking the students whether they noticed having any negative thoughts during the past week or whether they had any stressful experiences and worked through those examples in the group.

SESSION 5

Session 5 focused primarily on introducing *in vivo* exposure and creating a fear hierarchy. The clinician first provides a rationale for real-life exposure. Following the rationale, the remainder of the session is spent building a fear hierarchy with group members and assigning the group members items from the fear hierarchy to practice between group sessions. Items on the fear hierarchy include objectively safe situations, places, and people that the students are avoiding because they serve as trauma reminders. See Figure 9.1 for Lily's fear hierarchy. Following the hierarchy, homework was assigned (i.e., practice real-life exposures). Depending on the developmental stage and age of the child, parental involvement (e.g., a phone call) may be needed. For Lily's first assignment, she is asked to eat at the kitchen table with her mom at least three times instead of eating dinner in her room. Lily said this made her anxious (fear rating = 5) because "My mom think's differently about me now that I have gone through this and talking to her for a long time makes me uncomfortable." With Lily's permission, the clinician called Lily's mother to make sure that she is aware that this is part of Lily's treatment program and that she understands the importance of making sure they add dinner at the table to their weekly schedule.

INDIVIDUAL SESSION

After Session 5, Lily met with the clinician individually to complete a type of imaginal exposure. The clinician provided a rationale for imaginal exposure, then asked Lily to explain the trauma as if it were a movie projected onto a screen and to provide details such as how she was feeling and what she was thinking during the trauma (see the CBITS manual for the imaginal exposure rationale; Jaycox, 2004). The exercise was conducted for about 30 minutes.

LILY: The guy jumped out of the car and he ran right over to this girl who was listening to music on her headphones and just punched her. Then he took out a knife and stabbed her somewhere, like in the stomach.

[Clinician observation: Lily was furrowing her brow a bit and speaking softly. She seemed engaged with the memory, so I did not probe much.]

Real-Life Situation	Stress
Standing in front of school building at the end of the school day when buses are there	7
Riding in the bus with the other cheerleaders to the football game	9
Standing at a bus stop with a friend	8
Going to a crowded restaurant with my mom	6
Going to a non-crowded restaurant with my mom	5
Going to the mall on a weekend (crowded) with friends	8
Going to the mall on a weekday (not crowded) with friends	4
Hanging out with Jenny	7
Eat dinner at the table with my mom instead of eating in my room	5

FIGURE 9.1. Lily's fear hierarchy

LILY: She screamed *so* loud. It was so scary. Like I remember seeing red all over her dress and wondering what it was and then being, like, oh my God, it's blood. I felt, like, sick. But I just stood there, too, staring. Jenny grabbed my hand and yanked me, and we just started running away. I couldn't really think.

[Clinician observation: Lily started to tear up during this section so I provided gentle encouragement to Lily, praising her courage for sticking with this memory.]

LILY: Then, we just ran as fast as we could until we saw a restaurant. We ran in, called my mom, and just waited there until she picked us up.

[Clinician observation: Lily appeared very calm during this section and less engaged so I asked Lily, "What were you feeling when you were waiting for your mom to pick you up?"].

Lily repeated the trauma memory for about 25 minutes. Following this, the therapist asked Lily which parts of the memory were harder and which parts were easier. Lily identified the part where Jenny grabbed her hand and yanked her away, and they started running away together as a harder part. Lily stated that she would rate her fear at an 8 (on the thermometer) when thinking about that part of the memory. She stated that she wanted to work on that part in the group exposure sessions.

Clinically, it is important to gauge child engagement during the discussion of the memory. Although the therapist does not want the child to be overly upset in a school setting, he or she does want the child to experience some anxiety in order to process the memory (see the CBITS manual for suggestions on encouraging appropriate engagement; Jaycox, 2004). Following the exposure, the therapist asked Lily if she is still friends with Jenny, and Lily says, "Yes," but states that she does not think that Jenny was "bothered" by the trauma, and so she felt "stupid" talking to Jenny about it. The therapist reviewed cognitive strategies with Lily regarding her thoughts about Jenny's reactions (e.g., "How do you know that Jenny isn't bothered by the trauma? Are there other reactions that Jenny might have if she knew you were still upset about the trauma?"). The clinician also asked Lily what she would like to share with the group about her experience, and how she would like to show support to other group members. Lily said that she would like to tell group members, "Even though we all had different traumas, we are going through things together now and we can help each other."

SESSIONS 6 AND 7

At the beginning of Sessions 6 and 7 the clinician reviewed the real-life exposure assignments and took a few minutes to assign new homework, moving up the fear hierarchy for each group member. Lily reported that it was becoming easier to have dinner with her mom, and they had even decided to go to the mall together the upcoming weekend. She realized that her mom was not judging her or "thinking I'm being all weird now," and this reduced Lily's distress surrounding interactions with her mom. This example was used in the group to highlight that the more one engages in an activity, the less uncomfortable it becomes.

Following homework review, Sessions 6 and 7 focused on having group members either write, draw, or imagine their trauma for about 30 minutes. Following the exposure, each member was asked to share his or her reactions to the exposure. For example, the clinician asked the students to report how it felt to think/write/draw their memory during the session. Clinically, it is important to encourage the group members to be supportive of one another. Overall, these sessions are important not only to allow them to process the trauma but also to build trust and cohesion among the group members. The transcript from this session based on Lily's reactions to the exposure follows:

CLINICIAN: How did it feel to write/draw your trauma memory here in the group today?

LILY: It feels good. Like, I could never share any of this with other people at school. One time at lunch I heard these girls talking when they didn't know I was behind them. They were like "Lily is practically crazy now. I heard she has mental issues." It made me never want to talk to anyone about this.

CLINICIAN: Thank you for sharing, Lily. It's true that when we feel hurt by people, it makes it hard to trust. Other group members, if you had this experience that Lily just talked about, what could you tell yourself to make yourself feel better?

GROUP MEMBER: I would think, "They have no idea what I have been through, and they don't know the real story."

CLINICIAN: And how would that make you feel?

GROUP MEMBER: Well, maybe annoyed a little. But also easier to let it go because it's like I have been through something hard and maybe they haven't, so they don't know what it's like. So I wouldn't blame them maybe.

SESSIONS 8 AND 9

Similar to prior sessions, homework was reviewed at the beginning of the session, including real-life exposures, breathing exercises, and practice with cognitive strategies to reduce problematic thinking. Lily reported that she was sleeping better. In particular she reported that she liked listening to beach wave sounds while imagining she was lying on a beach prior to going to bed at night, and this helped her to sleep. In Session 7, her homework involved going on the bus with the other cheerleaders to and from the Friday night football game. This was higher on Lily's hierarchy (see Figure 9.1). She reported that she would discuss this assignment with her mother (who usually drove her to the football games). Also, if she was getting anxious while on the bus, she would text her mom or listen to relaxing music on her headphones. In Session 8, Lily came back and reported that she felt the most anxious right when she stepped on the bus (fear rating = 7). However, by the time she arrived at the football field, she became less nervous (fear rating = 4) because she began talking to her friends, listening to music, and "having a little fun, I guess." Lily said she felt like she needed to keep doing this exposure because it still made her "kinda nervous."

Following homework review, Sessions 8 and 9 focused on social problem solving. These sessions are particularly helpful for children with troubled social relationships. The clinician first provided a rationale for social problem solving by defining a problem and identifying the link between negative thoughts and potential actions (see the CBITS manual for Social Problem Solving Rationale and Model; Jaycox, 2004). During this session, it can be helpful to ask the group for recent conflicts or issues that they have had to demonstrate how problem solving works. The transcript from Session 9 based on a problem Lily brought up during the group follows:

> CLINICIAN: Last week we talked a lot about how to problem-solve by generating lots of solutions and deciding on how to pick the most helpful one. Since all of you are getting the hang of this now, let's go through some real examples. Has anyone had any conflicts that they would like to have the group help them problem-solve this week?
>
> LILY: Yeah, actually. Remember a couple of weeks ago I told you I overheard those girls saying that I "have mental problems." Well, ever since then, I feel like my friends have been ignoring me more.
>
> CLINICIAN: OK, this is a really good example. So the problem is that it seems like your friends are ignoring you. And your thought is that maybe they believe those girls. What are some other thoughts people might have if their friends are ignoring them?
>
> GROUP MEMBER 1: Maybe they are busy. It is around finals time, so maybe they are studying or something.
>
> GROUP MEMBER 2: I would start to think, "Maybe I am crazy" or wonder a lot that maybe those girls were right about me.
>
> GROUP MEMBER 3: I might think, like, "Are they actually ignoring me or am I just being overly paranoid?"
>
> CLINICIAN: What would you *do* if you thought, "Maybe they are just busy?"
>
> LILY: Nothing, really, but I guess I wouldn't feel as bad.
>
> CLINICIAN: What would you *do* if you started to think, "Maybe those girls were right."
>
> GROUP MEMBER 2: Probably just be alone and not want to be around anyone because I would feel bad about myself.

CLINICIAN: What would you *do* if you thought you might be overly paranoid?

GROUP MEMBER 3: I might just ask them if they were busy and wanted to hang out or something to test it out.

Following generation of these possible actions, the group brainstormed other possible solutions. At the end of the session, Lily realized that she did not have "real proof" that her friends were ignoring her, and she planned on asking one of her friends to go see a movie that weekend.

SESSION 10

Session 10 was geared toward discussing overall treatment progress and student reactions to the group. Lily reported that she felt closer to people, particularly the students in the group and also to Jenny [her best friend]. She also reported that getting on buses is "like, no big deal anymore." Lilly obtained a score of 9 on the CPSS and a CDI score of 7, indicating mild PTSD and depressive symptoms. Lily also reported that she wanted to continue to think about the pros and cons of "believing everything that goes through my head" and "shutting everyone out." She planned on continuing to have dinner with mom at least once a week and calling Jenny or another friend when got upset instead of "blocking out the world."

CONCLUSION

Unfortunately, the experience of trauma among children and adolescents is relatively common. For clinicians treating childhood disorders, special attention should be paid to symptoms of PTSD, as well as other symptoms that may be related to trauma. Understanding developmental models of PTSD onset is essential for implementing effective treatment for traumatized youth. Unique considerations, such as the child's ability to understand the traumatic event, accurately report symptoms, and rely on assistance from caretakers, require that evidence-based treatment be developmentally sensitive. Treatment efficacy trials have begun to identify important components of treatment that reduce symptoms of PTSD and comorbid pathology in children, including trauma narration, exposure, cognitive strategies, and parental involvement. Finally, it should be noted that children, like adults, often "bounce back" after a trauma. Natural resilience processes may be facilitated or hindered by factors such as parental or caregiver support. For those with persistent PTSD symptoms, treatment is often efficacious. Clinicians should therefore pay close attention to the presence or absence of these factors when they are considering treatment options for children and families exposed to trauma or violence.

REFERENCES

American Psychiatric Association. (2000). *Diagnostic and statistical manual of mental disorders* (4th ed.). Washington, DC: Author.
American Psychiatric Association. (2013). *Diagnostic and statistical manual of mental disorders* (5th ed.). Arlington, VA: Author.

American Psychological Association. (1995). *Template for developing guidelines: Interventions for mental disorders and psychosocial aspects of physical disorders.* Washington, DC: American Psychological Association, Task Force on Psychological Intervention Guidelines.

American Psychological Association. (2006). *Evidence-based practice in psychology.* Washington, DC: American Psychological Association, Presidential Task Force on Evidence-Based Practice.

Birmaher, B., Axelson, D., Goldstein, B., Monk, K., Kalas, C., Obreja, M., et al. (2010). Psychiatric disorders in preschool offspring of parents with bipolar disorder: The Pittsburgh Bipolar Offspring Study (BIOS). *American Journal of Psychiatry, 167*(3), 321–330.

Blake, D. D., Weathers, F. W., Nagy, L. M., Kaloupek, D. G., Gusman, F. D., Charney, D. S., et al. (1995). The development of a clinician-administered PTSD scale. *Journal of Traumatic Stress, 8*(1), 75–90.

Bremner, J. D., Randall, P., Scott, T. M., Bronen, R. A., Seibyl, J. P., Southwick, S. M., et al. (1995). MRI-based measurement of hippocampal volume in patients with combat-related posttraumatic stress disorder. *American Journal of Psychiatry, 152,* 973–981.

Brewin, C. R., Andrews, B., & Valentine, J. D. (2000). Meta-analysis of risk factors for posttraumatic stress disorder in trauma-exposed adults. *Journal of Consulting and Clinical Psychology, 68*(5), 748.

Brewin, C. R., & Holmes, E. A. (2003). Psychological theories of posttraumatic stress disorder. *Clinical Psychology Review, 23,* 339–376.

Briere, J. (1996). *Trauma Symptom Checklist for Children.* Odessa, FL: Psychological Assessment Resources.

Bruce, M. (2006). A systematic and conceptual review of posttraumatic stress in childhood cancer survivors and their parents. *Clinical Psychology Review, 26*(3), 233–256.

Carrion, V. G., Weems, C. F., Eliez, S., Patwardhan, A., Brown, W., Ray, R. D., et al. (2001). Attenuation of frontal asymmetry in pediatric posttraumatic stress disorder. *Biological Psychiatry, 50,* 943–951.

Carrion, V. G., Weems, C. F., Ray, R., & Reiss, A. L. (2002). Toward an empirical definition of pediatric posttraumatic stress disorder: The phenomenology of posttraumatic stress disorder symptoms in youth. *Journal of the American Academy of Child and Adolescent Psychiatry, 41,* 166–173.

Chaffin, M., & Shultz, S. K. (2001). Psychometric evaluation of the Children's Impact of Traumatic Events Scale—Revised, *Child Abuse and Neglect, 25*(3), 401–411.

Chambless, D. L., & Hollon, S. D. (1998). Defining empirically supported therapies. *Journal of Consulting and Clinical Psychology, 66,* 7–18.

Charmandari, E., Tsigos, C., Chrousos, G. (2005). Endocrinology of the stress response. *Annual Review of Physiology, 67,* 259–284.

Cisler, J. M., Sigel, B. A., Kramer, T. L., Smitherman, S., Vanderzee, K., Pemberton, J., et al. (2015). Amygdala response predicts trajectory of symptom reduction during trauma-focused cognitive behavioral therapy among adolescent girls with PTSD. *Journal of Psychiatric Research, 71,* 33–40.

Cloitre, M., Stovall-McClough, K., Miranda, R., & Chemtob, C. M. (2004). Therapeutic alliance, negative mood regulation, and treatment outcome in child abuse-related posttraumatic stress disorder. *Journal of Consulting and Clinical Psychology, 72*(3), 411–416.

Cohen, J. A., Bukstein, O., Walter, H., Benson, S., Chrisman, A., Farchione, T. R., et al. (2010). Practice parameter for the assessment and treatment of children and adolescents with posttraumatic stress disorder. *Journal of the American Academy of Child and Adolescent Psychiatry, 49*(4), 414–430.

Cohen, J. A., Deblinger, E., Mannarino, A. P., & Steer, R. A. (2004). A multisite, randomized controlled trial for children with sexual abuse-related PTSD symptoms. *Journal of the American Academy of Child and Adolescent Psychiatry, 43,* 393–402.

Cohen, J. A., & Mannarino, A. P. (1993). A treatment model for sexually abused preschoolers. *Journal of Interpersonal Violence, 8*(1), 115–131.

Cohen, J. A., & Mannarino, A. P. (1996). A treatment outcome study for sexually abused preschool children: Initial findings. *Journal of the American Academy of Child and Adolescent Psychiatry, 35,* 42–50.

Cohen, J. A., & Mannarino, A. P. (1997). A treatment study for sexually abused preschool children: Outcome during a one-year follow-up. *Journal of the American Academy of Child and Adolescent Psychiatry, 36*(9), 1228–1235.

Cohen, J. A., & Mannarino, A. P. (1998). Factors that mediate treatment outcome of sexually abused preschool children: Six- and 12-month follow-up. *Journal of the American Academy of Child and Adolescent Psychiatry, 37*(1), 44–51.

Cohen, J. A., & Mannarino, A. P. (2000). Predictors of treatment outcome in sexually abused children. *Child Abuse and Neglect, 24*(7), 983–994.

Cohen, J. A., Mannarino, A. P., Berliner, L., & Deblinger, E. (2000). Trauma-focused cognitive behavioral therapy for children and adolescents an empirical update. *Journal of Interpersonal Violence, 15*(11), 1202–1223.

Cohen, J. A., Mannarino, A. P., & Deblinger, E. (2006). *Treating trauma and traumatic grief in children and adolescents.* New York: Guilford Press.

Cohen, J. A., Mannarino, A. P., & Knudsen, K. (2005). Treating sexually abused children: 1 year follow-up of a randomized controlled trial. *Child Abuse and Neglect, 29*(2), 135–145.

Cohen, J. A., Mannarino, A. P., Murray, L. K., & Igelman, R. (2006). Psychosocial interventions for maltreated and violence-exposed children. *Journal of Social Issues, 62*(4), 737–766.

Cohen, J. A., Mannarino, A. P., Perel, J. M., & Staron, V. (2007). A pilot randomized controlled trial of combined trauma-focused CBT and sertraline for childhood PTSD symptoms. *Journal of the American Academy of Child and Adolescent Psychiatry, 46*(7), 811–819.

Copeland, W. E., Keeler, G., Angold, A., & Costello, J. (2007). Traumatic events and posttraumatic stress in childhood. *Archives of General Psychiatry, 64,* 577–584.

Cuffe, S., Addy, C., Garrison, C., Waller, J., Jackson, K., McKeown, R., et al. (1998). Prevalence of PTSD in a community sample of older adolescents. *Journal of the American Academy of Child and Adolescent Psychiatry, 37*(2), 147–154.

Dalgleish, T. (2004). Cognitive approaches to posttraumatic stress disorder: The evolution of multirepresentational theorizing. *Psychological Bulletin, 130*(2), 228–260.

De Bellis, M. D., Hall, J., Boring, A. M., Frustaci, K., & Moritz, G. (2001). A pilot longitudinal study of hippocampal volumes in pediatric maltreatment-related posttraumatic stress disorder. *Biological Psychiatry, 50,* 305–309.

De Bellis, M. D., & Zisk, A. (2014). The biological effects of childhood trauma. In S. J. Cozza, J. A. Cohen, & J. G. Dougherty (Eds.), *Child and adolescent psychiatric clinics of North America: Vol. 22. Disaster and trauma* (pp. 185–222). New York: Elsevier.

Deblinger, E., Mannarino, A. P., Cohen, J. A., & Steer, R. A. (2006). A follow-up study of a multisite, randomized, controlled trial for children with sexual abuse-related PTSD symptoms. *Journal of the American Academy of Child and Adolescent Psychiatry, 45*(12), 1474–1484.

Delahanty, D. L., Nugent, N. R., Christopher, N. C., & Walsh, M. (2005). Initial urinary epinephrine and cortisol levels predict acute PTSD symptoms in child trauma victims. *Psychoneuroendocrinology, 30*(2), 121–128.

De Young, A. C., Kenardy, J. A., Cobham, V. E., & Kimble, R. (2012). Prevalence, comorbidity and course of trauma reactions in young burn-injured children. *Journal of Child Psychology and Psychiatry, 53*(1), 56–63.

Ehlers, A., & Clark, D. M. (2000). A cognitive model of posttraumatic stress disorder. *Behaviour Research and Therapy, 38,* 319–345.

Ehlers, A., Mayou, R. A., & Bryant, B. (2003). Cognitive predictors of posttraumatic stress disorder in children: Results of a prospective longitudinal study. *Behaviour Research and Therapy, 41,* 1–10.

Erwin, B. A., Newman, E., McMackin, R. A., Morrissey, C., & Kaloupek, D. G. (2000). PTSD, malevolent environment, and criminality among criminally involved male adolescents. *Criminal Justice and Behavior, 27*(2), 196–215.

Feeny, N. C., Foa, E. B., Treadwell, K. R., & March, J. (2004). Posttraumatic stress disorder in youth: A critical review of the cognitive and behavioral treatment outcome literature. *Professional Psychology: Research and Practice, 35,* 466–476.

Finkelhor, D., Turner, H., Ormrod, R., & Hamby, S. (2009). Violence, abuse, and crime exposure in a national sample of children and youth. *Pediatrics, 124*(5), 1–13.

First, M. B., Spitzer, R. L., Gibbon, M., & Williams, J. B. (2002). *Structured Clinical Interview for DSM-IV-TR Axis I Disorders, research version, patient edition.* New York: Biometrics Research, New York State Psychiatric Institute.

Foa, E. B., Chrestman, K., & Gilboa-Schectman, E. (2008). *Prolonged exposure manual for children and adolescents suffering from PTSD.* New York: Oxford University Press.

Foa, E. B., Huppert, J. D., & Cahill, S. P. (2006). Emotional processing theory: An update. In B. O. Rothbaum (Ed.), *Pathological anxiety: Emotional processing in etiology and treatment* (pp. 3–24). New York: Guilford Press.

Foa, E. B., Johnson, K., Feeny, N., & Treadwell, K. (2001). The Child PTSD Symptom Scale (CPSS): Preliminary psychometrics of a measure for children with PTSD. *Journal of Clinical Child Psychology, 30*(3), 376–384.

Foa, E. B., & Kozak, M. J. (1986). Emotional processing of fear: Exposure to corrective information. *Psychological Bulletin, 99,* 20–35.

Foa, E. B., McLean, C. P., Capaldi, S., & Rosenfield, D. (2013). Prolonged exposure vs supportive counseling for sexual abuse-related PTSD in adolescent girls: A randomized clinical trial. *Journal of the American Medical Association, 310*(24), 2650–2657.

Foa, E. B., Riggs, D. S., Dancu, C. V., & Rothbaum, B. O. (1993). Reliability and validity of a brief instrument for assessing post-traumatic stress disorder. *Journal of Traumatic Stress, 6,* 459–473.

Ford, J. D., Racusin, R., Ellis, C. G., Daviss, W. B., Reiser, J., Fleischer, A., et al. (2000). Child maltreatment, other trauma exposure, and posttraumatic symptomatology among children with oppositional defiant and attention deficit hyperactivity disorders. *Child Maltreatment, 5*(3), 205–217.

Gilboa-Schectman, E., Foa, E. B., Shafran, N., Aderka, I. M., Powers, M. B., Rachamim, L., et al. (2010). Prolonged exposure versus dynamic therapy for adolescent PTSD: A pilot randomized controlled trial. *Journal of the American Academy of Child and Adolescent Psychiatry, 49*(10), 1034–1042.

Gwadz, M. V., Nish, D., Leonard, N. R., & Strauss, S. M. (2007). Gender differences in traumatic events and rates of post-traumatic stress disorder among homeless youth. *Journal of Adolescence, 30*(1), 117–129.

Heim, C., & Nemeroff, C. (2009). Neurobiology of posttraumatic stress disorder. *CNS Spectrums, 14,* 13–24.

Horowitz, M., Wilner, N., & Alvarez, W. (1979). Impact of Event Scale: A measure of subjective stress. *Psychosomatic Medicine, 41*(3), 209–218.

Institute of Medicine. (2008). *Treatment of PTSD: An assessment of the evidence.* Washington, DC: National Academies Press.

Jaycox, L. (2004). Cognitive behavioral intervention for trauma in schools. Longmont, CO: RAND Corporation.

Kassam-Adams, N., Garcia-Espana, J. F., Fein, J. A., & Winston, F. K. (2005). Heart rate and posttraumatic stress in injured children. *Archives of General Psychiatry, 62,* 335–340.

Kataoka, S. H., Stein, B. D., Jaycox, L. H., Wong, M., Escudero, P., Tu, W., et al. (2003). A school-based mental health program for traumatized latino immigrant children. *Journal of the American Academy of Child and Adolescent Psychiatry, 42*(3), 311–318.

Kaufman, J., Birmaher, B., Brent, D., Rao, U., Flynn, C., Moreci, P., et al. (1997). Schedule for Affective Disorders and Schizophrenia for School-Age Children—Present and Lifetime Version (K-SADS-PL): Initial reliability and validity data. *Journal of the American Academy of Child and Adolescent Psychiatry, 36*(7), 980–988.

Kilpatrick, D. G., Ruggiero, K. J., Acierno, R., Saunders, B. E., Resnick, H. S., & Best, C. L. (2003). Violence and risk of PTSD, major depression, substance abuse/dependence, and comorbidity: Results from the national survey of adolescents. *Journal of Consulting and Clinical Psychology, 71*(4), 692–700.

Kirsch, V., Wilhelm, F. H., & Goldbeck, L. (2011). Psychophysiological characteristics of PTSD in children and adolescents: A review of the literature. *Journal of Traumatic Stress, 24*(2), 146–154.

Kolko, D. J., Iselin, A. R., & Gully, K. J. (2011). Evaluation of the sustainability and clinical outcome of alternatives for families: A cognitive-behavioral therapy (AF-CBT) in a child protection center. *Child Abuse and Neglect, 35*(2), 105–116.

Kolko, D. J., & Swenson, C. C. (2002). *Assessing and treating physically abused children and their families: A cognitive-behavioral approach.* Thousand Oaks, CA: SAGE.

Kovacs, M. (1981). Rating scales to assess depression in school-aged children. *Acta Paedopsychiatrica, 46*(5–6), 305–315.

La Greca, A. M., Silverman, W. K., Vernberg, E. M., & Prinstein, M. J. (1996). Symptoms of posttraumatic stress in children after hurricane Andrew: A prospective study. *Journal of Consulting and Clinical Psychology, 64*(4), 712–723.

Lang, A. J., Craske, M. G., & Bjork, R. A. (1999). Implications of a new theory of disuse for the treatment of emotional disorders. *Clinical Psychology: Science and Practice, 6*, 80–94.

Lieberman, A. F. (2004). Child–parent psychotherapy: A relationship-based approach to the treatment of mental health disorders in infancy and early childhood. In A. J. Sameroff, S. C. McDonough, & K. L. Rosenblum (Eds.), *Treating parent–infant relationship problems: Strategies for intervention* (pp. 97–122). New York: Guilford Press.

Lieberman, A. F., & Van Horn, P. (2013). Infants and young children in military families: A conceptual model for intervention. *Clinical Child and Family Psychology Review, 16*(3), 282–293.

Lieberman, A. F., Van Horn, P., & Ippen, C. G. (2005). Toward evidence-based treatment: Child–parent psychotherapy with preschoolers exposed to marital violence. *Journal of the American Academy of Child and Adolescent Psychiatry, 44*(12), 1241–1248.

Macdonald, A., Danielson, C. K., Resnick, H. S., Saunders, B. E., & Kilpatrick, D. G. (2010). PTSD and comorbid disorders in a representative sample of adolescents: The risk associated with multiple exposures to potentially traumatic events. *Child Abuse and Neglect, 34*(10), 773–783.

Martin, D. J., Garske, J. P., & Davis, M. K. (2000). Relation of the therapeutic alliance with outcome and other variables: A meta-analytic review. *Journal of Consulting and Clinical Psychology, 68*(3), 438–450.

Masten, A. S. (2001). Ordinary magic: Resilience processes in development. *American Psychologist, 56*, 227–238.

McGloin, J. M., & Widom, C. S. (2001). Resilience among abused and neglected children grown up. *Developmental Psychopathology, 13*(4), 1021–1038.

Meiser-Stedman, R., Dalgleish, T., Glucksman, E., Yule, W., & Smith, P. (2009). Maladaptive cognitive appraisals mediate the evolution of posttraumatic stress reactions: A 6-month follow-up of child and adolescent assault and motor vehicle accident survivors. *Journal of Abnormal Psychology, 118*(4), 778–787.

Merikangas, K. R., He, J., Burstein, M., Swanson, S., Avenevoli, S., Cui, L., et al. (2010). Lifetime prevalence of mental disorders in US adolescents: Results from the National Comordity Study–Adolescent Supplement (NCS-A). *Journal of the American Academy of Child and Adolescent Psychiatry, 49*(10), 980–989.

Nader, K. O., Kriegler, J., Blake, D., Pynoos, R., Newman, E., & Weathers, F. (1996). *Clinician-Administered PTSD Scale for Children and Adolescents.* Boston: National Center for PTSD, Boston Veterans Administration Medical Center.

Nugent, N. R., Ostrowski, S., Christopher, N. C., & Delahanty, D. L. (2007). Parental posttraumatic stress symptoms as a moderator of child's acute biological response and subsequent posttraumatic stress symptoms in pediatric injury patients. *Journal of Pediatric Psychology, 32*(3), 309–318.

Ormhaug, S. M., Jensen, T. K., Wentzel-Larsen, T., & Shirk, S. (2014). The therapeutic alliance in treatment of traumatized youths: Relation to outcome in a randomized clinical trial. *Journal of Consulting and Clinical Psychology, 82*(1), 52–64.

Ormhaug, S. M., Shirk, S. R., & Wentzel-Larsen, T. (2015). Therapist and client perspectives on the alliance in the treatment of traumatized adolescents. *European Journal of Psychotraumatology, 6*, 27705.

Perrin, S., Meiser-Stedman, R., & Smith, P. (2005). The Children's Revised Impact of Event Scale (CRIES): Validity as a screening instrument for PTSD. *Behavioural and Cognitive Psychotherapy, 33*(4), 487–498.

Perrin, S., Smith, P., & Yule, W. (2000). Practitioner review: The assessment of post-traumatic stress disorder in children and adolescents. *Journal of Child Psychology and Psychiatry, 41*(3), 277–289.

Pynoos, R. S., Steinberg, A. M., & Piacentini, J. C. (1999). A developmental psychopathology model of childhood traumatic stress and intersection with anxiety disorders. *Biological Psychiatry, 46*, 1542–1554.

Reich, W. (2000). Diagnostic Interview for Children and Adolescents (DICA). *Journal of the American Academy of Child and Adolescent Psychiatry, 39*(1), 59–66.

Resick, P. A., & Schnicke, M. K. (1992). Cognitive processing therapy for sexual assault victims. *Journal of Consulting and Clinical Psychology, 60*(5), 748–756.

Robb, A. S., Cueva, J. E., Sporn, J., Yang, R., & Vanderburg, D. G. (2010). Sertraline treatment of children and adolescents with posttraumatic stress disorder: A double-blind, placebo-controlled trial. *Journal of Child and Adolescent Psychopharmacology, 20*(6), 463–471.

Saarni, C., & Harris, P. L. (1991). *Children's understanding of emotion.* Cambridge, UK: Cambridge University Press.

Salmon, K., & Bryant, R. A. (2002). Posttraumatic stress disorder in children: The influence of developmental factors. *Clinical Psychology Review, 22*, 163–188.

Saxe, G., MacDonald, H., & Ellis, H. (2007). Psychosocial approaches for children with PTSD. In M. J. Friedman, T. M. Keane, & P. A. Resick (Eds.), *Handbook of PTSD: Science and practice* (pp. 359–375). New York: Guilford Press.

Scheeringa, M. S., Weems, C. F., Cohen, J. A., Amaya-Jackson, L., & Guthrie, D. (2011). Trauma-focused cognitive-behavioral therapy for posttraumatic stress disorder in three- through six-year-old children: A randomized clinical trial. *Journal of Child Psychology and Psychiatry, 52*(8), 853–860.

Scheeringa, M. S., Wright, M. J., Hunt, J. P., & Zeanah, C. H. (2006). Factors affecting the diagnosis and prediction of PTSD symptomatology in children and adolescents. *American Journal of Psychiatry, 163*(4), 644–651.

Scheeringa, M. S., & Zeanah, C. H. (2001). A relational perspective on PTSD in early childhood. *Journal of Traumatic Stress, 14*(4), 799–815.

Scheeringa, M. S., & Zeanah, C. H. (2008). Reconsideration of harm's way: Onsets and comorbidity patterns of disorders in preschool children and their caregivers following hurricane Katrina. *Journal of Clinical Child and Adolescent Psychology, 37*(3), 508–518.

Scheeringa, M. S., Zeanah, C. H., & Cohen, J. A. (2011). PTSD in children and adolescents: Toward an empirically based algorithm. *Depression and Anxiety, 28,* 770–782.

Seedat, S., Lockhat, R., Kaminer, D., Zungu-Dirwayi, N., & Stein, D. J. (2001). An open trial of citalopram in adolescents with post-traumatic stress disorder. *International Clinical Psychopharmacology, 16*(1), 21–25.

Shaffer, D., Fisher, P., Lucas, C. P., Dulcan, M. K., & Schwab-Stone, M. E. (2000). NIMH Diagnostic Interview Schedule for Children Version IV (NIMH DISC-IV): Description, differences from previous versions, and reliability of some common diagnoses. *Journal of the American Academy of Child and Adolescent Psychiatry, 39*(1), 28–38.

Sharma-Patel, K., Filton, B., Brown, E. J., Zlotnick, D., Campbell, C., & Yedlin., J. (2011). Pediatric posttraumatic stress disorder. In D. McKay & E. Storch (Eds.), *Handbook of child and adolescent anxiety disorders* (pp. 303–321). New York: Springer.

Silverman, W. K., Ortiz, C. D., Viswesvaran, C., Burns, B. J., Kolko, D. J., Putnam, F. W., et al. (2008). Evidence-based psychosocial treatments for children and adolescents exposed to traumatic events. *Journal of Clinical Child and Adolescent Psychology, 37,* 156–183.

Silverman, W. K., Saavedra, L. M., & Pina, A. A. (2001). Test–retest reliability of anxiety symptoms and diagnoses with the Anxiety Disorders Interview Schedule for DSM-IV: Child and Parent versions. *Journal of the American Academy of Child and Adolescent Psychiatry, 40*(8), 937–944.

Smith, P., Perrin, S., Dyregrov, A., & Yule, W. (2003). Principal components analysis of the Impact of Event Scale with children in war. *Personality and Individual Differences, 34*(2), 315–322.

Stallard, P. (2003). A retrospectice analysis to explore the applicability of the Ehlers and Clark (2000) cognitive model to explain PTSD in children. *Behavioural and Cognitive Psychotherapy, 31,* 337–345.

Stallard, P., & Smith, E. (2007). Appraisals and cognitive coping styles associated with chronic post-traumatic symptoms in child road traffic accident survivors. *Journal of Child Psychology and Psychiatry, 48,* 194–201.

Stein, B. D., Jaycox, L. H., Kataoka, S. H., Wong, M., Tu, W., & Fink, A. (2003). A mental health intervention for schoolchildren exposed to violence: A randomized controlled trial. *Journal of the American Medical Assocation, 290*(5), 603–611.

Strawn, J. R., Keeshin, B. R., DelBello, M. P., Geracioti, T. D., Jr., & Putnam, F. W. (2010). Psychopharmacologic treatment of posttraumatic stress disorder in children and adolescents: A review. *Journal of Clinical Psychiatry, 71*(7), 932–941.

Teicher, M. H., Anderson, C. M., & Polcari, A. (2012). Childhood maltreatment is associated with reduced volume in the hippocampal subfields CA3, dentate gyrus, and subiculum. *Proceedings of the National Academy of Sciences USA, 109*(9), E563–E572.

Trickey, D., Siddaway, A. P., Meiser-Stedman, R., Serpell, L., & Field, A. (2012). A meta-analysis of risk factors for post-traumatic stress disorder in children and adolescents. *Clinical Psychology Review, 32,* 122–138.

Tupler, L. A., De Bellis, M. D. (2006). Segmented hippocampal volume in children and adolescents with posttraumatic stress disorder. *Biologcial Psychiatry, 59,* 523–529.

Valentino, K., Berkowitz, S., & Stover, C. S. (2010). Parenting behaviors and posttraumatic symptoms in relation to children's symptomatology following a traumatic event. *Journal of Traumatic Stress, 23*(3), 403–407.

van der Kolk, B. A. (2005). Developmental trauma disorder. *Psychiatric Annals, 35*(5), 401–408.

Vernberg, E. M., Silverman, W. K., L. A. Greca, A. M., & Prinstein, M. J. (1996). Prediction of posttraumatic stress symptoms in children after hurricane Andrew. *Journal of Abnormal Psychology, 105,* 237–248.

Wolfe, V., & Gentile, C. (1991). *Children's Impact of Traumatic Events Scale—Revised.* Unpublished assessment instrument, Department of Psychology, London Health Sciences Centre, London, ON, Canada.

Yelland, C., Robinson, P., Lock, C., La Greca, A. M., Kokegei, B., Ridgway, V., et al. (2010). Bushfire impact on youth. *Journal of Traumatic Stress, 23*(2), 274–277.

Yule, W., Bolton, D., Udwin, O., Boyle, S., O'Ryan, D., & Nurrish, J. (2000). The long-term psychological effects of a disaster experienced in adolescence: I. The incidence and course of PTSD. *Journal of Child Psychology and Psychiatry, 4,* 503–511.

Yule, W., Smith, P., Perrin, S., & Clark, D. M. (2013). Post-traumatic stress disorder. In C. Essau & T. Ollendick (Eds.), *The Wiley-Blackwell handbook of the treatment of childhood and adolescent anxiety* (pp. 451–470). West Sussex, UK: Wiley.

Zhang, N., Zhang, Y., Wu, K., Zhu, Z., & Dyregrov, A. (2011). Factor structure of the Children's Revised Impact of Event Scale among children and adolescents who survived the 2008 Sichuan earthquake in China. *Scandinavian Journal of Psychology, 52*(3), 236–241.

CHAPTER 10

Obsessive–Compulsive Disorder

Tara S. Peris and Benjamin N. Schneider

THE DSM-5 DEFINITION OF OBSESSIVE–COMPULSIVE DISORDER

Once thought rare in younger age groups, obsessive–compulsive disorder (OCD) is now recognized as relatively common condition in childhood and adolescence. The disorder is characterized by obsessions and/or compulsions that are distressing and time-consuming, leading to significant functional impairment. *Obsessions* are recurrent distressing thoughts, images, or urges; *compulsions* the repetitive behaviors or mental acts designed to reduce the distress that results from obsessions. Together, these symptoms create a self-reinforcing cycle that can be chronic and highly impairing.

Although OCD was conceptualized as an anxiety disorder in the fourth edition of the *Diagnostic and Statistical Manual of Mental Disorders* (DSM-IV; American Psychiatric Association, 2000), it is classified in DSM-5 in its own section of obsessive–compulsive and related disorders (American Psychiatric Association, 2013). This change stems from the growing body of research documenting biological, genetic, and phenomenological features that reliably distinguish OCD from other anxiety disorders (Bartz & Hollander, 2006; Rosenberg, Russell, & Fougere, 2005). Indeed, this body of work suggests that OCD clusters more closely with conditions such as hoarding, trichotillomania (hair-pulling disorder), and skin picking (Hajcak, Franklin, Simons, & Keuthen, 2006). Certainly, not all youngsters describe their symptoms as anxiety-related. Many youth report performing their rituals in an effort to alleviate feelings of disgust, discomfort, incompleteness, or the sense that something just does not feel right.

In this chapter, we begin by describing the phenomenology, prevalence, and course of child and adolescent OCD. We then describe the current state of the evidence base of the disorder, including a brief discussion of emerging new treatments. We follow with a description of best-practice strategies for the assessment and treatment of pediatric OCD, including illustrative examples of how they might be applied.

As with adult forms of the disorder, OCD presents as a relatively heterogeneous disorder in childhood and adolescence (Ivarsson & Valderhaug, 2006). Concerns regarding germs, contamination, illness, and other preoccupations related to fears of harm or other negative outcomes to self and others are among the most common youth obsessions (Moore et al., 2007). Sexual, religious, superstitious (e.g., lucky/unlucky numbers, colors, or words), and somatic obsessions, as well as obsessions related to scrupulosity, symmetry, and fear of humiliation, occur with relatively less frequency but are not uncommon (Geller et al., 2001; Swedo, Rapoport, Leonard, Lenane, & Cheslow, 1989).

Compulsions are correspondingly diverse. Excessive washing, cleaning, and checking are the most commonly seen behaviors among youth with OCD; however, arranging and ordering, confessing, reassurance seeking, and ritualized repeating occur frequently as well. Mental rituals/compulsions may also be observed, and these may include behaviors such as mental counting or arranging and praying. Symptoms can vary over time, with one compulsion potentially giving way to another. However, the absolute number of symptoms is thought to remain relatively constant (Rettew, Swedo, Leonard, Lenane, & Rapport, 1992). The vast majority of children and adolescents with OCD experience both obsessions and compulsions. In cases where only one domain of symptoms is reported, it is more common to see compulsions in the absence of obsessions than to see purely obsessional OCD.

Taken together, OCD symptoms frequently derail the normal developmental trajectory. They create functional impairment that extends across multiple domains, impacting academic performance, peer relationships, and family dynamics (Geller et al., 2001; Markarian et al., 2009; Piacentini, Bergman, Keller, & McCracken, 2003; Piacentini, Langley, & Roblek, 2007). The most common impairments are seen at home, with family members, and with daily living skills (e.g., doing chores, getting ready for bed, bathing and grooming, modifying family routines). The condition can take a significant toll on family functioning and is associated with high levels of conflict, blame, and distress for family members (Farrell & Barrett, 2007; Peris, Bergman, et al., 2008; Piacentini et al., 2003; Waters & Barrett, 2000), features that add to the burden of disease and complicate treatment (Peris et al., 2012). Difficulties at school (e.g., concentrating on schoolwork, completing homework and in-class assignments) and in social settings are also prominent for many youth (Piacentini et al., 2003; Piacentini, Langley, & Roblek, 2007).

OCD is a chronic condition and, in the absence of treatment, is likely not only to persist but also to place youth at risk for later poor outcomes (Moore et al., 2007). Follow-up studies of clinical samples support this view. Approximately 40% of youngsters with OCD will meet diagnostic criteria for the disorder up to 15 years after initial diagnosis, with another 20% evidencing subclinical disturbance (Stewart et al., 2004). Moreover, given that nearly one-half of adults with OCD report an onset of symptoms in childhood or adolescence (Rasmussen & Eisen, 1990), it is clear that pediatric OCD portends significant adult morbidity.

PREVALENCE AND COURSE

Epidemiological studies suggest that the prevalence of childhood OCD mirrors that of adult OCD, falling somewhere between 0.5 and 2% (Apter et al., 1993; Moore et al.,

2007; Rapoport et al., 2000; Valleni-Basile et al., 1994). However, children differ from their adult counterparts in that their insight into their symptoms may be more limited. Moreover, they may be prone to secrecy about their symptoms or lack the ability to report on them accurately. Collectively, these features may contribute to falsely lowered rates of OCD in children (Heyman et al., 2003).

The typical age of onset for youth meeting the criteria for OCD ranges from 8 to 11 years (Hanna, 1995; Chabane et al., 2005; Piacentini et al., 2003; Rapoport, Swedo, & Leonard, 1992), although children with onset as early as age 2–3 years have been reported, and there has been growing interest in early manifestations of the illness (Freeman et al., 2003; Garcia et al., 2009; Lewin, Park, et al., 2014). Boys are typically overrepresented in clinical samples by about a 3:2 ratio, although by adolescence, the gender distribution tends to equalize (Swedo et al., 1989; Rasmussen & Eisen, 1990).

COMMON COMORBID CONDITIONS

Childhood OCD frequently co-occurs with other psychiatric disorders, and comorbidity has been linked to worsened OCD symptom severity (Langley, Bergman, Lewin, Lee, & Piacentini, 2010; Storch, Larson, et al., 2008) and poorer response to cognitive-behavioral therapy (CBT; Storch, Stigge-Kaufman, et al., 2008). Reports suggest that up to 80% of children with OCD present with one or more additional comorbid disorders, most commonly tic disorders and Tourette's disorder (Geller et al., 2001; Hanna, 1995; Ivarsson, Melin, & Wallin, 2008; Piacentini et al., 2003; Rapoport et al., 2000; Storch, Larson, et al., 2008). There has been work suggesting that tic disorders and Tourette's disorder share neurobiological characteristics with OCD (de Mathis et al., 2009; Jaisoorya, Reddy, Srinath, & Thennarasu, 2008; Leckman et al., 1994–1995; Storch, Merlo, et al., 2008) and clinically, studies have shown that tics in childhood predict increased OCD symptoms in adolescents and young adults (Peterson, Pine, Cohen, & Brook, 2001). Indeed, tic comorbidity is associated with earlier onset of OCD symptoms (mean age 9 years 1 month vs. 10 years 5 months; Masi et al., 2010).

Although tic disorders may have higher rates of comorbidity with OCD, the comorbidity of OCD and attention-deficit/hyperactivity disorder (ADHD) appears to have a particularly significant negative impact on childhood academic and social functioning (Sukhodolsky et al., 2005). ADHD symptoms tend to present earlier than OCD (Geller et al., 2002), and rates of comorbid ADHD have been reported to be 25–30% (Geller, Biederman, Griffin, Jones, & Lefkowitz, 1996; Masi, Millepiedi, & Mucci, 2006). Anxiety disorders such as generalized anxiety disorder and social phobia also co-occur with OCD at rates of 38–60% (Diniz et al., 2004; Geller et al., 2001; Piacentini et al., 2003; Zohar, 1999).

ETIOLOGICAL/CONCEPTUAL MODELS OF OCD

Behavioral conceptualizations of OCD view obsessions as intrusive, unwanted thoughts, images, or urges that trigger a significant and rapid increase in anxiety. From this perspective, compulsions are overt behaviors or cognitions (also known as *covert behaviors*) designed to reduce ensuing negative feelings (Albano, March, & Piacentini, 1999). The learning theory that underlies this framework posits that compulsions become solidified via the negative reinforcement that occurs when compulsive behavior reduces obsession-triggered distress. The more effective the distress reduction, the more powerful the reinforcement. As an example, a child with an obsessive fear of contamination may experience distress when touching what he or she perceives to be an unclean surface, and the experienced distress triggers a compulsion to wash his or her hands, perhaps multiple times. Handwashing effectively reduces distress for the child, which then strengthens the urge to perform the handwashing ritual in the future.

Traditional learning theory posits that repeated exposure practice facilitates autonomic habituation that in turn leads to decreased anxiety (Foa & Kozak, 1986). Preventing individuals from engaging in compulsions (response prevention) is thought to promote extinction of the negative reinforcement properties of the compulsion. In combination, exposure and response prevention (ERP) is meant to help individuals foster and solidify new learning (Foa & Kozak, 1986): The child begins to see that the obsessional stimuli are in fact tolerable, and that their feared consequences of not engaging in compulsions do not materialize.

ERP remains the most effective and widely used form of behavior therapy for OCD in both children and adults (Freeman, Garcia, et al., 2014). ERP involves systematically triggering the child's obsessions, then prompting him or her to resist the urge to engage in compulsive behaviors that typically reduce distress (Kozak & Foa, 1997; Meyer, 1966). Consistent with exposure-based approaches to youth anxiety (e.g., Coping Cat; Kendall et al., 1997), therapist and client work collaboratively to develop a hierarchy of symptoms, ordered from least to most distressing, and exposure practice progresses through this hierarchy using a blend of *in vivo* and imaginal experiences.

Emerging research with adults suggests that habituation—either within or between sessions—does not underlie the success of exposure therapy (see Craske et al., 2008, for review). Rather, varying the intensity of exposure practice and mixing exposure tasks and targets within sessions may help to maximize extinction of fear associations in session, with better generalization of in-session gains to real-world functioning (e.g., Abramowitz, 2013; Kircanski & Peris, 2014; Kircanski, Wu, & Piacentini, 2014). From a practical perspective, this may involve combining two or more exposure targets into a single, larger exposure; practicing a more challenging exposure, followed by an easier exposure before returning again to a more difficult exposure; and focusing on distress tolerance rather than anxiety reduction as the goal of therapy. Recent research supports these approaches (designed to enhance variability in distress and combined exposure techniques) as predictors of more favorable CBT outcome for youth with OCD (Kircanski & Peris, 2014).

EVIDENCE-BASED TREATMENTS FOR OCD IN CHILDREN AND ADOLESCENTS

Exposure-based CBT is considered the front-line treatment for cases of mild to moderate childhood OCD according to expert consensus (Geller & March, 2012; March, Frances, Carpenter, & Kahn, 1997) and reviews of the literature (Abramowitz, Whiteside, & Deacon, 2006; Barrett, Farrell, Pina, Peris, & Piacentini, 2008; Freeman, Garcia, et al., 2014; Watson & Rees, 2008). Over 20 clinical trials document its efficacy, with between-group effect sizes ranging from 0.27 to 2.84 (Barrett et al., 2004; Pediatric OCD Treatment Study [POTS] Team, 2004; Piacentini et al., 2011). In the POTS Team, the largest clinical trial of youth OCD treatment to date, individual child CBT mono-therapy outperformed medication monotherapy (sertraline) and yielded comparable results to combined treatment (CBT + sertraline) on some outcome measures. Collec-tively, the existing evidence base supports both individual child CBT and individual family-focused CBT as "probably efficacious" interventions, and they are recommended as front-line treatments according to expert consensus and review of the literature (Free-man, Sapyta, et al., 2014).

The basic approach to individual child CBT for OCD is similar across protocols (March & Mulle, 1998; Piacentini, Langley, & Roblek, 2007). It outlines 12–16 weeks of treatment that include psychoeducation, cognitive restructuring, ERP, and behavioral rewards (March & Mulle, 1998; Piacentini et al., 2011; Valderhaug, Larsson, Gotestam, & Piacentini, 2007). Psychoeducation is designed to provide families with important information about the OCD cycle, the rationale for ERP, and what is known about the causes and prevalence of childhood OCD. Such education provides a critical foundation for treatment and can be a powerful tool for reducing stigma and blame associated with the condition. Cognitive restructuring is designed to address patterns of maladaptive thinking that may underlie compulsive behaviors. Indeed, in the adult literature, factors such as inflated sense of responsibility for harm, excessive self-doubt, and thought–action fusion have been implicated as important etiological and maintaining factors for OCD (Salkovskis, 1996). Although it remains unclear to what degree these cognitive vari-ables are specific to, or even applicable to, child and adolescent OCD (Barrett & Healy-Farrell, 2003), cognitive techniques directly addressing obsessional beliefs and/or aimed at enhancing compliance with ERP often are included in interventions for young people with OCD (Piacentini, Peris, March, & Franklin, 2012; Soechting & March, 2002).

As noted earlier, exposure exercises are considered the central treatment strategy, particularly in light of developmental considerations that may complicate practice with cognitive components of treatment. These same developmental factors call for the devel-opment of behavior reward systems designed to reward efforts to fight OCD. Such reward systems can be tailored to the developmental status of the child and are important tools for enhancing motivation and treatment adherence.

Finally, it is worth noting that virtually every CBT treatment for childhood OCD involves some degree of family involvement. Family therapy is encouraged as an adjunct to individual child treatment (Geller & March, 2012; March et al., 1997), although data demonstrating the incremental efficacy of this strategy have yet to emerge. Nonetheless, some degree of family involvement in child OCD treatment is now the norm, and it stems from the recognition that youth with OCD are embedded in their family context in a way that necessarily influences their access to and experience in treatment. It also ema-nates from growing recognition of the toll that OCD takes on the larger family system (Renshaw, Steketee, & Chambless, 2005; Stewart et al., 2011). Indeed, OCD is unique in the way that it pulls families into the illness, often prompting their direct participa-tion in rituals (accommodation). This involvement comes at a price, and most families report high levels of distress and disrupted family functioning (Piacentini et al., 2003; Piacentini, Langley, & Roblek, 2007; Storch et al., 2009). Rates of conflict, blame, and poor cohesion are high (Peris, Bergman, et al., 2008) and these factors have been found to predict poorer response to exposure-based CBT (Peris et al., 2012).

In many CBT treatments, family involvement is administered at the discretion of the therapist. There may be specific parent sessions with designated introductory content; however, typically the format thereafter is open ended and flexible, with instructions to include families "as needed" (Benazon, Ager, & Rosenberg, 2002; March & Mulle, 1998; Piacentini, Bergman, Jacobs, McCracken, & Kretchman, 2002). In recent years, efforts have been made to involve families in treatment in a more systematic manner (Freeman, Sapyta, et al., 2014; Lewin, Park, et al., 2014; Piacentini et al., 2011). These approaches differ in the degree of family involvement but are largely similar with regard to treatment techniques. They rely heavily on psychoeducation about OCD and its causes to help families adhere to treatment (Barrett et al., 2004; Piacentini et al., 2002; Storch et al., 2007). A smaller number of family treatments has employed parents as coaches or co-therapists (Freeman et al., 2008; Freeman, Sapyta, et al., 2014; Scahill, Vitulano, Brenner, Lynch, & King, 1996) or focused on basic behavior management techniques that have specific relevance for OCD (Freeman et al., 2008, 2014b; Lewin, McGuire, Murphy, & Storch, 2014). With few exceptions (e.g., Barrett et al., 2004), most of these "family" treatments focus on parents, requiring that at least one parent be present at each session (Storch et al., 2007) or identifying specific family sessions during which any willing family members participate (Piacentini et al., 2003). Treatments that involve the entire family system are few and far between (Peris & Piacentini, 2013), an unfortunate shortcoming of the field given the well-known impact of OCD on parents, siblings, and extended family alike. Certainly, the limited evidence that exists points to the value of inclusive family treatment, inasmuch as it improves outcomes for siblings, including reduction in sibling depressive symptoms and accommodation (Barrett et al., 2004).

Emerging Treatments

As research on the family correlates of OCD has proliferated and links have emerged between aspects of family functioning and poor CBT response (Garcia et al., 2010; Merlo, Storch, Adkins, Murphy, & Geffken, 2007; Peris et al., 2012; Peris & Piacentini, 2013; Piacentini et al., 2011), focus has shifted to the development of more targeted family treatments for childhood OCD. These treatments are designed to address specific aspects of family functioning (e.g., family conflict, blame) known to contribute to poor CBT response for youth with OCD (Peris & Piacentini, 2013, 2014). They move beyond basic psychoeducation and behavior management techniques to teach families strategies for regulating emotions and tolerating distress that may be caused by the illness. These skills are practiced in the service of more effective problem solving around OCD and disengaging from patterns of symptom accommodation that serve to maintain the illness over time. A recent pilot randomized controlled trial (RCT) comparing a targeted family treatment approach (positive family interaction therapy; PFIT) to individual child CBT with standard family involvement suggested that PFIT is both acceptable to families and feasible to administer. PFIT involves six sessions of family therapy designed to be used as an adjunct to individual child CBT, and it focuses on emotion regulation skills training and effective problem solving around difficult OCD situations. The goal is to teach family members to maintain a calm and constructive approach to supporting exposure therapy, while disengaging from patterns of symptom accommodation. Preliminary inspection of clinical outcomes suggests that it may have an advantage over standard CBT in families that present with high levels of dysfunction (Peris & Piacentini, 2013). Although encouraging, further work is needed to demonstrate the efficacy of this approach.

Other novel treatment strategies build on the large body of research documenting basic cognitive biases associated with OCD and anxiety. This work reveals a propensity to orient toward threat, to interpret neutral stimuli as threatening, and to demonstrate greater recall of threatening information among anxious individuals versus their healthy counterparts (see Pine, 2007, for a review). Similar alterations in how threat-related information is processed and regulated are evident among adults with OCD, and research with younger age groups is under way. Treatments directly targeting attention biases—frequently referred to as attention modification programs (AMPs)—use computerized protocols to systematically train attention away from negative stimuli and toward more neutral stimuli. They are innovative in their attempt to target underlying disease pathology directly and they offer the benefit of portable administration that may be delivered in the home to individuals who might typically lack access to quality treatment. Preliminary applications to youth with anxiety disorders show promise for reducing symptom severity and functional impairment (Bar-Haim, Morag, & Glickman, 2011; Eldar et al., 2012). Likewise, initial work with adults with OCD points to the potential value of this approach (Williams & Grisham, 2013). Although this work has yet to be extended to youth with OCD, the sound theoretical foundation and promising results from related strands of research make it worthy of further inquiry.

Pharmacological Interventions

There is a sound base of evidence supporting the use of pharmacological agents to treat OCD. Although CBT is recommended widely as the first-line treatment for mild to moderate OCD, recommendations from the American Academy of Child and Adolescent Psychiatry suggest a combination of CBT and pharmacotherapy with selective serotonin reuptake inhibitors (SSRIs) in cases of more severe OCD. Certainly, it is worth noting that outcomes for CBT monotherapy, while sometimes surpassing those of medication monotherapy (POTS, 2004; Watson & Rees, 2008), leave considerable room for improvement, with more than half achieving less than optimal response. In light of this, it is clear that a significant number of youth will require additional intervention aimed at reducing symptoms and related functional impairment.

In this section, we provide a brief review of the evidence in support of SSRI treatment in childhood OCD, information on standard medication decision-making approaches (i.e., algorithms), and adjunctive agents that may have utility. Detailed discussion of these topics is beyond the scope of this chapter; however, practicing clinicians are well advised to familiarize themselves with standards of practice given the frequency with which youth with OCD require medication treatment. Moreover, given that parents have a strong preference for the use of CBT over medication to treat OCD (Lewin et al., 2014), psychotherapists are likely to assume the role of educator when providing initial referrals for psychopharmacology.

There are several RCTs demonstrating the efficacy of SSRIs in pediatric OCD (Geller et al., 2001; POTS, 2004; Riddle et al., 2001). A 2009 Cochrane Review of pharmacotherapy of anxiety disorders found the greatest number of trials showing efficacy assessing the SSRIs in treating pediatric OCD (Ipser, Stein, Hawkridge, & Hoppe, 2009). These agents, which include sertraline (Zoloft), fluvoxamine (Luvox), fluoxetine (Prozac), escitalopram (Lexapro), and citalopram (Celexa), are most commonly used as first-line medications in the treatment of OCD. There are no head-to-head trials comparing different SSRIs, but a meta-analysis suggests similar efficacy across this medication class (Watson & Rees, 2008). Notably, OCD symptoms commonly require higher dosing than do other pediatric anxiety disorders. Thus, dosing should be considered in deciding whether a robust medication trial has actually been accomplished. It is worth mentioning that clomipramine, a tricyclic antidepressant, is also commonly used and supported by evidence, though its use as first-line agent is limited by its side effect profile, most saliently an increased risk for cardiovascular side effects, as well as common side effects, such as dry mouth, constipation, sedation, and dizziness (Flament et al., 1985). Still, multiple pediatric RCTs and meta-analyses show a greater effect size (ES = 0.8) for clomipramine than for SSRIs (Sánchez-Meca, Rosa-Alcázar, Iniesta-Sepúlveda, & Rosa-Alcázar, 2014; Watson & Rees, 2008).

Notably, even when medication is used in conjunction with CBT, outcomes often leave room for improvement. Indeed, in the POTS trial (2004), only 54% of youth achieved optimal response following combined treatment of sertraline and CBT. The current recommended approach, if an SSRI trial fails to garner adequate response (at adequate dose and 10-week trial) is first to try a second SSRI at adequate dose and duration. If this also fails to produce results, pharmacological augmentation may then be employed. Notably, some practitioners use clomipramine as not only a monotherapy but also an augmentation strategy. Alternative options include atypical antipsychotic medications, and strong consideration may be given to this approach for cases in which an evidence-base exists for treatment of comorbid symptoms (e.g., tics and externalizing symptoms).

Predictors of Treatment Response

Given that a significant portion of youth fails to respond to current treatments for OCD, an important area of focus is to understand factors that may contribute to poor clinical outcomes. Research in this area remains relatively scant. Although the number of carefully controlled clinical trials for CBT (Barrett et al., 2004; Freeman, Saptya, et al., 2014; Piacentini et al., 2011), SSRI monotherapy (Flament et al., 1985; Geller et al., 2004; Leonard et al., 1989; March & Mulle, 1998; Riddle et al., 2001) and their combination (POTS, 2004) is growing, predictors and moderators rarely are examined (Ginsburg, Kingery, Drake, & Grados, 2008). This is likely because the sample sizes in these trials remain relatively modest, thereby undermining statistical power. Nonetheless, the existing evidence base points to several features that may be important for treatment outcome.

Among both controlled and open-ended studies of exposure-based CBT for childhood OCD, higher levels of baseline symptom severity, functional impairment, and comorbidity have all emerged as predictors of treatment outcome (Barrett, Farrell, Dadds, & Boulter, 2005; Piacentini et al., 2002; Storch, Merlo, et al., 2008). This is not surprising given that these features reflect greater levels of acuity and sicker, more impaired patients face a significant set of challenges in treatment. In addition to these features, several family factors have been identified as important for CBT outcome among youth with OCD. The most widely studied family feature associated with poor CBT response for youth with OCD is accommodation, which occurs in many forms, including the provision of verbal reassurance in response to worries, participation in rituals, and enabling of avoidance behaviors. These accommodating responses are a defining feature of families of youth with OCD. They occur in virtually every family and, for many, are a part of daily life (Peris, Roblek, Langley, Benazon, & Piacentini, 2008; Storch et al., 2007). Research indicates that higher levels of baseline accommodation predict worse response to CBT (Garcia et al., 2010; Merlo, Lehmkuhl, Geffken, & Storch, 2009), which suggests that this pattern of responding to OCD is an important treatment target. To this end, a recent clinical trial indicated that changes in family accommodation of OCD temporally preceded decreases in obsessive–compulsive symptom severity (Piacentini et al., 2011). In addition to accommodation, poor baseline family functioning (Barrett et al., 2005) and parental stress both portend worse outcomes in CBT for OCD (Storch, Merlo, et al., 2008). Higher levels of family conflict, blame, and poor cohesion also are linked to poor CBT response, demonstrating both individual and additive effects (Peris et al., 2012).

Few studies to date have examined predictors and moderators of outcome among youth assigned to CBT, medication monotherapy with sertraline, or combined treatment (Garcia et al., 2010; March, Franklin, & Leonard, 2007). Analyzing data from the POTS trial (2004), they found that across conditions, higher levels of symptom severity, functioning impairment, externalizing comorbidity, and poor family accommodation predicted worse outcome across conditions (Garcia et al., 2010). However, two important moderators emerged. First, among youth with a family history of OCD, there was a sixfold decrease in the response to CBT (Garcia et al., 2010). Second, among youth with comorbid tic conditions, there was a diminished response to medication monotherapy (March et al., 2007). Together, these findings provide an important first step toward developing strategies that might serve to match children with OCD to optimal treatment approaches. They suggest that youngsters with a family history of OCD may be better served by combined treatment or by an approach that integrates parents more fully into the treatment process. Likewise, among youth who present with tic disorder, CBT monotherapy or a combination of CBT and medication may prove most efficacious. Similarly, research from Flessner and colleagues (2010) suggests neuropsychological factors that may influence treatment response; specifically, patients who demonstrated better recall abilities prior to treatment were more likely to respond well to behavioral interventions.

EVIDENCE-BASED ASSESSMENT AND TREATMENT IN PRACTICE

Assessment

A comprehensive evidence-based assessment provides a foundation for effective case conceptualization and treatment planning. Such assessment is necessary for diagnostic clarification; it accurately establishes the presence of OCD, distinguishes between phenomenologically similar conditions, and identifies comorbid mental health conditions that may be relevant for treatment planning (Langley, Bergman, & Piacentini, 2002). To that end, the initial evaluation should include careful assessment of both current and past OCD symptoms, the course and severity of the illness, and related functional impairment (March & Franklin, 2006). It should also evaluate comorbid psychopathology and, in light of the role of the family in OCD, family responses to managing the illness. Finally, in addition to collecting information about symptoms and associated interference, the evaluation should also consider the strengths of the child and his or her family.

In what follows, we describe several widely used instruments that are useful in the evidence-based assessment of child and adolescent OCD. Although each is manageable in its own right, it is worth noting that they often combine to create a potentially time-consuming assessment battery, particularly for younger clients. To ease this burden, it is often helpful to mail a packet of self-report questionnaires to the family in advance of the assessment visit. These measures may ascertain relevant medical and mental health history, including history of OCD symptoms and treatment, psychosocial functioning, and possible comorbid problems. If they are returned prior to the initial assessment, they may also be reviewed in advance to facilitate the identification of potential problem areas and allow for more careful evaluation during the intake process.

Assessment of OCD centers on established measures of OCD symptom severity. Although these measures have proliferated in recent years, by far the most established is the Children's Yale–Brown Obsessive–Compulsive Scale (CY-BOCS; Goodman, Price, Rasmussen, Riddle, & Rapoport, 1991; Scahill et al., 1997). The CYBOCS is a well-validated and psychometrically sound clinician interview that ascertains the profile of OCD symptoms and severity of the disorder (Lewin & Piacentini, 2010). In addition to the CY-BOCS, clinicians may benefit from using the Anxiety Disorders Interview Schedule for DSM-IV—Parent and Child Versions (ADIS-IV-C/P; Silverman & Albano, 1996), both to confirm the OCD diagnosis and to identify other diagnostic comorbidities. Beyond these two measures, several supplementary instruments developed specifically for use in child and adolescent OCD may be useful in forming a complete diagnostic picture. We detail several of them below and refer readers to Lewin and Piacentini (2010) for more extensive discussion of evidence-based assessment of childhood OCD.

Children's Yale–Brown Obsessive–Compulsive Scale

The CY-BOCS is a clinician-administered interview that assesses the full spectrum of obsessive–compulsive symptoms (Scahill et al., 1997). It is scored on the basis of combined information from observation and parent and child reports, asking respondents to indicate which symptoms have occurred in the previous week and which have occurred at any point in the child's history (Goodman et al., 1991). The initial section of the CY-BOCS uses a checklist format to ascertain the presence or absence of a comprehensive list of obsessions and compulsions. Notably, this checklist provides a valuable foundation for developing a symptom hierarchy once treatment has commenced. Following completion of the checklist, the clinician separately completes a summary section for both obsessions and compulsions. In each section, he or she rates the child's collective symptoms following five dimensions: time spent, interference, distress, resistance, and control. Each summary section yields subscale scores ranging from 0 to 20. These scores combine to produce a total score ranging from 0 to 40. As with its adult counterpart (Goodman et al., 1989), the CY-BOCS has been shown to possess favorable overall psychometric properties (Gallant et al., 2008; Scahill et al., 1997). Notably, it has shown reasonable treatment sensitivity (Merlo et al., 2009; POTS, 2004) and discriminant validity with measures of child depression and non-OCD anxiety (Gallant et al., 2008; Scahill et al.,

1997). However, questions remain about the factor structure of the instrument in children and adolescents, as well as the reliability of the resistance and control components (McKay et al., 2003). A total score of 16 or greater is typically used to indicate clinically significant OCD, and recent work has attempted to establish clinical norms for child and adolescent populations (Lewin, McGuire, et al., 2014).

Anxiety Disorders Interview Schedule for Children, Fourth Edition

The ADIS-IV is widely considered the "gold standard" instrument for assessing DSM-IV anxiety disorders and related conditions in children and adolescents (Silverman & Albano, 1996). Designed for youngsters ages 8–17 years, the ADIS-IV has parallel parent and child versions, both of which possess sound psychometric properties for the internalizing disorders relative to other available diagnostic instruments (Silverman, Saavedra, & Pina, 2001; Wood, Piacentini, Bergman, McCracken, & Barrios, 2002). The ADIS-IV uses a semi-structured interview format that allows the clinician considerable flexibility in integrating information from parents, children, and behavioral observations. In addition, it asks clinicians to complete an eight-point clinical severity rating (CSR) that provides a dimensional measure of severity/impairment for each positive diagnosis (Silverman & Albano, 1996). Higher scores reflect higher levels of acuity, with CSRs of four and higher indicating the presence of disorder. When more than one mental health condition is present, CSRs may be used to prioritize treatment planning based on the relative acuity of each disorder.

Child OCD Impact Scale—Revised

The Child OCD Impact Scale—Revised (COIS-R; Piacentini, Peris, Bergman, Chang, & Jaffer, 2007) is a self-report questionnaire assessing OCD-specific functional impairment. The COIS-R has parallel parent and child self-report formats that focus on impairment in family, academic, and social environments. From a treatment perspective, the COIS-R provides complementary information to the CY-BOCS by examining the extent to which changes in symptom severity translate into enhanced psychosocial functioning. It has specific utility, in that it anchors progress in the real-world impact of the condition. A total score is generated by summing the individual factor scores. The COIS-R has favorable psychometric properties, including internal consistency, test–retest reliability, and concurrent validity (Piacentini, Peris, et al., 2007).

Family Accommodation Scale

Given that family accommodation is common in child and adolescent OCD (Peris, Roblek, et al., 2008; Storch et al., 2007) and is known to predict poor outcome in CBT (Garcia et al., 2010; Merlo et al., 2009), it is often helpful to take stock of the ways in which family members respond to OCD symptoms at the outset of treatment. The Family Accommodation Scale (FAS; Calvocoressi et al., 1995) is a brief, clinician-administered interview that assesses 13 questions related to family accommodation. These questions evaluate the extent to which family members have modified routines and participated in OCD rituals over the last month. They also examine levels of familial distress surrounding accommodation and how the child responds when family members attempt to refrain from accommodation. The FAS demonstrates adequate psychometric properties and has also been administered successfully as a self-report questionnaire (Flessner et al., 2009; Peris, Roblek, et al., 2008; Stewart et al., 2008; Storch et al., 2007).

OCD Family Functioning Scale

The OCD Family Functioning Scale (OFF; Stewart et al., 2011) provides a more detailed assessment of the ways in which OCD affects family functioning, and it is a valuable complement to other measures of obsessive–compulsive-specific functional impairment (e.g., COIS-R). The OFF is a self-report measure with parallel patient and family member versions that assesses the impact of OCD across three domains: Daily Life, Social and Occupational, and Emotional. The OFF scale has demonstrated sound psychometric properties, including internal consistency, test–retest reliability, convergent and divergent validity (Stewart et al., 2011).

Treatment

As noted, exposure-based CBT is the psychosocial treatment of choice for child and adolescent OCD (Freeman, Garcia, et al., 2014). In the sections that follow, we provide a brief overview of the specific techniques that comprise this approach, including sample scripts to demonstrate how they might be used in practice. We then discuss developmental considerations that may influence how treatment is administered. We conclude with strategies for helping families to manage OCD symptoms.

As detailed in Table 10.1, treatment typically begins with psychoeducation about OCD and the CBT approach, followed by a session devoted to developing a symptom hierarchy. Exposure practice begins shortly thereafter, often as early as the second or third session. From there on, sessions typically proceed according to the following basic agenda: (1) check-in and homework review; (2) review of symptoms (including symptom hierarchy ratings); (3) exposure practice; (4) supplementary skills (e.g., cognitive restructuring, relaxation skills, problem solving); (5) review of session, homework, and rewards; and (6) family check-in.

Psychoeducation (Session 1)

During the initial treatment visit, the focus is on educating the child and family about the following topics: the prevalence and causes of OCD, the cognitive-behavioral conceptualization of OCD (including the OCD cycle), and what treatment will entail. It should also include some discussion of the role of the family in OCD treatment. Regardless of treatment format (individual or family), it is often useful to conduct this session jointly with the child and parents to ensure that all parties have a basic understanding of the treatment process at the outset. Although the primary goal of the session is to describe the rationale for using exposure-based CBT and to begin to build rapport, psychoeducation has valuable secondary benefits. In particular, it may be used to address feelings of stigma and embarrassment on the part of the child and feelings of anger, blame, or hopelessness on the part of the family. It may also help to establish the therapist's credibility

TABLE 10.1. Sample Treatment Schedule

Week	Session (ERP/family)	Child's ERP focus	Family treatment focus
1	1	Psychoeducation and ERP rationale	(n/a as session conducted jointly)
2	2/1	Symptom hierarchy	(n/a as session conducted jointly)
3	3	Beginning ERP/challenging negative assumptions	Exploring parental feelings and beliefs about OCD
4	4/2	Continued ERP, cognitive restructuring	Blame reduction
5	5	Continued ERP, dealing with obsessions	Understanding the range of responses to OCD
6	6/3	Continued ERP, review of progress	Child's responsibility in treatment
7	7	Continued ERP, troubleshooting obstacles	Barriers to treatment success
8	8/4	Continued ERP, differentiating OCD from non-OCD behaviors	What OCD is and is not
9	9	Addressing more difficult symptoms	Family self-care
10	10/5	Addressing more difficult symptoms	Family problem solving
12	11	Planning for termination	Review, relapse prevention
14	12/6	Review of progress, graduation	

Note. The individual child ERP content may vary. For illustrative purposes, we follow the treatment progression used in our clinic (Piacentini, Roblek, & Langley, 2007), which involves a taper of visits during the final weeks of treatment in order to promote generalization.

and to build confidence in his or her ability to manage care. Indeed, research suggests that beliefs about the value of therapy and its likelihood of success matter a great deal: Higher expectations of treatment success at the outset of treatment are linked not only to higher levels of clinical response but also to better adherence and lower attrition (Lewin, Peris, Bergman, McCracken, & Piacentini, 2011).

Often, psychoeducation begins with a discussion of OCD as a relatively common condition. It may be helpful to mention the size of the child's school when discussing prevalence rates in order to anchor estimates in meaningful reference points (Piacentini, Langley, & Roblek, 2007). That is, a prevalence rate of 1–2% suggests that 10–20 children in a school with 1,000 students will be affected, a discussion point that can help to reduce stigma about being different from others or "the only one in the world with this problem" (Piacentini & Langley, 2004). When discussing the causes of OCD, it is useful to describe the condition as a multidetermined neurobehavioral disorder. Emphasizing the many causes, both genetic and environmental, of OCD may reduce feelings of guilt and blame among family members who see themselves as having "given" the child the disorder. Likewise, this emphasis may begin to address beliefs that the child's symptoms are willful or intentional. Importantly, a neurobehavioral perspective does not attribute OCD entirely to organic causes; it recognizes well-documented environmental determinants that may play an important role in the development and/or expression of specific symptoms (March & Mulle, 1998; Piacentini, Langley, & Roblek, 2007).

> "Do you know anyone in your class who has asthma? What about diabetes? Do you know anyone who wears eyeglasses? These are pretty common problems, and we think of OCD as being really similar. Asthma is a condition that affects how you breathe and diabetes is something that happened when your body has problems handling sugar. OCD is a condition that affects your thoughts and feelings and behaviors; it makes you feel worried when you don't need to be. Just like those other medical problems, seeing a doctor can help you learn to manage your OCD."

In addition to normalizing the experience of OCD and framing it in terms that may be less stigmatizing for the child and family, this approach also allows the therapist to begin to discuss OCD as a stress-sensitive condition that will need ongoing management, a subject that is often covered in the later stages of treatment when discussing relapse prevention.

> "Just like your friends who have asthma or diabetes, I hope you will get to a point where you don't need to see the doctor all the time. You'll just go once in a while for checkups. Some people can go a long time in between checkups, so that OCD really isn't a big part of their lives. However, just like asthma or diabetes can sometimes act up, OCD can, too. There may be times when you are feeling stressed or under the weather that symptoms seem harder to manage. That's normal and it just means it's time for another checkup."

Metaphors can be valuable tools for helping youth to understand key components of psychoeducation, and a commonly used approach involves describing OCD as a "false alarm" (Piacentini, Langley, & Roblek, 2007).

> "We think of OCD as working a lot like a fire alarm. Do you ever have fire drills at school? What happens when you hear the alarm? That's right. You leave the building and line up on the field. Why do you do that? To stay safe if there's a fire, right? Well, has the fire alarm ever gone off by accident? Or have you ever heard of someone pulling it as a prank? What happened? You heard the alarm and reacted, right? But was there any need to? Were you actually in danger? That's right. It was a false alarm. We think of OCD as working the same way. When OCD thoughts pop into your head, it's like an alarm going off to scare you. But it's a false alarm because there's really nothing bad that will happen to you. Our job in treatment is to figure out when it's just a false alarm."

Once the prevalence, causes, and false alarm metaphor have been discussed, the main topic that remains is the rationale for CBT. The importance of this topic cannot be overstated given that CBT for childhood OCD by definition involves the practice of uncomfortable (and often unusual) tasks. There must be buy-in from both parent and child or treatment compliance may be compromised.

"Let's look more closely at how OCD works [refer to the OCD model; Figure 10.1. When you have an OCD thought, how does it make you feel? That's right, you feel anxious or uncomfortable. What do you do to feel better? Most people do a compulsion [reference the child's own symptoms] that makes them feel better, at least for a little bit. The problem is, that relief doesn't last long and it doesn't stop the uncomfortable thoughts from coming back. It also has the unintended effect of making OCD stronger. Because you felt a little relief, you learned that doing your compulsion makes it better, and next time, you may want to do it even more. So every time you do your rituals, OCD gets a little bit stronger. Our job is to stop that from happening. In our work together, we will practice resisting the urge to give in when OCD makes you want to do a compulsive behavior."

Additional psychoeducation may include a discussion of how exposure practice works. Such a discussion should serve to reassure the child that he or she will never be

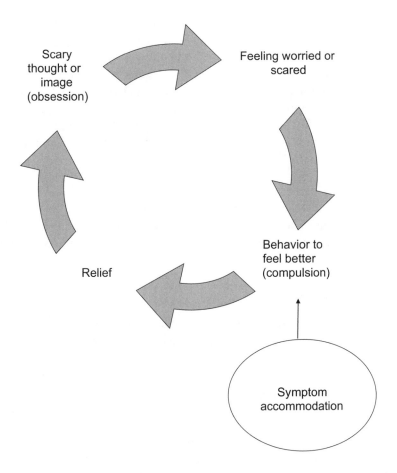

FIGURE 10.1. Model of the OCD cycle.

forced to do anything for which he or she is not ready. Rather he or she will work collaboratively with the therapist to decide what to practice. In addition, many tasks may get easier with practice (either through habituation or improved distress tolerance). Again, metaphors that reinforce the value of repeated practice may prove useful, and they may be tailored to the interests of the child (e.g., practicing a sport or instrument, swimming in a cold pool and noticing that it warms up with time).

The final topic in psychoeducation is the role of the family in treatment. Although not a standard component of most psychoeducation modules, and certainly, somewhat dependent on the treatment format (individual child vs. family), it is important to let parents know about their role in treatment. This includes introducing the concept of accommodation and discussing its role in the OCD cycle (Peris & Piacentini, 2013).

> "We know that OCD doesn't just affect the person who has it. It can affect everyone around them. One way that OCD creates trouble for everyone is by pulling family members into rituals. This may mean answering questions over and over when the person with OCD is worried, providing the things he or she needs to perform the rituals (like soap or towels), or helping him or her avoid things that make him or her uncomfortable. We call this accommodation, and we know that it happens in every family where someone has OCD, and that in most such families, it happens every single day. Most of the time, it happens because everyone is just trying to help make things better. But the problem is, accommodation is another thing that makes OCD stronger. When parents of the person with OCD answer his or her questions or wash their hands, it reinforces the OCD [reference Figure 10.1]. So in treatment, we'll also start to think about when and where accommodation shows up and what we can do to change that pattern."

Many parents ask whether they should immediately discontinue all involvement in accommodation of symptoms. This section of psychoeducation can encourage them simply to identify patterns of accommodation and bring them to treatment. Family members should be reminded that change—even on their end—will be gradual and proceed at a pace the child can tolerate.

Symptom Hierarchy (Session 2)

The development of the symptom hierarchy follows soon after psychoeducation. If the evidence-based approaches described earlier have been employed, the therapist already has a wealth of information about the child's current obsessive–compulsive symptoms, particularly as reported on the CY-BOCS. The goal of this session, then, is to get a sense of how distressing and disruptive each symptom is. The therapist can review the CY-BOCS, focusing on symptoms that have been currently endorsed and on obtaining a distress rating on a 0- to 10-point scale for each item. Each symptom/target may be placed on an individual index card alongside its distress rating, and the cards can be ordered from least to most distressing. Alternatively, symptoms may be placed along a picture of a ladder or pyramid to provide a visual for the child that conveys an approach of beginning with the easiest symptoms. Depending on the age of the child, parent involvement may be useful in identifying symptoms to target in treatment. Regardless of format, the symptom hierarchy is best viewed as a living document that will change shape over time as initial symptoms improve and others are discovered and addressed. The therapist should encourage parent and child to add to the list as needed or to let him or her know when certain symptoms are no longer problematic.

Exposure Practice (Sessions 3–14)

The course of ERP often starts with milder exposures to gain patient buy-in and to increase likelihood of early successes, and individuals gradually work up to addressing more difficult or distressing situations. The therapist should always model tasks first, demonstrating related coping skills before asking the child to practice.

> "We're going to get started today by doing some experiments to see how your OCD works. Just like we talked about earlier, your OCD works in a cycle that keeps you going round and round in circles. We're going to see if we can break the cycle with our exposure practice, and we'll treat it like an experiment to see what happens. We can observe whether you get stronger the more you practice resisting those OCD urges. And we can observe whether the bad outcomes you're expecting actually happen. Each week, we'll practice and see what we learn. Over time, you can decide for yourself whether this approach is helpful."

As a rule, exposures are first practiced in a therapy session, with the child subsequently given "homework assignments" to practice the same exposure on his or her own in a natural environment. When exposures cannot be recreated in the therapy setting, imaginal exposures can be used; for example, an adolescent with obsessional fears of running over pedestrians may be asked to imagine him- or herself doing that repeatedly. Imaginal exposures can also be useful as a stepping-stone toward *in vivo* exposures that a child perceives as too challenging, or to address obsessions that are not linked with a compulsive behavior (e.g., repeated obsessional thoughts about being a bad person), or to practice location- or situation-specific obsessions in the office setting. For both imaginal and *in vivo* exposures, the child's between-session practice of the exposure is a crucial component of ERP; this practice fosters robust consolidation of the gains initiated in session.

As noted earlier, traditional models of ERP have emphasized the importance of habituation; accordingly, many treatments encourage soliciting distress ratings at regular intervals and continuing a given exposure task until distress ratings have dropped by 50%. Given that youth ratings of distress may not be reliable, and that emerging evidence calls into question this approach (Craske et al., 2008), it may be more useful to think about exposure from the perspective of distress tolerance; that is, the child's ratings may or may not decrease over time, but his or her ability to cope with arousal and manage it effectively may be improving. In addition, rather than waiting for distress ratings to decline, it may also be useful to consider sustaining the exposure long enough to violate the child's assumptions about what will happen during the designated task. For example, the therapist might ask, "How long do you think you could tolerate touching the inside of the toilet?" If the child says 2 seconds, but is then able to remain in the task for 10 or 15 seconds, the therapist can use this as evidence that counters the child's expectations. Once an exposure task has been practiced successfully in session and at home, the expectation is that it will become part of more naturalistic everyday practice; that is, the task may no longer be viewed as homework but as something the child does as part of his or her usual routine.

Family members should be integrated into exposure practice systematically, and it is important to allow adequate time for their participation in sessions. In individually administered CBT, this involvement should, at the very least, include a check-in with parents at the end of session, during which a review of exposure targets, progress, and homework is conducted. It is ideal that the review of the session be directed by the child, so that he or she may take ownership of accomplishments and share material that is most comfortable for him or her. During this time, *in vivo* demonstration of an exposure practiced earlier in session may also be very useful. Such practice provides an opportunity for the therapist to coach parents on how to respond effectively in the moment, including optimal strategies for praise, containing their own anxiety, and modeling brave behavior. It also provides a valuable glimpse into family dynamics that may need further attention in treatment (e.g., conflict, blame, enmeshment).

Additional family involvement may focus on ongoing psychoeducation for family members (Piacentini, Langley, & Roblek, 2007). Families enter treatment highly distressed, and it may be difficult for them to process and retain the large amount of information that typically is presented in the first few psychoeducation sessions. Accordingly, the therapist should plan for frequent review, particularly of topics related to accommodation, and he or she should be sure to allot time each week to addressing additional relevant topics, such as family members' emotional responses to OCD, attributions about the illness, barriers to treatment success (e.g., motivation, secondary gain), and limit setting around oppositional or unsafe behavior.

In cases in which more advanced family work is needed or where time permits greater involvement, it can be useful to focus on helping family members to develop the skills they will need to problem-solve effectively around OCD situations. Because both OCD symptoms and the ERP interventions that address them may be very arousing for parents, these skills involve emotion regulation (i.e., recognizing, monitoring, and managing) and distress tolerance strategies such as relaxation or mindfulness (Peris & Piacentini, 2013). They may also involve the development of a step-by-step plan for responding to OCD in the moment, and guided help with disengaging from patterns of accommodation (Peris & Piacentini, 2013, 2014).

Obsessions

In some cases, ERP approaches require that the child directly address distressing thoughts rather than simply resisting the compulsive behaviors they trigger. Harm-related obsessions, including those that center on fears of harming someone/being harmed and sexual obsessions, may require more direct exposure techniques. In these situations, a number of creative strategies may be employed to solicit the distressing thoughts and practice tolerating them. These strategies may include the imaginal exposures described earlier, with the child repeatedly writing out the fearful thought (sometimes in a declarative statement; e.g., "Today I will get in a car accident"), and describing it to others, or listening to the child talk about it repeatedly. Other strategies that may work well to diffuse the intensity of the thought include singing about an obsessional thought, rapping or rhyming about the thought, or changing feared images into innocuous or humorous ones (Piacentini et al., 2012).

Developmental Considerations

Core treatment techniques in CBT for childhood OCD largely emanate from approaches used to treat adult OCD. However, virtually every child and adolescent protocol acknowledges the importance of thoughtful, developmentally sensitive adaptations of techniques implemented with adults (Freeman et al., 2008; Freeman, Garcia, et al., 2014; Lewin, Park, et al., 2014; March & Franklin, 2006). Children and adolescents differ from adults in specific ways that are likely to impact the success of exposure-based CBT approaches. First, developmental limitations may impede their ability to report on symptoms accurately or to understand the link between their obsessions and the compulsions they trigger; insight regarding the impact of OCD may be limited. Second, young children may not have a well-developed sense of time and may therefore be more present-oriented. This in turn may complicate efforts to motivate them to participate in tasks that are immediately distressing, with the promise of future improvements in anxiety. Third, as noted earlier, comorbid externalizing disorders are relatively common, creating a unique set of treatment challenges that may be best addressed with a flexible approach that integrates traditional behavior management techniques with ERP. Along these lines, poor frustration tolerance and coping abilities may be prominent (Piacentini et al., 2012). Despite these challenges, the evidence base overwhelmingly points to the ability of youth across the developmental spectrum to benefit from ERP treatment (Freeman, Sapyta, et al., 2014; Lewin, Park, et al., 2014; Piacentini et al., 2011; POTS, 2004). Certainly, there are likely to be salient individual differences in insight, motivation, and readiness for treatment irrespective of age, a fact that underscores the importance of systematic evaluation of these factors at the start of treatment.

Adaptation of exposure-based CBT protocols for younger age groups typically includes several basic modifications to address the previously discussed considerations. First, language is modified throughout to improve uptake by clients whose verbal abilities may still be developing. This includes the use of age-appropriate metaphors to understand key treatment concepts and to facilitate cognitive restructuring (Piacentini et al., 2012). Treatment content may also be introduced via hands-on activities that are more engaging for younger children. For example, to teach youngsters to externalize their OCD, it is often helpful to draw a picture of the "OCD bully" or to give OCD a nasty (or sometimes silly and ridiculing) name. Second, these protocols involve use of behavioral reward systems that are tailored to the child's specific needs. Younger children may require more frequent, concrete rewards, whereas older youth may be able to wait longer periods of time in the service of earning something they might not normally get, and reward systems are developed with these distinctions in mind. Third, these protocols call for systematic family involvement in treatment (Barrett, Healy-Farrell, & March, 2004; Freeman, Garcia, & Coyne, 2008; Freeman, Sapyta, et al., 2014; March & Mulle, 1998; Piacentini et al., 2011), and, in cases of younger clients, extensive training of parents as co-therapists and coaches (Freeman, Sapyta, et al., 2014; Lewin, Park, et al., 2014). Using this combination of techniques, ERP has been used to successfully treat preschool (Lewin, Park, et al., 2014) and early childhood (Freeman, Sapyta, et al., 2014) cases of OCD.

REFERENCES

Abramowitz, J. S. (2013). The practice of exposure therapy: Relevance of cognitive-behavioral theory and extinction theory. *Behavior Therapy, 44*(4), 548–558.

Abramowitz, J. S., Whiteside, S. P., & Deacon, B. J. (2006). The effectiveness of treatment for pediatric obsessive–compulsive disorder: A meta-analysis. *Behavior Therapy, 36*(1), 55–63.

Albano, A., March, J., & Piacentini, J. (1999). Cognitive behavioral treatment of obsessive–compulsive disorder. In R. E. Ammerman (Ed.), *Handbook of prescriptive treatments for children and adolescents* (pp. 193–213). Boston: Allyn & Bacon.

American Psychiatric Association. (2000). *Diagnostic and statistical manual of mental disorders* (4th ed.). Washington, DC: Author.

American Psychiatric Association. (2013). *Diagnostic and statistical manual of mental disorders* (5th ed.). Arlington, VA: Author.

Apter, A., Pauls, D. L., Bleich, A., Zohar, A. H., Kron, S., Ratzoni, G., et al. (1993). An epidemiologic study of Gilles de la Tourette's syndrome in Israel. *Archives of General Psychiatry, 50,* 734–738.

Bar-Haim, Y., Morag, I., & Glickman, S. (2011). Training to disengage attention from threat reduces vulnerability to stress in anxious children. *Journal of Child Psychology and Psychiatry, 52,* 861–869.

Barrett, P., Farrell, L., Dadds, M., "& Boulter, N. (2005). Cognitive-behavioral family treatment of childhood obsessive–compulsive disorder: Long-term follow-up and predictors of outcome. *Journal of the American Academy of Child and Adolescent Psychiatry, 44,* 1005–1014.

Barrett, P., Farrell, L., Pina, A., Peris, T. S., & Piacentini, J. (2008). Evidence-based psychosocial treatments for child and adolescent OCD. *Journal of Clinical Child and Adolescent Psychology, 37,* 131–155.

Barrett, P. M., & Healy-Farrell, L. J. (2003). Perceived responsibility in childhood obsessive–compulsive disorder: An experimental manipulation. *Journal of Clinical Child and Adolescent Psychiatry, 32,* 430–441.

Barrett, P., Healy-Farrell, L., & March, J. (2004). Cognitive-behavioral family treatment of childhood obsessive–compulsive disorder: A controlled trial. *Journal of the American Academy of Child and Adolescent Psychiatry, 43,* 46–62.

Bartz, J. A., & Hollander, E. (2006). Is obsessive–compulsive disorder an anxiety disorder? *Progress in Neuro-Psychopharmacology and Biological Psychiatry, 30*(3), 338–352.

Benazon, N. R., Ager, J., & Rosenberg, D. R. (2002). Cognitive behavior therapy in treatment-naïve children and adolescents with obsessive–compulsive disorder: An open trial. *Behaviour Research and Therapy, 40*(5), 529–539.

Calvocoressi, L., Lewis, B., Harris, M., Trufan, S. J., Goodman, W. K., McDougle, C. J., et al. (1995). Family accommodation in obsessive–compulsive disorder. *American Journal of Psychiatry, 152,* 441–443.

Chabane, N., Delome, R., Millet, B., Mouren, M. C., Leboyer, M., & Pauls, D. (2005). Early-onset obsessive–compulsive disorder: A subgroup with a specific clinical and familial pattern. *Journal of Child Psychology and Psychiatry, 46,* 881–887.

Craske, M. G., Kircanski, K., Zelikowsky, M., Mystkowsi, J., Chowdhury, N., & Baker, A. (2008). Optimizing inhibitory learning during exposure therapy. *Behaviour Research and Therapy, 46*(1), 5–27.

de Mathis, M. A., Diniz, J. B., Shavitt, R. G., Torres, A. R., Ferrao, Y. A., Fossaluza, V., et al. (2009). Early-onset obsessive compulsive disorder with and without tics. *CNS Spectrums, 14,* 362–370.

Diniz, J. B., Rosario-Campos, M. C., Shavitt, R. G., Curi, M., Hounie, A. G., Brotto, S. A., et al. (2004). Impact of age at onset and duration of illness on the expression of comorbidities in obsessive–compulsive disorder. *Journal of Clinical Psychiatry, 65,* 22–27.

Eldar, S., Apter, A., Lotan, D., Edgar, K. P., Naim, R., Fox, N. A., et al. (2012). Attention bias modification treatment for pediatric anxiety disorders: A randomized controlled trial. *American Journal of Psychiatry, 169,* 213–220.

Farrell, L. J., & Barrett, P. M. (2007). Prevention of childhood emotional disorders: Reducing the burden of suffering associated with anxiety and depression. *Child and Adolescent Mental Health, 12,* 58–65.

Flament, M. F., Rapoport, J. L., Berg, C. J., Sceery, W., Kilts, C., Mellstrom, B., et al. (1985). Clomipramine treatment of childhood obsessive–compulsive disorder. *Archives of General Psychiatry, 42,* 977–983.

Flessner, C., Allgair, A., Garcia, A., Freeman, J., Sapyta, J., Franklin, M., Foa, E., et al. (2010). The impact of neuropsychological functioning on treatment outcome in pediatric obsessive–compulsive disorder. *Depression and Anxiety, 27,* 365–371.

Flessner, C. A., Sapyta, J., Garcia, A., Freeman, J. B., Franklin, M. E., Foa, E., et al. (2009). Examining the psychometric properties of the Family Accommodation Scale–Parent-Report (FAS-PR). *Journal of Psychopathology and Behavioral Assessment, 31*(1), 38–46.

Foa, E., & Kozac, M. (1986). Emotional processing of fear: Exposure to corrective information. *Psychological Bulletin, 99,* 450–472.

Freeman, J., Garcia, A. M., & Coyne, L. (2008). Early childhood OCD: Preliminary findings from a family-based cognitive behavioral approach. *Journal of the American Academy of Child and Adolescent Psychiatry, 47,* 593–602.

Freeman, J., Garcia, A., Frank, H., Benito, K., Conelea, C., Walther, M., et al. (2014). Evidence base update for psychosocial treatments for pediatric obsessive–compulsive disorder. *Journal of Clinical Child and Adolescent Psychology, 43*(1), 7–26.

Freeman, J. B., Garcia, A. M., Fucci, C., Karitani, M. K., Miller, L., & Leonard, H. L. (2003). Family-based treatment of early-onset obsessive–compulsive disorder. *Journal of Child and Adolescent Psychopharmacology, 13,* 71–80.

Freeman, J., Sapyta, J., Garcia, A., Compton, C., Khanna, M., Flessner, C., et al. (2014). Family-based treatment of early childhood obsessive compulsive disorder: The Pediatric Obsessive Compulsive Disorder Study for Young Children (POTS Jr.)—a randomized clinical trial. *Journal of the American Medical Association, 71*(6), 689–698.

Gallant, J., Storch, E. A., Merlo, L. J., Ricketts, E. D., Geffken, G. R., Goodman, W. K., et al. (2008). Convergent and discriminant validity of the Children's Yale–Brown Obsessive Compulsive Scale–Symptom Checklist. *Journal of Anxiety Disorders, 22*(8), 1369–1376.

Garcia, A. M., Freeman, J. B., Himle, M. B., Berman, N. C., Ogata, A. K., Ng, J., et al. (2009). Phenomenology of early childhood onset obsessive compulsive disorder. *Journal of Psychopathology and Behavioral Assessment, 31,* 104–111.

Garcia, A. M., Sapyta, J. J., Moore, P. S., Freeman, J. B., Franklin, M. E., March, J. S., et al. (2010). Predictors and moderators of treatment outcome in the Pediatric Obsessive Compulsive Treatment Study (POTS I). *Journal of the American Academy of Child and Adolescent Psychiatry, 49,* 1024–1033.

Geller, D. A., Biederman, J., Faraone, S., Agranat, A., Cradock, K., Hagermoser, L., et al. (2001). Developmental aspects of obsessive compulsive disorder: Findings in children, adolescents, and adults. *Journal of Nervous and Mental Disease, 189,* 471–477.

Geller, D. A., Biederman, J., Faraone, S. V., Cradock, K., Hagermoser, L., Zaman, N., et al. (2002). Attention-deficit/hyperactivity disorder in children and adolescents with obsessive–compulsive disorder: Fact or artifact? *Journal of the American Academy of Child and Adolescent Psychiatry, 41*(1), 52–58.

Geller, D. A., Biederman, J., Griffin, S., Jones, J., & Lefkowitz, T. R. (1996). Comorbidity of juvenile obsessive compulsive disorder with disruptive behavior disorders. *Journal of the American Academy of Child and Adolescent Psychiatry, 35,* 1637–1646.

Geller, D. A., & March, J. (2012). Practice parameter for the assessment and treatment of children and adolescents with obsessive–compulsive disorder. *Journal of the American Academy of Child and Adolescent Psychiatry, 51*(1), 98–113.

Geller, D. A., Wagner, K. D., Emslie, G., Murphy, T., Carpenter, D. J., Wetherhold, E., et al. (2004). Paroxetine treatment in children and adolescents with obsessive–compulsive disorder: A randomized, multicenter, double-blind, placebo-controlled trial. *Journal of the American Academy of Child and Adolescent Psychiatry, 43,* 1387–1396.

Ginsburg, G. S., Kingery, J. N., Drake, K. L., & Grados, M. A. (2008). Predictors of treatment response in pediatric obsessive–compulsive disorder. *Journal of the American Academy of Child and Adolescent Psychiatry, 47,* 868–878.

Goodman, W., Price, L. H., Rasmussen, S. A., Mazure, C., Fleischmann, R. L., Hill, C. L., et al. (1989). The Yale–Brown Obsessive Compulsive Scale: Development, use and reliability. *Archives of General Psychiatry, 46,* 1006–1011.

Goodman, W. K., Price, L. H., Rasmussen, S. A., Riddle, M. A., & Rapoport, J. L. (1991). *Children's Yale–Brown Obsessive Compulsive Scale (CY-BOCS).* Providence, RI: Department of Psychiatry, Brown University School of Medicine.

Hajcak, G., Franklin, M. E., Simons, R. F., & Keuthen, N. J. (2006). Hair pulling and skin picking in relation to affective distress and obsessive compulsive symptoms. *Journal of Psychopathology and Behavioral Assessment, 28,* 179–187.

Hanna, G. (1995). Demographic and clinical features of obsessive–compulsive disorder in children and adolescents. *Journal of the American Academy of Child and Adolescent Psychiatry, 34,* 19–27.

Heyman, I., Fombonne, E., Simmons, H., Ford, T., Meltzer, H., & Goodman, R. (2003). Prevalence of obsessive–compulsive disorder in the British nationwide survey of child mental health. *International Review of Psychiatry, 15,* 178–184.

Ipser, J. C., Stein, D. J., Hawkridge, S., & Hoppe, L. (2009). Pharmacotherapy for anxiety disorders in children and adolescents. *Cochrane Database of Systematic Review, 3,* CD005170.

Ivarsson, T., Melin, K., & Wallin, L. (2008). Categorical and dimensional aspects of co-morbidity in obsessive–compulsive disorder (OCD). *European Child and Adolescent Psychiatry, 17,* 20–31.

Ivarsson, T., & Valderhaug, R. (2006). Symptom patterns in children and adolescents with obsessive–compulsive disorder (OCD). *Behaviour Research and Therapy, 44,* 1105–1116.

Jaisoorya, T. S., Reddy, Y. C., Srinath, S., & Thennarasu, K. (2008). Obsessive compulsive disorder with and without tic disorder: A comparative study from India. *CNS Spectrums, 13,* 705–711.

Kendall, P. C., Flannery-Schroeder, E., Panichelli-Mindel, S. M., Southam-Gerow, M., Henin, A., & Warman, M. (1997). Therapy for youths with anxiety disorders: A second randomized clinical trial. *Journal of Consulting and Clinical Psychology, 65*(3), 366–380.

Kircanski, K., & Peris, T. S. (2014). Exposure and response prevention process predicts treatment outcome in youth with OCD. *Journal of Abnormal Child Psychology, 43*(3), 543–552.

Kircanski, K., Wu, M., & Piacentini, J. (2014). Reduction of subjective distress in CBT for childhood OCD: Nature of change, predictors, and relation to treatment outcome. *Journal of Anxiety Disorders, 28,* 125–132.

Kozak, M. J., & Foa, E. B. (1997). *Mastery of obsessive–compulsive disorder: A cognitive-behavioral approach* (Therapist guide). San Antonio, TX: Psychological Corporation.

Langley, A., Bergman, R. L., Lewin, A., Lee, J. C., & Piacentini, J. (2010). Correlates of comorbid anxiety and externalizing disorders in childhood obsessive compulsive disorder. *European Child and Adolescent Psychiatry, 19*(8), 637–645.

Langley, A., Bergman, R. L., & Piacentini, J. (2002). Assessment of childhood anxiety. *International Review of Psychiatry, 14,* 102–113.

Leckman, J. F., Grice, O. E., & Barr, L. C., de Vries, A. L., Martin, C., Cohen, D. J., et al. (1994–1995). Tic-related versus non-tic-related obsessive compulsive disorder. *Anxiety, 1,* 208–215.

Leonard, H. L., Swedo, S. E., Rapoport, J. L., Koby, E. V., Lenane, M. C., Cheslow, D. L., et al. (1989). Treatment of obsessive–compulsive disorder with clomipramine and desipramine in children and adolescents. *Archives of General Psychiatry, 46,* 1088–109.

Lewin, A., & Piacentini, J. (2010). Evidence-based assessment of child obsessive compulsive disorder: Recommendations for clinical practice and treatment research. *Child and Youth Care Forum, 39*, 73–89.

Lewin, A. B., McGuire, J. F., Murphy, T. K., & Storch, E. A. (2014). The importance of considering parent's preferences when planning treatment for their children—the case of childhood obsessive–compulsive disorder. *Journal of Child Psychology and Psychiatry, 55*(12), 1314–1316.

Lewin, A. B., Park, J. M., Jones, A. M., Crawford, E. A., DeNadai, A. S., Menzel, J., et al. (2014). Family-based exposure and response prevention therapy for preschool-aged children with obsessive–compulsive disorder: A pilot randomized controlled trial. *Behaviour Research and Therapy, 56*, 30–38.

Lewin, A. L., Peris, T. S., Bergman, R. L., McCracken, J. T., & Piacentini, J. (2011). The role of treatment expectancy in youth receiving exposure-based CBT for obsessive compulsive disorder. *Behavior Research and Therapy, 49*, 536–543.

March, J., Frances, A., Carpenter, D., & Kahn, D. (1997). Expert consensus guidelines: Treatment of obsessive–compulsive disorder. *Journal of Clinical Psychiatry, 58*, 1–72.

March, J. S., & Franklin, M. E. (2006). Cognitive-behavioral therapy for pediatric OCD. In B. O. Rothbaum (Ed.), *Pathological anxiety: Emotional processing in etiology and treatment* (pp. 147–165). New York: Guilford Press.

March, J. S., Franklin, M. E., & Leonard, H. (2007). Tics moderate treatment outcome with sertraline but not cognitive-behavior therapy in pediatric obsessive–compulsive disorder. *Biological Psychiatry, 61*, 344–347.

March, J. S., & Mulle, K. (1998). *OCD in children and adolescents: A cognitive-behavioral treatment manual.* New York: Guilford Press.

Markarian, Y., Larson, M. J., Aldea, M. A., Baldwin, S. A., Good, D., Berkeljon, A., et al. (2009). Multiple pathways to functional impairment in obsessive compulsive disorder. *Clinical Psychology Review, 30*, 78–88.

Masi, G., Millepiedi, S., & Mucci, M. (2006). Comorbidity of obsessive compulsive disorder and attention-deficit/hyperactivity disorder in referred children and adolescents. *Comprehensive Psychiatry, 46*, 42–47.

Masi, G., Millepiedi, S., Perugi, G., Pfanner, C., Berloffa, S., Pari, C., et al. (2010). A naturalistic exploratory study of the impact of demographic, phenotypic and comorbid features in pediatric obsessive–compulsive disorder. *Psychopathology, 43*(2), 69–78.

McKay, D., Piacentini, J., Greisberg, S., Graae, F., Jaffer, M., Miller, J., et al. (2003). The Children's Yale–Brown Obsessive Compulsive Scale: Item structure in an outpatient setting. *Psychological Assessment, 15*, 578–581.

Merlo, L. J., Lehmkuhl, H. D., Geffken, G. R., & Storch, E .A. (2009). Decreased family accommodation associated with improved therapy outcome in pediatric obsessive compulsive disorder. *Journal of Consulting and Clinical Psychology, 77*, 355–360.

Merlo, L. J., Storch, E. A., Adkins, J. W., Murphy, T. K., & Geffken, G. R. (2007). Assessment of pediatric obsessive–compulsive disorder. In E. A. Storch, G. R. Geffken, & T. K. Murphy (Eds.), *Handbook of child and adolescent obsessive–compulsive disorder* (pp. 67–107). Mahwah, NJ: Erlbaum.

Meyer, V. (1966). Modification of expectations in cases with obsessive rituals. *Behavioural Research and Therapy, 4*, 270–280.

Moore, P. S., Mariaskin, A., March, J., Franklin, M. E., Storch, E., Geffken, G., et al. (2007). Obsessive–compulsive disorder in children and adolescents: Diagnosis, comorbidity, and developmental factors. In E. A. Storch, G. Geffken, & T. K. Murphy (Eds.), *Handbook of child and adolescent obsessive–compulsive disorder* (pp. 17–45). New York: Routledge.

Pediatric OCD Treatment Study Team. (2004). Cognitive-behavioral therapy, sertraline, and their combination for children and adolescents with obsessive–compulsive disorder: The Pediatric OCD Treatment Study (POTS) randomized controlled trial. *Journal of the American Medical Association, 292*, 1969–1976.

Peris, T. S., Bergman, R. L., Langley, A., Chang, S., McCracken, J. T., & Piacentini, J. (2008). Correlates of family accommodation of childhood obsessive compulsive disorder: Parent, child, and family characteristics. *Journal of the American Academy of Child and Adolescent Psychiatry, 47,* 1173–1181.

Peris, T. S., & Piacentini, J. (2013). Optimizing treatment for complex cases of childhood obsessive compulsive disorder: A preliminary trial. *Journal of Clinical Child and Adolescent Psychology, 42*(1), 1–8.

Peris, T. S., & Piacentini, J. (2014). Addressing barriers to change in the treatment of childhood obsessive compulsive disorder. *Journal of Rational Emotive and Cognitive Behavior Therapy. Special Issue: The Evolution of CBT with Youth.* [Epub ahead of print]

Peris, T. S., Roblek, T., Langley, A., Benazon, N., & Piacentini, J. (2008). Parental responses to obsessive compulsive disorder: Development and validation of the Parental Attitudes And Behaviors Scale (PABS). *Child and Family Behavior Therapy, 30,* 199–214.

Peris, T. S., Sugar, C. A., Bergman, L. R., Chang, S., Langley, A., & Piacentini, J. (2012). Family factors predict treatment outcome for pediatric obsessive–compulsive disorder. *Journal of Consulting and Clinical Psychology, 80,* 255–263.

Peterson, B. S., Pine, D. S., Cohen, P., & Brook, J. S. (2001). Prospective, longitudinal study of tic, obsessive–compulsive, and attention-deficit/hyperactivity disorders in an epidemiological sample. *Journal of the American Academy of Child and Adolescent Psychiatry, 40,* 685–695.

Piacentini, J., Bergman, R. L., Chang, S., Langley, A., Peris, T., Wood, J. J., et al. (2011). Controlled comparison of family cognitive behavioral therapy and psychoeducation/relaxation training for child obsessive–compulsive disorder. *Journal of the American Academy of Child and Adolescent Psychiatry, 50,* 1149–1161.

Piacentini, J., Bergman, R. L., Jacobs, C., McCracken, J., & Kretchman, J. (2002). Cognitive-behaviour therapy for childhood obsessive–compulsive disorder: Efficacy and predictors of treatment response. *Journal of Anxiety Disorders, 16,* 207–219.

Piacentini, J., Bergman, R. L., Keller, M., & McCracken, J. (2003). Functional impairment in children and adolescents with obsessive compulsive disorder. *Journal of Child and Adolescent Psychopharmacology, 13,* 61–70.

Piacentini, J., & Langley, A. K. (2004). Cognitive-behavioral therapy for children who have obsessive–compulsive disorder. *Journal of Clinical Psychology, 60*(11), 1181–1194.

Piacentini, J., Langley, A., & Roblek, T. (2007). *Cognitive-behavioral treatment of childhood OCD.* New York: Oxford University Press.

Piacentini, J., March, J., & Franklin, M. (2006). Cognitive-behavioral therapy for youngsters with obsessive–compulsive disorder. In P. C. Kendall (Ed.), *Child and adolescent therapy: Cognitive-behavioral procedures* (3rd ed., pp. 297–321). New York: Guilford Press.

Piacentini, J., Peris, T. S., Bergman, R. L., Chang, S., & Jaffer, M. (2007). The Child Obsessive Compulsive Impact Scale—Revised (COIS-R): Development and psychometric properties. *Journal of Clinical Child and Adolescent Psychology, 36,* 645–653.

Piacentini, J. C., Peris, T. S., March, J. S., & Franklin, M. E. (2012). Obsessive–compulsive disorder. In P. C. Kendall (Ed.), *Child and adolescent therapy: Cognitive-behavioral procedures* (4th ed., pp. 259–282). New York: Guilford Press.

Pine, D. S. (2007). Research review: A neuroscience framework for pediatric anxiety disorders. *Journal of Child Psychology and Psychiatry, 48,* 631–648.

Rapoport, J., Inoff-Germain, G., Weissman, M. M., Greenwald, S., Narrow, W. E., Jensen, P. S., et al. (2000). Childhood obsessive–compulsive disorder in the NIMH MECA Study: Parent versus child identification of cases. *Journal of Anxiety Disorders, 14,* 535–548.

Rapoport, J., Swedo, S. E., & Leonard, H. L. (1992). Childhood obsessive–compulsive disorder. *Journal of Clinical Psychiatry, 53,* 11–16.

Rasmussen, S., & Eisen, J. (1990). Epidemiology of obsessive compulsive disorder. *Journal of Clinical Psychiatry, 51*(2, Suppl.), 10–13.

Renshaw, K. D., Steketee, G., & Chambless, D. L. (2005). Involving family members in the treatment of OCD. *Cognitive Behavior Therapy, 34,* 164–175.

Rettew, D., Swedo, S. E., Leonard, H. L., Lenane, M. C., & Rapport, J. L. (1992). Obsessions and compulsions across time in 79 children and adolescents with obsessive–compulsive disorder. *Journal American Academy of Child and Adolescent Psychiatry, 31,* 1050–1056.

Riddle, M. A., Reeve, E. A., Yaryura-Tobias, J. A., Yang, H. M., Claghorn, J. L., Gaffney, G., et al. (2001). Fluvoxamine for children and adolescents with obsessive–compulsive disorder: A randomized, controlled multicenter trial. *Journal of the American Academy of Child and Adolescent Psychiatry, 40,* 222–229.

Rosenberg, D. R., Russell, A., & Fougere, A. (2005). Neuropsychiatric models of OCD. In J. S. Abramowitz & A. C. Houts (Eds.), *Concepts and controversies in obsessive–compulsive disorder* (pp. 209–228). New York: Springer.

Salkovskis, P. M. (1996). Cognitive-behavioural approaches to the understanding of obsessional problems. In R. M. Rapee (Ed.), *Current controversies in the anxiety disorders* (pp. 191–200). New York: Guilford Press.

Sánchez-Meca, J., Rosa-Alcázar, A., Iniesta-Sepúlveda, M., & Rosa-Alcázar, A. (2014). Differential efficacy of cognitive-behavioral therapy and pharmacological treatments for pediatric obsessive–compulsive disorder: A meta-analysis. *Journal of Anxiety Disorders, 28,* 31–44.

Scahill, L., Riddle, M. A., McSwiggan-Hardin, M. T., Ort, S. I., King, R. A., Goodman, W. K., et al. (1997). Children's Yale–Brown Obsessive–Compulsive Scale: Reliability and validity. *Journal of the American Academy of Child and Adolescent Psychiatry, 36,* 844–852.

Scahill, L., Vitulano, L. A., Brenner, E. M., Lynch, K. A., & King, R. A. (1996). Behavioral therapy in children and adolescents with obsessive–compulsive disorder: A pilot study. *Journal of Child and Adolescent Psychopharmacology, 6,* 191–202.

Silverman, W., & Albano, A. M. (1996). *Anxiety Disorders Interview Schedule for DSM-IV: Parent Version.* San Antonio, TX: Graywing.

Silverman, W., Saavedra, L., & Pina, A. (2001). Test–retest reliability of anxiety symptoms and diagnoses with Anxiety Disorders Interview Schedule for DSM-IV: Child and Parent versions. *Journal of the American Academy of Child and Adolescent Psychiatry, 40,* 937–944.

Soechting, L., & March, J. (2002). Cognitive aspects of obsessive compulsive disorder in children. In R. Frost & G. Steketee (Eds.), *Cognitive approaches to obsessions and compulsions: Theory, assessment, and treatment* (pp. 299–314). Amsterdam: Pergamon/Elsevier Science.

Stewart, S., Geller, D., Jenike, M., Pauls, D., Shaw, D., Mullin, B., et al. (2004). Long-term outcome of pediatric obsessive–compulsive disorder: A meta-analysis and qualitative review of the literature. *Acta Psychiatrica Scandinavica, 110,* 4–13.

Stewart, S. E., Geller, D. A., Leckman, J. F., Illmann, C., Scharf, J. M., Brown, T. A., et al. (2008). Four-factor structure of obsessive–compulsive disorder symptoms in children, adolescents, and adults. *Journal of the American Academy of Child and Adolescent Psychiatry, 47*(7), 763–772.

Stewart, S. E., Hu, Y. P., Hezel, D. M., Proujansky, R., Lamstein, A., Walsh, C., et al. (2011). Development and psychometric properties of the OCD Family Functioning (OFF) scale. *Journal of Family Psychology, 25,* 434–443.

Storch, E. A., Geffken, G. R., Merlo, L. J., Mann, G., Duke, D., & Munson, M. (2007). Family-based cognitive-behavioral therapy for pediatric obsessive–compulsive disorder: Comparisons of intensive and weekly approaches. *Journal of the American Academy of Child and Adolescent Psychiatry, 46,* 469–478.

Storch, E. A., Khanna, M., Merlo, L. J., Leow, B. A., Franklin, M., Reid, J. M., et al. (2009). Children's Florida Obsessive Compulsive Inventory: Psychometric properties and feasibility of a self-report measure of obsessive–compulsive symptoms in youth. *Child Psychiatry and Human Development, 40*(3), 467–483.

Storch, E. A., Larson, M. J., Merlo, M. J., Keeley, M. L., Jacob, M. L., Geffken, G. R., et al. (2008). Cormorbidity of pediatric obsessive compulsive disorder and anxiety disorders:

Impact on symptom severity and impairment. *Journal of Psychopathology and Behavioral Assessment, 30,* 111–120.

Storch, E. A., Merlo, L. J., Larson, M. J., Geffken, G. R., Lehmkuhl, H. D., & Jacob, M. L. (2008). Impact of comorbidity on cognitive-behavioral therapy response in pediatric obsessive–compulsive disorder. *Journal of the American Academy of Child and Adolescent Psychiatry, 47,* 583–592.

Storch, E. A., Stigge-Kaufman, D., Marien, W. E., Sajid, M., Jacob, M. L., Geffken, G. R., et al. (2008). Obsessive–compulsive disorder in youth with and without a chronic tic disorder. *Depression and Anxiety, 25,* 761–767.

Sukhodolsky, D. G., do Rosario-Campos, M. C., Scahill, L., Katsovich, L., Pauls, D. L., Peterson, B. S., et al. (2005). Adaptive, emotional, and family functioning of children with obsessive–compulsive disorder and comorbid attention deficit hyperactivity disorder. *American Journal of Psychiatry, 162*(6), 1125–1132.

Swedo, S., Rapoport, J., Leonard, H., Lenane, M., & Cheslow, D. (1989). Obsessive–compulsive disorder in children and adolescents: Clinical phenomenology of 70 consecutive cases. *Archives of General Psychiatry, 46,* 335–341.

Valderhaug, R., Larsson, B., Gotestam, K. G., & Piacentini, J. (2007). An open clinical trial of cognitive-behavior therapy in children and adolescents with obsessive–compulsive disorder administered in regular outpatient clinics. *Behaviour Research and Therapy, 45,* 577–589.

Valleni-Basile, L., Garrison, C., Jackson, K., Waller, J., McKeown, R., Addy, C., et al. (1994). Frequency of obsessive–compulsive disorder in a community sample of young adolescents. *Journal of the American Academy of Child and Adolescent Psychiatry, 33,* 782–791.

Waters, T., & Barrett, P. (2000). The role of the family in childhood obsessive–compulsive disorder. *Clinical Child and Family Psychology Review, 3,* 173–184.

Watson, H. J., & Rees, C. S. (2008). Meta-analysis of randomized, controlled treatment trials for pediatric obsessive–compulsive disorder. *Journal of Child Psychology and Psychiatry, 49,* 489–498.

Williams, A. D., & Grisham, J. R. (2013). Cognitive bias modification (CBM) of obsessive compulsive beliefs. *BMC Psychiatry, 13*(1), 256.

Wood, J., Piacentini, J., Bergman, R. L., McCracken, J., & Barrios, V. (2002). Concurrent validity of the anxiety disorders section of the Anxiety Disorders Interview Schedule for DSM-IV: Child and Parent version. *Journal of Clinical Child Psychology, 31,* 335–342.

Zohar, A. H. (1999). The epidemiology of obsessive–compulsive disorder in children and adolescents. *Child and Adolescent Psychiatric Clinics of North America, 8,* 445–460.

CHAPTER 11

Disruptive Behavior Disorders

John E. Lochman, Caroline Boxmeyer,
Nicole Powell, Casey Dillon,
Cameron Powe, and Francesca Kassing

DSM-5 DEFINITIONS OF DISRUPTIVE BEHAVIOR DISORDERS

Conduct disorder (CD) and the related disruptive behavior disorder, oppositional defiant disorder (ODD), are grouped under the disruptive, impulse-control, and conduct disorders category in DSM-5 (American Psychiatric Association, 2013) and develop during the childhood years. ODD, involving frequent and persistent angry and irritable mood and argumentative and defiant behavior, is a common precursor to CD. Four of the eight ODD symptoms must last at least 6 months for ODD to be diagnosed. The severity level of ODD increases when the symptoms occur in multiple settings ("severe" when symptoms are present in three or more settings; "mild" if only in one setting). The symptoms are often part of a pattern of problematic interactions with others. ODD has a prevalence of 3.3%, and is more prevalent in boys than girls (1.4:1). The first symptoms of ODD typically develop during the preschool years.

PREVALENCE AND COURSE

CD is prevalent in 4% of youth and includes four sets of symptoms involving aggression toward others, destruction of property, covert behaviors such as lying and stealing, and serious violations of rules (running away from home, truant from school; American Psychiatric Association, 2013). There are three levels of CD severity, with the most severe involving primarily the aggressive symptoms. CD is a repetitive and persistent pattern of behavior that violates societal norms or the basic rights of others. These serious conduct problems are differentiated from ODD, which does not include aggressive behavior, property destruction, deceitfulness, or theft. Most children who meet criteria for childhood-onset CD also meet criteria for ODD. DSM-5 criteria allow both diagnoses to be given when indicated. In the United States, rates of CD are estimated to be in the range of 6–16% for boys and 2–9% for girls (American Psychiatric Association, 1994), and to be more prevalent in boys than girls at a rate of about three to one.

Youth with CD are at risk for later mood disorders, anxiety disorders, posttraumatic stress disorder, impulse control disorders, and psychotic disorders, as well as substance-related disorders as adults (American Psychiatric Association, 2013). Longitudinal research has indicated that CD is often a precursor of antisocial personality disorder (APD) in adulthood (Myers, Stewart, & Brown, 1998). It is estimated that approximately half of children with CD develop significant APD symptomatology. Two factors that predict the development of APD are the number of CD symptoms the child exhibits and early age of onset of symptoms (American Psychiatric Association, 2013). In addition, children with CD who show pervasive symptoms in a variety of settings (e.g., home, school, community) and who develop "versatile" forms of antisocial behavior, including both overt (assaults, direct threats) and covert (theft) behaviors by early to midadolescence, are at risk for a wide range of negative outcomes in adolescence, including truancy, substance use, early teenage parenthood, and delinquency (Lochman & Wayland, 1994).

One specifier for CD indicates whether the youth has limited prosocial emotions; if present, the youth is expected to be less responsive to intervention and to be at greater risk for APD disorder in adulthood. To receive this specifier, the individual must exhibit two of the following four characteristics for at least 12 months: lack of remorse or guilt; callous, with lack of empathy; unconcerned about performance; and shallow or deficient affect. Since youth may not provide valid self-reports related to this specifier, multiple informants are necessary to assess limited prosocial emotions. Individuals with limited prosocial emotions are expected to have more persistent conduct problems and may be less responsive to treatment.

Another specifier exists for the age of onset of CD. Childhood-onset CD begins prior to age 10 years, and adolescent-onset CD is asymptomatic until after age 10. The latter form of CD is expected to remit by adulthood for most of these adolescents. In contrast, youth with childhood-onset CD have a worse prognosis, with increased and persistent rates of criminal behavior and substance-related disorders throughout adolescence and adulthood. Children classified as childhood-onset type are typically more aggressive, with more behavior problems than children classified as adolescent-onset type. This subset typically has more difficulty with peer relationships than children diagnosed with adolescent-onset CD. Childhood-onset CD is also associated with prolonged aggressive and antisocial behavior into adulthood. Because of this outcome, the childhood-onset type has also been called the life-course-persistent CD subtype (Moffitt, 2003). Conversely, children classified as adolescent-onset type typically display disruptive behaviors, particularly in the company of peers, but do not usually exhibit severe behavior problems or continued conduct problems into adulthood.

The distinction between childhood- and adolescent-onset CD is consistent with Moffitt's (1993) identification of youth with life-course-persistent antisocial behavior, in contrast to other delinquent youth who have adolescence-limited antisocial behavior. The youth with life-course-persistent antisocial behavior are at early risk because of combined biological and family factors.

Some longitudinal studies suggest that among the children with childhood-onset CD, some lack the continuity of conduct problems from childhood to adulthood; these children therefore have been termed the "childhood-limited conduct problem group" (Moffitt, 2003). However, to date, there is not enough evidence to further divide the childhood-onset type into a life-course-persistent versus a childhood-limited group (Moffitt et al., 2008).

COMMON COMORBID CONDITIONS

ODD commonly precedes CD (especially in the childhood-onset subtype), causing these diagnoses to co-occur in many cases. In addition, attention-deficit/hyperactivity disorder (ADHD) is common in children with ODD and/or CD (American Psychiatric Association, 2013). Having these comorbities is linked to worse outcomes later in life. Children with ODD are also at increased risk for anxiety disorders and major depressive disorder, as well as substance-related disorders later in adolescence and adulthood. Children with CD may also have these disorders along with a specific learning disorder and bipolar disorder.

The symptoms of ODD and CD are part of a more general construct of externalizing behavior problems. Externalizing behaviors include aggressive and conduct problem behaviors. *Aggression* is generally defined as a behavioral act that results in harming or hurting others. Because aggressive behavior and treatment of aggression vary greatly according to the intentions and conditions surrounding the aggression, it is typically categorized according to the different types. Aggression can be physical or verbal; relational, proactive, or reactive; and overt or covert. The literature often differentiates between proactive and reactive aggression because such a framework allows for explanation and description of the aggression (Dodge, Lochman, Harnish, Bates, & Pettit, 1997). Children engaging in proactive aggression typically use aggression to meet a goal. When the aggressive behavior yields the desired reward, the child is more likely to engage in proactive aggression the next time he or she intends to meet a goal. Conversely, reactively aggressive children do not seek to meet goals through their aggressive behavior. Instead, these children react quickly and impulsively to perceived or actual threats and may become intensely irritated.

ETIOLOGICAL/CONCEPTUAL MODEL OF DISRUPTIVE BEHAVIOR DISORDERS

As children develop, they may experience an accumulation and "stacking" of risk factors increasing the probability that they will eventually display serious antisocial behavior. Risk factors may be involved in the development or maintenance of problem behaviors, or may influence the effectiveness of interventions. These risk factors can be conceptualized as falling within five categories: biological and temperamental child factors, family context, neighborhood context, peer context, and later-emerging child factors involving social-cognitive processes and related emotion regulation abilities.

Biological and Temperament Factors

Many biological factors have been found to affect affect childhood aggression directly. One such factor is genetic heritability. Some studies have shown heritability estimates as high as 82% for aggressive behavior in young children (Arseneault et al., 2003). For children with ODD and CD, it is important to note that antisocial behavior has been found to be more heritable in children with callous–unemotional traits than in children without them (Viding, Blair, Moffitt, & Plomin, 2005).

When considering genetic factors, it is important to understand how genetic and environmental factors influence each other through gene–environment interaction. Research indicates that children with certain genetic predispositions (e.g., monoamine oxidase A [MAOA] expression) combined with certain environmental factors are more likely to develop adolescent-onset CD and adult antisocial behavior than children without these genetic predispositions. These results have been found specifically in children who have experienced maltreatment, parental neglect, interparental violence, and inconsistent discipline (e.g., Foley et al., 2004).

Another interaction effect may be seen when environmental factors influence individual biological characteristics that predict childhood aggression. For example, maternal exposure to substances such as alcohol, methadone, and cocaine has been found to affect neurological functioning of children, in turn increasing their risk for aggressive behavior (Wakschlag, Pickett, Kasza, & Loeber, 2006).

Autonomic arousal is another biological factor that has consistently been related to aggressive behavior in children and adults. The autonomic nervous system (ANS) comprises two branches: the sympathetic nervous system (SNS) and the parasympathetic nervous system (PNS). The SNS prepares the body for fight or flight, while the PNS conserves and restores energy. In a meta-analysis, Lorber (2004) found that children with aggressive behavior had resting heart rates 0.51 standard deviations lower than controls. This meta-analysis also indicated lower baseline skin conductance levels (an indicator of SNS activity) in children with conduct problems and other disruptive behaviors. Other ANS indicators that have been found to predict aggressive behavior in children include respiratory sinus arrhythmia and preejection period.

Temperament, while referring to behavioral traits rather than biological processes, is believed to be a more innate part of an individual's personality. Therefore, several studies have examined how child temperament predicts aggressive behavior later in life. One dimension of temperament, "lack of control," when present in early childhood, predicted antisocial behavior and CD in later childhood and early adolescence (Caspi, Henry, McGee, Moffitt, & Silva, 1995). Similarly, infant fussiness, activity level, unpredictability, and positive affect all predicted conduct problems in childhood and adolescence (Lahey et al., 2008).

There are many other biological factors associated with child aggressive behavior, including birth complications, cortisol reactivity, testosterone, and serotonin levels. However, these, along with the risk factors discussed earlier, only predict conduct problems in individuals when additional environmental risk factors such as harsh punishment or low socioeconomic status are also present (Foley et al., 2004).

Community and Neighborhood Contextual Factors

Neighborhood problems have been associated with childhood aggression, separate from their influence on family functioning. Specifically, deprived neighborhoods (characterized by high unemployment rates, dense public housing, social isolation, crime, and violence) have been found to account for 5% of the variance in teacher-reported emotional and conduct problems (Boyle & Lipman, 2002). However, mediators such as less supervision, more deviant social influences, and greater opportunity to engage in risky behaviors may help to explain these neighborhood influences.

Exposure to community violence has been found to uniquely increase children's aggressive behavior (Fite, Winn, Lochman, & Wells, 2009). However, the presence of community violence may influence proactive aggression more than reactive aggression. While the development of reactive aggression may be influenced by experiences such as child abuse and harsh punishment, the development of proactive aggression appears more strongly related to exposure to and encouragement of aggressive behavior (Dodge, 1991). Therefore, exposure to neighborhood disadvantage appears to affect proactive rather than reactive aggression, and modeling of aggressive behavior may be an important mechanism for this relationship (Fite et al., 2009).

School characteristics such as low-quality classroom contextual factors have been found to act cumulatively with child predispositions (e.g., aggressive behavior at home) to increase children's risk of disruptive behaviors at school (Thomas, Bierman, Thompson, Powers, & the Conduct Problems Prevention Research Group, 2009). More specifically, children in classrooms with a larger proportion of aggressive students were found to be more aggressive themselves. A high density of aggressive students may elicit changes in teacher behavior, such as the use of more punitive discipline, which may in turn increase antisocial behavior (Barth, Dunlap, Dane, Lochman, & Wells, 2004). These classroom contextual factors tend to undermine a classroom's learning environment, and without positive models from teachers, children may be more likely to continue the cycle of aggressive behavior.

Family Contextual Factors

Many different family factors influence the presentation of aggressive behavior in children. These factors range from poverty to more specific stresses within the family structure. Children from low-income homes have been found to exhibit more behavioral problems (e.g., Boyle & Lipman, 2002). However, the relationship between poverty and aggressive behavior may be mediated by other family factors. One study found that poverty itself did not directly affect children's aggression, but economic stress did affect paternal depression, marital conflict, and parental hostility, which led to higher levels of conduct problems in children (Conger, Ge, Elder, Lorenz, & Simmons, 1994).

More specific family factors such as parent criminality, substance use and depression, stressful life events, marital conflict, and single and teenage parenthood have also been linked to child aggression (Lochman et al., 2012). Many of these family factors are highly correlated with one another, and most influence child behavior through their effect on parental processes rather than through direct links. For example, maternal depression predicts the use of inconsistent discipline, which in turn predicts child aggression (Barry, Dunlap, Lochman, & Wells, 2009).

Some specific parenting processes linked to child aggressive behavior include nonresponsive parenting, harsh and inconsistent discipline, unclear directions and commands, lack of warmth and involvement, and lack of supervision or monitoring (e.g., Reid, Patterson, & Snyder, 2002). Harsh parenting may create cognitive distortions in children, which may facilitate continued aggressive behavior. Physical abuse, in particular, has also been found to predict child aggression and other antisocial outcomes, independent of parental history of criminality and risk of genetic transmission (Jaffee, Caspi, Moffitt, & Taylor, 2004).

Conversely, maternal affection and positive parenting have been related to lower levels of behavioral problems. One study found that supportive parenting (defined by mother-to-child warmth, proactive teaching, and positive involvement) predicted children's adjustment even after researchers controlled for harsh parenting. The same study also found that supportive parenting acted as a protective factor against more forceful parental behaviors and even risk factors such as low socioeconomic status and single-parent households (Pettit, Bates, & Dodge, 1997).

While it is important to examine parenting practices as risk and protective factors for child aggression, the directionality of this relationship must also be addressed. There is often a bidirectional relationship between parenting practices and children's behavior, creating a cycle between parents and children that contributes to the development and maintenance of children's aggressive behaviors. Research findings support both the importance of parental influence on child behavior and, conversely, the role of children's behavior in influencing parental practices (Fite, Colder, Lochman, & Wells, 2006).

Peer Contextual Factors

Children with disruptive behaviors are at risk for peer rejection (Cillessen, van IJzendoorn, Van Lieshout, & Hartup, 1992) and for having inflated perceptions of their levels of peer acceptance (Pardini, Barry, Barth, Lochman, & Wells, 2006). Aggressive children who are also socially rejected exhibit more severe antisocial behavior than do children who are either aggressive only or rejected only (Lochman & Wayland, 1994; Miller-Johnson, Coie, Maumary-Gremaud, Bierman, & the Conduct Problems Prevention Research Group, 2002). The match between students' race and that of their peers in a classroom influences the degree of social rejection that students experience (Jackson, Barth, Powell, & Lochman, 2006), and race and gender appear to moderate the relation between peer rejection and negative adolescent outcomes. For example, Lochman and Wayland (1994) found that peer rejection ratings of African American children within a mixed-race classroom did not predict subsequent externalizing problems in adolescence, whereas peer rejection ratings of European American children were associated with future disruptive behaviors. Similarly, while peer rejection can predict serious delinquency in boys, it may fail to do so with girls (Miller-Johnson, Coie, Maumary-Gremaud, Lochman, & Terry, 1999).

As children with conduct problems enter adolescence they tend to associate with deviant peers (Warr, 2002). Adolescents who have been continually rejected from more prosocial peer groups because they lack appropriate social skills turn to antisocial cliques for social support (Miller-Johnson et al., 1999). The tendency for aggressive children to associate with one another increases the probability that their antisocial behavior will escalate (e.g., Dishion, Andrews, & Crosby, 1995; Fite, Colder, Lochman, & Wells, 2007).

Social Cognition

Based on children's temperament and biological dispositions, and on their contextual experiences with family, peers, and community, they begin to form stable patterns of processing social information and of regulating their emotions. The contextual social-cognitive model (Lochman & Wells, 2002) stresses the reciprocal interactive relationships among children's initial cognitive appraisal of problem situations, their efforts to think about solutions to the perceived problems, and their physiological arousal and behavioral response. The level of physiological arousal depends on the individual's biological predisposition to become aroused, and it varies depending on their interpretation of the event (Williams, Lochman, Phillips, & Barry, 2003). The level of arousal further influences social problem solving, operating either to intensify the fight-or-flight response or to interfere with the generation of solutions. Because of the ongoing and reciprocal nature of interactions, it may be difficult for children to extricate themselves from aggressive behavior patterns.

Aggressive children have cognitive distortions at the appraisal phases of social-cognitive processing because of difficulties in encoding incoming social information, partially due to neurocognitive difficulties in their executive functions (Ellis, Weiss, & Lochman, 2009), and in accurately interpreting social events and others' intentions. In the appraisal phases of information processing, aggressive children have been found to recall fewer relevant nonhostile cues about events (Lochman & Dodge, 1994) and to misperceive the levels of aggressive behavior that they and peers emit in dyadic interactions (Lochman & Dodge, 1998). Reactively aggressive children have a hostile attributional bias and excessively infer that others are acting toward them in a provocative and hostile manner (Dodge et al., 1997; Lochman & Dodge, 1994; Orobio de Castro, Veerman, Koops, Bosch, & Monshouwer, 2002).

Aggressive children also have cognitive deficiencies at the problem solution phases of social-cognitive processing. They have dominance- and revenge-oriented social goals (Lochman, Wayland, & White, 1993), which guide the maladaptive action-oriented and nonverbal solutions they generate for perceived problems (Dunn, Lochman, & Colder, 1997; Lochman & Dodge, 1994). Aggressive children frequently have low verbal skills, and this contributes to their difficulty in accessing and using competent verbal assertion and compromise solutions. At the next processing step, they identify consequences for each of the solutions generated and decide how to respond to the situation. Aggressive children tend to evaluate aggressive behavior in a positive way (Crick & Werner, 1998) and they expect that aggressive behavior will lead to positive outcomes for them (Lochman & Dodge, 1994). Deficient beliefs at this stage of information processing are especially characteristic of children with proactive aggressive behavior patterns (Dodge et al., 1997) and for youth who have callous–unemotional traits consistent with early phases of psychopathy (Pardini, Lochman, & Frick, 2003). Children's schematic beliefs and expectations affect each of these information-processing steps (Lochman & Dodge, 1998; Zelli, Dodge, Lochman, Laird, & the Conduct Problems Prevention Research Group, 1999).

EVIDENCE-BASED TREATMENTS FOR DISRUPTIVE BEHAVIOR DISORDERS

Disruptive behavior disorders are among the most challenging and treatment-resistant mental health problems in youth. However, decades of research on risk factors have informed the development of treatment protocols, and outcome studies have established the effectiveness of several such interventions. Eyberg, Nelson, and Boggs (2008) conducted a review of treatment outcome studies focused on disruptive behavior in children and adolescents. Based on criteria established by Chambless and colleagues (1998), the review identified one evidence-based treatment as "well established," along with 15 "probably efficacious" and nine "possibly efficacious" evidence-based treatments. Several of these are reviewed below.

One of the "probably efficacious treatments," the Anger Coping Program (Lochman, Barry, & Pardini, 2003), is the predecessor of the Coping Power Program, which we describe in detail later in this chapter. The Coping Power Program is an expanded version of the Anger Coping Program, retaining all of the original program's therapeutic elements while including additional material for children, and a separate 16-session intervention for parents. Empirical support for the Coping Power Program has been demonstrated through several large-scale, longitudinal studies in which positive effects on youth aggression, substance use, and delinquency have been found (Lochman et al., 2009, 2014; Lochman & Wells, 2003, 2004; Lochman, Wells, & Lenhart, 2008; Lochman, Wells, Qu, & Chen, 2013; Muratori Bertacchi, Giuli, Nocentini, & Lochman, in press; Mushtaq, Lochman, Tariq, & Sabih, in press; Zonnevylle-Bender, Matthys, van de Wiel, & Lochman, 2007).

Well-Established Treatments

There is a substantial body of evidence supporting the effectiveness of individually administered parent management training in reducing children's disruptive behaviors. Parent Management Training—Oregon Model (PMTO; Patterson, Reid, Jones, & Conger, 1975) was developed based on a social interaction learning (SIL) model that reflects the importance of interpersonal relationships in establishing patterns of behavior, and behavioral and social learning principles are used to explain how these patterns are maintained over time (Forgatch & Patterson, 2010). Parenting processes are conceptualized as instrumental in the development of disruptive behaviors, but also, with intervention, as potentially powerful mechanisms of change. PMTO focuses predominantly on teaching five dimensions of positive parenting practices. Parents learn to break desired behaviors into steps for their children, and to use positive reinforcement to support their successive approximations of developing skills (scaffolding). Parents also learn to use limit setting with mild punishment to discourage their children's negative behaviors. Monitoring children's activities and whereabouts is encouraged, as are family problem solving and positive parental involvement with children.

Over 40 years of research support the PMTO model (Forgatch & Patterson, 2010) in addressing disruptive behaviors in toddlers, children, and adolescents. PMTO has been shown to improve parents' use of positive parenting strategies, with resulting reductions in child behavior problems (e.g., DeGarmo, Patterson, & Forgatch, 2004; Forgatch, Patterson, & DeGarmo, 2006; Kazdin, 1997). In addition, positive effects for PMTO have been demonstrated up to 9 years posttreatment, with boys whose parent received PMTO later reporting lower rates of arrest and delinquency than untreated youth of similar risk status (Forgatch, Patterson, DeGarmo, & Beldavs, 2009). Other research has identified the importance of fidelity to the treatment model in effecting reductions in children's disruptive behavior (Hukkelberg & Ogden, 2013).

Probably Efficacious Treatments

Other high-quality interventions supported by rigorous outcome research are considered "probably efficacious treatments" and include programs for preschoolers, children, and adolescents. Some of these include protocols for parents and children; others target one or the other. Several of these interventions are described below (see Eyberg et al., 2008, for review of all programs).

Parent–Child Interaction Therapy

Parent–child interaction therapy (PCIT; Zisser & Eyberg, 2010), most often implemented with families of preschoolers (i.e., between ages 3 and 6 years), was designed to teach an authoritative parenting style that combines a high degree of nurturance with firm control. Sessions include both parents and children, and are focused on coaching parents to use skills such as labeled praise and to deliver effective directions. Treatment outcome studies have demonstrated significant improvements in children's behavior, reduction of parenting stress, and positive parent–child interactions in families receiving PCIT relative to families in a wait-list control group (Schumann, Foote, Eyberg, Boggs, & Algina, 1998). Long-term follow-up research has revealed maintenance of treatment gains up to 6 years posttreatment (Hood & Eyberg, 2003).

Problem-Solving Skills Training

Problem-solving skills training (PSST; Kazdin, 2010) is a manualized, cognitive-behavioral intervention for 7- to 13-year-old children with disruptive behaviors. Across 25 weekly sessions, children learn to apply a five-step problem-solving model to challenging situations, with a goal of increasing prosocial responses in their daily lives. PSST can also be combined with a 12-session parent management training (PMT) component encompassing behavioral parenting skills such as positive reinforcement, shaping new behaviors, and administering mild punishment. When PSST and PMT are administered as stand-alone interventions, each significantly reduces children's disruptive behaviors and increases prosocial behaviors; together, the two components produce stronger effects (Kazdin, Siegel, & Bass, 1992).

Multidimensional Treatment Foster Care

Multidimensional treatment foster care (MTFC; Smith & Chamberlain, 2010), a community-based, comprehensive intervention, was originally developed as an alternative to incarceration or residential care for delinquent adolescents. The program has also been successfully applied to youth with serious emotional and mental health issues. In the MTFC model, the youth is placed with trained foster parents for 6–9 months while his or her biological family (or others identified to provide posttreatment care) also receives instruction in effective parenting strategies to support the adolescent's transition back to the home. MTFC foster homes provide a high degree of structure and supervision, and the adolescent also receives individual therapy, psychiatric services, and academic support as needed.

Three randomized trials have demonstrated MTFC's superiority over usual care practices for adolescent boys (Chamberlain & Reid, 1998) and girls (Chamberlain, Leve, & DeGarmo, 2007) with histories of chronic delinquency, and in youth with severe mental health problems (Chamberlain, Moreland, & Reid, 1992; Chamberlain & Reid, 1991). Positive results have been reported relative to delinquent behavior and arrests, school attendance, and pregnancy rates.

Possibly Efficacious Treatments

RECAP

Another program that has shown promise in the treatment of child and adolescent disruptive behavior disorders is RECAP (Reaching Educators, Children, and Parents; Weiss, Catron, Harris, & Han, 2000) though it has less empirical support than do the aforementioned treatments. This manualized treatment (Weiss, 1998) was developed for use with children with concurrent externalizing and internalizing behavior problems. The program lasts one academic year and involves individual and small-group sessions with RECAP participants, classroom groups with the peer group, and parents and teachers. The child component targets social skills, reattribution training, communication skills, self-monitoring and self-control, emotion recognition and expression, and relaxation, while the parent and teacher components target appropriate use of praise and punishment, adult–child communication, improvement of the adult–child relationship, and support of children in their use of learned RECAP skills (Weiss, Harris, Catron, & Han, 2003). In a study of 93 children with a mean age of 9.7 years, Weiss and colleagues (2003) found a significant treatment effect, though the treatment group did not show reliable change. However, this treatment effect appeared to represent a prevention effect because the control group did show reliable change, such that externalizing symptoms worsened. Also of note, despite a significant treatment effect, approximately half of the participants were still functioning in the disordered range at the end of treatment. Although it may be unrealistic to expect a high percentage of high-risk children to score in the normal range of functioning following treatment, these findings still suggest that there is room for improvement in the efficacy of the RECAP program.

Parenting with Love and Limits

Although group PMT has considerable support as an effective treatment when paired with problem-solving skills training for children and adolescents, few studies have offered support for its effectiveness as a stand-alone treatment (Eyberg et al., 2008). One such study (Baruch, Vrouva, & Wells, 2011) examined treatment outcomes for 10- to 17-year-olds with conduct problems, whose parents completed the Parenting with Love and Limits (PLL) program (Sells, 1998). This manualized treatment, although developed for use with both parents and adolescents present, can be administered to parent groups alone. In this manner, treatment comprises six 2-hour sessions that target parent–adolescent interactions, praise, behavioral expectations, appropriate consequences, and use of outside support (Baruch et al., 2011). Following treatment administration, findings indicated that children and adolescents experienced significant reduction of externalizing behaviors.

However, these results must be treated with caution, since analyses were only completed with approximately half of the sample because the remaining half did not complete follow-up data measures. Studies such as that of Baruch and colleagues (2011) indicate potential for group PMT as a stand-alone treatment for child and adolescent disruptive behaviors. However, further research is needed to evaluate whether these treatment programs can be as efficacious as previously discussed treatments.

Pharmacological Interventions

Psychotherapy, typically in the form of individual PMT, is generally the front-line treatment for child and adolescent disruptive behavior disorders (Eyberg et al., 2008). Presently, there is no medication that solely targets aggression. However, given the high comorbidity rates between ODD and CD with ADHD, medication may often be an appropriate supplemental treatment to therapy (Althoff, Rettew, & Hudziak, 2003). For example, some children with ADHD struggle to benefit from psychotherapy due to inattention- and hyperactivity-related challenges. In these cases, a trial with psychostimulant medication to treat the ADHD is often appropriate. Furthermore, research has indicated that in children with comorbid disruptive behavior disorders and ADHD, stimulant medications have led to decreases in aggression, though this effect is somewhat diminished in the presence of CD (Connor, Glatt, Lopez, Jackson, & Melloni, 2002). In the cases in which stimulant medications fail to reduce aggressive behavior, evidence suggests that the addition of clonidine to the treatment regimen can be effective (Connor, Barkley, & Davis, 2000). Alternatively, atomoxetine, a nonstimulant medication, has been shown to decrease ODD symptoms in children with comorbid ADHD (Newcorn, Spencer, Biederman, Milton, & Michelson, 2005). Finally, data have begun to support the use of antipsychotics, particularly the newer atypical agents, in the treatment of disruptive behavior disorders. Specifically, risperidone has been shown to significantly reduce aggressive behavior and conduct problems (Althoff et al., 2003). However, given limited knowledge regarding the impact of antipsychotics on child and adolescent physiology, this class of medications is typically reserved for cases in which psychotherapy and other pharmacological treatments have proven ineffective.

Predictors of Treatment Response

Although there is substantial empirical support for treatments of child and adolescent disruptive behavior disorders, few studies have offered explanations for the poor treatment response that is seen in approximately one-third to one-half of cases (Beauchaine, Webster-Stratton, & Reid, 2005). One often considered variable is comorbidity because research has shown ODD and CD to be highly comorbid with ADHD, anxiety, and depression (Greene et al., 2002; Nock, Kazdin, & Hiripi, 2007). However, despite speculation that children with these comorbid disorders may require more intensive treatments and be less responsive to intervention, data indicate that ADHD, anxiety, and depression have little to no effect on treatment response (Ollendick, Jarrett, Grills-Taquechel, Hovey, & Wolff, 2008). In fact, several studies have provided evidence indicating that any predictive effect of comorbidity on treatment response is positive, such that children and adolescents with disruptive behavior disorders and comorbid ADHD, depression, or anxiety show a greater reduction of ODD and CD symptoms following intervention (Beauchaine et al., 2005; Costin & Chambers, 2007; Kazdin & Whitley, 2006).

Research has demonstrated that several additional family- and child-level factors may impact treatment response for children and adolescents with disruptive behavior disorders. For instance, the Conduct Problems Prevention Research Group (2002) found that lower rates of caretaker depression, two-parent households, and higher socioeconomic status predicted greater reductions in teacher-rated aggressive behavior. Additionally, their findings indicated that higher levels of cognitive ability and reading achievement predicted larger drops in teacher-rated aggressive behavior, while lower levels of initial antisocial behavior predicted greater reductions in parent-rated aggressive behavior. Dadds, Cauchi, Wimalaweera, Hawes, and Brennan (2012) found similar results: More antisocial children showed a poorer treatment response than their less antisocial counterparts. However, their findings also indicated that adding emotion recognition training (ERT) to the intervention led to reductions in aggressive behavior and conduct problems for these children.

ASSESSMENT OF EXTERNALIZING BEHAVIOR PROBLEMS

When evaluating a child for externalizing behavior problems, a wide variety of evidence-based assessments from multiple informants and across multiple domains of functioning are often used to gather information about that child. Behavior rating scales and structured interviews are often used to assist mental health professionals. For information on a child's overall emotional and behavioral functioning, teachers and parents can complete the Behavior Assessment System for Children, Second Edition (BASC-2, Reynolds & Kamphaus, 2004) or the Child Behavior Checklist (CBCL, Achenbach & Rescorla, 2001). The BASC-2 is designed to measure symptoms typically associated with both externalizing and internalizing problems, as well as adaptive skills. The CBCL is designed to provide information related to various diagnoses and symptomatology, including anxiety, depression, somatic complaints, social problems, thought problems, attention problems, rule-breaking behavior, and aggressive behavior. The Strengths and Difficulties Questionnaire (SDQ; Goodman, 1997; Goodman, Meltzer, & Bailey, 1998) is also a free resource that assesses children's prosocial behaviors, hyperactivity, emotional problems, conduct problems, and peer problems. Children who score in the clinical range for externalizing/conduct problems on one of these standardized measures are likely to meet diagnostic criteria for ODD or CD, especially if confirmed by the clinical interview, and may benefit from an intervention such as the Coping Power Program.

THE COPING POWER TREATMENT PROGRAM: PROCEDURES, CONTENT, AND STRUCTURE

The Coping Power program consists of separate child and parent components that are designed to run concurrently and that differ in the content presented; however, both present information designed to reduce aggressive and disruptive behavior in school-age children. Typically, children and parents attend sessions in small groups across a period of 16–18 months. The following sections describe in detail the structure, content, and procedures used within the components.

Child Component

The child component of the Coping Power Program (Lochman et al., 2008) is an extension of the Anger Coping Program (Larson & Lochman, 2011). The child component consists of 34 weekly sessions, normally delivered to five to seven fourth- to sixth-grade children (ages 9–12 years). These sessions typically last 45 minutes to 1 hour and are led by two leaders. One leader takes the primary responsibility of delivering the session's content, whereas the other primarily focuses on behavior management. While the Coping Power Program was originally designed for implementation in school settings, it can be used in a variety of other settings, including clinics and community centers. Leaders may also modify the program to deliver it to individual students or children who are slightly older or younger than the target age group.

Session Structure

The sessions are very structured and organized around teaching the children targeted cognitive-behavioral skills. Each session follows a consistent format, including standard opening and closing activities. During the main part of the sessions, the leader uses active teaching methods, including discussions, games, and role plays to help deliver the specific material required in each session. In addition to the group sessions, the children are each seen individually on a monthly basis to increase leader–student rapport and to help the leader individualize the program while still maintaining the group format.

Behavior Management

The program has a behavior management system built in, and the leader employs positive reinforcement for appropriate and prosocial behaviors and consequences for negative and/or disruptive behaviors. By positively participating in activities and following group rules, which are clearly established during the first meeting and posted for all subsequent sessions, students have the opportunity to earn points during each group meeting. The students may also earn up to five additional points each week through the program's goal-setting system, which is described below. Several sessions also give children the opportunity to earn extra points by completing homework assignments or by demonstrating their knowledge of the program's concepts through quizzes. Each week the students are allowed to spend their accumulated points at the prize box, where tangible rewards range from small, inexpensive items (e.g., stickers or pencils) to larger items (e.g., basketballs or video games). The larger rewards are included to help encourage children to delay gratification and work toward the goal of a highly desired object.

The majority of children who are referred to the Coping Power Program demonstrate both oppositional and disruptive conduct problems, and the program accounts for this by including a standard plan for delivering consequences. When it is appropriate, the leader can use differential reinforcement to reinforce appropriate behavior and ignore negative behaviors that occur within group meetings. If the problem behavior continues, the leader may deliver warnings or "strikes" verbally (e.g., "Jamal, you earned a strike for calling Mikayla a name") or may choose to deliver a strike in writing with the use of a whiteboard or strike board. The leader uses the term "strike" in reference to American baseball, as in three strikes and the batter is out. Therefore, children can receive up to three strikes during each group meeting, but once they receive their third strike, they no longer earn their point for following the group rules. Some students may have a hard time with this consequence and may be asked to leave the group with one of the group leaders to process what has occurred, while the other group leader continues to lead the group.

Goal Sheets

Another main feature of the program is the use of weekly "goal sheets." These goal sheets are used to set, monitor, and reward students' progress toward their own individual goals. Each of the students sets an operationally defined behavioral goal each week, with assistance from the group leaders, as well as input from parents and teachers. These goals are recorded on the goal sheet; for example, "I will complete and turn in my math homework" or "I will use respectful words with teachers and peers." The student is responsible for keeping track of his or her goal sheet during the week and for eliciting feedback on his or her performance from his or her teacher. The students can earn one point for each day that they meet their individualized goal. A main function of the goal sheet is to promote the generalization of treatment effects to environments outside of group sessions.

Opening Activities

The group meetings all begin with a review of the students' goal sheets. Each child is asked to identify the factors that contributed to his or her successes and difficulties in attempting to attain his or her goal. If the child was easily able to meet the goal, the goal can be modified, or a new goal can be established. If the child experienced some difficulty when trying to meet his or her goal, the leader can help the child problem-solve and adapt the goal accordingly. Next, the leader reviews the previous session's content and asks the children to provide an example of one thing they learned from the past week. This allows the leader to assess the students' retention and comprehension, and to provide additional instruction where it is needed.

Closing Activities

At the end of the session, students need to have completed three activities. First, students provide positive feedback to one another about the appropriate or prosocial behavior. This behavior can be demonstrated within group, in the classroom, or on the playground. Each student gives and receives this feedback, which acts as a reinforcer for positive behaviors and enhances feelings of self-esteem and self-efficacy. Second, students are informed of their point totals and are allowed to spend these points at the prize box. Finally, if there is enough time, students who have demonstrated appropriate in-session behavior by either following the rules or earning a positive participation point will earn 5–10 minutes of free time. During this period they may play games or visit with other group members. This free-time period not only acts as a reinforcer but also gives the leader an opportunity to observe and evaluate the students' social skills and their abilities to navigate any conflicts that may arise. The students who did not demonstrate appropriate in-session behavior spend this time processing their behavior with the leaders. If the leaders determine that a child is too upset to engage actively in this conversation, they may choose to meet with that student individually prior to the next meeting.

Content

The Coping Power Program child component has seven main foci, including goal setting, organization and study skills, emotional awareness, anger management, perspective taking, social problem solving, and handling peer pressure. Table 11.1 provides an overview of the child program, and the major intervention units are described below.

GOAL-SETTING UNIT

The goal-setting unit comprises activities that are designed to assist students in identifying personally meaningful long-term goals (e.g., "I will improve my grades so that I can be part of the cheerleading team"), then breaking those long-term goals into more easily accomplished short-term goals (e.g., "I will read from my textbook for 30 minutes each evening"). The leader often uses a staircase analogy to help students comprehend the steps they need to take before they can accomplish their long-term goals. The short-term goals that the students identify can then be used as their weekly goal on their individual goal sheets.

TABLE 11.1. Overview of the Coping Power Program Child Component

Unit	Typical number of sessions	Overview of session content
Goal Setting	Three sessions	Identifying long-term goals and short-term personal goals
Organizational and Study Skills	Two sessions	Organizing backpack and school–home folders, study skills
Emotional Awareness	Three sessions	Identifying and verbalizing emotions, physical cues of anger
Anger Management	Five sessions	Recognizing and coping with different levels of anger
Perspective Taking	Three sessions	Learning to see situations from others' points of view
Social Problem Solving	Twelve sessions	Automatic responding versus thinking ahead, valuing affiliative versus aggressive solutions, PICC model
Peer Relationships	Six sessions	Developing adaptive/prosocial relationships with peers, resisting peer pressure

ORGANIZATIONAL AND STUDY SKILLS UNIT

The organization and study skills unit is included due to the fact that problems in these areas frequently accompany disruptive behaviors that take place in a school setting, and because the difficulties in these areas are often sources of conflict between students and their parents and teachers. The leader uses games and activities to address this subject and make it interesting for the students. Though some games are designed to be more competitive in nature, if the leader believes that his or her group will respond negatively to competitive games, he or she may modify the games and activities. For example, students can complete the activities individually and then compete again against their own personal time rather than against one another in the group. In one activity, students compete against one another to find a common object (e.g., pencil, assignment sheet) in their personal book bags. The leader then gives the children the opportunity to reorganize their book bags and they repeat the activity. In another activity, students are required to organize a set of cards with the names of objects printed on them, then each student competes against the group to see who can find a specific card in the least amount of time. The students who have organized the cards most effectively are the "winners" and are asked to explain their method of organization to the rest of the group. In addition to having students complete the games and activities in session, requiring them to keep track of their own personal goal sheet encourages the development of good organization skills.

EMOTIONAL AWARENESS UNIT

The emotional awareness unit helps students develop the abilities to identify their feelings and teaches them how to verbalize those feelings in a constructive manner. The leaders accomplish this by using a feelings thermometer. This analogy works by placing words describing low levels of emotion (e.g., "irritated" or "down") at the bottom of the thermometer and those describing more intense levels (e.g., "enraged" or "depressed") higher up on the thermometer. This helps to demonstrate to students that emotions come in varying degrees of intensity, which is an important concept for children who often think their feelings are similar to a light switch, and are either on or off. In addition to the feelings thermometer, there are other activities designed to help children recognize the thoughts, physiological sensations, and behaviors that come with other emotions. Children are also taught to recognize "triggers" that can lead to feeling a certain emotion.

ANGER MANAGEMENT UNIT

The anger management unit builds on the skills the children learned in the emotional awareness unit. The first step is to teach students how to recognize their anger at the earliest stage, when anger management strategies are more likely to be successful. The children then learn various anger management strategies, including distraction techniques, relaxation exercises, and coping statements. The students learn how to use distraction techniques effectively when they are required to take part in a memorization or construction task while they are being taunted and teased by another peer. This helps students understand that by directing their focus somewhere else, their emerging feelings of anger can be decreased and controlled. Another set of activities involves the use of coping self-statements (e.g., "I'll grow up, not blow up"; "What he says doesn't matter, he doesn't know me anyway"; "I won't be a fool, I'll keep my cool") in response to peer teasing. During the first activities, the students practice adaptive self-talk by using puppets. After they have mastered this skill, they move on to a more real-life scenario in which their ingroup peers tease them directly rather than teasing the puppet. The student who is being teased practices using coping statements to maintain self-control.

PERSPECTIVE-TAKING UNIT

The perspective-taking unit helps to address the deficits in perspective that are commonly experienced by children who have conduct problems. Several activities are designed to challenge the students' tendencies to make hostile attributions and to encourage students to consider alternative explanations for others' behavior. The students' role play of hypothetical and actual ingroup situations that they may experience helps them become engaged in the topic and effectively illustrate the lesson. Given that these students will likely experience conflicts with their teachers, other activities are specifically designed to help improve the children's understanding of their teachers' viewpoints. For example, one such activity is designed as a "Family Feud" game. The students guess the top 10 things that teachers expect from their students in the classroom, and in most cases are surprised by what the teachers actually expect. The students also conduct an interview with one of their teachers, which gives the teachers a chance to explain the reasons behind disciplinary procedures in a nonconfrontational setting and fosters a positive connection between the student and teacher by having the teacher talk about things they like about teaching.

SOCIAL PROBLEM-SOLVING UNIT

The next unit, social problem-solving training, helps students overcome their deficiencies in this area. The PICC model, which is essential to this unit, has three main steps: (1) Problem Identification, (2) Choices that the children have in response to the problem situation, and (3) Consequences that are associated with each choice. To begin, the children learn how to correctly identify what the problem is in a given situation. For example, if a child comments that his or her mom is not being fair, then the leader prompts and guides the child to restate this as "My mom wants me to clean my room but I want to go play basketball with my friends."

One activity that is a favorite gives students the opportunity to write a script, act it out, and videotape their own skit illustrating the PICC model. This serves a variety of purposes. It gives the children a chance to be active participants in the lesson, and helps to reinforce their understanding of and ability to use the PICC model. It also introduces children to the ambiguous problems that they encounter in the real world. Because these sessions are much less structured than the typical Coping Power Program session, there is also the opportunity for real problems to develop; the leader is there to facilitate the use of the PICC model, which helps to further students' internalization of the problem-solving process.

The problem-solving unit is expanded by introducing the idea of deliberate versus automatic responding in social problem situations. The students are introduced to this topic when asked to quickly list possible choices for a hypothetical problem situation, then are asked to respond to the same situation, but this time, they are told to think about the potential consequences of their choices before responding. This activity helps children to understand that by stopping to think, they are likely to come up with better solutions to their problems and are more likely to achieve the outcome that they desire. Other concepts that are addressed within this unit involve identifying good times to approach another person to solve a problem, the importance of being persistent when working on solving a problem, and applying social problem solving to potential conflicts with teachers, siblings, and peers.

PEER RELATIONSHIP UNIT

The last unit in the Coping Power Program child component involves responding to peer pressure adaptively and promoting prosocial peer relationships. The students learn a variety of skills to handle peer pressure (e.g., making a joke, leaving the situation), and to practice the skills in the group during role plays. The students are also encouraged to identify positive peer groups and associate with those positive peers. Other concepts include teaching the students to recognize their personal strengths and the positive leadership qualities that they have to offer in a friendship.

The Coping Power Program concludes with a review session in which students demonstrate the knowledge they have gained during the course of the program. They do this by playing a board game that asks questions about key program content. Often the leaders also hold a party for students, with snacks and fun activities to promote closure and to help end the program on a positive note.

Parent Component

The parent component of the Coping Power Program is intended to run concurrently with the child program. Parent and child sessions are held separately, typically at different times and locations. The Coping Power parent component includes 16 sessions, designed to last 60–90 minutes each. Ideally, parent groups are led by two co-leaders and include up to 12 parents or parent dyads. Efforts are made to include all of the primary caregivers in each child's family, to promote a consistent approach to caring for the child.

Start-Up Considerations

Prior to beginning a Coping Power Program parent group, there are a number of start-up considerations. A first consideration is to identify a regular meeting time and location. While the child sessions are typically held at school during the school day, parent sessions can be held at the school or at an alternative location that is convenient for the parent participants (e.g., mental health clinic, public library, or community center). Leaders are advised to survey parents about their availability before selecting a regular meeting time. Common meeting times that tend to be popular include early morning, after school drop off; during lunch break; the last hour before school pick-up; or in the evening. Meetings held during the evening typically allow more working parents to attend, but they are also more likely to require parents to obtain child care.

Providing refreshments and child care can be important for fostering parent engagement. Other critical factors for maximizing parent engagement include contacting parents individually and inviting them to participate in the group, and taking time to learn about each family and describing how the program will address their specific needs and concerns. During initial parent contacts, it can also be helpful to identify and problem-solve specific barriers to attendance (e.g., assist in developing a ride-sharing arrangement to address transportation concerns, prepare a work excuse note, offer a supervised study hall or recreation activity during the parent meeting). Once the parent program is under way, providing reminder calls and flyers prior to each session and contacting each parent who misses a session can also be important to fostering parent engagement. When planning the parent meeting schedule, it is also advisable to allot time for parents to socialize with one another in an unstructured way.

Content

Many elements of the Coping Power parent program derive from well-established behavioral parent training programs and focus on nurturing positive parenting skills. Parent sessions also include a focus on stress management, building family cohesion and communication, and family problem solving. Moreover, an additional aim of the parent sessions is to teach parents how to reinforce the skills their children are learning in their Coping Power child groups. While new content is introduced to parents in each session, all sessions include a review of prior content and activities to facilitate the generalization of skills (e.g., interactive worksheets, role plays, homework). Leaders deliver this intervention in a flexible manner, with an eye toward adapting session activities to best address the specific problems and issues that group members present. Sessions are run in an interactive discussion style rather than as a didactic "parenting class." The leaders do use an agenda to guide the discussion, which is displayed visually on a whiteboard or easel and can be adapted to incorporate parent input and needs. What follows is a description of the substantive intervention foci of the Coping Power parent component. Table 11.2 also provides an overview of the parent program content.

ACADEMIC SUPPORT IN THE HOME

Because the Coping Power child group typically takes place at school, and school is a very significant aspect of children's lives, the parent program begins with a discussion of strategies that parents can use to support their child's academic learning. Parents are encouraged to be proactive about communicating with their child's teacher (rather than waiting until specific problems arise). Parents are provided with potential questions they might ask during a parent–teacher conference. Role plays are used to help parents practice communicating with their child's teacher in a positive and proactive way, including during parent–teacher conferences.

Next, the idea of a "homework completion system" is introduced. This system allows for increased parent–teacher communication about homework assignments and homework completion, to promote children's academic success. Time during the parent meeting is spent to discuss any existing homework completion systems and how well they seem to be working. For parents without an existing system, time is spent brainstorming

TABLE 11.2. Overview of the Coping Power Program Parent Component

Unit	Typical number of sessions	Overview of session content
Academic Support at Home	Three	Ways that parents can support children's academic success
Stress Management	Two	Taking care of yourself as a parent
Praise and Ignoring	Two	Using praise and positive reinforcement to increase positive child behavior, ignoring minor disruptive behavior
Giving Effective Instructions and Household Rules	Two	Giving effective instructions to children, setting and enforcing household rules and expectations
Discipline and Punishment	Two	Time-out, assigning work chores, privilege removal
Family Cohesion, Family Problem Solving, and Family Communication	Three	Strategies for increasing family bonding and communication, and solving family-level problems
Long-Term Planning	Two	Planning for your child's future

possibilities (e.g., an assignment notebook in which the teacher places his or her initials by each homework assignment, communication via a classroom blog or e-mail list). The leader emphasizes that additional support structures are still needed at this age to ensure children's homework completion. Parents are encouraged to strategize about what support structures might be useful (e.g., a "protected homework time," in which phone calls are not accepted and the television is off). Parents are also encouraged to discuss how they might monitor their child's progress. It is important to acknowledge parents' concerns about the level of time and energy required to implement these strategies. Efforts should be made to help parents create a system that will work well for them given their particular family and scheduling demands. Parents are encouraged to involve their child in the process of establishing a homework system and signing a homework contract.

STRESS MANAGEMENT

The next unit of the parent program focuses on defining stress and leading parents through a discussion of how stress can undermine their positive parenting behaviors. Parents engage in a "pie of life" activity that helps them evaluate their current commitments, priorities, and time set aside for their own self-care. This typically leads to acknowledgment of how difficult it is for parents to make time for themselves, yet how important it is to do so, in order to take time to relax on a regular basis so they can be the kind of parents they wish to be. Parents share ideas about how they might take care of themselves to reduce stress (e.g., exercise, taking a bath, listening to music, talking to a supportive friend or family member, shopping, having alone time). Parents then spend time planning how they will schedule time to engage in one or more of these activities on a regular basis.

Next, the practice of active relaxation is introduced as a way to reduce stress. During the session, parents are led in activities that teach them deep, diaphragmatic breathing and physical relaxation strategies. To the extent that parents feel comfortable, the meeting room can be modified to create a relaxing scene, such as rearranging the chairs so that participants can put their feet up, dimming the lights, playing soothing background music, or lighting a candle. In addition to practicing deep breathing and relaxation during the session, parents are encouraged to practice between sessions and provided with a written guide they can use to do so.

In a second session on stress management, skills for managing one's time are provided as another way to reduce stress. Parents practice saying "no" to unnecessary commitments, using a planner, and setting priorities for their time. Additionally, a cognitive model of stress and mood management is introduced. In reviewing this model, parents are encouraged to identify and discuss how internal thoughts can contribute to feelings and subsequent behaviors in parenting situations (e.g., "My child is driving me crazy by tapping his pencil like that over and over again. He is doing that just to bother me" [this thought is immediately followed by the parent angrily yelling at her son]). During the group session, parents engage in role plays modeling stressful parent–child situations. For each situation, the parents identify the thoughts and feelings that resulted in a behavioral overreaction by the parent. They also practice generating alternative thoughts that can help them remain calm in parent–child interactions.

BASIC SOCIAL LEARNING THEORY, PRAISE, AND IMPROVING
THE PARENT–CHILD RELATIONSHIP

In this unit, basic social learning theory is presented to parents using an ABC Chart to introduce the concepts of antecedents (A), behavior (B), and consequences (C). The leader facilitates a discussion of how parents might modify children's behavior by rewarding good behavior with positive consequences. Parents learn the concept of "catching your child being good" and identify desired target behaviors that they will make an extra effort to notice. Parents then spend time identifying positive consequences (e.g., allowing the child to select the dinner menu, providing labeled praise) and introduce a tracking system whereby they become more aware of their child's positive and negative behaviors. To facilitate positive parent–child attachment, parents are reminded of the importance of setting aside parent–child "special time" for simply connecting and enjoying each other. The leaders then help parents set personal goals for "special time" (e.g., the number of times per week they engage with their child in a certain activity, and what the activity might be) for the coming week. Parents are given tips for keeping "special time" special (e.g., avoid conflictual topics, engage in more listening than talking, ignore issues that arise, or wait to address them).

Common questions and concerns that arise during this portion of the parent program include "Shouldn't my child just do what I say without having to get a reward or special praise?"; "Won't it just spoil my child to be giving prizes and compliments all the time?" Also, parents often wish to discuss how to discipline their child or handle misbehavior right away, rather than focusing on reinforcement strategies first. To address these concerns, the leader explains that the program intentionally starts with strategies that can help the parent and child reconnect in a positive way (especially since disruptive behavior problems can adversely affect the parent–child relationship), while also meeting the goal of improving the child's behavior. The leader reassures parents that the goal is to give rewards strategically only to increase a limited number of target behaviors, and that the rewards can be phased out as soon as the child begins to demonstrate the target behavior consistently. The leader also informs parents that later in the program they will discuss setting behavior rules and expectations for the household that can be enforced without rewards or warnings, and also discuss effective punishment strategies for addressing child misbehavior.

IGNORING MINOR DISRUPTIVE BEHAVIOR

The focus in this session is on managing children's minor disruptive behaviors by ignoring them. First, the concept of "minor" disruptive behavior is defined (e.g., the child repeatedly making an annoying noise or changing the television channel), and these behaviors are distinguished from more serious transgressions that cannot be ignored (e.g., hitting a sibling, violating a safety rule). The leader then facilitates discussion of how to appropriately "ignore" (e.g., saying nothing to the child about the annoying behavior and looking away). While these discussions lay important groundwork, the centerpiece of this work is role play. Leaders should first model a parent–child interaction in which the parent ignores the child's escalating behavior. Parents should then role-play a similar scenario. After these role plays, the leader engages parents in a debriefing discussion about what they think about "ignoring" and how they felt about the role plays. The leader should be prepared to address negative reactions parents might have to the concept of ignoring. The leader makes it clear that giving the child attention is very important in general for maintaining a strong parent–child connection, but brief periods of strategic ignoring (ranging from a few seconds to a few minutes) can be a useful strategy for reducing minor disruptive behavior and preventing conflictual parent–child interchanges.

This topic often generates further discussion about how parents' own moods and stress levels can affect how they interact with their children. The leader tries to create an environment in which parents feel comfortable sharing examples of times they handled situations with their children more or less well, depending on their own mood state. The leader tries to normalize that even the most caring parents do not handle every parenting situation in an ideal way. Then, the leader tries to illustrate how parents can stay calm and ignore minor irritating child behaviors, even when parents are feeling short-tempered (e.g., by taking time to calm down and assess how problematic the behavior truly is before deciding whether to address it or ignore it; by taking time to think about the type of relationship they want to have with their child and ways of handling the situation that will best maintain this type of relationship).

ANTECEDENT CONTROL: GIVING EFFECTIVE INSTRUCTIONS AND ESTABLISHING RULES AND EXPECTATIONS

The ABC Chart is revisited, and the leader points out the ways in which parental instructions can be antecedents to compliant or noncompliant child behaviors. Ineffective instructions often precede child noncompliance, whereas clear instructions often precede child compliance. Identify the qualities of "good" and "bad" instructions and work with parents to identify specific examples (e.g., avoid overly vague or complicated instructions, or shouting instructions from another room; instead, politely provide a specific, single-step command). Parents often enjoy sharing and laughing with each other about some of the ineffective instructions they tend to give (e.g., "Tim, would you like to go clean up your room now?"), then practice giving more effective instructions and following through to monitor whether the child subsequently complies.

Parents also spend time generating rules and expectations for their household, so that all family members have a clear picture of the behaviors that are valued and expected in their family. A distinction is made between household rules and expectations. Behavior rules establish the behaviors that children should decrease (e.g., hitting, arguing), whereas behavior expectations establish the behaviors that children should increase (e.g., making the bed daily, treating others nicely). In discussing rules and expectations with parents, the importance of labeling rule violations (e.g., "Tommy, you just hit your sister and that is against our family's behavior rules") is emphasized, so that children are made more aware of the rules. The importance of keeping expectations age-appropriate is also emphasized (e.g., assign two or three age-appropriate household chores to each child in the family). Parents are coached in how to establish behavior rules and expectations at home, and how to involve their children in this process. Then parents are encouraged to track their child's compliance, their positive reinforcement of the child's compliance, and their labeling of noncompliance.

DISCIPLINE AND PUNISHMENT

The concept of punishment is then introduced and a definition of *punishment* is provided (i.e., a response that will decrease the problem behavior the child has exhibited). The leader solicits parents' ideas regarding appropriate and effective punishment strategies. Often, one or more parents will express that they believe in spanking and other forms of physical punishment, since their own parents engaged in this practice and it seemed to work out well. The leader tries to acknowledge this perspective without making parents feel judged, explain why physical punishment is often ineffective in curbing children's misbehavior, then seeks to "devalue" physical forms of punishment (by explaining that it models the very behavior that the child needs to decrease and can adversely affect the parent–child relationship). The leader indicates that the goal of the program is to expand parents' toolboxes for addressing noncompliant child behavior, by practicing several alternative punishment strategies.

Parents are ultimately taught a system for increasing child compliance without engaging in excessively harsh or conflictual parent–child interchanges. The key is for parents to enact the steps calmly and systematically, which is practiced via a variety of role plays in session. The first step is for the parents to gain their child's attention and provide clear instruction. Parents then waits briefly to assess whether the child complies with the instruction. If the child complies, the parents provide labeled praise to show that they noticed and appreciate the child's compliance. If the child does not comply, the parents give one reminder, with a warning that informs the child of the consequences if he or she does not comply with the parents' initial instruction. If the child then complies, the parents express their appreciation. If the child does not comply, the parents informs the child that he or she will now have to face the consequence and will also still be required to follow through with the original instruction. These steps continue until the child complies with the initial instruction. Parents are taught to follow these steps in a calm, consistent manner, even in the presence of escalating emotions in the child. The goal of this approach is to increase the child's compliant behavior without excessively harsh or angry parent–child interchanges.

Parents are then taught a menu of options that can be used as consequences for noncompliant behavior. First, the "time-out" procedure is introduced and the steps for implementing a time-out effectively are rehearsed. Discussion focuses on parents' prior experiences implementing time-out and how important it is to follow a specific system in order for this approach to be effective. Parents discuss how to handle child misbehavior before and during the time-out, and discuss parents' reactions and attitudes toward the time-out procedure. Parents then generate examples of child behaviors that will result in time-out and to name their time-out procedures (e.g., location, length, strategies they will put in place).

Other disciplinary techniques are then introduced, such as the removal of privileges and the assignment of additional work chores. Role plays are utilized to allow parents to practice implementing these disciplinary techniques calmly, even amid strong child emotionality and protests. These role plays give parents additional practice and aid in the generalization of skills. Parents are also engaged in an open-ended conversation about punishment for major misbehavior, with an eye toward helping them find alternatives to physical punishment and lengthy, unspecified grounding.

FAMILY COHESION BUILDING, FAMILY PROBLEM SOLVING, AND FAMILY COMMUNICATION

If both parents have not been attending the parent meetings, extra effort is made to encourage group members to invite their spouse, significant other, or other important caretakers in their child's life to this session. The focus of this session is on discussing parents' hopes and concerns for their child as he or she matures. The discussion is guided to underscore that having a positive, healthy parent–child relationship will become increasingly important as the child grows older. Parents are led in brainstorming strategies for how families can build or strengthen their cohesiveness, both in the home (e.g., family game nights) and outside the home (e.g., going to a park, taking a family vacation). Parents are encouraged to plan and follow through with family cohesion-building activities.

Next, parents are exposed to the PICC problem-solving model that the children have learned. The group leaders describe (and show) the parents how the children have been coached in this problem-solving model—through worksheets and videotaped role plays. This is a good opportunity to show parents the videos that their children made to illustrate the PICC model in action. Often this is a nice time to have a conjoint child–parent group meeting, if possible, to allow children to "show off" their video and have an opportunity to teach their parents about the PICC model for solving problems. Parents are then encouraged to use this model to resolve family conflicts and to involve their child(ren) in the family problem-solving process.

Finally, parents are encouraged to plan ahead for the future. As peer relationships and autonomy become increasingly important to their child, it will be critically important to have family communication structures for making decisions, talking with each other about issues and concerns, and negotiating the child's involvements and activities.

Discussion questions explore whether the family members have a way of talking with each other about their concerns; how they go about negotiating when someone wants to change a preestablished rule; and whether they are satisfied with the way they currently communicate and make decisions in their family. The notion of the "family meeting" is introduced as one way to preserve positive parent involvement in children's lives and tackle potential problems before they arise. Parents are guided through a discussion of how they might establish family meetings at home. A communication system is also presented to help parents monitor their child's activities and whereabouts, especially their outings with peers.

While parents often see the value in these family communication strategies, they also express concerns about whether they will be able to get their child to participate, especially as their child becomes older, more interested in friends, and may even grow physically larger than their parents. The leader empathizes with this important concern and assures parents that they will continue to be the most important figures in their child's life. The leader also uses this concern to emphasize to parents the importance of creating a strong bond with their child now, and to teach their child to respect adults and to comply with rules and instructions, before their child becomes an adolescent.

TERMINATION

To conclude the parent group on a positive note, the last group meeting is structured as a celebration. Parents spend time sharing what they have appreciated about the group and how it has impacted their family. The leaders share their regard with the parents, and the group members are given an opportunity to share their regards with each other. Sharing of contact information is encouraged, to facilitate parents' continued communication with each other after the group ends. Parents are then presented with a certificate documenting their completion of the Coping Power Program for parents.

REFERENCES

Achenbach, T. M., & Rescorla, L. A. (2001). *Manual for the ASEBA school-age forms and profiles*. Burlington: University of Vermont Research Center for Children, Youth, and Families.

Althoff, R. R., Rettew, D. C., & Hudziak, J. J. (2003). Attention-deficit/hyperactivity disorder, oppositional defiant disorder, and conduct disorder. *Psychiatric Annals, 33*(4), 245–252.

American Psychiatric Association. (1994). *Diagnostic and statistical manual of mental disorders* (4th ed.). Washington, DC: Author.

American Psychiatric Association. (2013). *Diagnostic and statistical manual of mental disorders* (5th ed.). Arlington, VA: Author.

Arseneault, L., Moffitt, T. E., Caspi, A., Taylor, A., Rijsdijk, F. V., Jaffee, S. R., et al. (2003). Strong genetic effects on cross-situational antisocial behaviour among 5-year-old children according to mothers, teachers, examiner-observers, and twins' self-reports. *Journal of Child Psychology and Psychiatry, 44*, 832–848.

Barry, T. D., Dunlap, S., Lochman, J. E., & Wells, K. C. (2009). Inconsistent discipline as a mediator between maternal distress and aggression in boys. *Child and Family Behavior Therapy, 31*, 1–19.

Barth, J. M., Dunlap, S. T., Dane, H., Lochman, J. E., & Wells, K. C. (2004). Classroom environment influences on aggression, peer relations, and academic focus. *Journal of School Psychology, 42*, 115–133.

Baruch, G., Vrouva, I., & Wells, C. (2011). Outcome findings from a parent training programme for young people with conduct problems. *Child and Adolescent Mental Health, 16*(1), 47–54.

Beauchaine, T., Webster-Stratton, C., & Reid, M. (2005). Mediators, moderators, and predictors of one-year outcomes among children treated for early-onset conduct problems: A latent growth curve analysis. *Journal of Consulting and Clinical Psychology, 73*, 371–388.

Boyle, M. H., & Lipman, E. L. (2002). Do places matter?: Socioeconomic disadvantage and behavioral problems of children in Canada. *Journal of Consulting and Clinical Psychology, 70*, 378–389.

Caspi, A., Henry, B., McGee, R. O., Moffitt, T. E., & Silva, P. A. (1995). Temperamental origins of child and adolescent behavior problems: From age three to age fifteen. *Child Development, 66*, 55–68.

Chamberlain, P., Leve, L. D., & DeGarmo, D. S. (2007). Multidimensional treatment foster care for girls in the juvenile justice system: 2-year follow-up of a randomized clinical trial. *Journal of Consulting and Clinical Psychology, 75*(1), 187–193.

Chamberlain, P., Moreland, S., & Reid, K. (1992). Enhanced services and stipends for foster parents: Effects on retention rates and outcomes for children. *Child Welfare, 71*(5), 387–401.

Chamberlain, P., & Reid, J. B. (1991). Using a specialized foster care community treatment model for children and adolescents leaving the state mental hospital. *Journal of Community Psychology, 19*(3), 266–276.

Chamberlain, P., & Reid, J. B. (1998). Comparison of two community alternatives to incarceration for chronic juvenile offenders. *Journal of Consulting and Clinical Psychology, 66*(4), 624–633.

Chambless, D. L., Baker, M. J., Baucom, D. H., Beutler, L. E., Calhoun, K. S., Crits-Christoph, P., et al. (1998). Update on empirically validated therapies: II. *Clinical Psychologist, 51*(1), 3–16.

Cillessen, A. H., van IJzendoorn, H. W., Van Lieshout, C. F., & Hartup, W. W. (1992). Heterogeneity among peer-rejected boys: Subtypes and stabilities. *Child Development, 63*, 893–905.

Conduct Problems Prevention Research Group. (2002). Predictor variables associated with positive Fast Track outcomes at the end of third grade. *Journal of Abnormal Child Psychology, 30*(1), 37–52.

Conger, R. D., Ge, X., Elder, G. H., Lorenz, F. O., & Simmons, R. L. (1994). Economic stress, coercive family process and developmental problems of adolescents. *Child Development, 65*, 541–561.

Connor, D. F., Barkley, R. A., & Davis, H. T. (2000). A pilot study of methylphenidate, clonidine, or the combination in ADHD comorbid with aggressive oppositional defiant or conduct disorder. *Clinical Pediatrics, 39*(1), 15–25.

Connor, D. F., Glatt, S. J., Lopez, I. D., Jackson, D., & Melloni, R. H. (2002). Psychopharmacology and aggression: I. A meta-analysis of stimulant effects on overt/covert aggression-related behaviors in ADHD. *Journal of the American Academy of Child and Adolescent Psychiatry, 41*(3), 253–261.

Costin, J., & Chambers, S. (2007). Parent management training as a treatment for children with oppositional defiant disorder referred to a mental health clinic. *Clinical Child Psychology and Psychiatry, 12*, 511–524.

Crick, N. R., & Werner, N. E. (1998). Response decision processes in relational and overt aggression. *Child Development, 69*, 1630–1639.

Dadds, M., Cauchi, A., Wimalaweera, S., Hawes, D., & Brennan, J. (2012). Outcomes, moderators, and mediators of empathic-emotion recognition training for complex conduct problems in childhood. *Psychiatry Research, 199*(3), 201–207.

DeGarmo, D. S., Patterson, G. R., & Forgatch, M. S. (2004). How do outcomes in a specified parent training intervention maintain or wane over time? *Prevention Science, 5*(2), 73–89.

Dishion, T. J., Andrews, D. W., & Crosby, L. (1995). Antisocial boys and their friends in early adolescence: Relationship characteristics, quality, and interactional process. *Child Development, 66*, 139–151.

Dodge, K. A. (1991). The structure and function of reactive and proactive aggression. In D. J. Pepler & K. H. Rubin (Eds.), *Development and treatment of childhood aggression* (pp. 201–218). Hillsdale, NJ: Erlbaum.

Dodge, K. A., Lochman, J. E., Harnish, J. D., Bates, J. E., & Pettit, G. S. (1997). Reactive and proactive aggression in school children and psychiatrically impaired chronically assaultive youth. *Journal of Abnormal Psychology, 106,* 37–51.

Dunn, S. E., Lochman, J. E., & Colder, C. R. (1997). Social problem-solving skills in boys with conduct and oppositional defiant disorders. *Aggressive Behavior, 23,* 457–469.

Ellis, M. L., Weiss, B., & Lochman, J. E. (2009). Executive functions in children: Associations with aggressive behavior and social appraisal processing. *Journal of Abnormal Child Psychology, 37,* 945–956.

Eyberg, S. M., Nelson, M. M., & Boggs, S. R. (2008). Evidence-based psychosocial treatments for children and adolescents with disruptive behavior. *Journal of Clinical Child and Adolescent Psychology, 37*(1), 215–237.

Fite, P. J., Colder, C. R., Lochman, J. E., & Wells, K. C. (2006). The mutual influence of parenting and boys' externalizing behavior problems. *Journal of Applied Developmental Psychology, 27,* 151–164.

Fite, P. J., Colder, C. R., Lochman, J. E., & Wells, K. C. (2007). Pathways from proactive and reactive aggression to substance use. *Psychology of Addictive Behaviors, 21,* 355–364.

Fite, P. J., Winn, P., Lochman, J. E., & Wells, K. C. (2009). The effect of neighborhood disadvantage on proactive and reactive aggression. *Journal of Community Psychology, 37,* 542–546.

Foley, D. L., Eaves, L. J., Wormley, B., Silberg, J. L., Maes, H. H., Kuhn, J., et al. (2004). Childhood adversity, monoamine oxidase A genotype, and risk for conduct disorder. *Archives of General Psychiatry, 61,* 738–744.

Forgatch, M. S., & Patterson, G. R. (2010). Parent Management Training—Oregon Model. In J. R. Weisz & A. E. Kazdin (Eds.), *Evidence-based therapies for children and adolescents* (2nd ed., pp. 159–178). New York: Guilford Press.

Forgatch, M. S., Patterson, G. R., & DeGarmo, D. S. (2006). Evaluating fidelity: Predictive validity for a measure of competent adherence to the Oregon model of parent management training. *Behavior Therapy, 36*(1), 3–13.

Forgatch, M. S., Patterson, G. R., DeGarmo, D. S., & Beldavs, Z. G. (2009). Testing the Oregon delinquency model with 9-year follow-up of the Oregon Divorce Study. *Development and Psychopathology, 21*(02), 637–660.

Goodman, R. (1997). The Strengths and Difficulties Questionnaire: A research note. *Journal of Child Psychology and Psychiatry, 38,* 581–586.

Goodman, R., Meltzer, H., & Bailey, V. (1998). The Strengths and Difficulties Questionnaire: A pilot study on the validity of the self-report version. *European Child and Adolescent Psychiatry, 7,* 125–130.

Greene, R., Biederman, J., Zerwas, S., Monuteaux, M., Goring, J. C., & Faraone, S. (2002). Psychiatric comorbidity, family dysfunction, and social impairment in referred youth with oppositional defiant disorder. *American Journal of Psychiatry, 159,* 1214–1224.

Hood, K. K., & Eyberg, S. M. (2003). Outcomes of parent–child interaction therapy: Mothers' reports of maintenance three to six years after treatment. *Journal of Clinical Child and Adolescent Psychology, 32*(3), 419–429.

Hukkelberg, S. S., & Ogden, T. (2013). Working alliance and treatment fidelity as predictors of externalizing problem behaviors in parent management training. *Journal of Consulting and Clinical Psychology, 81*(6), 1010–1020.

Jackson, M. F., Barth, J. M., Powell, N., & Lochman, J. E. (2006). Classroom contextual effects of race on children's peer nominations. *Child Development, 77,* 1325–1337.

Jaffee, S. R., Caspi, A., Moffitt, T. E., & Taylor, A. (2004). Physical maltreatment victim to antisocial child: Evidence of an environmentally mediated process. *Journal of Abnormal Psychology, 113,* 44–55.

Kazdin, A. E. (1997). Parent management training: Evidence, outcomes, and issues. *Journal of the American Academy of Child and Adolescent Psychiatry, 36*(10), 1349–1356.

Kazdin, A. E. (2010). Problem-solving skills training and parent management training for oppositional defiant disorder and conduct disorder. In J. R. Weisz & A. E. Kazdin (Eds.), *Evidence-based psychotherapies for children and adolescents* (2nd ed., pp. 211–226). New York: Guilford Press.

Kazdin, A. E., Siegel, T. C., & Bass, D. (1992). Cognitive problem-solving skills training and parent management training in the treatment of antisocial behavior in children. *Journal of Consulting and Clinical Psychology, 60*(5), 733–747.

Kazdin, A., & Whitley, M. (2006). Comorbidity, case complexity, and effects of evidence-based treatment for children referred for disruptive behavior. *Journal of Consulting and Clinical Psychology, 74,* 455–467.

Lahey, B. B., Van Hulle, C. A., Keenan, K., Rathouz, P. J., D'Onofrio, B. M., Rodgers, J. L., et al. (2008). Temperament and parenting during the first year of life predict future child conduct problems. *Journal of Abnormal Child Psychology, 36*(8), 1139–1158.

Larson, J., & Lochman, J. E. (2011). *Helping school children cope with anger: A cognitive-behavioral intervention* (2nd ed.). New York: Guilford Press.

Lochman, J. E., Baden, R. E., Boxmeyer, C. L., Powell, N. P., Qu, L., Salekin, K. L., et al. (2014). Does a booster intervention augment the preventive effects of an abbreviated version of the Coping Power Program for aggressive children? *Journal of Abnormal Child Psychology 42,* 367–381.

Lochman, J. E., Barry, T. D., & Pardini, D. (2003). Anger control training for aggressive youth. In A. E. Kazdin & J. R. Weisz (Eds.), *Evidenced-based psychotherapies for children and adolescents* (pp. 263–281). New York: Guilford Press.

Lochman, J. E., Boxmeyer, C., Powell, N., Qu, L., Wells, K., & Windle, M. (2009). Dissemination of the Coping Power Program: Importance of intensity of counselor training. *Journal of Consulting and Clinical Psychology, 77,* 397–409.

Lochman, J. E., Boxmeyer, C. L., Powell, N. P., Qu, L., Wells, K., & Windle, M. (2012). Coping Power dissemination study: Intervention and special education effects on academic outcomes. *Behavioral Disorders, 37,* 192–205.

Lochman, J. E., & Dodge, K. A. (1994). Social-cognitive processes of severely violent, moderately aggressive and nonaggressive boys. *Journal of Consulting and Clinical Psychology, 62,* 366–374.

Lochman, J. E., & Dodge, K. A. (1998). Distorted perceptions in dyadic interactions of aggressive and nonaggressive boys: Effects of prior expectations, context, and boys' age. *Development and Psychopathology, 10,* 495–512.

Lochman, J. E., & Wayland, K. K. (1994). Aggression, social acceptance and race as predictors of negative adolescent outcomes. *Journal of the American Academy of Child and Adolescent Psychiatry, 33,* 1026–1035.

Lochman, J. E., Wayland, K. K., & White, K. J. (1993). Social goals: Relationship to adolescent adjustment and to social problem solving. *Journal of Abnormal Child Psychology, 21,* 135–151.

Lochman, J. E., & Wells, K. C. (2002). Contextual social-cognitive mediators and child outcome: A test of the theoretical model in the Coping Power Program. *Development and Psychopathology, 14,* 971–993.

Lochman, J. E., & Wells, K. C. (2003). Effectiveness study of Coping Power and classroom intervention with aggressive children: Outcomes at a one-year follow-up. *Behavior Therapy, 34,* 493–515.

Lochman, J. E., & Wells, K. C. (2004). The Coping Power program for preadolescent aggressive boys and their parents: Outcome effects at the one-year follow-up. *Journal of Consulting and Clinical Psychology, 72,* 571–578.

Lochman, J. E., Wells, K. C., & Lenhart, L. A. (2008). *Coping Power child group program facilitator guide*. New York: Oxford University Press.

Lochman, J. E., Wells, K. C., Qu, L., & Chen, L. (2013). Three year follow-up of Coping Power intervention effects: Evidence of neighborhood moderation? *Prevention Science, 14*, 364–376.

Lorber, M. F. (2004). Psychophysiology of aggression, psychopathy, and conduct problems: A meta-analysis. *Psychological Bulletin, 130*, 531–552.

Miller-Johnson, S., Coie, J. D., Maumary-Gremaud, A., Bierman, K., & Conduct Problems Prevention Research Group. (2002). Peer rejection and aggression and early starter models of conduct disorder. *Journal of Abnormal Child Psychology, 30*, 217–230.

Miller-Johnson, S., Coie, J. D., Maumary-Gremaud, A., Lochman, J., & Terry, R. (1999). Relationship between childhood peer rejection and aggression and adolescent delinquency severity and type among African American youth. *Journal of Emotional and Behavioral Disorders, 7*, 137–146.

Moffitt, T. E. (1993). Adolescence-limited and life-course-persistent antisocial behavior: A developmental taxonomy. *Psychological Review, 100*(4), 674–701.

Moffitt, T. E. (2003). Life-course-persistent and adolescence-limited antisocial behaviour: A 10-year research review and a research agenda. In B. J. Lahey, T. E. Moffitt, & A. Caspi (Eds.), *Causes of conduct disorder and juvenile delinquency* (pp. 49–75). New York: Guilford Press.

Moffitt, T. E., Arseneault, L., Jaffee, S. R., Kim-Cohen, J., Koenen, K. C., Odgers, C. L., et al. (2008). Research review: DSM-V conduct disorder: Research needs for an evidence base. *Journal of Child Psychology and Psychiatry, 49*, 3–33.

Muratori, P., Bertacchi, I., Giuli, C., Nocentini, A., & Lochman, J. E. (in press). Implementing Coping Power adapted as an universal prevention program in Italian primary schools: A randomized control trial. *Prevention Science*.

Mushtaq, A., Lochman, J. E., Tariq, P. N., & Sabih, F. (in press). Preliminary effectiveness study of Coping Power program for aggressive children in Pakistan. *Prevention Science*.

Myers, M. G., Stewart, D. G., & Brown, S. A. (1998). Progression from conduct disorder to antisocial personality disorder following treatment for adolescent substance abuse. *American Journal of Psychiatry, 155*, 479–485.

Newcorn, J. H., Spencer, T. J., Biederman, J., Milton, D. R., & Michelson, D. (2005). Atomoxetine treatment in children and adolescents with attention-deficit/hyperactivity disorder and comorbid oppositional defiant disorder. *Journal of the American Academy of Child and Adolescent Psychiatry, 44*(3), 240–248.

Nock, M., Kazdin, A., & Hiripi, E. (2007). Lifetime prevalence, correlates and persistence of oppositional defiant disorder: Results from the National Comorbidity Survey Replication. *Journal of Child Psychology and Psychiatry, 48*, 703–713.

Ollendick, T. H., Jarrett, M. A., Grills-Taquechel, A. E., Hovey, L. D., & Wolff, J. C. (2008). Comorbidity as a predictor and moderator of treatment outcome in youth with anxiety, affective, attention deficit/hyperactivity disorder, and oppositional/conduct disorders. *Clinical Psychology Review, 28*(8), 1447–1471.

Orobio de Castro, B., Veerman, J. W., Koops, W., Bosch, J. D., & Monshouwer, H. J. (2002). Hostile attribution of intent and aggressive behavior: A meta-analysis. *Child Development, 73*, 916–934.

Pardini, D. A., Barry, T. D., Barth, J. M., Lochman, J. E., & Wells, K. C. (2006). Self-perceived social acceptance and peer social standing in children with aggressive–disruptive behaviors. *Social Development, 15*, 46–64.

Pardini, D. A., Lochman, J. E., & Frick, P. J. (2003). Callous/unemotional traits and social cognitive processes in adjudicated youth. *Journal of the American Academy of Child and Adolescent Psychiatry, 42*, 364–371.

Patterson, G. R., Reid, J. B., Jones, R. R., & Conger, R. E. (1975). *A social learning approach to family intervention.* Eugene, OR: Castalia.

Pettit, G. S., Bates, J. E., & Dodge, K. E. (1997). Supportive parenting, ecological context, and children's adjustment: A seven year longitudinal study. *Child Development, 68,* 908–923.

Reid, J. B., Patterson, G. R., & Snyder, J. (2002). *Antisocial behavior in children and adolescents: A developmental analysis and model of intervention.* Washington, DC: American Psychological Association.

Reynolds, C. R., & Kamphaus, R. W. (2004). *Behavior Assessment System for Children, Second Edition (BASC-2).* Bloomington, MN: Pearson Assessments.

Schumann, E. M., Foote, R. C., Eyberg, S. M., Boggs, S. R., & Algina, J. (1998). Efficacy of parent–child interaction therapy: Interim report of a randomized trial with short-term maintenance. *Journal of Clinical Child Psychology, 27*(1), 34–45.

Sells, S. (1998). *Treating the tough adolescent: A family-based, step-by-step guide.* New York: Guilford Press.

Smith, D. K., & Chamberlain, P. (2010). Multidimensional treatment foster care for adolescents: Processes and outcomes. In J. R. Weisz & A. E. Kazdin (Eds.), *Evidence-based therapies for children and adolescents* (2nd ed., pp. 243–258). New York: Guilford Press.

Thomas, D. E., Bierman, K. L., Thompson, C., Powers, C. J., & the Conduct Problems Prevention Research Group. (2009). Double jeopardy: Child and school characteristics that predict aggressive–disruptive behavior in the first grade. *School Psychology Review, 37,* 516–532.

Viding, E., Blair, J. R., Moffitt, T. E., & Plomin, R. (2005). Psychopathic syndrome indexes strong genetic risk for antisocial behaviour in 7-year-olds. *Journal of Child Psychology and Psychiatry, 46,* 592–597.

Wakschlag, L. S., Pickett, K. E., Kasza, K. E., & Loeber, R. (2006). Is prenatal smoking associated with a developmental pattern of conduct problems in young boys? *Journal of the American Academy of Child and Adolescent Psychiatry, 45,* 461–467.

Warr, M. (2002) *Companions in crime: The social aspects of criminal conduct.* Cambridge, UK: Cambridge University Press.

Weiss, B. (1998). *RECAP manuals.* Unpublished manuscript, Vanderbilt University, Nashville, TN.

Weiss, B., Catron, T., Harris, V., & Han, S. (2000, October). *Effectiveness of an intervention program for children with concurrent internalizing and externalizing problems.* Paper presented at the Kansas Conference in Clinical Child Psychology, University of Kansas, Lawrence, KS.

Weiss, B., Harris, V., Catron, T., & Han, S. S. (2003). Efficacy of the RECAP intervention program for children with concurrent internalizing and externalizing problems. *Journal of Consulting and Clinical Psychology, 71*(2), 364–374.

Williams, S. C., Lochman, J. E., Phllips, N. C., & Barry, T. (2003). Aggressive and nonaggressive boys' physiological and cognitive processes in response to peer provocations. *Journal of Clinical Child and Adolescent Psychology, 32,* 568–576.

Zelli, A., Dodge, K. A., Lochman, J. E., Laird, R. D., & the Conduct Problems Prevention Research Group. (1999). The distinction between beliefs legitimizing aggression and deviant processing of social cues: Testing measurement validity and the hypothesis that biased processing mediates the effects of beliefs on aggression. *Journal of Personality and Social Psychology, 77,* 150–166.

Zisser, A., & Eyberg, S. M. (2010). Parent–child interaction therapy and the treatment of disruptive behavior disorders. In J. R. Weisz & A. E. Kazdin (Eds.), *Evidence-based therapies for children and adolescents* (2nd ed., pp. 179–193). New York: Guilford Press.

Zonnevylle-Bender, M. J. S., Matthys, W., van de Wiel, N. M. H., & Lochman, J. (2007). Preventive effects of treatment of DBD in middle childhood on substance use and delinquent behavior. *Journal of the American Academy of Child and Adolescent Psychiatry, 46,* 33–39.

CHAPTER 12

Attention-Deficit/ Hyperactivity Disorder

Amy Altszuler, Fiona Macphee, Brittany Merrill,
Anne Morrow, William E. Pelham, Jr.,
and Nicole K. Schatz*

THE DSM-5 DEFINITION OF ATTENTION-DEFICIT/HYPERACTIVITY DISORDER

Attention deficit/hyperactivity disorder (ADHD) is a chronic neurodevelopmental disorder with childhood onset characterized by core deficits including inattention (e.g., distractibility, disorganization, poor time management), hyperactivity/impulsivity (e.g., fidgetiness, restlessness, acting without thinking), or both (American Psychiatric Association, 2013). According to DSM-5 (American Psychiatric Association, 2013), to meet criteria for an ADHD diagnosis, children under the age of 17 must exhibit six out of nine inattentive symptoms for a predominantly inattentive presentation, six out of nine hyperactive/impulsive symptoms for a predominantly hyperactive/impulsive presentation, or both for a diagnosis of the combined presentation (for individuals ages 17 and older, only five symptoms within a category are required for diagnosis). In addition to symptom counts, there must be evidence of symptoms across multiple settings, onset of symptoms prior to age 12, and clear evidence of significant impairment associated with symptoms. Furthermore, symptoms and impairment must not be better explained by the presence of another condition. ADHD is associated with pervasive impairment across home, academic, and social settings (Pelham, Fabiano, & Massetti, 2005). Children with ADHD experience greater conflict with parents and siblings (Johnston & Chronis-Tuscano, 2014), significant academic impairment (Kuriyan et al., 2013), and difficulties interacting with peers (Hoza et al., 2005).

*Author order is alphabetical. All authors contributed equally to the writing of this chapter.

PREVALENCE AND COURSE

According to the American Academy of Pediatrics (2011), ADHD is a chronic disorder among the most prevalent mental disorders for children and adolescents with an estimated prevalence rate of 8–12% (Visser et al., 2014). Prevalence and presentation vary across gender, with a 2:1 male-to-female ratio in children and adolescents and females more likely than males to present as inattentive type (American Psychiatric Association, 2013). The majority of children with ADHD continue to have symptoms and impairment during adolescence (Sibley et al., 2012) and adulthood (Barkley, Murphy, & Fischer, 2010). ADHD is associated with a variety of impairments in daily life functioning that result from the core problems in symptomatology (Pelham, Fabiano, et al., 2005), including low academic achievement and behavior problems in school (DuPaul & Jimerson, 2014; Loe & Feldman, 2007); conflict with parents, teachers, and other adults (Johnston & Chronis-Tuscano, 2014); problems with peers and siblings; and associated comorbidities that impact these domains (Pelham & Bender, 1982). Parents of youth with ADHD endorse marked caregiver strain (Anastopoulos, Sommer, & Schatz, 2009) and have high associated rates of marital distress and divorce (Wymbs et al., 2008) and stress-related alcohol consumption (Pelham et al., 1998). ADHD is also associated with peer rejection (Hoza et al., 2005) due to impulsive (e.g., interrupting in the classroom, butting in line, not taking turns or following rules in games) and negative verbal and aggressive behaviors (McQuade & Hoza, 2008; Nijmeijer et al., 2008; Pelham & Bender, 1982). Notably, these functional impairments associated with the disorder—not the DSM symptomatology—constitute the most important areas to be targeted in intervention for ADHD (Pelham, Fabiano, et al., 2005).

For the vast majority of individuals with ADHD, significant impairment persists into adulthood, marked by a lesser likelihood than those without the disorder to pursue higher education, hold a steady job, manage their finances, and maintain adaptive social relationships, and a greater likelihood to have difficulties with substance use and abuse (Altszuler et al., 2016; Barkley et al., 2010; Lee, Humphreys, Flory, Liu, & Glass, 2011; Molina & Pelham, 2014). Adults with ADHD also routinely report lower self-esteem and poorer overall quality of life (Danckaerts et al., 2010). Notably, individuals identified as having ADHD in childhood rarely self-identify as having ADHD in adulthood and underreport their symptoms and impairments (Altszuler et al., 2016; Sibley et al., 2012).

COMMON COMORBID CONDITIONS

As many as 80% of children and adults with ADHD have at least one other psychiatric disorder (Barkley et al., 2010). In the large Multimodal Treatment Study of Children with ADHD (MTA; Jensen et al., 2001), 40 to 60% of the children diagnosed with ADHD also met criteria for comorbid oppositional defiant disorder (ODD), 25% for an anxiety disorder, 20–25% for conduct disorder (CD), 10% for a tic disorder, and 5% for an affective disorder. Furthermore, approximately one child in three with ADHD meets criteria for a learning disorder, and an additional portion function below expected levels academically (DuPaul & Stoner, 2014).

ETIOLOGICAL/CONCEPTUAL MODELS OF ADHD

Most conceptualizations view ADHD as being biologically based. With an approximate broad heritability rate of 70% (Nikolas & Burt, 2010), ADHD is among the most genetically influenced of all psychiatric disorders (Barkley, 2015). A decade ago, molecular genetics researchers had begun to identify specific genes that may contribute to the development of ADHD (Faraone & Mick, 2011); however, more recent approaches have argued that single-candidate genes are unlikely to have a large effect on presence of ADHD, and researchers are beginning to focus on groups of genes as they relate to neural networks (Barkley, 2015). Accumulating neuroimaging evidence supports the claim that the pathophysiology of ADHD is related to abnormalities in multiple neural systems and their interactions spanning high-level cognitive functions, sensorimotor processes, and default mode networks (Cortese et al., 2012). The observed diversity in brain dysfunction may contribute to the noted heterogeneity in cognitive behavioral performance (Nigg, Willcutt, Doyle, & Sonuga-Barke, 2005). Children with ADHD demonstrate deficits of moderate to large magnitude across several areas of cognitive functioning, including working memory, behavioral inhibition, temporal estimation, processing speed, and reaction time variability; however, recent advancements in analytic techniques reveal significant heterogeneity across multiple levels of analysis (i.e., emotional, cognitive, and neurobiological), suggesting that different impaired cognitive processes (at the individual level) contribute to a similar behavioral phenotype characteristic of ADHD (at the group level) (Baroni & Castellanos, 2015; Willcutt, Doyle, Nigg, Faraone, & Pennington, 2005).

From an epigenetic standpoint, biological risk for ADHD interacts with adverse environmental factors such as low socioeconomic class, maternal psychopathology, and family conflict to affect presentation and severity of ADHD symptoms and impairment (Biederman, Faraone, & Monuteaux, 2002).

Despite the findings suggesting brain and genetic bases for ADHD and the development of devices that putatively measure neurological aspects of ADHD, to date no research has successfully documented that any biological or genetic measure is useful in diagnosis or treatment of children with ADHD. Similarly, psychological tasks that measure various aspects of cognition have not yet been shown to have clinical utility in ADHD diagnosis or treatment response (Pelham & Fabiano, 2008; Pelham, Fabiano, et al., 2005). One reason for this may be that studies of cognition and neurological functioning in ADHD have only rarely examined the relationship between performance on these laboratory tasks/measures and behavioral functioning in the natural environment. As studies of these relationships occur, light will be shed on the brain and cognitive processes involved in ADHD.

Finally, it is worth noting that although not considered to be a cause of ADHD, the three domains of associated impairments—parenting, functioning in the classroom, and peer relationships—have long been known to be important predictors of long-term outcomes in both epidemiological populations and in clinical samples of children with disruptive behavior, including ADHD. Considerable research demonstrates that these domains of dysfunction are also arguably the mediators through which improvement in outcomes must be attained (Pelham, Fabiano et al., 2005). Thus, while these important domains are not causally implicated in the development of ADHD, they are major influences on children's outcomes in later life and are therefore the most critical areas to assess and modify in treating ADHD children.

EVIDENCE-BASED TREATMENTS FOR ADHD

ADHD is a chronic disorder requiring ongoing treatment and monitoring. Currently, according to American Psychological Association Division 12 Task Force guidelines (Lonigan, Elbert, & Johnson, 1998) behavioral interventions, pharmacological treatment, and their combination are the only evidence-based, acute interventions for ADHD and are discussed in turn below.

Behavioral Interventions

Three cumulative, systematic reviews of behavioral treatments have been conducted since the Task Force guidelines were developed (Evans, Owens, & Bunford, 2014; Pelham & Fabiano, 2008; Pelham, Wheeler, & Chronis, 1998) and all three have documented the increasing evidence for the effectiveness of behavioral parent training, behavioral school interventions, and behavioral social skills training programs. There is some variability in the number of studies and strength of the evidence across the age ranges from young children through adolescence, and we review this below. In contrast, there is not support for the efficacy of cognitive treatments in improving the symptoms or functioning of children with ADHD (Melby-Lervåg & Hulme, 2013; Rapport, Orban, Kofler, & Friedman, 2013), and we do not discuss such treatments (e.g., working memory training) in this chapter. Other treatments for ADHD such as play therapy, office-based psychotherapy, biofeedback, and dietary restrictions do not have empirical support and are not discussed further.

Behavioral Parent Training

Behavioral parent training (BPT) has been used for children with disruptive behavior disorders for more than 50 years, and it has strong empirical support and meets criteria for a well-established treatment according to multiple systematic reviews of psychosocial treatments for childhood and adolescent ADHD (Evans et al., 2014; Pelham & Fabiano, 2008; Pelham, Wheeler, et al., 1998) with moderate to large treatment effects (Fabiano et al., 2009; Kaminski, Valle, Filene, & Boyle, 2008). Many manualized BPT interventions (e.g., Abikoff et al., 1994; Barkley, 2013; Cunningham, Bremner, & Secord-Gilbert, 1993; Eyberg et al., 2001; McMahon & Forehand, 2005; Sanders, 2012; Webster-Stratton, Reid, & Beauchaine, 2011) have been studied and have been found to be effective with ADHD. They include programs that can be delivered in group or individual sessions, or a mixture of the two. All have similar core components (see Table 12.1 and discussion below) based on social learning theory and decades of research in which parents learn strategies to modify the antecedents and consequences of their child's misbehavior. BPT programs that focus on increasing parent–child positive interactions, teaching time-out, and/or include practicing skills with the child have been shown to be associated with larger improvements in child behavior (e.g., for ages 5–11) and parenting practices (Kaminski et al., 2008). Because BPT requires active participation of parents, some families may struggle with engaging in the treatment and adhering to implementation of the strategies. To address this issue, traditional BPT programs have been modified to address common barriers to treatment such as single-parent households and parental psychopathology (Chronis, Chacko, Fabiano, Wymbs, & Pelham, 2004).

BPT programs also have strong, empirical support for preschool-age children (ages 3–5). Some, such as parent–child interaction therapy (Eyberg et al., 2001), were originally developed for this young but more diagnostically diverse population—including disruptive behavior problems in general. Because most BPT outcomes studies focused on children, the efficacy of behavioral interventions for adolescents remains unclear (Evans et al., 2014; Sibley, Kuriyan, Evans, Waxmonsky, & Smith, 2014). BPT models originally developed for children have been adapted for use with adolescents with some success (Barkley, Edwards, Laneri, Fletcher, & Metevia, 2001) by incorporating problem-solving and communication skills building for parents and teens (Robin & Foster, 1989). Other interventions focus on particular areas of impairment for adolescents with ADHD such as academics (Evans, Schultz, Demars, & Davis, 2011; Sibley et al., 2013) and driving (Fabiano et al., 2011). In the practice sections below, we describe modifications of BPT for younger children and adolescents when indicated.

Behavioral Classroom Management

School-based interventions for ADHD, variously labeled in systematic reviews as behavioral school interventions (BSIs) or behavioral classroom management (BCM) have 50 years of strong empirical support and meet criteria for a well-established treatment for children with ADHD (DuPaul, Eckert, & Vilardo, 2012; Evans et al., 2014). As with BPT, BCM studies with children began prior to the widespread use of ADHD as a diagnostic classification and generally focused on children with on-task and/or behavior problems in classroom settings. In the DSM classification scheme, these have always included children with ADHD, ODD, and CD. The texts, manuals, and websites that provide descriptions of these interventions are too numerous to cite (for a review, see Gutkin & Reynolds, 2009). Effective classroomwide behavioral strategies and interventions for elementary

TABLE 12.1. Parent Training Session Topics

Session	Topic
1	Overview of social learning theory and behavior management principles
2	Establishing house rules and routines
3	Effective commands and rewarding compliance
4	Contingent attention
5	Time-out and loss of privileges
6	Home reward systems
7	Daily Report Card
8	Generalizing strategies to other settings
9	Maintaining gains after program ends

school-age students include developing clear classroom rules, providing differential positive attention, implementing class lotteries, providing contingent rewards based on group
behavior, and implementing comprehensive response cost systems (DuPaul & Stoner,
2014). Notably, as with BPT, all are based on similar principles and are in widespread use
in classrooms throughout the United States (Gutkin & Reynolds, 2009; Sugai & Horner,
2009; Hart et al., 2016). On an individual level, developing and implementing a daily
report card (DRC) is a solidly evidence-based intervention for children with ADHD that
positively affects observed classroom behavior and teacher ratings of academic productivity and disruptive behavior (Fabiano et al., 2010). DRCs are school–home notes that list
specific behavioral or academic targets (e.g., work completion and accuracy, interruptions, classroom rule violations) and include a clear goal for each target (e.g., completes
work *with three or fewer reminders*). Classroom teachers monitor success throughout
the day and rewards are provided at home, in school, or in both places (for guidelines on
implementation, see Volpe & Fabiano, 2013, and *www.ccf.fiu.edu*).

As with BPT, BCI has been documented as effective with elementary school-age children, but studies also show strong support with preschool-age children. The preschool
classroom is a critical setting for treatment, especially in light of the disproportionate
expulsion rate in preschool, primarily due to behavioral problems (13 times the national
average for elementary and secondary school years; Gilliam & Shahar, 2006). Teacher
trainings, such as The Incredible Years program, and continuing consultation services,
are effective with this age range (Brennan, Bradley, Allen, & Perry, 2008; Gorman-Smith
& Metropolitan Area Child Study Research Group, 2003; Raver, Jones, & Li-Grining,
2008). As we discuss below, specific strategies differ from elementary age interventions
primarily in reward salience and frequency.

Classroom-based problems for adolescents with ADHD are typically addressed
through BPT approaches given the difficulties inherent in implementing teacher-driven
behavioral interventions in middle school and high school settings. Secondary school
teachers may see hundreds of students a day and are unable to provide individualized
support (Eccles & Roeser, 2004). Furthermore, the majority of children with ADHD no
longer exhibit severely disruptive behaviors in adolescence (Sibley & Yeguez, 2014; Sibley
et al., 2012). Therefore, conventional classroom behavioral management as a treatment
strategy is not a good fit for the secondary school environment or the presenting problems of poor organization or time management outside of the classroom. Instead, organizational training, in which youth learn skills to address specific areas of impairment,
is a well-established treatment that may work better for adolescents (Evans et al., 2014).

Behavioral Peer Interventions

In clinical and often in school settings, interventions for the problems of children with
ADHD and their peers typically occur in weekly, clinic-based (or school counselor-based)
social skills training groups. However, such approaches are not considered evidence-
based and have not been found to improve social functioning deficits of children with
ADHD (Evans et al., 2014; Mikami, Jia, & Na, 2014; Pelham & Fabiano, 2008; Pelham,
Wheeler, et al., 1998). Alternatively, more intensive interventions targeting peer interac-
tions in group recreational settings, such as a therapeutic summer treatment program
(STP), meet criteria for the well-established status and have been shown to positively

affect observed social behavior (both reductions in negative behavior and increases in positive), sports skills, and staff-rated impairments in the peer domain (O'Connor et al., 2014; Pelham & Fabiano, 2008; Pelham et al., 2010, 2014). Peer intervention strategies used in the STP include brief social skills training discussions, modeling of appropriate social skills by counselors, social reinforcement and a DRC for using appropriate skills, and a point/token system implemented throughout the day to provide consequences for positive and negative social behaviors. These interventions are implemented in a group setting, along with intensive sports skills training and practice while playing common children's sports (baseball, basketball, and soccer). The STP and similar programs are well-established treatments for childhood ADHD. At the same time, they are intensive and therefore more costly than typical BPT and BCI interventions, and because of the cost are less available than other behavioral treatment modalities.

The STP has been modified to target school readiness and social–emotional skills among preschool- and kindergarten-age children at risk for externalizing behavior problems with initial success (STP-PreK; Graziano, Slavec, Hart, Garcia, & Pelham, 2014). The peer-specific components of the STP-PreK were training in social skills (e.g., participation, encouragement) and emotional states (e.g., happy, sad, and disgusted) in which counselors used puppets, modeling, and role play, and provided positive reinforcement for use of strategies throughout the camp day. These same modifications have been employed in school-based programs for children with ADHD and disruptive behavior disorders that integrate a focus on social skills and classroom management (e.g., Webster-Stratton et al., 2011).

Few studies have assessed BPI for adolescents with ADHD. Two preliminary studies have assessed treatment components from the STP modified for use with adolescents with mixed results (Evans et al., 2011; Sibley, Pelham, Gnagy, Ross, & Greiner, 2011). More research is needed to accurately determine the efficacy of BPI for youth in this age range.

Finally, many aspects of BCM include interventions to improve peer relationships, and a number of these have been used with children with ADHD and have a solid evidence base. These programs include RECESS (Walker, Hops, & Greenwood, 1981) and CLASS (Hops et al., 1978) for elementary school-age children, and the Coping Power Program (Lochman, Boxmeyer, Powell, Barry, & Pardini, 2010). Among other classroom-based behaviors, these programs target negative behaviors directed toward peers in classroom settings (e.g., teasing, interruptions, and aggression) and have been shown to have substantial beneficial effects on these target behaviors even though they have not typically been employed as stand-alone interventions in studies limited to ADHD students.

Summary

BPT, BCI, and BPI for ADHD meet the standard criteria for whether an intervention is evidence-based or not according to the criteria employed in this chapter; however, there are several caveats to this conclusion. First, although authors of the reviews and meta-analyses cited earlier (Evans et al., 2014; Pelham & Fabiano, 2008; Pelham, Wheeler, et al., 1998) suggest that these are effective treatments, there are others who state the opposite (e.g., Sonuga-Barke et al., 2013). Meta-analyses with null or negative findings for behavioral treatments with ADHD should be interpreted with caution given that some reviews include only randomized controlled trials, excluding the wealth of studies employing other designs (e.g., single-subject designs), which may bias the results (Fabiano, Schatz, Aloe, Chacko, & Chronis-Tuscano, 2015).

Additionally, there is considerably more research on elementary school–age children than on young children and adolescents—by at least a factor of 10. This means that the strength of the evidence varies across ages, as discussed in the systematic reviews and meta-analyses we cited earlier (Evans et al., 2014; Pelham & Fabiano, 2008; Pelham, Wheeler, et al., 1998). Second, the majority of studies have employed packages of interventions rather than unique components in the evaluations of effectiveness. For example, the frequently cited MTA (MTA Cooperative Group, 1999) simultaneously employed all three of the interventions we cited earlier as evidence-based for parent training, school intervention, and peer problems. Similarly, the STP incorporates BPT (Cunningham et al., 1993) and a classroom BCI, including DRC follow-up, along with the intensive BPI implemented in all of the studies in which STP effectiveness is demonstrated. Finally, most BPT programs teach parents how to implement DRCs in school settings and often implement simultaneous classroom- and peer-based interventions while implementing parent training (e.g., Webster-Stratton et al., 2011). As others have noted (Evans et al., 2014), few studies, however, have disentangled the effects of these separable components of treatment, and it is therefore difficult to rule out that one component might have contributed to the impact of another. As we discuss below in our discussion of treatment in practice, one reason for this is that BPT, BCI, and BPI are often, if not always, inextricably linked when interventions are implemented in practice. For example, the typical targets for behaviors of a child with ADHD in the classroom include academic work, teacher–child interactions, and peer interactions, with a feedback and reward system (a DRC) typically implemented by the child's parents. Thus, although evaluated separately for the purposes of making decisions for evidence-based lists, in practice, BPT, BCI, and BPI are typically integrated, with the specific components of each tailored to the presenting problems of the referred child. Thus, the fact that they have often not been separated in treatment studies reflects the way they are used in practice.

Pharmacological Interventions

Stimulant medications are the most widely used treatment for children diagnosed with ADHD and are recommended as first-line treatment for all but the youngest children with ADHD (American Academy of Pediatrics, 2011). Recent reports indicate that over 80% of youth with ADHD are prescribed stimulants in a given year (Visser et al., 2015). They consistently produce acute ameliorative effects of ADHD symptoms for most children and adolescents (Faraone & Buitelaar, 2010; Pliszka, 2007). The two primary psychostimulant medications are methylphenidate and amphetamine, and each produces large, immediate, acute effects on classroom behavior (e.g., observed rule violations), daily seatwork productivity, and teacher ratings of ADHD symptoms and behavior (Evans et al., 2001; Faraone & Buitelaar, 2010). Most children experience benefits at relatively low to moderate doses, and the incremental benefit of higher doses is often small and may be outweighed by potential side effects (e.g., decreased appetite; Fabiano et al., 2007; Pelham, Manos, et al., 2005). In addition to their impact on school behavior, when long-acting versions of stimulants are employed, parent ratings of ADHD symptoms and behavior are also acutely more positive (e.g., Pelham et al., 2001). Stimulant effects are apparent for a child only as long as the medication has a pharmacological effect—4 to 12 hours, depending on the formulation and type of medication, after which the benefits are completely gone (Pelham et al., 2001). Despite 50 years of research documenting their acutely beneficial effects, evidence of long-term, functional benefits of stimulant medication (that is, improvement in problematic functioning in adolescence and adulthood) continue to be absent from the literature even when the acute effects have been documented in the same sample (Langberg et al., 2011; Molina et al., 2009). Given the very poor outcomes that characterize individuals with ADHD in adolescence and adulthood, this is the single largest limitation of pharmacological treatments for ADHD and the single largest justification for use of psychosocial treatment in addition to stimulants with children with ADHD.

The American Academy of Pediatrics (2011) does not recommend pharmacological treatment as a first-line treatment for young children diagnosed with ADHD, though the American Academy of Child and Adolescent Psychiatry (2007) does not differentiate between different ages in its recommendation that stimulants should be a first-line treatment for ADHD. A major, National Institute of Mental Health (NIMH)–funded multisite trial examining stimulant effects among preschool-age children with ADHD showed that the efficacy and tolerability of stimulant medications are more variable in preschoolers than in older children (Vitiello et al., 2007; Wigal et al., 2006), leading to the recommendation of the American Academy of Pediatrics and the recent Centers for Disease Control and Prevention (2016) report urging the use of behavioral intervention as a first-line treatment for young children.

Stimulant treatment has a small to moderate effect on symptoms and impairment among adolescents with ADHD (Evans et al., 2001; Faraone & Buitelaar, 2010; Sibley et al., 2014) and both pediatric and psychiatric guidelines recommend medication as first-line treatment for adolescents with ADHD (American Academy of Child and Adolescent Psychiatry, 2007; American Academy of Pediatrics, 2011). Controlled studies document that adolescents with ADHD exhibit improvement in the same domains as children when receiving low to moderate doses of stimulant medication, but the incremental gains of higher doses are small and may not outweigh the additional side effects (Evans et al., 2001; Smith et al., 1998). The major problem with stimulant therapy in adolescents with ADHD is nonadherence driven by some teenagers' refusal to take medication. Treatment decisions for this population must take into account the individual teen's motivation and willingness of the parent to enforce and monitor medication compliance (Biswas, Gnagy, Molina, & Pelham, 2009; McCarthy et al., 2009; Molina et al., 2009).

Finally, over the past decade, a handful of nonstimulant medications have been approved for treatment of ADHD. However, their effects are substantially smaller than those produced by stimulants, their side effect profiles are no better, and there is similarly no evidence of long-term benefit (Faraone, Biederman, Spencer, & Aleardi, 2006; Waxmonsky, 2005).

Combined Pharmacological and Behavioral Interventions

As independent treatment modalities, behavioral interventions and stimulant treatments have clear limitations. As we discussed earlier, high-intensity behavioral treatment can be costly and difficult to implement consistently. On the other hand, stimulants are effective only when the medication is active in the child's central nervous system; higher doses are associated with side effects, and long-term medication use does not lead to improved long-term outcomes.

Optimal improvement and adherence may often be achieved by combining low doses of both of these treatments. In fact, low-intensity behavioral modification in combination with a low dose of methylphenidate (e.g., 0.15–0.3 mg/kg) produces behavioral change similar to that of a high dose of either treatment modality (Fabiano et al., 2007; Pelham, Manos, et al., 2005; Pelham et al., 2014). Combining low doses of both interventions allows the behavioral intervention to be sufficiently simple to facilitate teacher and parent administration of behavior management skills without prolonged consultation or intensive interventions. Furthermore, parents may be more likely to comply with lower doses of medication due to attenuated side effects. Additionally, parents tend to prefer treatment programs that include behavioral intervention over stimulant treatment alone (Schatz et al., 2015; Waschbusch et al., 2011). Therefore, a low dose of each treatment modality addresses adherence and maintenance concerns, increasing the likelihood that treatment will be consistently implemented over time.

At the same time, most parents prefer not to medicate their children with ADHD unless it is necessary. Some children are sufficiently responsive to an inexpensive and practical level of behavioral approach that they do not need medication—one-third of referred children in a recent study (Pelham et al., 2016). Since there is no way to predict in advance who these children are, it makes logical sense to begin with behavioral treatment and add medication (or more intensive behavioral treatment, depending on parent preference) for the two-thirds of referred children with ADHD who need more treatment. Furthermore, as we discuss in our conclusion, sequencing of administration of combined treatments may have important implications for outcome.

Other Treatments Considered

In the most recent review of evidence-based treatments, neurofeedback met Task Force criteria for a possibly efficacious treatment (Evans et al., 2014). Neurofeedback training involves a computer game in which children receive rewards for successfully regulating their own electrical neurological activity. In one study, neurofeedback was shown to have a significant effect on neural activity (Gevensleben et al., 2009). However, other studies show that, when parents and teachers are blind to treatment conditions, neurofeedback has smaller, and typically nonsignificant, effects on symptoms and problems in daily life functioning—particularly in classroom settings in which children with ADHD show highest levels of impairment and need for treatment (Chacko et al., 2014; Holtmann, Sonuga-Barke, Cortese, & Brandeis, 2014). Neurofeedback-related increases in the nature of a child's electroencephalographic (EEG) functioning is conceptually interesting but has no practical relevance for the children, their families, or their teachers. We do not believe that the evidence for neurofeedback is sufficiently strong to recommend it as an effective treatment for ADHD, despite its having met criteria in the Evans and colleagues (2014) review.

Predictors and Moderators of Treatment Response

Despite the routine search for predictors and moderators of treatment response, no variable has been consistently identified in treatment studies of children with ADHD as a predictor/moderator of treatment response (Fabiano et al., 2004; Owens et al., 2003).

When dozens of predictors have been employed in major trials, a few findings have been reported. For example in the MTA study, the presence of comorbid anxiety was found to be a small predictor of a positive response to behavioral intervention, but it is noteworthy that it was included in the study because it was hypothesized to predict (negatively) response to medication, which it did not (MTA Cooperative Group, 1999). We are not aware of any study that has replicated this finding. In general, children with ADHD respond to various behavioral treatments independent of comorbidities or other child characteristics. In part, this may be a reflection of how behavioral treatments are implemented both in studies and in practice. Target behaviors, or the child's difficulties that are most in need of treatment, are identified for all components of intervention (e.g., those involving parents, teachers, or peers). Those domains might have otherwise predicted response to treatment; however, over the course of treatment, such areas are typically uniquely identified to receive more targeted treatment (e.g., higher intensity or additional components) that, if successful, eliminates the effect of the moderating variable, thus limiting the ability to determine whether response would have otherwise been moderated.

The one area of exception is related to parent rather than child characteristics. Parental ADHD, parental depression, substance use, and family socioeconomic status appear to be associated with more parenting problems in families with children with ADHD (Johnston & Chronis, 2014). However, findings are mixed as to whether such variables moderate response to parent training (McMahon, Forehand, Griest, & Wells, 1981; Sonuga-Barke, Daley, & Thompson, 2002). Studies that have targeted these domains for unique variations in treatment have demonstrated some success (Chronis, Chacko, et al., 2004).

EVIDENCE-BASED ASSESSMENT AND TREATMENT IN PRACTICE

Assessment

Diagnostic Classification

The unifying principle of evidence-based ADHD assessment for childhood mental health disorders is the multimethod approach: Information is gathered from multiple informants, using multiple formats, about multiple domains of the child's life (Kamphaus & Frick, 2005; Mash & Hunsley, 2009). This approach also applies to the assessment of ADHD (Anastopoulos & Shelton, 2002; Barkley, 2015; Pelham, Fabiano, et al., 2005). The goal of assessment for ADHD extends much further than establishing a DSM diagnosis. A clinician must also select treatment targets, make a treatment plan, and monitor progress.

Initial Evaluation

Diagnosis is often necessary for administrative reasons, such as eligibility for school-based services, and health care reimbursement and inclusion in research studies (Pelham, Fabiano, et al., 2005), whereas the other components of assessment are crucial for conceptualizing the child's problems and developing a treatment plan that involves the three major domains of dysfunction discussed earlier: problems in the family, the school, and with peers. In this view, the goal of assessment is to provide effective treatment (Pelham, Fabiano, et al., 2005). The four steps of the initial ADHD evaluation are (1) systematically to gather symptom and impairment rating scales from key adults in the child's life, (2) interview primary caretakers to gather historical, contextual, and additional information regarding the child's presenting problems and the environmental factors that influence them; and (3) gather additional key information (e.g., the child's individualized educational plan [IEP], if applicable) and history of the problem, and select and administer additional measures suggested by Steps 1 and 2; and (4) synthesize the information, make a diagnosis, and develop a treatment plan.

Step 1: Gather Rating Scales of Symptoms and Impairment

This includes rating scales from multiple informants—always parents and teachers. Rating scales are easy and inexpensive to administer and score, take minimal rater and clinician time, and allow for comparison to normative samples (Pelham, Fabiano, et al., 2005). Narrowband rating scales allow efficient assessment of the presence and severity of DSM ADHD symptoms so that a DSM diagnosis can be reached. There are numerous commercially available ADHD rating scales (e.g., the ADHD Rating Scale; Power, Anastopoulos, & Reid, 1998), two that are freely available on the Internet: the Disruptive Behavior Disorders Rating Scale (DBD; downloadable at *www.ccf.fiu.edu*) and the Swanson, Nolan, and Pelham Rating Scale (SNAP; downloadable at *www.adhd.net*). A third scale derived from the DBD and the SNAP is widely available in pediatric settings at no cost (the Vanderbilt Rating Scale). All three of these list the DSM symptoms of ADHD and all (the DBDRS) or some of the DSM CD and ODD symptoms—the two most common comorbidities with ADHD. These DSM-based scales are typically implemented using the either–or rule; that is, if a symptom is indicated on the scale in the "pretty much" or "very much" columns by *either* the parent *or* the teacher, the symptom is counted as present. If the number of symptoms required by the DSM (discussed earlier) is present and the other inclusionary criteria for the diagnosis (discussed earlier) are met, then the diagnosis is considered present.

In addition to DSM-based scales, brief rating scales for identifying ADHD have been available for many years—for example, the Inattention/Overactivity with Aggression (IOWA) Conners Rating Scale (Loney & Milich, 1982) and the Attention Problems subscale of the CBCL (Achenbach & Rescorla, 2001). Pelham, Fabiano, and colleagues (2005) reviewed these non-DSM-based scales and concluded that they were as accurate as the DSM-based scales but considerably shorter and therefore easier for parents and teachers to complete.

These DSM-based scales ask only about the symptoms of ADHD—not impairment. Since impairment in multiple settings is required, rating scales assessing that construct have been developed. The simplest to use and lowest cost (free) scale is the Impairment Rating Scale (IRS; Fabiano et al., 2006). This scale asks about impairment across a variety of domains (e.g., parent–child relationship, academic, self-esteem), has good psychometric properties, and differentiates between clinical and nonclinical samples (Fabiano et al., 2006). Normative data are available for children (Fabiano et al., 2006) and adolescents (Evans et al., 2012). Following our logic regarding the goal of assessment, the IRS and other ratings of impairment are far more useful than the DSM symptom checklist because they identify the degree to which those symptoms cause problems in daily life functioning that warrant intervention.

In contrast to ADHD-specific scales, broadband rating scales allow normative comparison on a wide range of behaviors and assist with differential diagnosis of concurrent problems by serving as screening tools for comorbid conditions. The two most widely used are the CBCL and the accompanying Teacher Report Form (Achenbach & Rescorla, 2001) and the Behavioral Assessment System for Children (BASC; Reynolds & Kamphaus, 1998). These age- and gender-norm-referenced scales assess presence and severity of behaviors associated with a range of common childhood disorders (e.g., mood, anxiety, and disruptive behaviors). Using age and gender norms, these measures yield t-scores that allow clinicians to determine the extent to which reported symptoms are developmentally deviant. Furthermore, these measures serve as screeners for other disorders, informing differential diagnoses. Both of these rating scales include some items that assess impairment in various domains. Assessing impairment not only informs diagnoses but also identifies treatment targets.

It is worth noting that, for research purposes, many child psychologists and psychiatrists do not rely solely on rating scales, believing that interviews with the parents are necessary to confirm the presence of the child's ADHD symptoms. These interviews involve systematic questioning of the parents regarding the child's ADHD and comorbid symptoms to confirm a diagnosis. Two broad types of interviews have been developed and standardized—structured and semistructured. Fully structured interviews, such as the Computerized Diagnostic Interview Schedule for Children (C-DISC; Shaffer, Fisher, Lucas, Dulcan, & Schwab-Stone, 2000) and the Diagnostic Interview for Children and Adolescents (DICA; Reich, 2000) may be administered by lay interviewers. Semistructured interviews such as the Kiddie Schedule of Affective Disorders (K-SADS; Kaufman, Birmaher, Brent, Rao, & Ryan, 1996) and the DBD Parent Interview (Hartung, McCarthy, Milich, & Martin, 2005) are less rigid and more conversational but rely on the clinical judgment of experienced clinicians. Both types of interviews are very time consuming, taking 1–2 hours of parent and clinician time. Importantly, although more time consuming, these interviews do not provide any information that cannot be obtained through 15 minutes of parent time completing a narrowband symptom checklist.

Structured and semistructured interviews are the standard in the field for confirming a research diagnosis of ADHD. Pelham, Fabiano, and colleagues (2005) carefully reviewed the literature examining whether semistructured or structured diagnostic interviews added incremental utility to diagnoses made with rating scales alone, and whether the significant additional time and costs were justified by improvements in the validity of diagnosis of ADHD. They concluded that there was no incremental utility provided by these interviews. We therefore do not recommend them for use in clinical settings.

Step 2: Interview the Primary Caretakers

The cornerstone of the multimethod assessment approach is the clinical interview (Anastopoulos & Shelton, 2002; Mash & Hunsley, 2009). By reviewing written information collected in Step 1 and relying on that for making a diagnosis, clinicians will be able to devote their time during the clinical interview to providing a comprehensive history and description of the problems that have prompted the parents to seek treatment for their child, leading directly to a functional analysis of behavior, thus facilitating development of a treatment plan.

The traditional first question of a clinical interview (i.e., "What brings you here today?") initiates a conversation with parents about their child's difficulties in a way that flows naturally into a Functional Behavior Assessment (FBA; see Figure 12.1). Through the FBA, parents and the clinician clarify how environmental factors (parents, teachers, setting, time of day, etc.) interact to influence child behaviors and associated impairment (Bronfenbrenner, 1979; Kanfer & Grimm, 1977). The FBA allows the clinician to identify the antecedents and consequences of the primary behaviors contributing to impairment. Informed by ratings scales and the diagnostic interview, the parent and clinician work together to generate a list of presenting problems at home, at school, and with peers. Parents rank problem behaviors in terms of importance and select the most important target behaviors to explore more thoroughly (Kanfer & Grimm, 1977; Watson & Skinner, 2001). These target behaviors, which almost never coincide with DSM symptoms (Pelham, Fabiano, et al., 2005), are the treatment targets for intervention.

Together, clinician and parent discuss possible antecedents of the target behavior; the details of the behavior, including the overall severity, and variability in presence or severity of the behavior based on the time of day or environment; and the current consequences (including parenting practices) of the behavior. This exercise helps the parent and clinician elucidate the function of the behavior—what is maintaining the child's behavior and what can be changed to modify it. By discussing presenting problems in terms of the FBA, parents are set up to think in terms of social learning theory rather than in terms of DSM-5 symptoms. Additionally, using FBA during the clinical interview reduces diagnostic errors (Pelham, Fabiano, et al., 2005): For example, if a clinician focuses on symptom counts, he or she may misdiagnose children with many symptoms but no impairment—that is, children whose parents cannot identify problem behaviors to modify. For an extended review of FBA, we refer interested readers to Watson and Skinner (2001) and to *www.ccf.buffalo.edu* for assistance setting up an FBA.

After the FBA portion of the clinical interview, the following additional relevant information is collected to inform diagnosis and treatment planning: household composition, including primary caretakers and disciplinarians; current classroom functioning; past and present school placement, including history of special placements and accommodations; past and present grades; relationship with teachers and school personnel; purpose and results of any previous evaluations; and treatment history, including any past or present psychosocial or pharmacological treatment. It is also helpful to discuss the child's strengths. Much of the interview process focuses on a child's weaknesses and difficulties. Clinicians can use a discussion of strengths to develop a more complete picture of the child, leverage child and family strengths in treatment, and build rapport.

Step 3: Determine if Additional Information is Necessary

Following a comprehensive clinical interview, the clinician reviews the information gathered and determines what additional information is needed. Additional relevant information for a child with ADHD should include whether the child has a 504 plan or an IEP—two federal laws governing special services available to children with ADHD—and copies, if applicable, past academic records, records of medication history and other

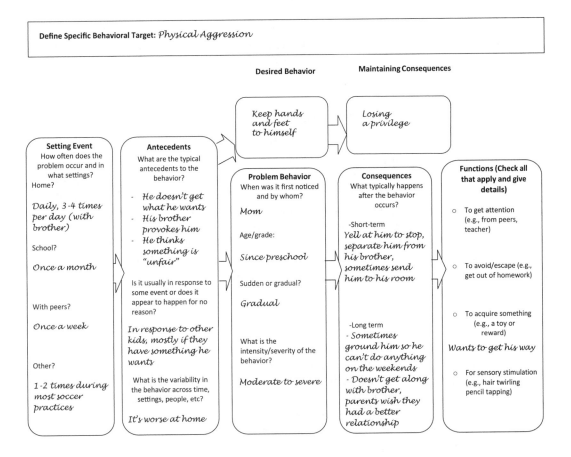

FIGURE 12.1. Functional analysis of behavior.

relevant medical problems, copies of previous evaluations, and other relevant information regarding child functioning or history that is indicated. Based on information collected in Steps 1 and 2, additional assessment may be necessary to clarify diagnoses. If broadband rating scales indicate elevated levels of symptoms of other disorders (e.g., mood or anxiety disorders) additional questionnaires or interviewing may be useful for differential diagnosis. For challenging cases, clinicians may also consider obtaining the ratings/impressions of additional caregivers in the child's life (e.g., babysitters, grandparents).

Despite the temptation, especially in medical settings, to add neurological evaluation or neuropsychological assessment, all of the guidelines for assessment of ADHD, most notably the American Academy of Pediatrics (2011) recommendations, note that no medical (e.g., neurological exam) or psychological (e.g., Wechsler Intelligence Scale for Children [WISC], Continuous Performance Test [CPT], neuropsychological battery) test or task is useful in ruling in (as opposed to ruling out) a diagnosis of ADHD (Pelham, Fabiano, et al., 2005). Even in the case of a comorbid learning disorder (LD), intelligence testing is not necessarily recommended (Fletcher, Francis, Morris, & Lyon, 2005), given the emphasis on a response to intervention (Sugai & Horner, 2009) model for identifying learning problems and resulting accommodations for children with academic difficulties in school. When differentiating between ADHD and LD, patterns of academic impairment often matter most. The academic impairment associated with ADHD is typically nonspecific rather than limited to one particular content area, as is frequently the case for specific LDs (Vile Junod, DuPaul, Jitendra, Volpe, & Cleary, 2006).

Step 4: Synthesize Information, Make a Diagnosis, and Develop a Treatment Plan

A comprehensive written report tells the story from the referral question to the treatment recommendations (Anastopoulos & Shelton, 2002) and serves as documentation of a diagnosis. State the reason for referral, history of presenting problems, developmental/ social/medical history, diagnostic impressions, and treatment recommendations. Use language that is easily interpretable, and define treatment recommendations very specifically. Ultimately, the role of the clinician during ADHD assessment is to be a detective. What is the diagnosis? What are the impairments? Why is this impairment occurring? What can be done to minimize the impairments and maximize adaptive functioning? When assessment revolves around impairment, treatment planning follows naturally.

Treatment

Behavioral Parent Training

The goal of BPT is to develop a comprehensive home behavior management plan individualized to the family's needs, abilities, resources, and preferences. This is typically accomplished over eight to 12 group or individual sessions using behavioral strategies from any one of a number of manuals (e.g., Barkley, 2013; Cunningham et al., 1993; McMahon & Forehand, 2005). As we noted earlier, the manuals all derive from a common set of principles—in fact, from the same parent training manual at the University of Oregon (Reitman & McMahon, 2013). Parents complete homework assignments throughout treatment to track child behavior and practice behavioral techniques at home. Therapist contact begins weekly and fades over time, and plans for maintenance (e.g., booster treatment sessions) after contact ends are made, so that parents are able to implement strategies effectively over the long-term. Common strategies from evidence-based manuals for a 10-session course of BPT are described below, from mildest to most intensive, which is the order in which they are presented in most manuals. These strategies need to be modified for young children (ages 3–5) and adolescents (age 12 and above), as described below and as indicated in the manuals available for those ages.

ESTABLISHING HOUSE RULES AND ROUTINES

Household routines and rules are antecedent control methods that help to create a structured environment, reducing the likelihood of problem behavior. Parents break routines and chores into manageable steps and set time limits for completion appropriate to children's developmental level. House rules represent expected behaviors, that is, behaviors that children should (or should not) do without parent prompts. Thus, parents do not give warnings when house rules are violated; rather, children receive an immediate consequence (e.g., time-out or other loss of privileges). Rules are also more effective when phrased in positive terms (e.g., "Obey adults") rather than negative (e.g., "Don't ignore parents"), teaching children what *to do* rather than what *not to do*. Once rules are established, parents discuss the rules with their children, and provide several examples to ensure that children understand. The rules are posted prominently to remind children of the rules and to help parents remember to monitor rules and apply consequences for violating the rules consistently.

EFFECTIVE COMMANDS AND REWARDING COMPLIANCE

Effective commands maximize the likelihood of compliance. Parents issue commands only when (1) they are willing to follow through with a consequence if the child does not comply and (2) the child has the ability and the attention span to complete the task. When giving commands, parents make eye contact and use the child's name to obtain his or her attention. The parent then gives a brief, direct, and specific command in a firm but neutral tone of voice, such as, "Johnny, please brush your teeth." After giving a command, the parent waits a few moments to give the child the opportunity to comply. Establishing a time limit (e.g., "10-second rule") for the child to begin to comply will help both parents and the child be consistent. Parents praise compliance and give a reprimand or time-out for instances of noncompliance. Some common ineffective commands are listed below:

- *"Let's" commands.* If a parent says, "Let's clean up the toys" when he or she means "Please clean up the toys," the child may expect the parent to help and therefore be less likely to comply.
- *Chain commands.* When parents link several instructions together (e.g., "Go upstairs, brush your teeth, put on your pajamas, and put your clothes in the hamper"), children—especially younger ones—are likely to lose track after the first or second command.
- *Vague commands.* Vague instructions (e.g., "Be good," "Stop that") are confusing to a child because they do not specifically tell the child *what to do*.
- *Buried commands.* Providing too much dialogue before and after the command makes it difficult for a child to attend to the command (e.g., "It's going to rain all day today so you need to go and get your umbrella before you leave the house. I don't want you coming home sopping wet like you did last time it rained!").

CONTINGENT ATTENTION

The function of many behaviors of children with behavioral problems is to gain parental attention (whether it be positive or negative). Therefore, providing and removing parental attention contingent on child behavior is likely to increase the frequency of appropriate behaviors and decrease the frequency of minor inappropriate behaviors. When praising appropriate behaviors, parents provide immediate, specific feedback about the behavior in a genuine and enthusiastic tone: "Thank you for sitting at the table so nicely!" Parents provide more frequent praise for new behaviors and refrain from "overdoing" it for routine behaviors. Parents can also use praise to gradually shape behaviors to the desired level. To help remind parents to "catch their child being good," encourage parents to praise at a rate of three positive comments for every one reprimand.

Conversely, active ignoring involves removing all verbal and nonverbal attention in response to minor inappropriate behavior. Active ignoring is often difficult for parents to implement consistently because when parents begin to target a behavior with planned ignoring, they may find that children initially escalate the frequency and intensity of the behavior (i.e., an *extinction burst*). With consistent implementation of active ignoring, children learn that the behavior no longer has the desired effect (e.g., getting their way, getting out of an undesirable activity) and the behaviors typically decrease over time.

TIME-OUT AND LOSS OF PRIVILEGES

During a time-out, all forms of positive reinforcement (e.g., parental attention, toys) are removed in response to serious negative behavior, such as aggression, destruction of property, or noncompliance to adult commands. Detailed descriptions for implementing time-outs are available in the BPT treatment manuals listed previously. In general, effective time-outs are held in an assigned location, away from reinforcing people or activities and last 2–3 minutes for preschool children and 5–10 minutes for elementary school–age children. Minor disruptive behaviors should be ignored during time-outs, and major rule violations may result in additional time on the clock or other consequences. Parents should look for opportunities to praise children as soon as possible after a time-out.

Time-outs are not appropriate for adolescents. For adolescents (age 12 and older), the removal of a privilege (e.g., use of the cell phone, hanging out with friends) is a more salient consequence than a time-out. If parents find that removing a privilege is not sufficient to manage serious negative behavior, they may also consider adding chores or other undesirable activities. Ideally, parents and teens discuss and agree on punishments ahead of time. If the consequence involves the removal of a privilege, parents must also specify time limits ahead of time to avoid restricting access for longer than is feasible (e.g., in the heat of the moment telling the adolescent he or she cannot play video games for 6 months).

HOME POINT SYSTEMS: REWARD AND RESPONSE COST METHODS

This low-cost intervention is designed to shape the frequency of target behaviors by rewarding children for meeting incremental behavioral goals. These reward systems integrate well with the home–school daily report card discussed below and can help bridge the gap between behavior at school and consequences at home. Home reward systems vary in complexity depending on individual needs. Premack contingencies, or "when–then" contingencies, are low-intensity reward systems that use desirable activities as rewards for completing tasks. Parents can use natural reinforcers (i.e., things children already get "for free" or noncontingently) as motivation to complete less desirable tasks such as homework and chores: For example, "*When* you have finished your homework, *then* you may watch TV for 30 minutes." Some children may require more intensive reward systems such as token economies or point systems that pair clear rules and expectations with frequent reinforcement for meeting expectations. Consequences for targeted behaviors involve tangible objects (e.g., marbles, poker chips, stickers) that may be traded in for rewards (e.g., screen time, access to a preferred toy).

Daily Report Card

	Special	Language Arts	Math	Reading	SS/Science	Special
1. Follows class rules with 3 or fewer rule violations per period	☺ ☹	☺ ☹	☺ ☹	☺ ☹	☺ ☹	☺ ☹
2. Completes assignments within the designated time	☺ ☹	☺ ☹	☺ ☹	☺ ☹	☺ ☹	☺ ☹
3. Completes assignments with 80% accuracy	☺ ☹	☺ ☹	☺ ☹	☺ ☹	☺ ☹	☺ ☹
4. Complies with teacher requests with three or fewer reminders	☺ ☹	☺ ☹	☺ ☹	☺ ☹	☺ ☹	☺ ☹

Other:

1. Follows recess rules with 3 or fewer reminders   ☺   ☹

Total number of yeses ____20____   Total number of nos ____5____   Percentage of yeses ____80% (20 yeses /25 total)____

Comments: *Johnny was daydreaming and had a hard time finishing work. He did a great job following classroom rules and listening to teachers today!*

FIGURE 12.2. Daily Report Card.

Token economies and point systems are most effective when they are tied to a home–school DRC (see Figure 12.2) and when they begin as a rewards program with response costs implemented only if needed, and only after an initial period of time with rewards only. The number of points children earn for engaging in target behaviors may vary according to the difficulty of the behavior and the frequency with which the child typically does the behavior without a problem. For point systems using response cost, points lost for undesirable behaviors should be comparable to the severity of the behavior. An effective response cost system will emphasize positive behaviors over negative behaviors, so that children earn more tokens than they lose.

Behavioral Classroom Management

The same behavioral principles employed in behavioral parenting intervention also apply to behavioral classroom management; however, there are important distinctions that necessitate using a different approach with teachers from that used with parents. Parents typically initiate the request for school-based services; yet teachers are the ones who are asked to implement the interventions. Teachers may not be adequately prepared to intervene with students with ADHD (Arcia, Frank, Sanchez-LaCay, & Fernandez, 2000; Reinke et al., 2011), especially in the general education classrooms in which most students with ADHD are placed. Furthermore, general education teachers often have many students, making it difficult to implement and monitor behavioral interventions effectively in the classroom. Given these challenges, we recommend a school consultation model, in which a consultant works together with teachers and, in some cases, parents to identify and analyze problem behaviors, implement treatment, and evaluate the effectiveness of treatment (Kratochwill & Bergan, 1990). For in-depth guides to clinician–teacher consultation models, the reader is referred to Kratochwill and Bergan (1990) and DuPaul and Stoner (2014), and for a description of the conjoint consultation model, in which the consultant works with both teachers and parents, the reader is referred to Sheridan and Kratochwill (2008).

Treatment planning and evaluation must be collaborative in nature, balancing the consultant's expertise in psychopathology and evidence-based behavioral interventions, the teacher's expertise in curriculum and classroom procedures, and the parents' expertise on their child (Sheridan & Kratochwill, 2008). Taking a collaborative approach helps to ensure that the intervention is viewed as feasible and acceptable to consultees, thereby increasing treatment engagement and potentially the fidelity with which treatment procedures are followed (Han & Weiss, 2005). To help increase consultee engagement, we recommend initiating a consultation by interviewing teachers to understand preferences regarding behavioral interventions and which strategies teachers already use in their classroom. The amount and frequency of consultation varies depending on the teacher's existing behavior management skills, classroom composition, and the complexity of the case. See *www.ccf.buffalo.edu* for an example teacher interview.

Begin with less-intensive strategies such as a home–school DRC. The DRC (described in detail below) has been rated favorably by teachers (Chafouleas, Riley-Tillman, & Sassu, 2006) and is effective as a stand-alone intervention (O'Leary, Pelham, Rosenbaum, & Price, 1976). If problems persist despite effective implementation of less-intensive strategies, more intensive interventions (as described below) may be added as resources allow.

If consultees are unfamiliar with any of the strategies selected, the consultant provides appropriate training. The number of sessions held between the consultant and teacher therefore depend on the teacher's experience with behavioral intervention and the specific treatment plan developed.

Regardless of the treatment plan developed, ongoing consultation is crucial to success of any behavioral program. An effective consultant maintains regular contact with consultees (by phone/e-mail or in person) to monitor the frequency of problem behaviors and the fidelity with which interventions are implemented. Together, the consultant and consultees use data to determine whether interventions are working to reduce problem behaviors and modify the program as necessary. Alternatively, consultants can train parents to take over treatment monitoring and evaluation (Wells et al., 2000).

In addition to the components listed below, interventions targeting academic success for students with ADHD may also include organizational and study skills training, and strategies for homework success. These strategies are not described in detail here, but interested readers are referred to the Homework, Organization and Planning Skills (HOPS) Intervention (Langberg, 2011) and the Homework Success for Children with ADHD program (Power, Karustis, & Habboushe, 2001) for older elementary school students and the Challenging Horizons Program (Evans et al., 2011) for adolescents.

CLASSROOM RULES

Organized and predictable classrooms reduce the likelihood of off-task and disruptive behavior (Paine, Radicchi, Deutchman, & Darch, 1983). Like house rules, classroom rules target behaviors that students are expected to do without prompts from the teacher (e.g., "Raise your hand," "Keep your hands to yourself"). Teachers should make frequent reference to the classroom rules and expected behaviors, and provide regular feedback regarding behaviors that are consistent and inconsistent with rules.

EFFECTIVE CLASSROOM INSTRUCTION

Teachers may use a number of strategies to promote student engagement, including the following: maintain a brisk pace of instruction, use verbal and nonverbal cues (e.g., putting fingers to lips for quiet, gently tapping on an off-task student's desk) to redirect inappropriate behavior, maintain eye contact to monitor student behavior and attention, and circulate through the classroom. When assigning independent work, teachers should check to see that students understand instructions and should communicate clear expectations for the use of class time. Additionally, teachers should cue children when transitioning from one activity to another, making clear the expectations related to the next activity.

CONTINGENT ATTENTION

Just as discussed with parents, one thing to emphasize with teachers is to catch children being good and provide praise for appropriate behaviors (DuPaul & Stoner, 2014). Active ignoring procedures differ from those in the home setting; however, disruptive students are often reinforced by both peer and teacher attention, making the removal of teacher attention alone an ineffective strategy. Instead, encourage teachers to praise "positive opposites," or behaviors that are incompatible with disruptive behavior. Once the disruptive child demonstrates appropriate behavior, the teacher should provide positive attention.

APPROPRIATE COMMANDS AND PRIVATE REPRIMANDS

Teachers should use the same procedures for giving effective commands as described earlier for parents. Private reprimands that are brief, unemotional, and given immediately following behavior are also an effective means of increasing compliance. Teachers should avoid public, emotional reprimands, as students may find the teacher's negative attention reinforcing, leading to an increase in disruptive behavior. The reader is referred to Abramowitz and O'Leary (1991) for a review of effective reprimands.

PREMACK CONTINGENCIES

As described earlier for parents, teachers can use preferred activities as motivators for children to complete less desired tasks (e.g., "When you finish your math worksheet, then you can go to recess").

DAILY REPORT CARDS

Teachers implement the intervention during the day and send the DRC home with the student, so that the parents are able to provide home-based reinforcement (using the reward systems described previously). A step-by-step guide for setting up a DRC can be found at *www.ccf.fiu.edu*. Much like the home-based reward system described earlier, parents and teachers (and sometimes also a clinician or consultant) meet to choose target behaviors (e.g., following classroom rules, academic productivity, peer and teacher relationships) and develop specific behavioral goals. During the class period, the DRC is kept on the student's desk. Each time the child exhibits a target behavior (e.g., interrupts), the teacher or the student marks the behavior on the DRC. Success at meeting goals should be evaluated periodically throughout the day according to the classroom schedule and the child's developmental level, with younger children requiring more frequent feedback. At the end of the day, children take the DRC home. This informs parents of the day's classroom behavior, and parents then provide the agreed-upon reward, if earned. Some children may require rewards during the school day as well.

As recommended for the home setting, token economies and response cost programs (described below for the school setting) are more effective means than are DRCs for shaping behavior in children younger than age 6. Initialing the agenda is an alternative to the home–school DRC that tends to be more agreeable to middle and high school students. The student is responsible for copying down homework assignments and for bringing the agenda to the teacher to sign. The teacher signs the agenda to confirm its accuracy and, if necessary, writes a note to parents regarding the student's behavior that day. The parents then use the agenda to monitor the teen's homework that evening and sign to indicate that the teen has completed the homework for the agenda, which is returned to the teacher the following day.

POINT SYSTEM/RESPONSE COST FOR THE INDIVIDUAL CHILD

As with the home setting, some children may require more immediate and tangible reinforcement in the form of a classroom token economy system (DuPaul & Stoner, 2014). The implementation of the token economy in the classroom setting is similar to that in the home setting and should be tied to classroom rules, so that students earn tokens (e.g., stickers, poker chips, tickets) for following classroom rules and meeting other predetermined expectations. Response cost procedures that deduct tokens for violating classroom rules may also be necessary for some children to meet classroom expectations (Chronis, Fabiano, et al., 2004; Fabiano et al., 2007). At the end of evaluation periods, tokens are tallied and exchanged for school-based rewards. Many teachers use point systems for all students in the classroom for following class rules, and a child with ADHD may need only a slight modification of this. If the teacher does not have a system like this, then setting up an individual point system for the child with ADHD may be needed and should be integrated with the DRC.

CLASSROOMWIDE INTERVENTIONS

Classroomwide interventions are designed to improve the learning and behavior of the entire class and are often implemented when a large portion of the students display inappropriate behavior or when students reinforce each other's negative behavior. See Pfiffner (2011) for a review.

- *Class-wide token economy.* When used with an entire class, teachers may use a public point board or a simplified color system to keep track of child behavior. Additionally, *ClassDojo* is a free, Internet-based program that allows teachers to award and deduct points in response to student behavior using a computer or mobile device. Points are displayed visually for students and shared with parents at the end of the day. As with point systems for individual children, tokens are exchanged for school- and/or home-based rewards.

- *Classroom lotteries.* In a classroom lottery system (Witt & Elliot, 1982), the teacher scans the room at preselected (but unannounced) 10- to 15-second intervals and records on the board the names of the students who were violating classroom rules. This procedure is repeated several times throughout the day, and at the end of the day, any students who followed the rules above the preselected criterion level (e.g., four of the five evaluated intervals) are entered into the lottery. The teacher should select five to 10 lottery winners, so that students who follow the rules the majority of the time have a reasonable chance of being rewarded. The reinforcers should be naturally occurring, such as the student jobs common in most classrooms (e.g., line leader, homework collector).

- *Good Behavior Game.* The "Good Behavior Game" (GBG; Barrish, Saunders, & Wolf, 1969; *www.interventioncentral.org/behavioral-intervention-modification*) divides the class into two teams, and the team with fewer classroom rule violations earns a group reward. Other group contingencies may involve earning a special Friday activity if the class has under a certain amount of rule violations, or earning daily free time based on the number of points the class has earned.

Behavioral Peer Interventions

One of the most difficult to treat domains of dysfunction in children with ADHD is their problems in peer relationships. Importantly, as we discussed earlier, this is one of the key domains that, arguably, moderates and mediates long-term outcome for children with ADHD. The home- and school-based contingency management strategies outlined earlier may be used to target and intervene with negative, peer-directed behaviors (e.g., teasing, annoying, interrupting, aggression) but are unlikely to be sufficient to maximally improve peer relationships. Additionally, decades of research indicate that pharmacological treatment does not normalize peer relationships among children with ADHD (e.g., Hinshaw, Henker, Whalen, Erhardt, & Dunnington, 1989; Pelham & Bender, 1982). Therefore, children with ADHD who experience impaired peer relationships need an effective behavioral peer intervention—usually combining a contingency management system applied at home through BPT and, as discussed earlier, in the classroom through BCM with a peer-relationship-focused component (see also Mikami et al., 2014).

These interventions are most effective when delivered in naturalistic group settings such as schools, afterschool programs, and summer camps (e.g., the STP; Pelham et al., 2010) and in the context of other activities in children's daily lives and through which their peer skills and relationships develop (e.g., sports, recess, games). We describe below a number of the components of the STP that can be incorporated in peer-relationship-focused interventions across a variety of settings.

The STP is an 8-week, 9 hours per day, packaged intervention that includes components of BPT, BCM and BPI (Pelham et al., 2010). Children are assigned to age-based groups with a dozen ADHD peers and four or five trained counselors who implement the treatment. The groups of children cycle through typical camp activities that include common children's sports (baseball, basketball, and soccer), art, swimming, classroom, recess, and transition periods. Peer intervention strategies used in the STP include brief (5-minute) social skills training discussions that occur at the beginning and end of each hour's activity, modeling of appropriate social skills by counselors, social reinforcement, a DRC to parents for using appropriate skills and individualized target behaviors, and a point/token system implemented throughout the day to provide point gain for prosocial behaviors and point loss for negative social behaviors. During recreational periods (4 hours daily), the focus is on teaching the rules and providing the intensive practice necessary to improve the sports skills of children with ADHD to a level that will help raise their status among peers and (we hope) generalize to neighborhood and school game activities. Such delivery models minimize misbehavior and allow for *in vivo* practice and coaching with peers to maximize the generalizability of learned skills. Teaching parents to reinforce peer relationship skills at home can help improve social outcomes (Pfiffner & McBurnett, 1997), and this is an integral component of STPs, school-based, and other peer-relationship-focused programs.

SOCIAL SKILLS TRAINING

Social skills training (SST) is a major component of behavioral peer interventions for ADHD. As noted earlier in this chapter and elsewhere (Evans et al., 2014; Mikami et al., 2014), traditional 1-hour SST sessions in clinics or therapist's offices have not been shown to be effective interventions for children with ADHD. At the same time, brief versions of SST that occur more frequently (e.g., multiple times daily in STP settings, daily in school-based programs) are ubiquitous in programs focused on social skills. SST involves teaching children to use general social skills, such as communication, participation, cooperation, and validation (Oden & Asher, 1977) and other more specific skills that vary depending on the particular program employed. In the STP, daily sessions begin with brief (i.e., 10-minute) discussions during which the group leader introduces the day's social skill. Children generate and role-play positive and negative examples of how the social skill can be used in the day's activities. The use of action figures or puppets often helps engage young children in social skills discussions and is incorporated in many social skills programs (e.g., Webster-Stratton et al., 2011). Similar but shorter and more targeted discussions occur at the beginning of each recreational activity, with children discussing how they will exhibit the daily social skill during the recreational activity. Throughout the activity, counselors model appropriate social behavior, provide positive reinforcement when children use appropriate social skills with peers, and coach children on how to use appropriate skills when opportunities arise. Following the recreational activity, the group participates in a short discussion to summarize how skills were used in the activity.

PROBLEM-SOLVING SKILLS

These are common aspects of many social-skills-based interventions, particularly those implemented in school settings (e.g., Lochman et al., 2010). In the STP, as conflicts arise, individual, small-group, and whole-group problem-solving discussions facilitate development of problem-solving skills (Spivack, Platt, & Shure, 1976). Group leaders begin discussions by identifying the problem and hearing all sides of the conflict. Next, participants generate solutions, identify pros and cons of solutions, and choose a solution. The group then writes the solution into a contract that is signed by all group members and includes the consequences that individuals or the group will experience if the contract is honored or broken. The selected solution is evaluated for effectiveness regularly and modified if necessary.

Another approach to problem solving is through peer-mediated conflict resolution in school settings (Cunningham et al., 1998). In this model, trained peer mediators are stationed in specific areas where conflict is likely to occur (e.g., hallways, playground). When conflicts arise, mediators approach disputants and engage in problem-solving discussions. This approach has been beneficial in several studies with elementary school-age students and can be incorporated in any group setting.

The general approach that we outlined earlier for an STP-based approach to BPI for children with ADHD has been adapted in a number of ways, some studied and validated, and others not. For example, the approach has been implemented in inner-city park programs (Frazier, Chacko, Van Gessel, O'Boyle, & Pelham, 2011), an inner-city, afterschool summer school program (O'Connor et al., 2012), and a Saturday Treatment Program (weekly groups for 8 weeks).

Monitoring and Modifying BPT, BCM, and BPI

Implicit throughout our discussion has been that assessment of the treated child's functioning continues throughout intervention and is the basis for treatment modification, addition, or deletion. Ongoing monitoring of function was discussed in a number of the texts we cited earlier regarding assessment of ADHD—particularly with respect to BCM. For a number of years, our clinic has used a simple and effective approach to monitoring children's function at home and at school during treatment—a modified version of the IRS (Fabiano et al., 2006). As noted earlier, this scale assesses functioning in several key domains of treatment and asks parents and teachers explicitly whether additional treatment is needed. We have added to that question an open-ended inquiry about what type of additional treatment is needed. We have parents and teachers complete the brief IRS monthly via telephone, e-mail, or on paper. If a child is receiving a DRC, which we ask parents and teachers to save, we also examine that to see how often a child is meeting his or her daily goals at school—an idiographic measure of the child's functioning (Pelham, Fabiano, et al., 2005). The therapist checks these sources monthly to determine whether additional treatment is needed and contacts parents and teachers as necessary. This process takes very little time on the part of parents, teachers, and therapists, but it provides important information regarding response to treatment and need for ongoing modification.

Case Example

The following abridged dialogue is from a fictionalized treatment case. Lucas is a first grader recently diagnosed with ADHD combined type. Lucas's mother, Ms. Garcia, has met with a clinician to review the results of the assessment and discuss treatment options. Ms. Garcia decided to start treatment with individual parent training sessions and a school consultation. Portions of these sessions are presented below.

SESSION 1: SOCIAL LEARNING THEORY

The goal of the first session is to review the child's major presenting problems, the parent's goals for treatment, and to introduce social learning theory. After establishing rapport, the therapist and Ms. Garcia discuss problem behaviors highlighted during assessment.

> THERAPIST: You said that the biggest problems at home are that he does not listen when you ask him to do something, morning and bedtime routines, finishing homework, and fighting with his sister.
>
> MS. GARCIA: That's the story of my life. Morning, noon, and night. Plus, I'm constantly getting calls from his teacher.
>
> THERAPIST: Your biggest concerns for Lucas at school were completing his work, calling out in class, and getting out of his seat.
>
> MS. GARCIA: Yeah, those are the big things. He got sent to the principal's office in April because he was singing and running around the classroom.
>
> THERAPIST: It's frustrating because these behaviors affect his grades, and make it hard for him to make friends.
>
> MS. GARCIA: Yeah, I feel bad for the little guy.
>
> THERAPIST: Has anything changed, or is there anything else you want to add to the problems list?

MS. GARCIA: There are a million things I'd like to fix, but I think this is a good place to start.

THERAPIST: Me, too. Before we go over solutions, I would like to know what you're hoping the result of all this change will be. What are some of the goals you have for treatment?

MS. GARCIA: I really want him to pass first grade. He's such a smart kid and I know he can do it. I guess I hope that he doesn't get in trouble at school, and that he finds a friend to hang out with on the weekends.

THERAPIST: We have a lot of work to do, but you know Lucas can succeed this year.

MS. GARCIA: Definitely. I just have no idea what I'm supposed to be doing.

THERAPIST: There are a lot of strategies that have been helpful for the other families we have worked with and we'll go over these strategies over the course of about 8 weeks or so.

They then discuss social learning theory and the ABC (antecedents, behaviors, and consequences) model, tying the discussion to the FBA conducted during the assessment. For homework, Ms. Garcia will begin to track Lucas's home target behaviors (noncompliance and fighting with his sister) using the ABC Tracking Sheet (Figure 12.3).

SESSION 2: ESTABLISHING HOUSE RULES AND ROUTINES

Each session begins with a review of the previous week's homework. At the start of the second session, the clinician and Ms. Garcia review the ABC Tracking Sheet, looking for patterns over the previous week that help explain Lucas's problem behaviors.

THERAPIST: You did an excellent job of tracking Lucas's behavior this week! Let's start with noncompliance. What patterns did you notice?

MS. GARCIA: Well, Lucas had the most trouble with listening to what I said when he was getting ready for school in the morning or when it was time to go to bed. Oh, and homework time, but that's always rough.

THERAPIST: What specifically about those times seems to make it tough for him to obey adults?

MS. GARCIA: He kept forgetting what he was supposed to be doing! In the morning, he starts to get dressed but then he gets distracted by the TV, or starts eating breakfast instead. I feel like a broken record because I just have to repeat myself over and over and he never listens!

THERAPIST: One thing that makes getting ready for school difficult is that Lucas has a tough time remembering everything he is supposed to do. What do you think might help him remember better?

The clinician then facilitates a conversation about establishing house rules and routines as a way to change the antecedents, or the settings in which unwanted behaviors occur. The clinician helps Ms. Garcia develop house rules that address target behaviors.

Operational definition of behavior being tracked: _____

Date/Time	Antecedents	Behavior	Consequences	Possible function	My thoughts/emotions

FIGURE 12.3. ABC Tracking Sheet.

For example, Ms. Garcia's house rules may include "Obey adults" and "Be respectful of others." Additionally, they discuss manageable routines for Lucas and role-play how Ms. Garcia might introduce the new procedures to Lucas and his sister. For homework, Ms. Garcia will use the ABC Tracking Sheet to record the frequency of rule violations. For now, Ms. Garcia will do whatever she normally does in response to those behaviors (as long as typical practices do not endanger the child).

SESSION 3: EFFECTIVE COMMANDS AND REWARDING COMPLIANCE

After reviewing homework and looking for patterns, the clinician and Ms. Garcia discuss effective commands as another antecedent strategy for increasing Lucas's compliance. The therapist and Ms. Garcia role-play using effective commands and discuss the importance of rewarding compliance.

> THERAPIST: We talked about giving good commands as one way of getting Lucas to listen to directions more often. Another way to increase compliance is to change what happens after his behavior. What currently happens when Lucas does what he's told?
>
> MS. GARCIA: Well, I spend most of the time yelling at him because he didn't follow directions. I've never really thought about what happens when he actually does it.
>
> THERAPIST: When Lucas doesn't listen he gets a lot of negative attention. What do you think you could do when he does listen?
>
> MS. GARCIA: I guess I could give him attention for that, too, so I'm not just yelling at him all the time.
>
> THERAPIST: What if you say something positive to him when he listens? What do you think will happen over time?
>
> MS. GARCIA: Well, if I keep giving him attention for doing the right thing, he might do that more.
>
> THERAPIST: Paying attention to positive behavior might make it happen more often. And what would it look like to give him attention for listening?
>
> MS. GARCIA: Well, after he does what he's told, instead of just asking him to do something else, I could say "Thank you" or "Nice job."

For homework, Ms. Garcia will track the commands she gives Lucas, his response (i.e., compliance or noncompliance), and the consequences (e.g., praise for listening).

SESSION 4: CONTINGENT ATTENTION

After reviewing homework, the clinician explains that the same strategy (i.e., praise) can be used to increase any positive behavior. The clinician and Ms. Garcia practice using praise in response to appropriate behaviors, then create a list of Lucas's behaviors to try to increase with praise, including compliance and getting along with his sister. The clinician should also introduce the removal of parent attention to decrease unwanted behaviors.

THERAPIST: When you didn't look at Lucas or talk to him when he tried to interrupt you while you were on the phone, it happened less often. How do you think you could use this strategy with behaviors you want to see less of?

MS. GARCIA: I guess I could ignore those things like you said. It would be really hard though. And what if I ignored the whining? He would probably just keep doing it until I gave in!

THERAPIST: You bring up a really important point. When you first start ignoring these behaviors, things could get worse before they get better.

MS. GARCIA: Yeah! He might learn that he just has to annoy me even more to get what he wants.

THERAPIST: What if you didn't give in, what would happen over time?

MS. GARCIA: Hmm, I hadn't thought of that. I usually always end up giving in. I guess if I didn't give in he might try a few more times, but eventually he would probably get sick of trying, like what happened with the phone. He would probably learn that complaining and begging aren't going to get him his way.

THERAPIST: So if you use ignoring, his behavior might get worse at first, but over time, as long as you stay consistent, it is likely to go away.

MS. GARCIA: Hopefully!

After discussing the strategy of planned ignoring, the therapist and Ms. Garcia develop a list of behaviors she would like to decrease by using ignoring. For homework, Ms. Garcia will track her use of praise and ignoring.

SESSION 5: TIME-OUT AND LOSS OF PRIVILEGE

While reviewing homework, Ms. Garcia reports that Lucas has become much more compliant since she has been implementing home routines, working on her commands, and praising him for his efforts. However, she has noticed that he still fights with his sister very frequently. This week, the therapist introduces time-out as another strategy for reducing the frequency of unwanted behaviors.

THERAPIST: You want to help Lucas get along better with his sister. What are some consequences that you could use when Lucas breaks the house rule to be respectful?

MS. GARCIA: Well, for his older sister, we ground her when she breaks the rules. No phone, no TV—just school and homework. She is different, though. If we grounded Lucas, it would be like that every weekend.

THERAPIST: You feel like you're not disciplining Lucas enough right now, but you don't like the other options you have.

MS. GARCIA: None of it really works. We tried time-out last year, but like we talked about last week, he complains so much.

THERAPIST: What was good about using time out at your house?

Ms. Garcia: Well it was easier to control him when we weren't in public. I could see his time-out chair from our kitchen and I could keep doing other things while he was in time-out.

Therapist: Even though Lucas whined, time-outs let you get things done.

Ms. Garcia: Yeah, time went by much quicker when I ignored the whining.

Therapist: There are some behaviors you're willing to ignore during time-out, and you're getting better at using that skill. What are some things you think shouldn't be ignored during time-out?

Ms. Garcia: Well, if he's bleeding. Or, if he runs away from the time-out area.

Therapist: Only safety concerns and major rule violations should get attention during time-out. What are some behaviors you are willing to ignore?

Ms. Garcia: I know I need to ignore that "Is it over, Mommy?" routine. I hate to say it, but I should probably ignore his crying and whimpering, too.

Therapist: You know what you need to ignore, but sometimes it's hard to follow through.

Ms. Garcia: Especially at the end of a long day at work, it's just so tough to deal with him. Sometimes he gets in two time-outs in a row. It's easier if he just watches TV while I cook dinner.

Therapist: It must be really hard when Lucas has two time-outs in a row. What does it look like when that happens?

Ms. Garcia: Well, he just cries and whines and one time-out just blends right in to the next one.

Therapist: What do you think you could do differently to help with this problem?

Ms. Garcia: I guess I could wait until he calms down.

Therapist: Some of the families we have worked with have found that it helps to wait until there is about a minute of quiet.

Ms. Garcia: I could try that.

Therapist: What else is a problem when Lucas gets into a couple of time-outs in a row?

Ms. Garcia: I don't know. He just keeps doing the bad behavior, I guess. By the end of it all, we both forget what the time-out even started for.

Therapist: What do you think you could do to change that?

Ms. Garcia: I guess I could remind him why he had the time-out.

Therapist: What would that look like?

Ms. Garcia: I could say something like, "Lucas, you're done with time-out now; you were in time-out because you hit your sister."

Therapist: So briefly explaining why he was in time-out in a calm tone of voice. What do you think you could do next?

The therapist and Ms. Garcia also role-play how Ms. Garcia will discuss time-outs with Lucas and his sister. For homework, Ms. Garcia will explain the time-out procedure and practice giving time-outs in response to serious negative behaviors.

SESSION 6: HOME REWARD SYSTEM

Time-out is typically a challenging strategy for parents to implement; therefore, the therapist carefully reviews the time-out homework and troubleshoots any issues from the previous week. Next, the clinician and Ms. Garcia discuss behaviors that continue to be a problem for Lucas. The clinician discusses strategies for rewarding behaviors at home, such as Premack contingencies and the home reward systems described in detail earlier. Ms. Garcia and the therapist establish appropriate behavioral targets and a home reward system. Lucas's behavioral targets include follows house rules with two or fewer reminders, completes homework assignments within the specified time, and completes morning and evening routines according to his checklists. For homework, Ms. Garcia implements the new system. Ms. Garcia will try out the reward system for a few weeks before the next session. In between sessions, the clinician will call Ms. Garcia to monitor implementation.

SESSION 7: SCHOOL–HOME DRC

Ms. Garcia reports that the combination of the home reward system, time-out, and the antecedent control procedures have been working well to manage Lucas's home behavior. However, his teacher is still complaining that he is disruptive in class and is constantly getting out of his seat, which is making it difficult for him to complete assignments. The clinician introduces the concept of a school–home DRC (described in detail earlier) to address school behaviors with at home rewards and consequences. The clinician talks with Ms. Garcia about strategies to work with Lucas's teacher to develop and implement a DRC, including options for school consultations. Ms. Garcia and the clinician also plan how the DRC will be incorporated into the existing home reward system. Following this session, at Ms. Garcia's request, the clinician meets with Lucas's teacher for a school consultation to set up the DRC.

SESSION 8: GENERALIZING STRATEGIES TO OTHER SETTINGS

After reviewing implementation of the DRC, the therapist works with Ms. Garcia to generalize strategies discussed in previous sessions to other settings outside the home. In particular, they discuss strategies for implementing time-out in public, something Ms. Garcia has found challenging in the past.

SESSION 9: MAINTAINING GAINS AFTER THE PROGRAM ENDS

Ms. Garcia and the therapist develop a plan for maintaining behavioral gains. This may involve coming back to the clinic for "booster" sessions or developing a plan to tackle new behaviors as they arise. The goal of treatment is to hand the reigns over to the parents, but the clinician must be careful not to do so prematurely. While parent training typically occurs over eight to 10 sessions, this is just a guideline. Some parents master skills in fewer sessions, while others require more sessions to be able to apply strategies competently on their own. Therefore, the therapist encourages the parent to try techniques independently, but should be available if there are difficulties.

CONCLUSION: SEQUENCING, DOSING, AND COMBINING TREATMENTS IN CLINICAL PRACTICE

We have discussed in some detail the three components of evidence-based psychosocial treatment for ADHD—BPT, BCM, and BPI—and have described how to implement these interventions for children with ADHD when indicated. We have only briefly discussed pharmacological and combined/multimodal treatments for ADHD because the focus of this text is on psychosocial treatments. However, ADHD is a special case among child mental health problems. It is the only diagnosis in which the majority of the diagnosed population in the United States is treated with a psychoactive drug as the first-line treatment. Other diagnostic categories of child mental health problems do not even come close to this percentage. Thus, it is not only prudent but also necessary to discuss the ways in which evidence-based psychological interventions can be implemented in conjunction with pharmacological approaches.

Prominent psychiatric and pediatric guidelines recommend combining treatment modalities (American Academy of Child and Adolescent Psychiatry, 2007; American Academy of Pediatrics, 2011; American Psychological Association [APA] Working Group on Psychoactive Medications for Children and Adolescents, 2006). However, they provide little guidance surrounding the sequencing and intensity of treatments. What is the best dose and combination of treatments for a child with ADHD in clinical practice? Should treatment begin with behavioral intervention or with medication? What is the best "dose" of initial treatment? Should the other modality be added or should the initial treatment be intensified if initial response is insufficient? In the most prominent combined treatment study in the literature (MTA Cooperative Group, 1999), high starting "doses" of both treatments were employed, all treatments began simultaneously, and the combined treatment group received high doses of both modalities. Thus, the cost of behavioral treatment was very high, and concerning side effects (a loss in rate of growth) occurred with medication. In addition, there were few advantages of the combined treatment condition over the component conditions.

Over the past decade, a number of studies have explored (1) whether lower doses of each modality of treatment than employed in the MTA Study might be effective and (2) whether combinations of low doses of each might have incremental benefit over higher doses (e.g., stronger effects, lower side effects, and lower costs). These tightly controlled, within-subject studies have suggested that much of the benefit of behavioral treatments (BPT, BCM, and BPI) and medication occur at relatively low-dose levels for a substantial percentage of children, and that combining these low-dose components yields an intervention with larger main effects and a lower rate of adverse effects of medication (i.e., side effects) compared to unimodal treatments (Fabiano et al., 2007; Pelham, Fabiano, et al., 2005; Pelham et al., 2014, 2016). Therefore, this research suggests that beginning treatment with a low dose of behavioral intervention might be the best approach to treating ADHD, with medication or more intensive behavioral treatment added as necessary.

The most recent study in this series (Page, Pelham, et al., 2016; Pelham et al., 2016) employed a unique sequential, multiple-assignment, randomized trial (SMART) to compare starting treatment with random assignment to a low dose of behavioral intervention (BFirst; eight sessions of group BPT and three brief teacher consultations to establish a DRC) or a low dose of MPH (MFirst; .15 mg/kg per dose twice a day) on school days only. Response was monitored in the classroom and at home, and children whose functioning showed a need for more treatment were rerandomized to receive either a higher dose of the modality with which they began, or the addition of an adaptive version of the other modality. Treatment continued for a school year. Thus, this study asked which treatment is best to start, and if intervention is insufficient, what is the best strategy for second-stage treatment?

The results had important implications for the questions we posed earlier regarding behavioral treatments in practice. First, a substantial number of children did not require rerandomization in school in the BFirst (33%) and MFirst (53%) groups. Children who began treatment with a low dose of BPT/BCM had significantly better primary endpoint outcome scores than did children who started with medication. Furthermore, children who followed the BFirst protocol that began with BPT/BCM and had medication added if necessary had substantially better outcomes than children in the MFirst protocol with the opposite sequence. The reason for this difference appeared to be that parents assigned to BPT as a second-stage treatment when needed had extremely poor uptake of BPT and therefore never actually received a multimodal treatment intervention. Furthermore, the BFirst intervention had substantially lower costs compared to the MFirst condition.

Thus, these studies addressed the questions we posed earlier regarding treatment of ADHD in clinical practice, demonstrating that beginning treatment with a low dose of behavioral treatment or medication treatment—lower doses than typical in the literature—was sufficient for a large percentage of both starting groups. However, starting with BPT/BCM was superior to starting with medication in outcome and cost. Furthermore, for children who were not sufficiently responsive to low doses, adding a low dose of medication to initial behavioral treatment was a far more effective and less expensive treatment than the opposite protocol.

Several years ago, we proposed a Buffalo Treatment Algorithm (Pelham, 2008) advocating this approach to treatment. The only variable we outlined in that article that has not yet been discussed is parent preference for treatment. We suggest that if additional intervention is needed following initial BPT/BCM/BPI, then parents should be presented with the choice of whether to add more intensive behavioral treatment or to add a low dose of medication, and that the risks and benefits of each approach be discussed with parents. Notably, in the SMART trial described earlier, adding more intensive behavioral intervention was as effective as adding medication to initial low-dose behavioral treatment and was in fact less costly than adding medication.

Thus, parents have a choice to make, based on how much effort they would like to invest or have their child's school/agency/insurer invest in their child's treatment—additional sessions of BPT and prompting the school or agency to engage in additional BCM/BPI or moving to medication. On the one hand, behavioral interventions require more effort on everyone's part; on the other hand, no evidence of a long-term benefit of adding medication to treatment has ever been documented. An effective therapist will lay out the facts for parents, encourage them to consider their short- and long-term goals and circumstances, and support them in their choice (practitioners and parents are referred to *www.ccf.fiu.edu* and *www.indices4kids.com* for a wealth of information on implementing evidence-based treatments). If routinely implemented, this approach would have important consequences for treatment of children with ADHD in the United States. Many fewer children would be medicated, more parents would be actively engaged in their children's treatment, and societal costs for treatment of children with ADHD would be substantially reduced.

REFERENCES

Abikoff, H., Abramowitz, A., Courtney, M., Cousins, L., Del Carmen, R., Eddy, M., et al. (1994). *Parent training manual: MTA study.* Unpublished manuscript.

Abramowitz, A. J., & O'Leary, S. G. (1991). Behavioral interventions for the classroom: Implications for students with ADHD. *School Psychology Review, 20*(2), 220–235.

Achenbach, T. M., & Rescorla, L. (2001). *ASEBA school-age forms and profiles.* Burlington, VT: ASEBA.

Altszuler, A. R., Page, T. F., Gnagy, E. M., Coxe, S., Arrieta, A., Molina, B. S. G., et al. (2016). Financial dependence of young adults with ADHD. *Journal of Abnormal Child Psychology, 44*(6), 1217–1229.

American Academy of Child and Adolescent Psychiatry. (2007). Practice parameter for the assessment and treatment of children and adolescents with attention-deficit/hyperactivity disorder. *Journal of the American Academy of Child and Adolescent Psychiatry, 46*(7), 894–921.

American Academy of Pediatrics: Subcommittee on Attention-Deficit/Hyperactivity Disorder, Steering Committee on Quality Improvement and Management. (2011). ADHD: Clinical practice guideline for the diagnosis, evaluation, and treatment of attention-deficit/hyperactivity disorder in children and adolescents. *Pediatrics, 128*(5), 1007–1022.

American Psychiatric Association. (2013). *Diagnostic and statistical manual of mental disorders* (5th ed.). Arlington, VA: Author.

Anastopoulos, A. D., & Shelton, T. L. (2002). *Assessing attention-deficit/hyperactivity disorder.* Boston: Springer.

Anastopoulos, A. D., Sommer, J. L., & Schatz, N. K. (2009). ADHD and family functioning. *Current Attention Disorders Reports, 1,* 167–170.

APA Working Group on Psychoactive Medications for Children and Adolescents. (2006). *Report of the Working Group on Psychoactive Medications for Children and Adolescents: Psychopharmacological, psychosocial, and combined interventions for childhood disorders: Evidence base, contextual factors, and future directions.* Washington, DC: American Psychological Association. Available at *www.apa.org/pi/cyf/childmeds/pdf.*

Arcia, E., Frank, R., Sanchez-LaCay, A., & Fernandez, M. C. (2000). Teacher understanding of ADHD as reflected in attributions and classroom strategies. *Journal of Attention Disorders, 4*(2), 91–101.

Barkley, R. A. (2013). *Defiant children: A clinician's manual for assessment and parent training* (2nd ed.). New York: Guilford Press.

Barkley, R. A. (Ed.). (2015). *Attention-deficit hyperactivity disorder: A handbook for diagnosis and treatment* (4th ed.). New York: Guilford Press.

Barkley, R. A., Edwards, G., Laneri, M., Fletcher, K., & Metevia, L. (2001). The efficacy of problem-solving communication training alone, behavior management training alone, and their combination for parent–adolescent conflict in teenagers with ADHD and ODD. *Journal of Consulting and Clinical Psychology, 69*(6), 926–941.

Barkley, R. A., Murphy, K. R., & Fischer, M. (2010). *ADHD in adults: What the science says.* New York: Guilford Press.

Baroni, A., & Castellanos, F. X. (2015). Neuroanatomic and cognitive abnormalities in attention-defict/hyperactivity disorder in the era of "high definition" neuroimaging. *Current Opinion in Neurobiology, 30,* 1–8.

Barrish, H. H., Saunders, M., & Wolf, M. M. (1969). Good behavior game: Effects of individual contingencies for group consequences on disruptive behavior in a classroom. *Journal of Applied Behavior Analysis, 2*(2), 119–124.

Biederman, J., Faraone, S. V., & Monuteaux, M. C. (2002). Differential effect of environmental adversity by gender: Rutter's index of adversity in a group of boys and girls with and without ADHD. *American Journal of Psychiatry, 159*(9), 1556–1562.

Biswas, A., Gnagy, E., Molina, B., & Pelham, W. (2009). *Examining the decline in treatment usage in adolescents with attention deficit hyperactivity disorder.* Poster presented at the annual meeting of the Association of Behavioral and Cognitive Therapies, New York.

Brennan, E. M., Bradley, J. R., Allen, M. D., & Perry, D. F. (2008). The evidence base for mental health consultation in early childhood settings: Research synthesis addressing staff and program outcomes. *Early Education and Development, 19*(6), 982–1022.

Bronfenbrenner, U. (1979). *The ecology of human development: Experiments by nature and design.* Cambridge, MA: Harvard University Press.

Centers for Disease Control and Prevention. (2016). ADHD in young children: Use recommended treatment first. Retrieved from *www.cdc.gov/vitalsigns/pdf/2016–05-vitalsigns.pdf.*

Chacko, A., Bedard, A. C., Marks, D. J., Feirsen, N., Uderman, J. Z., Chimiklis, A., et al. (2014). A randomized clinical trial of Cogmed Working Memory Training in school-age children with ADHD: A replication in a diverse sample using a control condition. *Journal of Child Psychology and Psychiatry, 55*(3), 247–255.

Chafouleas, S. M., Riley-Tillman, T. C., & Sassu, K. A. (2006). Acceptability and reported use of daily behavior report cards among teachers. *Journal of Positive Behavior Interventions, 8*(3), 174–182.

Chronis, A. M., Chacko, A., Fabiano, G. A., Wymbs, B. T., & Pelham, W. E. (2004). Enhancements to the behavioral parent training paradigm for families of children with ADHD: Review and future directions. *Clinical Child and Family Psychology Review, 7*(1), 1–27.

Chronis, A. M., Fabiano, G. A., Gnagy, E. M., Onyango, A. N., Pelham, W. E., Lopez-Williams, A., et al. (2004). An evaluation of the summer treatment program for children with attention-deficit/hyperactivity disorder using a treatment withdrawal design. *Behavior Therapy, 35*(3), 561–585.

Cortese, S., Kelly, C., Chabernaud, C., Proal, E., Di Martino, A., Milham, M. P., et al. (2012). Toward systems of neuroscience of ADHD: A meta-analysis of 55 fMRI studies. *American Journal of Psychiatry, 169,* 1038–1055.

Cunningham, C. E., Bremner, R., & Secord-Gilbert, M. (1993). *A school-based family systems oriented course for parents of children with disruptive behavior disorders (Leader's manual).* Hamilton, ON, Canada: McMaster University.

Cunningham, C. E., Cunningham, L. J., Martorelli, V., Tran, A., Young, J., & Zacharias, R. (1998). The effects of primary division, student-mediated conflict resolution programs on playground aggression. *Journal of Child Psychology and Psychiatry and Allied Disciplines, 39*(5), 653–662.

Danckaerts, M., Sonuga-Barke, E. J. S., Banaschewski, T., Buitelaar, J., Döpfner, M., Hollis, C., et al. (2010). The quality of life of children with attention deficit/hyperactivity disorder: A systematic review. *European Child and Adolescent Psychiatry, 19*(2), 83–105.

DuPaul, G. J., Eckert, T. L., & Vilardo, B. (2012). The effects of school-based interventions for attention deficit hyperactivity disorder: A meta-analysis 1996–2010. *School Psychology Review, 41*(4), 387–412.

DuPaul, G. J., & Jimerson, S. R. (2014). Assessing, understanding, and supporting students with

ADHD at school: Contemporary science, practice, and policy. *School Psychology Quarterly,* *29*(4), 379–384.

DuPaul, G. J., & Stoner, G. (2014). *ADHD in the schools: Assessment and intervention strategies* (3rd ed.). New York: Guilford Press.

Eccles, J. S., & Roeser, R. W. (2004). Schools, academic motivation, and stage-environment fit. In R. M. Lerner & L. Steinberg (Eds.), *Handbook of adolescent psychology* (2nd ed., pp. 125–153). Hoboken, NJ: Wiley.

Evans, S. W., Brady, C. E., Harrison, J. R., Bunford, N., Kern, L., State, T., et al. (2012). Measuring ADHD and ODD symptoms and impairment using high school teachers' ratings. *Journal of Clinical Child and Adolescent Psychology, 42*(2), 197–207.

Evans, S. W., Owens, J. S., & Bunford, N. (2014). Evidence-based psychosocial treatments for children and adolescents with attention-deficit/hyperactivity disorder. *Journal of Clinical Child and Adolscent Psychology, 43*(4), 527–551.

Evans, S. W., Pelham, W. E., Smith, B. H., Bukstein, O., Gnagy, E. M., Greiner, A. R., et al. (2001). Dose–response effects of methylphenidate on ecologically valid measures of academic performance and classroom behavior in adolescents with ADHD. *Experimental and Clinical Psychopharmacology, 9*(2), 163–175.

Evans, S. W., Schultz, B. K., Demars, C. E., & Davis, H. (2011). Effectiveness of the Challenging Horizons After-School Program for young adolescents with ADHD. *Behavior Therapy, 42*(3), 462–474.

Eyberg, S. M., Funderburk, B. W., Hembree-Kigin, T. L., McNeil, C. B., Querido, J. G., & Hood, K. K. (2001). Parent–child interaction therapy with behavior problem children: One- and two-year maintenance of treatment effects in the family. *Child and Family Behavior Therapy, 23*(4), 1–20.

Fabiano, G. A., Hulme, K., Linke, S., Nelson-Tuttle, C., Pariseau, M., Gangloff, B., et al. (2011). The Supporting a Teen's Effective Entry to the Roadway (STEER) program: Feasibility and preliminary support for a psychosocial intervention for teenage drivers with ADHD. *Cognitive and Behavioral Practice, 18*(2), 267–280.

Fabiano, G. A., Pelham, W. E., Coles, E. K., Gnagy, E. M., Chronis-Tuscano, A., & O'Connor, B. C. (2009). A meta-analysis of behavioral treatments for attention-deficit/hyperactivity disorder. *Clinical Psychology Review, 29*(2), 129–140.

Fabiano, G. A., Pelham, W. E., Gnagy, E. M., Burrows-MacLean, L., Coles, E. K., Chacko, A., et al. (2007). The single and combined effects of multiple intensities of behavior modification and methylphenidate for children with attention deficit hyperactivity disorder in a classroom setting. *School Psychology Review, 36*(2), 195–216.

Fabiano, G. A., Pelham, W. E., Manos, M. J., Gnagy, E. M., Chronis, A. M., Onyango, A. N., et al. (2004). An evaluation of three time-out procedures for children with attention-deficit/hyperactivity disorder. *Behavior Therapy, 35,* 449–469.

Fabiano, G. A., Pelham, W. E., Jr., Waschbusch, D. A., Gnagy, E. M., Lahey, B. B., Chronis, A. M., et al. (2006). A practical measure of impairment: Psychometric properties of the Impairment Rating Scale in samples of children with attention deficit hyperactivity disorder and two school-based samples. *Journal of Clinical Child and Adolescent Psychology, 35*(3), 369–385.

Fabiano, G. A., Schatz, N. K., Aloe, A. M., Chacko, A., & Chronis-Tuscano, A. (2015). A systematic review of meta-analyses of psychosocial treatment for attention-deficit/hyperactivity disorder. *Clinical Child and Family Psychology Review, 18,* 77–97.

Fabiano, G., Vujnovic, R. K., Pelham, W. E., Waschbusch, D. A., Massetti, G. M., Pariseau, M. E., et al. (2010). Enhancing the effectiveness of special education programming for children with attention deficit hyperactivity disorder using a daily report card. *School Psychology Review, 39*(2), 219–239.

Faraone, S. V., Biederman, J., Spencer, T. J., & Aleardi, M. (2006). Comparing the efficacy of medications for ADHD using meta-analysis. *Medscape General Medicine, 8*(4), 4.

Faraone, S. V., & Buitelaar, J. (2010). Comparing the efficacy of stimulants for ADHD in children and adolescents using meta-analysis. *European Child and Adolescent Psychiatry, 19*(4), 353–364.

Faraone, S. V., & Mick, E. (2011). Molecular genetics of attention deficit hyperactivity disorder. *Psychiatric Clinics of North America, 33*(1), 1–20.

Fletcher, J. M., Francis, D. J., Morris, R. D., & Lyon, G. R. (2005). Evidence-based assessment of learning disabilities in children and adolescents. *Journal of Clinical Child and Adolescent Psychology, 34*(3), 506–522.

Frazier, S. L., Chacko, A., Van Gessel, C., O'Boyle, C., & Pelham, W. E. (2012). The summer treatment program meets the south side of Chicago: Bridging science and service in urban after-school programs. *Child and Adolescent Mental Health, 17*(2), 86–92.

Gevensleben, H., Holl, B., Albrecht, B., Schlamp, D., Kratz, O., Studer, P., et al. (2009). Distinct EEG effects related to neurofeedback training in children with ADHD: A randomized controlled trial. *International Journal of Psychophysiology, 74*(2), 149–157.

Gilliam, W. S., & Shahar, G. (2006). Preschool and child care expulsion and suspension: Rates and predictors in one state. *Infants and Young Children, 19*(3), 228–245.

Gorman-Smith, D., & Metropolitan Area Child Study Research Group. (2003). Effects of teacher training and consultation on teacher behavior toward students at high risk for aggression. *Behavior Therapy, 34*, 437–452.

Graziano, P. A., Slavec, J., Hart, K., Garcia, A., & Pelham, W. E. (2014). Improving school readiness in preschoolers with behavior problems: Results from a summer treatment program. *Journal of Psychopathology and Behavioral Assessment, 36*(4), 555–569.

Gutkin, T. B., & Reynolds, C. R. (Eds.). (2009). *The handbook of school psychology* (4th ed.). Hoboken, NJ: Wiley.

Han, S. S., & Weiss, B. (2005). Sustainability of teacher implementation of school-based mental health programs. *Journal of Abnormal Child Psychology, 33*(6), 665–679.

Hart, K. C., Fabiano, G. A., Pelham, W. E., Jr., Evans, S. W., Manos, M. J., Hannah, J. N., et al. (2016). Elementary and middle school teachers' self-reported use of positive behavioral supports for children with ADHD: A national survey. *Journal of Emotional and Behavioral Disorders.* [Epub ahead of print]

Hartung, C., McCarthy, D., Milich, R., & Martin, C. (2005). Parent–adolescent agreement on disruptive behavior symptoms: A multitrait–multimethod model. *Journal of Psychopathology and Behavioral Assessment, 27*(3), 159–168.

Hinshaw, S. P., Henker, B., Whalen, C. K., Erhardt, D., & Dunnington, R. E. (1989). Aggressive, prosocial, and nonsocial behavior in hyperactive boys: Dose effects of methylphenidate in naturalistic settings. *Journal of Consulting and Clinical Psychology, 57*(5), 636–643.

Holtmann, M., Sonuga-Barke, E., Cortese, S., & Brandeis, D. (2014). Neurofeedback for attention-deficit/hyperactivity disorder. *Child and Adolescent Psychiatric Clinics of North America, 23*, 789–806.

Hops, H., Walker, H. M., Fleischman, D. H., Nagoshi, J. T., Omura, R. T., Skindrud, K., et al. (1978). CLASS: A standardized in-class program for acting-out children: II. Field test evaluations. *Journal of Educational Psychology, 70*(4), 636–644.

Hoza, B., Mrug, S., Gerdes, A. C., Hinshaw, S. P., Bukowski, W. M., Gold, J. A., et al. (2005). What aspects of peer relationships are impaired in children with attention-deficit/hyperactivity disorder? *Journal of Consulting and Clinical Psychology, 73*(3), 411–423.

Jensen, P. S., Hinshaw, S. P., Kraemer, H. C., Lenora, N., Newcorn, J. H., Abikoff, H. B., et al. (2001). ADHD comorbidity findings from the MTA study: Comparing comorbid subgroups. *Journal of the American Academy of Child and Adolescent Psychiatry, 40*(2), 147–158.

Johnston, C., & Chronis-Tuscano, A. (2014). Families and ADHD. In R. A. Barkley (Ed.), *Attention-deficit hyperactivity disorder: A handbook for diagnosis and treatment* (pp. 191–209). New York: Guilford Press.

Kaminski, J. W., Valle, L. A., Filene, J. H., & Boyle, C. L. (2008). A meta-analytic review of components associated with parent training program effectiveness. *Journal of Abnormal Child Psychology, 36*(4), 567–589.

Kamphaus, R. W., & Frick, P. J. (2005). *Clinical assessment of child and adolescent personality and behavior* (2nd ed.). New York: Springer.

Kanfer, F. H., & Grimm, L. G. (1977). Behavioral analysis selecting target behaviors in the interview. *Behavior Modification, 1*(1), 7–28.

Kaufman, J., Birmaher, B., Brent, D., Rao, U., & Ryan, N. (1996). *Kiddie-SADS—Present and Lifetime version (K-SADS-PL)*. Pittsburgh, PA: University of Pittsburgh, School of Medicine.

Kazdin, A. E. (2005). *Parent management training: Treatment for oppositional, aggressive, and antisocial behavior in children and adolescents*. New York: Oxford University Press.

Kratochwill, T. R., & Bergan, J. (1990). *Behavioral consultation in applied settings: An individual guide*. New York: Plenum Press.

Kuriyan, A. B., Pelham, W. E., Molina, B. S. G., Waschbusch, D. A., Gnagy, E. M., Sibley, M. H., et al. (2013). Young adult educational and vocational outcomes of children diagnosed with ADHD. *Journal of Abnormal Child Psychology, 41*(1), 27–41.

Langberg, J. M. (2011). *Homework, organization and planning skills (HOPS) intervention: A treatment manual*. Bethesda, MD: National Association of School Psychologists.

Langberg, J. M., Molina, B. S. G., Arnold, L. E., Epstein, J. N., Altaye, M., Hinshaw, S. P., et al. (2011). Patterns and predictors of adolescent academic achievement and performance in a sample of children with attention-deficit/hyperactivity disorder. *Journal of Clinical Child and Adolescent Psychology, 40*(4), 519–531.

Lee, S. S., Humphreys, K. L., Flory, K., Liu, R., & Glass, K. (2011). Prospective association of childhood attention-deficit/hyperactivity disorder (ADHD) and substance use and abuse/dependence: A meta-analytic review. *Clinical Psychology Review, 31*(3), 328–341.

Lochman, J. E., Bierman, K. L., Coie, J. D., Dodge, K. A., Greenberg, M. T., McMahon, R. J., et al. (2010). The difficulty of maintaining positive intervention effects: A look at disruptive behavior, deviant peer relations, and social skills during the middle school years. *Journal of Early Adolescence, 30*(4), 593–624.

Lochman, J. E., Boxmeyer, C. L., Powell, N. P., Barry, T. D., & Pardini, D. A. (2010). Anger control training for aggressive youths. In J. R. Weisz & A. E. Kazdin (Eds.), *Evidence-based psychotherapies for children and adolescents* (2nd ed., pp. 227–242). New York: Guilford Press.

Loe, I. M., & Feldman, H. M. (2007). Academic and educational outcomes of children with ADHD. *Journal of Pediatric Psychlogy, 32*(6), 643–654.

Loney, J., & Milich, R. (1982). Hyperactivity, inattention, and aggression in clinical practice. *Advances in Developmental and Behavioral Pediatrics, 3*, 113–147.

Lonigan, C. J., Elbert, J. C., & Johnson, S. B. (1998). Empirically supported psychosocial interventions for children: An overview. *Journal of Clinical Child Psychology, 27*(2), 138–145.

Mash, E. J., & Hunsley, J. (2009). Assessment of child and family disturbance: A developmental-systems approach. In E. J. Mash & R. A. Barkley (Eds.), *Assessment of childhood disorders* (4th ed., pp. 3–52). New York: Guilford Press.

McCarthy, S., Asherson, P., Coghill, D., Hollis, C., Murray, M., Potts, L., et al. (2009). Attention-deficit hyperactivity disorder: Treatment discontinuation in adolescents and young adults. *British Journal of Psychiatry, 194*(3), 273–277.

McMahon, R. J., & Forehand, R. (2005). *Helping the noncompliant child: Family-based treatment for oppositional behavior*. New York: Guilford Press.

McMahon, R. J., Forehand, R., Griest, D. L., & Wells, K. C. (1981). Who drops out of treatment during parent behavioral training? *Behavioral Counseling Quarterly, 1*, 79–85.

McQuade, J. D., & Hoza, B. (2008). Peer problems in attention deficit hyperactivity disorder: Current status and future directions. *Developmental Disabilities Research Reviews, 14*(4), 320–324.

Melby-Lervåg, M., & Hulme, C. (2013). Is working memory training effective?: A meta-analytic review. *Developmental Psychology, 49*(2), 270–291.

Michelson, L., Sugai, D., Wood, & Kazdin, A. E. (1983). *Social skills assessment and training with children: An empirically based handbook.* New York: Plenum Press.

Mikami, A. Y., Jia, M., & Na, J. J. (2014). Social skills training. *Child and Adolescent Psychiatric Clinics of North America, 23,* 775–788.

Molina, B. S. G., Hinshaw, S. P., Swanson, J. M., Arnold, L. E., Vitiello, B., Jensen, P. S., et al. (2009). The MTA at 8 years: Prospective follow-up of children treated for combined-type ADHD in a multisite study. *Journal of the American Academy of Child and Adolescent Psychiatry, 48*(5), 484–500.

Molina, B. S., & Pelham, W. E., Jr. (2014). Attention-deficit/hyperactivity disorder and risk of substance use disorder: Developmental considerations, potential pathways, and opportunities for research. *Annual Review of Clinical Psychology, 10,* 607–639.

MTA Cooperative Group. (1999). 14-month randomized clinical trial of treatment strategies for attention deficit hyperactivity disorder. *Archives of General Psychiatry, 56,* 1073–1086.

Nigg, J. T., Willcutt, E. G., Doyle, A. E., & Sonuga-Barke, E. J. S. (2005). Causal heterogeneity in attention-deficit/hyperactivity disorder: Do we need neuropsychologically impaired subtypes? *Biological Psychiatry, 57,* 1224–1230.

Nijmeijer, J. S., Minderaa, R. B., Buitelaar, J. K., Mulligan, A., Hartman, C. A., & Hoekstra, P. J. (2008). Attention-deficit/hyperactivity disorder and social dysfunctioning. *Clinical Psychology Review, 28*(4), 692–708.

Nikolas, M. A., & Burt, S. A. (2010). Genetic and environmental influences on ADHD symptom dimensions of inattention and hyperactivity: A meta-analysis. *Journal of Abnormal Psychology, 119*(1), 1–17.

O'Connor, B. C., Fabiano, G. A., Waschbusch, D. A., Belin, P. J., Gnagy, E. M., Pelham, W. E., et al. (2014). Effects of a summer treatment program on functional sports outcomes in young children with ADHD. *Journal of Abnormal Child Psychology, 42*(6), 1005–1017.

O'Connor, B. C., Tresco, K. E., Pelham, W. E., Waschbusch, D. A., Gnagy, E. M., & Greiner, A. R. (2012). Modifying an evidence-based summer treatment program for use in a summer school setting: A pilot effectiveness evaluation. *School Mental Health, 4*(3), 143–154.

Oden, S., & Asher, S. R. (1977). Coaching children in social skills for friendship making. *Child Development, 48*(2), 495–506.

O'Leary, D. K., Pelham, W. E., Rosenbaum, A., & Price, G. H. (1976). Behavioral treatment of hyperkinetic children. *Clinical Pediatrics, 15*(6), 510–515.

Owens, E. B., Hinshaw, S. P., Kraemer, H. C., Arnold, L. E., Abikoff, H. B., Cantwell, D. P., et al. (2003). Which treatment for whom for ADHD?: Moderators of treatment response in the MTA. *Journal of Consulting and Clinical Psychology, 71*(3), 540–552.

Page, T. F., Pelham, W. E., III, Fabiano, G. A., Greiner, A. R., Gnagy, E. M., Hart, K. C., et al. (2016). Comparative cost analysis of sequential, adaptive, behavioral, pharmacological, and combined treatments for childhood ADHD. *Journal of Clinical Child and Adolescent Psychology, 45*(4), 416–427.

Paine, S. C., Radicchi, J., Deutchman, L., & Darch, C. B. (1983). *Structuring your classroom for academic success.* Champaign, IL: Research Press.

Pelham, W. E. (2008). Against the grain: A proposal for a psychosocial-first approach to treating ADHD—the Buffalo treatment algorithm. In K. McBurnett & L. Pfiffner (Eds.), *Attention deficit/hyperactivity disorder: Concepts, controversies, new directions* (pp. 301–316). New York: Informa Healthcare.

Pelham, W. E., & Bender, M. E. (1982). Peer relationships in hyperactive children: Description and treatment. In K. D. Gadow & J. Bialer (Eds.), *Advances in learning and behavioral disabilities* (pp. 365–436). Greenwich, CT: JAI Press.

Pelham, W. E., Burrows-Maclean, L., Gnagy, E. M., Fabiano, G. A., Coles, E. K., Wymbs, B. T., et al. (2014). A dose-ranging study of behavioral and pharmacological treatment in social settings for children with ADHD. *Journal of Abnormal Child Psychology, 42*(6), 1019–1031.

Pelham, W. E., & Fabiano, G. A. (2008). Evidence-based psychosocial treatments for attention-deficit/hyperactivity disorder. *Journal of Clinical Child and Adolescent Psychology, 37*(1), 184–214.

Pelham, W. E., Fabiano, G. A., & Massetti, G. M. (2005). Evidence-based assessment of attention deficit hyperactivity disorder in children and adolescents. *Journal of Clinical Child and Adolescent Psychology, 34*(3), 449–476.

Pelham, W. E., Fabiano, G. A., Waxmonsky, J. G., Greiner, A. R., Gnagy, E. M., Pelham, W. E., et al. (2016). Treatment sequencing for childhood ADHD: A multiple-randomization study of adaptive medication and behavioral interventions. *Journal of Clinical Child and Adolescent Psychology, 45*(4), 396–415.

Pelham, W. E., Gnagy, E. M., Burrows-MacLean, L., Williams, A., Fabiano, G. A, Morrisey, S. M., et al. (2001). Once-a-day Concerta methylphenidate versus three-times-daily methylphenidate in laboratory and natural settings. *Pediatrics, 107*(6), E105.

Pelham, W. E., Gnagy, E. M., Greiner, A. R., Waschbusch, D. A., Fabiano, G. A., & Burrows-MacLean, L. (2010). Summer treatment programs for attention deficit/hyperactivity disorder. In A. E. Kazdin & J. R. Weisz (Eds.), *Evidence-based psychotherapies for children and adolescents* (pp. 277–292). New York: Guilford Press.

Pelham, W. E., Lang, A. R., Atkeson, B., Murphy, D. A., Gnagy, E. M., Greiner, A. R., et al. (1998). Effects of deviant child behavior on parental alcohol consumption: Stress-induced drinking in parents of ADHD Children. *American Journal on Addictions, 7*(2), 103–114.

Pelham, W. E., Manos, M. J., Ezzell, C. E., Tresco, K. E., Gnagy, E. M., Hoffman, M. T., et al. (2005). A dose-ranging study of a methylphenidate transdermal system in children with ADHD. *Journal of the American Academy of Child and Adolescent Psychiatry, 44*(6), 522–529.

Pelham, W. E., Wheeler, T., & Chronis, A. (1998). Empirically supported psychosocial treatments for attention deficit hyperactivity disorder. *Journal of Clinical Child Psychology, 27*(2), 190–205.

Pfiffner, L. J. (2011). *All about ADHD: The complete practical guide for classroom teachers* (2nd ed.). New York: Scholastic Teaching Resources.

Pfiffner, L. J., & McBurnett, K. (1997). Social skills training with parent generalization: Treatment effects for children with attention deficit disorder. *Journal of Consulting and Clinical Psychology, 65*(5), 749–757.

Pliszka, S. R. (2007). Pharmacologic treatment of attention-deficit/hyperactivity disorder: Efficacy, safety and mechanisms of action. *Neuropsychology Review, 17*, 61–72.

Power, T. J., Anastopoulos, A. D., & Reid, R. (1998). *ADHD Rating Scale–IV: Checklists, norms, and clinical interpretation.* New York: Guilford Press.

Power, T. J., Karustis, J. L., & Habboushe, D. F. (2001). *Homework success for children with ADHD: A family–school intervention program.* New York: Guilford Press.

Rapport, M. D., Orban, S. A., Kofler, M. J., & Friedman, L. M. (2013). Do programs designed to train working memory, other executive functions, and attention benefit children with ADHD?: A meta-analytic review of cognitive, academic, and behavioral outcomes. *Clinical Psychology Review, 33*(8), 1237–1252.

Raver, C. C., Jones, S. M., & Li-Grining, C. P. (2008). Improving preschool classroom processes: Preliminary findings from a randomized trial implemented in Head Start settings. *Early Childhood Research Quarterly, 23*(1), 10–26.

Reich, W. (2000). Diagnostic Interview for Children and Adolescents (DICA). *Journal of the American Academy of Child and Adolescent Psychiatry, 39*(1), 59–66.

Reinke, W. M., Stormont, M., Herman, K. C., Puri, R., & Goel, N. (2011). Supporting children's mental health in schools: Teacher perceptions of needs, roles, and barriers. *School Psychology Quarterly, 26*(1), 1–13.

Reitman, D., & McMahon, R. J. (2013). Constance "Connie" Hanf (1917–2002): The mentor and the model. *Cognitive and Behavioral Practice, 20*, 106–116.

Reynolds, C. R., & Kamphaus, R. W. (1998). *BASC: Behavior Assessment System for Children: Manual.* Circle Pines, MN: American Guidance Service.

Robin, A. L., & Foster, S. L. (1989). *Negotiating parent–adolescent conflict: A behavioral-family systems approach.* New York: Guilford Press.

Sanders, M. R. (2012). Development, evaluation, and multinational dissemination of the Triple P-Positive Parenting Program. *Annual Review of Clinical Psychology, 8*(1), 345–379.

Schatz, N. K., Fabiano, G. A., Cunningham, C. E., DosReis, S., Waschbusch, D. A., Jerome, S., et al. (2015). Systematic review of patients' and parents' preferences for ADHD treatment options and processes of care. *The Patient, 8*(6), 483–497.

Shaffer, D., Fisher, P., Lucas, C., Dulcan, M., & Schwab-Stone M. (2000). NIMH Diagnostic Interview Schedule for Children, Version IV (NIMH DISC-IV): Description, differences from previous versions, and reliability of some common diagnoses. *Journal of the American Academy of Child and Adolescent Psychiatry, 39,* 28–38.

Sheridan, S. M., & Kratochwill, T. R. (2008). *Conjoint behavioral consultation: Promoting family-school connections and interventions* (2nd ed., Vol. 40). New York: Springer-Verlag.

Sibley, M. H., Kuriyan, A. B., Evans, S. W., Waxmonsky, J. G., & Smith, B. H. (2014). Pharmacological and psychosocial treatments for adolescents with ADHD: An updated systematic review of the literature. *Clinical Psychology Review, 34*(3), 218–232.

Sibley, M. H., Pelham, W. E., Derefinko, K. J., Kuriyan, A. B., Sanchez, F., & Graziano, P. A. (2013). A pilot trial of Supporting Teens' Academic Needs Daily (STAND): A parent–adolescent collaborative intervention for ADHD. *Journal of Psychopathology and Behavioral Assessment, 35*(4), 436–449.

Sibley, M. H., Pelham, W. E., Gnagy, E. M., Ross, J. M., & Greiner, A. R. (2011). An evaluation of a summer treatment program for adolescents with ADHD. *Cognitive and Behavioral Practice, 18*(4), 530–544.

Sibley, M. H., Pelham, W. E., Molina, B. S. G., Gnagy, E. M., Waschbusch, D. A., Garefino, A. C., et al. (2012). Diagnosing ADHD in adolescence. *Journal of Consulting and Clinical Psychology, 80*(1), 139–150.

Sibley, M. H., & Yeguez, C. E. (2014). The impact of DSM-5 A-criteria changes on parent ratings of ADHD in adolescents. *Journal of Attention Disorders.* [Epub ahead of print]

Smith, B. H., Pelham, W. E., Evans, S., Gnagy, E., Molina, B., Bukstein, O., et al. (1998). Dosage effects of methylphenidate on the social behavior of adolescents diagnosed with attention-deficit hyperactivity disorder. *Experimental and Clinical Psychopharmacology, 6*(2), 187–204.

Sonuga-Barke, E. J. S., Brandeis, D., Cortese, S., Daley, D., Ferrin, M., Holtmann, M., et al. (2013). Nonpharmacological interventions for ADHD: Systematic review and meta-analyses of randomized controlled trials of dietary and psychological treatments. *American Journal of Psychiatry, 170*(3), 275–289.

Sonuga-Barke, E. J. S., Daley, D., & Thompson, M. (2002). Does maternal ADHD reduce the effectiveness of parent training for preschool children's ADHD? *Journal of the American Academy of Child and Adolescent Psychiatry, 41*(6), 696–702.

Spivack, G., Platt, J. J., & Shure, M. B. (1976). *The problem-solving approach to adjustment.* San Fransisco: Jossey-Bass.

Sugai, G., & Horner, R. H. (2009). Responsiveness-to-intervention and school-wide positive behavior supports: Integration of multi-tiered system approaches. *Exceptionality, 17,* 223–237.

Vile Junod, R. E., DuPaul, G. J., Jitendra, A. K., Volpe, R. J., & Cleary, K. S. (2006). Classroom observations of students with and without ADHD: Differences across types of engagement. *Journal of School Psychology, 44*(2), 87–104.

Visser, S. N., Bitsko, R. H., Danielson, M. L., Ghandour, R. M., Blumberg, S. J., Schieve, L. A., et al. (2015). Treatment of attention deficit/hyperactivity disorder among children with special health care needs. *Journal of Pediatrics, 166*(6), 1423–1430.

Visser, S. N., Danielson, M. L., Bitsko, R. H., Holbrook, J. R., Kogan, M. D., Ghandour, R. M., et al. (2014). Trends in the parent-report of health care provider–diagnosed and medicated attention-deficit/hyperactivity disorder: United States, 2003–2011. *Journal of the American Academy of Child & Adolescent Psychiatry, 53*(1), 34–46.

Vitiello, B., Abikoff, H. B., Chuang, S. Z., Kollins, S. H., McCracken, J. T., Riddle, M. A., et al. (2007). Effectiveness of methylphenidate in the 10-month continuation phase of the Preschoolers with Attention-Deficit/Hyperactivity Disorder Treatment Study (PATS). *Journal of Child and Adolescent Psychopharmacology, 17*(5), 593–604.

Volpe, R. J., & Fabiano, G. A. (2013). *Daily behavior report cards: An evidence-based system of assessment and intervention.* New York: Guilford Press.

Walker, H. M., Hops, H., & Greenwood, C. R. (1981). RECESS: Research and development of a behavior management package for remediating social aggression in the school setting. In P. S. Strain (Ed.), *The utilization of classroom peers as behavior change agents* (pp. 261–303). New York: Springer.

Waschbusch, D. A., Cunningham, C. E., Pelham, W. E., Rimas, H. L., Greiner, A. R., Gnagy, E. M., et al. (2011). A discrete choice conjoint experiment to evaluate parent preferences for treatment of young, medication naive children with ADHD. *Journal of Clinical Child and Adolescent Psychology, 40*(4), 546–561.

Watson, T. S., & Skinner, C. H. (2001). Functional behavioral assessment: Principles, procedures, and future directions. *School Psychology Review, 30*(2), 156–172.

Waxmonsky, J. G. (2005). Non-stimulant therapies for pediatric and adult ADHD. *Essential Psychopharmacology, 6*(5), 262–276.

Webster-Stratton, C. H., Reid, M. J., & Beauchaine, T. (2011). Combining parent and child training for young children with ADHD. *Journal of Clinical Child and Adolescent Psychology, 40*(2), 191–203.

Wells, K. C., Pelham, W. E., Kotkin, R. A., Hoza, B., Abikoff, H. B., Abramowitz, A., et al. (2000). Psychosocial treatment strategies in the MTA study: Rationale, methods, and critical issues in design and implementation. *Journal of Abnormal Child Psychology, 28*(6), 483–505.

Wigal, T., Greenhill, L. L., Chuang, S., McGough, J., Vitiello, B., Skrobala, A., et al. (2006). Safety and tolerability of methylphenidate in preschool children with ADHD. *Journal of the American Academy of Child and Adolescent Psychiatry, 45*(11), 1294–1303.

Willcutt, E. G., Doyle, A. E., Nigg, J. T., Faraone, S. V., & Pennington, B. F. (2005). Validity of the executive function theory of attention-deficit/hyperactivity disorder: A meta-analytic review. *Biological Psychiatry, 57,* 1336–1346.

Witt, J. C., & Elliot, S. N. (1982). The response cost lottery: A time efficient and effective classroom intervention. *Journal of School Psychology, 20*(2), 155–161.

Wymbs, B. T., Pelham, W. E., Molina, B. S. G., Gnagy, E. M., Wilson, T. K., et al. (2008). Rate and predictors of divorce among parents of youths with ADHD. *Journal of Consulting and Clinical Psychology, 76*(5), 735–744.

Zentall, S. S. (1993). Research on the educational implications of attention deficit hyperactivity disorder. *Exceptional Children, 60*(2), 143–153.

CHAPTER 13

Eating Disorders

Dawn M. Eichen, Anna M. Karam,
and Denise E. Wilfley

DSM-5 DEFINITIONS OF EATING DISORDERS

The fifth edition of the *Diagnostic and Statistical Manual of Mental Disorders* (DSM-5; American Psychiatric Association, 2013) includes diagnoses for three specific threshold eating disorders (EDs): anorexia nervosa (AN), bulimia nervosa (BN) and binge-eating disorder (BED). DSM-5 identifies three features of AN: (1) significantly low body weight; (2) pronounced fear of becoming fat or gaining weight and/or actively avoiding weight gain regardless of a low body weight; and (3) self-evaluation highly influenced by weight and/or shape, disturbance in how one's weight or shape is perceived, or denial of the severity of the current low weight. For children and adolescents, calculating a body mass index (BMI) percentile may be useful to determine whether body weight is significantly low. Significantly low body weight is considered less than what is minimally expected given the child's age, sex, physical health, and developmental trajectory. Accordingly, this may include children who fail to maintain their expected growth trajectory but are not necessarily under the fifth BMI percentile, designated as underweight by the Centers for Disease Control and Prevention. Current symptoms (over the past 3 months) may be described by meeting one of two subtypes: (1) restricting type—whereby the individual does not engage in bingeing or purging or (2) binge-eating/purging type for individuals who have engaged in recurrent binge-eating and purging (American Psychiatric Association, 2013).

Three defining features also characterize BN: (1) recurrent episodes of binge eating (eating an objectively large amount of food while experiencing loss of control); (2) recurrent inappropriate compensatory behaviors (e.g., purging; misuse of laxatives, diuretics or other medications; fasting; or excessive exercise) to prevent weight gain; and (3) undue influence of shape and/or weight on self-evaluation. The bingeing and compensatory behaviors must occur, on average, at least once per week, for 3 months. The diagnosis of BN excludes individuals meeting criteria for AN (American Psychiatric Association, 2013).

Last, BED is defined by regular binge eating (at least once a week over the past 3 months). Additionally, the binge eating must cause marked distress and include three of the following five features: (1) eating much more rapidly than normal; (2) eating until feeling uncomfortably full; (3) eating when not feeling physically hungry; (4) eating alone because of embarrassment over how much one is eating; and (5) feeling disgusted, depressed, or guilty afterward. The category other specified feeding or eating disorder (OSFED) has been distinguished to include those who exhibit ED symptoms that are clinically distressing but do not fully meet criteria of AN, BN or BED. Finally, avoidant/restrictive food intake disorder (ARFID) distinguishes criteria for a restrictive/avoidant eater that is distinct from AN because shape and weight concerns are not causing the food restriction or avoidance (American Psychiatric Association, 2013).

PREVALENCE AND COURSE

In the few studies that report the prevalence rates for DSM-5 EDs in female children and adolescents, the range for AN is 0.3–2.0%; that for BN is 0.8–2.6%; that for BED is 1.4–4.1%; and that for OSFED is 2.7–11.5% (Allen, Byrne, Oddy, & Crosby, 2013; Fairweather-Schmidt & Wade, 2014; Smink, van Hoeken, Oldehinkel, & Hoek 2014; Stice, Marti, & Rohde, 2013). Although little information is available specifically regarding males, some studies estimate the prevalence of any ED (including OSFED) ranges from 1.2 to 2.9% (Allen et al., 2013; Smink et al., 2014).

AN typically begins in adolescence or young adulthood, but some cases of early onset, prior to puberty commencing, have been identified. The course of AN varies, with some individuals recovering after one episode, while others maintain a chronic course or periods of recovery and relapse (American Psychiatric Association, 2013). BN also generally begins in adolescence or young adulthood, but typically has a later age of onset than AN. As with AN, the course may be chronic or intermittent, with the individual experiencing periods of recovery and relapse. Some individuals diagnosed with BN may convert to a diagnosis of AN; however, most return to a diagnosis of BN or continue to switch between these disorders. Some cease using inappropriate compensatory behaviors, resulting in a crossover to a diagnosis of BED or OSFED. Children who experience loss of control (LOC) eating, regardless of amount of food, are more likely to develop disordered eating and BED or subclinical BED (now OSFED; Tanofsky-Kraff et al., 2011). It is thought that LOC eating or instances of binge eating are a precursor for developing BED for some adolescents. BED can begin in adolescence, but is more likely than the other EDs to develop later in life.

Some longitudinal studies have explored the change in ED symptoms, known risk factors, and diagnoses throughout adolescence into young adulthood (Fairweather-Schmidt & Wade, 2014; Rohde, Stice, & Marti, 2015; Stice et al., 2013). These studies demonstrated that the presence of known risk factors, such as thin ideal internalization and body dissatisfaction, in early adolescence in the absence of an ED, predicted the development of an ED by age 20, providing support for a likelihood of the development of

EDs during adolescence. Many early adolescents with OSFED developed full-syndrome EDs into late adolescence/young adulthood, and substantial diagnostic crossover was seen between EDs with binge eating (Stice et al., 2013). Less is known about the progression and potential crossover of AN, whose prevalence was very low in this sample. Changes in diagnoses make it difficult to describe the course of individual ED diagnoses, but they may provide some evidence for the predictive validity of DSM-5 diagnoses and demonstrate improvement over the previous version.

COMMON COMORBID DISORDERS

Individuals with EDs often present with at least one other comorbid disorder and even more have met lifetime criteria for another DSM disorder. Using DSM-IV criteria, one study demonstrated that among adolescents with BN or BED, respectively, 50 or 45% had a lifetime history of a mood disorder, 66 or 65% had a lifetime history of an anxiety disorder, and 20 or 27% had alcohol and/or drug abuse or dependence (Swanson, Crow, Le Grange, Swendsen, & Merikangas, 2011). In contrast, adolescents with AN were only significantly associated with having a lifetime diagnosis of oppositional defiant disorder, which contradicts the high rates of comorbidity in studies of adults with AN; however, nearly 60% of adolescents with subthreshold AN had a lifetime anxiety disorder, and 30% had a lifetime history of major depressive disorder (Swanson et al., 2011). In a clinical sample, nearly 50% of adolescents with AN met criteria for at least another lifetime psychiatric disorder, with mood and anxiety disorders being the most common comorbid disorders (Bühren et al., 2014). Individuals with AN binge–purge subtype were more likely to have a comorbid disorder than those with the restricting subtype. Similarly, rates of substance abuse were higher among those with binge–purge subtypes (Root et al., 2010). Taken together, EDs with binge and/or purge behaviors may be related to greater psychiatric comorbidity, or it is possible that AN predates the onset of other comorbid diagnoses. Although prospective longitudinal studies are needed, retrospective studies indicate that many individuals with AN or BN had at least one anxiety disorder prior to the onset of their ED (Godart, Flament, Lecrubier, & Jeammet, 2000; Kaye et al., 2004).

There is growing evidence that EDs may be comorbid with attention-deficit/hyperactivity disorder (ADHD). Girls with ADHD were 3.6 times more likely to meet criteria for an ED than those without ADHD (Biederman et al., 2007). Furthermore, among girls with ADHD, those with a comorbid ED were more likely to have additional comorbidities, including major depression, anxiety, and disruptive behavior disorders, compared to girls with ADHD without a comorbid ED. A nationally representative study found that adolescents who reported having been diagnosed with ADHD by a health professional were more likely to have experienced a clinical ED as diagnosed by a health professional (Bleck, DeBate, & Olivardia, 2015). All in all, EDs are often comorbid with other disorders. Although a better understanding of whether the onset of an ED causes additional comorbid conditions is needed through longitudinal studies, the impact of comorbid disorders is seen in the impairment individuals with EDs experience.

ETIOLOGICAL/CONCEPTUAL MODELS OF EDs

Many factors are thought to contribute to the development and maintenance of EDs (Polivy & Herman, 2002). Significant evidence that EDs should be classified as biologically based, serious mental illnesses exists (Klump, Bulik, Kaye, Treasure, & Tyson, 2009). Growing neurobiological evidence examining neural circuitry, neurotransmitters, and heredity suggests a biological component to EDs (Adan & Kaye, 2011). The heritability rates of EDs (AN, BN, and BED) range from 50 to 83% (Klump et al., 2009). Disturbances in the serotonin and dopamine systems affecting neurocircuits (e.g., reward circuit) have been demonstrated in individuals with EDs through imaging and molecular genetic studies, and may predispose the disorder, although the state of starvation in AN can alter neurofunctioning further (Kaye, 2008).

A host of psychological and social factors also appear to increase the risk that an individual will develop an ED. It is believed that body dissatisfaction, negative emotion, and low self-esteem are precursors to the development of an ED (Polivy & Herman, 2002). Furthermore, environmental stressors, cognitive distortions (e.g., obsessive thoughts), and personality traits (e.g., need for control) may contribute to the development of EDs. Additionally, perfectionism, interpersonal difficulties, family influence, and criticism (high expressed emotion), dieting, and a history of abuse are also thought to contribute to the development of an ED (Polivy & Herman, 2002).

Cognitive-behavioral theories describing the development and maintenance of EDs are relatively well accepted. More recently, an adopted transdiagnostic perspective has posited that there are similar, overlapping mechanisms across EDs (Fairburn, Cooper, & Shafran, 2003). The central mechanism proposed is that overevaluation of shape and weight leads to dietary restraint, which then results in either low weight (AN) or binge eating with or without compensatory behaviors (BN or BED). This theory also includes four mechanisms that may contribute to the maintenance of the disorder: clinical perfectionism, core low self-esteem, mood intolerance, and interpersonal difficulties (Fairburn et al., 2003). Taken together, it is evident that EDs are complex mental disorders that can develop due to a variety of biopsychosocial issues.

EVIDENCE-BASED TREATMENTS FOR EDs IN ADOLESCENTS

Although some studies of young adolescents exist, there are no controlled treatment studies of children with EDs, likely due to its low incidence rate (Keel & Haedt, 2008). Research suggests that evidence-based treatments for adults with EDs are not necessarily efficacious for children and adolescents, and vice versa (e.g., Russell, Szmukler, Dare, & Eisler, 1987). Therefore, only treatments that have been evaluated for children and adolescents are presented.

Treatments were evaluated and categorized as interventions that are "well established" or "probably efficacious" based on guidelines set forth by the American Psychological Association Task Force on Promotion and Dissemination of Psychological Procedures (1995), or "possibly efficacious" (Chambless & Ollendick, 2001). "Well-established" treatments are (1) superior to a pill, or a psychological placebo or alternative treatment, or (2) equivalent to an already established treatment, in studies with adequate statistical power in at least two well-conducted group design studies by different investigators (American Psychological Association Task Force on Promotion and Dissemination of Psychological Procedures, 1995). "Probably efficacious" treatments are (1) more effective than a no-treatment wait-list control group in at least two good group design studies conducted by different investigators or (2) they meet criteria for a well-established treatment but only in two studies conducted by the same investigators (American Psychological Association Task Force on Promotion and Dissemination of Psychological Procedures, 1995). "Possibly efficacious" treatments are superior to a no-treatment wait-list control group in a least one well-conducted study (Chambless & Ollendick, 2001).

Treatments for Adolescents with AN

Family-based treatment (FBT) is the most well-established treatment for adolescents with AN (Kass, Kolko, & Wilfley, 2013; Stiles-Shields, Hoste, Doyle, & Le Grange, 2012). FBT is often referred to as the "Maudsley method" to pay homage to the original development and testing of FBT that was initiated at Maudsley Hospital in London. FBT was found to be statistically superior to individual therapy in two early studies (Robin et al., 1999; Russell et al., 1987). Additionally, a recent meta-analysis of randomized controlled trials (RCTs) for adolescent EDs found that FBT was superior to individual therapies in treating adolescent AN (Couturier, Kimber, & Szatmari, 2013).

There is one treatment manual for FBT that is widely used by clinicians (Lock & Le Grange, 2012). Although manuals are used flexibly, there are a few principles of FBT that should remain constant: (1) Family is not blamed as the cause of the illness from the perspective of treatment; (2) parents are tasked with taking charge and facilitating weight gain in their malnourished child; (3) the entire family is an important part of treatment success and ED recovery; (4) the acknowledgment that the adolescent's need for control and independence in areas other than weight must be respected (Lock & Le Grange, 2012).

FBT includes all members of the family living in the household and anyone who has a significant role in caring for the adolescent. FBT is marked by three phases. Phase I entails weight restoration of the patient, in which the therapist supports and reinforces parents' efforts to refeed their child. In Phase II, control of food and weight is transitioned back to the adolescent, with therapist and parental oversight. Phase III establishes that ED symptoms no longer need to be a central topic of conversation, and treatment is concluded. Greater detail on the phases of FBT for adolescent anorexia nervosa (FBT-AN), accompanied by sample therapy scripts, is discussed later in this chapter.

Although FBT has proven to be the most well-established treatment for adolescent AN, it is important to note its limitations. FBT requires all family members to be present throughout treatment, which can be challenging due to family members' often busy and conflicting schedules. Additionally, FBT is labor intensive and therefore costly (Lock, 2011). Therefore, alternatives to treating adolescent AN are necessary.

Two RCTs have found adolescent-focused therapy (AFT), or ego-oriented individual therapy, to be successful for adolescents with AN (Lock et al., 2010; Robin et al., 1999), which means that AFT is designated as probably efficacious. AFT is a psychodynamically informed individual psychotherapy that focuses on enhancing adolescent autonomy, self-efficacy, individuation, and assertiveness. AFT also includes meetings with parents to support individual treatment (Fitzpatrick, Moye, Hoste, Lock, & Le Grange, 2010). In Phase 1 of treatment, the therapist builds rapport and assesses motivation and the patient's psychological concerns. The therapist actively encourages the patient to stop dieting and to gain weight by setting weight goals and putting an emphasis on the importance of changing these behaviors (Lock et al., 2010). Additionally, weight gain is discussed and encouraged until the patient's weight is restored. The therapist interprets behavior, emotions, and motives to help the patient distinguish emotional states from bodily needs. AFT holds the patient responsible for gaining weight and eating (Lock et al., 2010). Phase 2 of AFT encourages separation, individuation, and increasing the patient's ability to tolerate negative affect. Phase 3 focuses on terminating treatment. In an RCT comparing AFT to FBT, both treatments led to significant improvement and were similarly effective in producing full remission at the end of treatment (Lock et al., 2010); however, FBT was more effective in maintaining full remission at 6- and 12-month follow-up.

Though currently there is insufficient evidence for it to be considered a well-established or probably efficacious treatment, cognitive-behavioral therapy–enhanced (CBT-E; Dalle Grave, Calugi, Doll, & Fairburn, 2013; Fairburn, 2008) and cognitive remediation therapy (CRT; Dahlgren, Lask, Landrø, & Rø, 2013; Pretorius et al., 2012; Wood, Al-Khairulla, & Lask, 2011) show promise for treating adolescents with AN and should be studied further.

CBT-E, a treatment for individuals with ED pathology, emphasizes the core psychopathology of overvaluation of body weight and shape (Fairburn, 2008). With adolescent patients with AN, CBT-E has three phases. In Phase 1, emphasis is on helping the patient to think about his or her current state and the process of maintaining his or her life as it is. This is followed by analyzing the advantages and disadvantages of addressing the ED. Progression to Phase 2, if the patient is willing, emphasizes weight restoration, while addressing other psychopathology. Phase 3 focuses on helping patients maintain the changes they have made. CBT-E for adolescents with AN involves routine involvement of the patient's parents. A detailed, published treatment manual for CBT-E (Fairburn, 2008) includes adaptations for adolescents. Adolescents with AN treated with CBT-E demonstrated substantial increases in weight and a marked decrease in ED psychopathology (Dalle Grave et al., 2013). Follow-up conducted over 60 weeks posttreatment showed little change among the patients. Accordingly, CBT-E should be considered a possibly efficacious treatment for adolescent AN, and a potentially good alternative to FBT.

CRT for AN addresses neuropsychological deficits, such as set shifting difficulties, weak central coherence, and visuospatial deficits (Wood et al., 2011). CRT uses cognitive exercises to increase cognitive flexibility and addresses the disabling attention to detail that is commonly seen in adolescents with AN through exercises that promote "big-picture" thinking. CRT does not focus explicitly on eating or weight; rather, it targets general cognitive functioning. Therefore, CRT is considered an adjunctive treatment with the aim of increasing motivation and cognitive skills in the hope of better utilizing other treatments (Baldock & Tchanturia, 2007; Whitney, Easter, & Tchanturia, 2008). Preliminary studies indicated that CRT for adolescents with AN was acceptable, feasible, and led to improvements in some of the targeted domains, such as cognitive flexibility and increased ability on specific cognitive tasks (Dahlgren et al., 2013; Pretorius et al., 2012; Wood et al., 2011).

Treatments for Adolescents with BN

Compared to the treatment research for adolescents with AN, treatment outcomes for adolescents with BN is quite limited. Although there are no well-established or probably efficacious treatments for adolescents with BN, there are two possibly efficacious treatments: family-based therapy for bulimia nervosa (FBT-BN; Le Grange & Lock, 2007) and cognitive-behavioral therapy–guided self-help (CBTgsh). Of note, there is evidence that CBT represents a well-established treatment for late adolescent/young adult females with BN (Keel & Haedt, 2008; Wilfley, Kolko, & Kass, 2011).

FBT, modified for the treatment of BN, may be efficacious for adolescents with BN (Couturier et al., 2013; Le Grange, Crosby, Rathouz, & Leventhal, 2007; Schmidt et al., 2007; Stiles-Shields et al., 2012). The first phase of FBT-BN focuses on regulating eating and eliminating binge-eating and purging behaviors instead of weight restoration, as in AN. Additionally, control of eating is never put entirely in the parents' hands in FBT-BN, as it is in FBT-AN.

CBTgsh, sometimes referred to as CBT self-care, appears to have at least similar efficacy to, and perhaps a slight advantage over, FBT-BN (Schmidt et al., 2007). Delivery of CBTgsh utilizes a workbook for patients and others who can provide support and a guide for therapists. The workbook was adapted from a self-help treatment for adult patients with BN (Schmidt & Treasure, 1997). CBTgsh includes 10 weekly sessions, three monthly follow-up sessions, and two optional sessions with someone close to the patient (Schmidt et al., 1997). The beginning of treatment focuses on the function of BN in the patient's life and facilitates motivation to change. Self-monitoring of thoughts, feelings, and behaviors provides the patient with information about how ED symptoms are being maintained. Problem solving with behavioral experiments and goal setting help patients recognize and change the cycle of bulimic symptoms. The case formulation is developed collaboratively by therapist and client. Homework is assigned throughout treatment. The sessions with the individual close to the patient focus on how this individual can help. At the end of the 10 weekly sessions, the therapist writes a "good-bye letter," and follow-up sessions detail relapse prevention. In one study, CBTgsh performed similarly to FBT, even reducing binge eating significantly faster than FBT (Schmidt et al., 2007). CBTgsh is more cost-effective than FBT, highlighting another advantage of this treatment.

Treatments for Adolescents with BED

There are currently no well-established probably efficacious or possibly efficacious treatments for children and adolescents with BED. However, preliminary studies support the use of interpersonal psychotherapy (IPT) for this population and demonstrated positive results for the prevention of excessive weight gain in overweight adolescents (Tanofsky-Kraff et al., 2011).

IPT, a brief, focused treatment originally developed for depression, has been adapted for BED (Wilfley et al., 1993; Wilfley, MacKenzie, Welch, Ayres, & Weissman, 2000). IPT has been adapted for the prevention of excess weight gain in adolescent females (IPT-WG; Tanofsky-Kraff et al., 2010) based on IPT for BED and the *Manual for Interpersonal Psychotherapy–Adolescent Skills Training* (Young & Mufson, 2003) for the prevention of depression. The treatment is delivered in a 12-session (75–90 minutes) group format with an introductory 90-minute individual meeting prior to starting group sessions. IPT-WG includes psychoeducation and skills that apply to various relationships within the interpersonal problem areas. Focus is placed on linking LOC eating to interpersonal functioning. This treatment resulted in reduced LOC eating and weight gain in overweight adolescents in a pilot trail (Tanofsky-Kraff et al., 2010). IPT-WG, which is delivered in a group format, is currently being adapted for rural African American girls and their parents/guardians, with preliminary findings suggesting that adapting IPT-WG may be an acceptable treatment concept to rural African American families (with recommendations for cultural adaptations, behavioral components, and parent components). Due to evidence in successfully treating adults with BED (Wilfley et al., 2002), IPT should be studied more in children and adolescents with BED.

In one study, group CBT, adapted for adolescent girls with recurrent binge eating, was tested in a pilot study compared to treatment as usual, followed by delayed CBT (Debar et al., 2013). All adolescents achieved remission from objective binge eating following receipt of CBT. Taken together, adapted group forms of IPT and CBT may be effective in treating BED in adolescents, but more controlled trials are necessary.

Summary of Evidence-Based Psychological Treatments for EDs in Adolescents

In summary, FBT is the most well-established treatment for adolescents with AN, followed by AFT, which is considered probably efficacious. For adolescents with BN, FBT and CBTgsh are considered possibly efficacious. Last, preliminary IPT-WG and CBT results show promise for treating adolescents with BED.

Pharmacological Interventions for EDs

Currently there are no evidence-based or U.S. Food and Drug Administration (FDA)-approved pharmacological treatments for children and adolescents with EDs (Couturier & Lock, 2007). Treatment guidelines suggest that medication should not be used as the primary treatment of children and adolescents with AN (Powers & Cloak, 2012). A retrospective study comparing 19 adolescent patients with AN taking selective serotonin reuptake inhibitors (SSRIs) to 13 patients with AN not being treated with SSRIs showed no significant differences between groups before treatment, after treatment, or at 1-year follow-up (Holtkamp et al., 2005). Although SSRIs are not effective in treating AN, they may be effective in treating comorbidities (Powers & Cloak, 2012). Many medications, primarily antidepressants and atypical antipsychotics, have been studied for adults with AN (Crow, Mitchell, Roerig, & Steffen, 2009). While initial findings were thought to be hopeful, further research suggests that neither class of drug appears to be helpful in improving symptoms (Powers & Cloak, 2012).

Although fluoxetine is not FDA-approved for treatment of BN in children and adolescents, it is approved for adults with BN. However, fluoxetine is FDA-approved to treat depression and obsessive–compulsive disorder (OCD) in children and adolescents; therefore, it should be the first-choice pharmacological treatment considered for children and adolescents with BN (Powers & Cloak, 2012). Additionally, one open trial found support for its use in children and adolescents with BN (Kotler, Devlin, Davies, & Walsh, 2003).

All participants were treated with fluoxetine (60 mg daily) in combination with supportive psychotherapy, and decreased episodes of both bingeing and purging were seen.

Topiramate may be a good alternative to fluoxetine given that it has been shown to be effective in adults with BN, and it has FDA approval for treating seizure disorders in children and adolescents (Hoopes et al., 2003; Nickel et al., 2005). However, topiramate should be used for the treatment of BN with caution because of its association with appetite suppression and weight loss.

Currently, there are no FDA-approved medications for children, adolescents, or adults with BED. Small trials with adult patients with BED have shown promising results with duloxetine and atomoxetine (Guerdjikova et al., 2012), which are approved by the FDA for children and adolescents with ADHD (Powers & Cloak, 2012).

In conclusion, evidence-based pharmacological treatments for children and adolescents with EDs do not yet exist due to lack of scientific evidence. More research is needed before conclusive decisions can be made about medications used to treat this population.

Predictors of Treatment Response

Research has shown that parental criticism of the adolescent with AN can have a negative impact on the family's ability to remain in treatment and the overall outcome (Eisler et al., 2000; Le Grange, Eisler, Dare, & Russell, 1992). Parental warmth (the opposite of family criticism) may increase chances for better treatment outcome (Le Grange, Hoste, Lock, & Bryson, 2011). High levels of expressed emotion (EE), a marker of parental criticism, in mothers predicted early dropout from family therapy but not from individual treatment (Szmukler, Eisler, Russell, & Dare, 1985). Criticism of the adolescent by either parent at the onset of treatment is highly predictive of poor treatment outcome. Therefore, it is critical to address family criticism during therapy sessions, and seek to facilitate family warmth. Additionally, adolescents with AN who come from highly critical families may benefit from separated family therapy (in which parents are seen separately from the patient) (Le Grange et al., 1992).

Studies that examined potential moderators in treatment response have found that higher scores on the Yale–Brown–Cornell Eating Disorder Scale (YBC-EDS; Mazure, Halmi, Sunday, Romano, & Einhorn, 1994), which represent greater food and body obsessions/compulsions, are associated with more weight gain in long-term than in short-term family therapy conditions (Lock, Agras, Bryson, & Kraemer, 2005). Additionally, patients from nonintact families demonstrated more decreases in global ED pathology in the long-term than in the short-term family therapy condition (Lock et al., 2005). Le Grange and colleagues (2012) preliminary results indicated the presence of binge-eating and purging behaviors, and predicted more success in FBT for those with high global ED pathology scores at the beginning of treatment compared to those without such high scores or behaviors.

In a study that evaluated predictors of treatment in a sample of adolescents with BN in FBT or individual supportive psychotherapy (Le Grange, Crosby, & Lock, 2008), researchers found that individuals treated with FBT-BN who presented with less severe ED symptoms (as measured by the Eating Disorder Examination [EDE] global score at the start of treatment), were more likely to have refrained from binge eating and purging at follow-up. These findings suggest that lower eating concerns are the best predictor of remission for adolescents with BN, and FBT-BN may be most helpful for individuals with less severe ED pathology (Le Grange et al., 2008).

ASSESSMENT OF EDs IN CHILDREN AND ADOLESCENTS

Assessment of EDs in children and adolescents presents several challenges. First, the main diagnostic classification system does not provide specific criteria for children and adolescents; however, DSM-5 is more sensitive to age differences than previous DSM versions and elucidates some differences that may be seen for children and adolescents (American Psychiatric Association, 2013). Second, denial of symptoms is more common among children and adolescents, particularly among restrictors and those with AN (Couturier & Lock, 2006). It is unknown whether this is due to developmental limitations in cognitive ability or because children do not experience symptoms in the same way as adults (Micali & House, 2011). Subthreshold presentation in children and adolescents may be significant enough to have a negative impact during a time when children are meant to experience significant cognitive and developmental growth and maturation. Third, many assessment tools used with children and adolescents have been adapted from instruments originally designed for adult populations. As such, less information about the psychometric properties of these adapted versions tends to be available, and more research is necessary to understand whether assessment tools need to be different for children (Micali & House, 2011).

Differential Diagnosis

A thorough medical assessment is necessary to confirm the ED diagnosis and rule out any potential medical causes for the ED symptoms (e.g., type 1 diabetes mellitus; Zucker, Merwin, Elliott, Lacy, & Eichen, 2009). Additionally, it is important to determine that the patient is presenting with an ED and not ARFID, which also is characterized by significant weight loss and nutritional deficiency; the distinguishing feature is that the avoidance or restriction is not explained by concerns about body weight or shape. Presentations may include avoidance due to sensory characteristics of food, or fear of a negative consequence such as choking or vomiting.

Medical Assessment

In addition to ruling out a medical condition as being responsible for the symptoms, a medical assessment provides the patient's current medical status and informs what physical effects the ED may have already caused (e.g., dehydration, bradycardia), and which ones are likely to occur if the ED continues. It is important for the therapist to know the medical sequelae so that he or she can educate the family and patient about the grave nature of the ED to demonstrate the need for treatment. Furthermore, a medical evaluation determines whether outpatient treatment is appropriate or if immediate medical attention is needed. Particularly for those with AN, the physician can help determine the patient's current percentage of ideal body weight (Lock & Le Grange, 2012). Due to the potentially severe effects of an ED, it is recommended that a medical assessment occur prior to beginning the psychological assessment and that the physician remain involved throughout the course of treatment.

Clinical Interview

It is important to involve multiple informants in the assessment of EDs (Lock & Le Grange, 2012; Micali & House, 2011; Zucker et al., 2009). Adolescents may lack insight into the severity of their problem (Couturier & Lock, 2006) or they may want to actively deny symptoms if they want to continue these behaviors. Parents may be able to provide a more accurate account; however, they also may have difficulties accepting that their child has a problem (Zucker et al., 2009). Lock and Le Grange (2012) suggest conducting separate interviews with the adolescent and the parents because the parents may be reluctant to be open in the presence of their child. This also serves to involve the family in treatment from the outset.

An essential part of assessment is a complete psychiatric history of the patient, which can be facilitated by the use of a semistructured interview such as the Schedule for Affective Disorders and Schizophrenia for School-Age Children–Present and Lifetime Version (K-SADS-PL). The K-SADS-PL has demonstrated good psychometric properties and is recommended because it allows the integration of parent and child reports to gather a comprehensive history (Kaufman, Birmaher, Brent, & Rao, 1997). Gathering information from both informants again helps ensure that the history is complete, since the adolescent may have concealed some behaviors or symptoms from his or her parents, or the parents may endorse the presence of symptoms that the adolescent denies. It is also recommended that the therapist obtain a family psychiatric history to understand the history of mental illness among family members.

A more thorough semistructured interview focusing on the ED symptoms may also be used to gather more information. The EDE (Fairburn & Cooper, 1993) is touted as the "gold-standard" assessment measure for adult ED symptoms. It has been adapted for use in children and adolescents (ChEDE; Bryant-Waugh, Cooper, Taylor, & Lask, 1996). Additionally, the Structured Interview for Anorexic and Bulimic Disorders (SIAB-EX; Fichter, Herpertz, Quadflieg, & Herpertz-Dahlmann, 1998) is another widely used interview for ED assessment. The YBC-ED, a clinician-rated assessment, provides information related to the preoccupations and ritualistic behaviors in individuals with ED to help understand symptom severity (Mazure et al., 1994).

Self- and Parent-Report Measures

The Eating Disorder Examination Questionnaire (EDE-Q; Fairburn & Beglin, 1994) adapted from the semistructured EDE interview may be better suited for screening purposes. Although some norms have been published for use in adolescents, the EDE-Q has been adapted to be used in youth (YEDE-Q; Goldschmidt, Doyle, & Wilfley, 2007), but further validation is needed. Additional self-report measures that may be used to help screen for ED symptoms include the child version of the Eating Disorder Inventory (EDI-C; Garner, 1991) and the Eating Attitude Test for children (Maloney, McGuire, & Daniels, 1988). The Questionnaire for Eating and Weight Patterns is available in adolescent self-report and parent-report versions, and may be helpful in assessing for binge eating and compensatory behaviors. Of note, these questionnaires should not be used as diagnostic measures.

EVIDENCE-BASED TREATMENT IN PRACTICE: FBT

At present, FBT is the only well-established treatment for adolescents with AN (Keel & Haedt, 2008). Furthermore, it is the only well-established treatment for any ED in adolescents. FBT has three phases and is characterized by parents' active involvement in treatment in order to help restore their child's weight to normal levels (taking into account the age and height of the adolescent), give control over eating back to their child, and encourage normal adolescent development (Lock & Le Grange, 2012).

The treatment usually includes 15–20 sessions and lasts about 1 year. However, many families can complete FBT in as few as 10 sessions over 6 months. The FBT approach conceptualizes the problem, or eating pathology, as belonging to the entire family, and the parents' involvement in the therapy process is critically important for treatment success. This therapy is most appropriate for adolescents with AN who are living at home with their families because it works on the premise that family members are in close contact, routinely interact with each other, and eat together. However, it has also been shown to be effective in nonintact families, including single-parent households (Lock et al., 2005). FBT requires a strong commitment from the family because sacrifices may need to be made to ensure that the adolescent gets better, including the youth missing school or the parents missing work to be able to maintain control over what the child is eating. Table 13.1 outlines the main goals of the three phases of FBT.

In Phase I of FBT, emphasis is placed on weight restoration. Prior to the beginning of each session in treatment, the therapist must weigh the patient. Weighing the patient encourages tracking the patient's weight over the course of treatment, and helps to strengthen the therapeutic relationship, with the therapist comforting the patient through a potentially difficult process. The patient's weekly weight steers the direction of the therapy session; if the patient's weight has increased, the therapist will praise the parents on their efforts and reinforce continued success. If the patient's weight has stayed the same or dropped, the therapist should use this information to attempt to motivate the parents' efforts to increase their child's weight. Lock and Le Grange (2012) urge plotting the patient's weight so that the therapist, patient, and patient's family can see weight changes and patterns over time, and to demonstrate that weight (and weight change) drives the focus of each session. To highlight the importance of weight restoration, the therapist will psychoeducate the family on how life threatening AN is, likening it to a severe medical illness such as cancer. As such, the parents must do everything they can to restore their child's health. Just as they would ensure that their child received chemotherapy or whatever medicine needed, in the case of AN, parents must make sure that their child eats because food is akin to medicine. If progress is not seen, the therapist will reiterate the severity of the illness to demonstrate a sense of urgency and try to increase motivation and action from the parents. Emphasis on the parent taking complete charge over the adolescent's food intake is seen throughout Phase I.

TABLE 13.1. Outline of FBT Goals

Phase I: Weight restoration

Session 1

Main goals for Session 1:
- Involve the entire family in therapy.
- Get a history of how the adolescent's eating disorder is influencing the family.
- Charge the family with task of refeeding adolescent.
- Emphasize seriousness of the disorder.
- Separate adolescent from the disorder.
- Learn helpful information about how the family functions to better understand familial dynamics (i.e., conflicts, power structure, roles).
- Plan for next session's family meal.

Session 2

Main goals for Session 2:
- Continue to collect information about the family structure.
- Give parent's an opportunity to guide their child in normal eating and gaining weight.
- Evaluate the family's strengths and weaknesses regarding controlling the adolescent's eating.

Sessions 3–10

Main goals for the remaining sessions of Phase 1:
- Ensure family remains focused on the adolescent's eating disorder.
- Continue to focus on adolescent's weight restoration.
- Continue to reduce criticism and separate patient from the disorder.
- Empower parents to take responsibility of their son's/daughter's eating.
- Encourage siblings to support their ill family member.

Phase II: Transitioning control of eating back to the adolescent

Main goals of Phase II:
- Retain parental management of adolescent's eating until the patient proves he or she is able to implement normal eating and weight gain on his or her own.
- Transfer control of food and weight to the adolescent.
- Examine the association between adolescent developmental issues and AN.

Phase III: Adolescent issues and termination

Main goals of Phase III:
- Establish that eating disorder symptoms no longer have to be a central topic of conversation within the family, specifically between the parents and patient.
- Evaluate and review adolescent issues with the family and problem-solve best practices for dealing with these issues.
- Conclude treatment.

Case Example

Patty, a 16-year-old female, was diagnosed 2 months ago with AN, when she was hospitalized due to fainting at soccer practice. Patty's parents, Mary (mother) and Frank (father), have been concerned about Patty's weight loss for the past 6 months. Patty is the middle child; her older sister, Stacy, is a freshman in college and lives out of the home, and her brother, Brandon, is 12. Patty and her family are seeking therapy because Patty has lost the weight that she regained while in the hospital, and her parents are afraid she will need to be admitted again if she continues to lose weight. Fictional scripts to demonstrate the core aspects of FBT are provided.

Session 1

Session 1 Outline

1. Weigh the patient.
2. Greet the family and build rapport but make sure to maintain a sense of authority to demonstrate the seriousness of the illness.
3. Engage every family member present in session to gather the patient history/history of illness.
4. Distinguish the patient from his or her illness.
5. Highlight the gravity of the illness and how difficult recovery will be.
6. Provide authority to the parents to control weight restoration and take complete charge of the adolescent's eating.
7. Introduce and prepare for the family meal, which will take place as part of the next therapy session.

The therapist should greet the family and take the adolescent away to be weighed. This provides a crucial time for the therapist to support the adolescent and hear any concerns he or she may have.

THERAPIST: Thank you all for coming here today. Before we get started, I am going to take Patty with me to get her weight. This will be how we start each session moving forward, as it is important for us to keep track and to know how her weight is progressing as a starting point for discussion. So, Patty, will you please come with me?

PATTY: Umm. Okay—I guess if I have to. (*Gets up and follows the therapist out of the waiting room.*)

THERAPIST: I've been doing this for a while and I know that it can be really hard to be weighed at each session. But it really is important. How are you feeling about getting weighed?

PATTY: Well, I already weighed myself today, so I won't be surprised, but I get really upset if I see my weight going up, and I know that is why I am here.

THERAPIST: I will be here each week with you to discuss any concerns you have over the scale or your weight, and anything else you might want to let me know about before we start the session. How do you feel about starting therapy?

PATTY: Well, I don't want to go back to the hospital, but I also don't want to gain weight. They try to hide it, but I know my parents are constantly watching my every move around the house, especially when I am eating.

THERAPIST: Yeah, I know that must be really hard feeling like everyone is watching you. We will talk about this more in session, but at the beginning it is important for your parents to take charge of your eating. As we move through treatment, you will work to gain your independence back. Can you take your shoes off and hop on the scale, please? (*Records Patty's weight. They return to the family and move to the therapist's office to start the session.*)

The therapist makes a point of taking a few minutes to get to know each family member by having everyone introduce themselves. He or she should greet the family in a genuine, warm, but solemn manner, as it is important for the family to feel comfortable in the therapeutic setting while realizing the seriousness of the situation. This sets the stage for everyone's involvement in the treatment and continues as the therapist engages each family member to understand the history of the disorder and how it affects each family member.

THERAPIST: So, all of you are here for the same reason, but it would really help me gain a better understanding if you all could tell me about what has been going on and how having this eating disorder in the family has affected each of you.

MARY: I guess I can start—I was the one who said we needed to see a therapist. Frank and I were worried about Patty before she was hospitalized. We noticed she was losing weight, but we thought it was just a phase. After Patty was hospitalized, she promised us she was OK and things would be different. But clearly things aren't. It seems like Patty made it her mission to lose the weight she gained.

THERAPIST: So it sounds like you were worried about Patty before she was hospitalized. How do you feel now?

MARY: I am terrified—do you know what it is like seeing your daughter attached to all these tubes? I don't want to see that again—I just don't know what to do—I can't sit there and force food down her throat.

THERAPIST: Yes, that would be terrifying, and it is possible that Patty could end up back in the hospital if things don't change. Frank, how has the eating disorder affected you?

FRANK: Well, actually, I feel guilty. At first, I complimented Patty for losing some weight. I didn't think she needed to lose weight but she kept going. I also travel quite a bit for work and was out of town when Patty was hospitalized. I came back as soon as I could, but I can't help but wonder if I had been around more, maybe this wouldn't have happened.

THERAPIST: It sounds like you did the best you could, getting back as soon as possible. Plus, you made it here, which is a great step.

FRANK: Yeah—I have an arrangement with work to be able to plan my travel around these appointments.

THERAPIST: That is great—it is important for everyone to be involved. Brandon, how has the eating problem affected you?

BRANDON: Well, I don't really get why I have to come here—all of my friends go to the park after school. I don't need help—Patty does. If she would just eat more, she would be fine. Plus my parents are always worried about her—it isn't fair—Mom is always crying and everyone is always stressed, so it's not fun being home anymore.

THERAPIST: So it sounds like you, too, are upset by the eating disorder. What about you, Patty?

PATTY: I feel like everyone thinks I should just "eat more"—I know I should, and I know I need to in order to get better. But it is so hard. Every time I think about eating, it stresses me out. I don't want everyone to have to be worried about me all the time and feel like they need to watch me, but if I don't watch what I eat, I am afraid I will gain too much weight and not be a good soccer player.

Involving the entire family in taking the history of AN shows how the illness is affecting the family, while helping the therapist learn about how the family functions to better understand familial dynamics, such as power and authority structures, roles, and conflicts (Lock & Le Grange, 2012). Engaging each family member demonstrates that everyone is involved in the recovery process. The therapist should address the seriousness of the disorder and educate the family on the severe consequences of the disorder. The therapist must externalize the illness, taking the blame for the illness away from the patient by saying something like:

THERAPIST: So I just told you how serious anorexia nervosa is and some of the consequences. But I need you to understand how necessary it is for all of you to help Patty with this. And even though she is 16, and most 16-year-olds can survive without the help of anyone, this illness is affecting her ability to take care of herself. Patty, have you noticed this?

PATTY: Yeah, like I said, I am trying, but it is hard. I know I should eat, but sometimes I just can't.

THERAPIST: It is really important to separate the illness from Patty. Many people at times feel like the disorder has taken over, to the point where they are the disorder. Patty, do you find it hard to separate yourself from it sometimes?

PATTY: (*Nods.*)

THERAPIST: You want to be able to play soccer and you don't want everyone else to worry about you. That is coming from you, Patty. But sometimes the eating disorder takes over and makes you do things you wouldn't want to do if you didn't have the disorder. Or your thoughts focus on what the eating disorder wants you to and not on what you would want to.

The therapist must consistently highlight that the patient must not be identified with the illness. He or she continues to emphasize the serious nature of AN and educates family members on the often challenging recovery process. The therapist presents the parents with the responsibility of weight restoration, but the parents must work to figure out how to take control of this:

> "So when Patty and Brandon were younger and got sick and needed to take antibiotics, you, as parents, were responsible for making sure they would take their medicine. As we just discussed, the illness is taking over and Patty can't quite take care of herself. So, as her parents, you must figure out how to help feed her. I can't tell you exactly what to do, but as her parents, who know her and love her, you can figure out how help to her best. It isn't about Patty; it is about focusing on getting rid of the anorexia—so until Patty can reach a reasonable weight and separate herself more from the anorexia, you need to be on top of her, until we see that Patty can be trusted to take responsibility back over herself."

The therapist ends the session by telling the parents that they should bring a meal for everyone in the family to eat next time, highlighting how this should be what the parents feel their daughter needs to eat to get well because they are in charge of her getting better, not what the anorexia wants her to eat. The therapist concludes by summarizing the session and reiterates getting to know the family, the gravity of anorexia, and reinforcing everyone's concern for Patty, separating the disorder from Patty and restating the importance of the parents taking control of their daughter's eating.

Session 2

Session 2 Outline

1. Weigh the patient.
2. While the family eats the meal, gather information on typical patterns of food preparation, serving, and discussions about eating. Observe dynamics that may help or hinder treatment and pay attention to alliances.
3. Aid the parents in convincing their child to eat a bit more than she wants in order to help promote weight gain.
4. Encourage the sibling to provide support outside of mealtimes; if there is no sibling, encourage a friend or an extended family member of similar age to fill this role.

As in every session, the therapist begins Session 2 begins by weighing the patient, separate from the family. This should take about 5–10 minutes. The therapist should judge the patient's reaction to weight change and use this time to develop a relationship with the patient by understanding her struggles and assessing her reaction to her parents' attempts to take control of the eating. They then join the rest of the family, and the therapist encourages family members to serve the meal and start eating. Because eating while someone else is watching can be awkward at first, the therapist engages family members in conversation about their eating patterns and habits based on what he or she is observing in session.

[Mary takes out a serving bowl of spaghetti with tomato sauce and meatballs. She puts some spaghetti and two meatballs on her plate and passes it to Brandon, who puts a healthy portion of spaghetti and meatballs on his plate. Patty puts a small portion of spaghetti and no meatballs on her plate. Meanwhile, Frank sliced up some garlic bread and takes some for himself and passes some to Mary and Brandon but does not offer any to Patty.]

THERAPIST: So when you typically eat at home, is this how meals are typically served—with everyone mostly taking their own portion and some parts being passed around?

MARY: Umm, it depends really on what we are eating—for stuff that is served in bowls, typically, we just pass it around. If things are already separated like slices of pizza, I might leave the box in the kitchen and just bring people plates with their food on it.

THERAPIST: Has this always been the case that you mostly serve yourselves?

FRANK: No—we used to all get the same thing, no matter what. At some point, Brandon was always asking for more and Patty wasn't finishing her food, so we just started passing it around so the kids could take what they want.

THERAPIST: (to Frank) I noticed that you didn't give Patty any garlic bread—do you usually avoid giving her certain foods?

BRANDON: Sometimes I will ask Patty if I can have hers instead, and she almost always lets me!

FRANK: Well, I know she wouldn't want to eat the garlic bread, so I just didn't want to watch it sit there until Brandon asked to take it.

THERAPIST: Patty, do you usually eat what your family does, or do you ever have something different?

PATTY: Nobody makes me a special meal or anything. Sometimes I just don't eat everything they are serving, and usually I take a smaller portion.

THERAPIST: Brandon, do you always eat dinner together at home as a family?

The therapist uses these observations to engage in dialogue to understand the family members' behaviors around eating, as well as their dynamics. The therapist continues to ask about who prepares the food, shops for the food, decides the menu, and whether anyone else is present at mealtime, in order to understand what patterns may need to change and how the ED might have changed previous patterns. The therapist can later use this information to help the parents with Patty's weight restoration if they are met with resistance. The therapist also notices the alliances. In this example, the therapist should notice how the father does not give the daughter a piece of bread to avoid causing stress, but doing so is counterproductive to the weight restoration. Throughout the discussion, whenever possible, the therapist continues to educate the family members about anorexia and corrects any misinformation about eating/digestion and nutrition they may have. Then, after some time passes, the therapist attempts to help the parents to encourage their daughter to eat "one more bite," to demonstrate how they must help her gain weight.

THERAPIST: So, Mary and Frank, do you think that the food Patty put on her plate is what she needs to eat in order to get healthy?

FRANK: Well, I am sure she could eat more, but it is a good start that she is eating anything at all.

MARY: But she didn't even take a meatball or get any garlic bread. She still has food on her plate, and she had less than everyone else started with.

THERAPIST: It sounds like it is pretty common that Patty doesn't eat as much or eat the same things as everyone else. Remember, last week, when we talked about how anorexia has many serious consequences, like weakening of the heart, potential fertility problems, and how the body is in a chronic state of malnutrition? Patty is starving and could die from this. You must provide her with the food she needs to eat to get back to a healthy state.

FRANK: Yes. (*to Patty*) How about a piece of garlic bread?

THERAPIST: Is there anything else you can do besides offer her the garlic bread?

MARY: (*Puts bread on Patty's plate.*) You have to eat the bread, Patty. You need to get better.

THERAPIST: (*Looks at Frank.*)

FRANK: Yeah, Patty, you need to eat that.

The therapist watches to see whether the patient eats the added food. In Session 2, the therapist tries to help the parents see that they can get their adolescent to eat at least "one more bite." This empowers the parents to ensure that their child eats as much as she needs to in order to gain the weight. The therapist consistently tries to promote parental alliances and works to prevent one parent from taking the patient's side. Meanwhile, the therapist encourages the sibling to align with the patient, so that the patient begins to develop an important social support system. However, the sibling is not to align in a way that interferes with the parents' attempts at weight restoration. Rather, the sibling can listen and try to understand the struggles of the patient but should not counteract any of the parents' efforts. Finally, the therapist concludes on a positive note by praising the efforts of the family and instilling success in the parents, so that they leave feeling hopeful that they can continue their efforts at home.

Remainder of Phase I (Sessions 3–10)

The length of Phase I is determined by the progress. Some individuals may not need 10 sessions, while others may need more before progressing to Phase II. The remaining sessions of Phase I are less structured than Sessions 1 and 2. Rather than focus on an outline, therapists are encouraged to maintain three targets: (1) Ensure that the family remains focused on the adolescent's ED; (2) empower parents to take responsibility for their daughter's eating; and (3) encourage siblings to provide continued support to the patient (Lock & Le Grange, 2012). These targets are accomplished by five interventions that may be used as applicable in the rest of Phase I. Regardless, each session starts with weighing the patient, and the weight should be plotted on a chart in front of all family members to set the stage for the session. While it is important to highlight progress, it is still important to emphasize that the patient still remains at a very low weight, to ensure that parents continue to keep control of the weight restoration and do not allow the ED to wedge back into the picture. Weight gain is the primary goal in Phase I. The transition to Phase II occurs when the adolescent is less resistant to eating and has achieved at least 90% of her expected body weight.

Interventions in Phase I (Sessions 3–10)

1. Weigh the patient.*
2. Focus discussions on food and eating behaviors to promote weight gain.
3. Ensure that parental alliance is maintained and that the parents continue to work as a team in weight restoration.
4. Evaluate the sibling's effort to support the patient and encourage continued help.
5. Reduce criticism of the patient.
6. Maintain the distinction between the ED and the adolescent.
7. Reiterate progress.*

Aside from reducing criticism, these other interventions were introduced in Sessions 1 and 2. Criticism has been shown to affect treatment outcome negatively (Le Grange et al., 1992). The therapist should continue to model positive praise to maintain focus on the progress rather than criticize and point out what still needs improvement. To that effect, sessions always end by reviewing progress that has been made with the family to reinforce continued improvement.

Transition to Phase II

Indicators that the patient and family are ready to transition to Phase II include steady weight gain of the adolescent (~90% of developmentally expected weight) accompanied by increased food consumption on a regular basis without resistance, and parental comfort with having control over adolescent's ED.

Interventions in Phase II

1. Weigh the patient.
2. Help the parents continue controlling the adolescent's eating, until she can eat well without much assistance.
3. Aid in the transition of control of eating back to the adolescent.
4. Maintain a middle ground and begin to explore other adolescent issues that have been pushed aside to manage the ED, while highlighting the need to continue to focus on eating.
5. Continue to reduce criticism, especially regarding transitioning control back to the adolescent.

---

*These should be done in each session.

6. Continue to encourage the adolescent's sibling to support her.

7. Maintain a distinction between the adolescent's ideas and the ED.

8. Reiterate progress.

The main goals of Phase II are to retain parental control over eating until the patient proves that she is able to implement normal eating and weight gain on her own, transfer control of food and weight to the adolescent, and examine the association between adolescent developmental issues and AN (Lock & Le Grange, 2012). Similar to Phase I, the therapist should continue to weigh the patient at the beginning of each session. In the beginning of Phase II, sessions are similar to those in Phase I, with continued focus on the parents' management of the ED symptoms. As in Phase I, it is important to make sure the parents do not relax too much, interfering with weight restoration. The therapist's role begins to shift from coaching the parents to instilling confidence that the parents know what they need to do to help their adolescent. It is crucial to support the parents in knowing when and how to return control over eating to their adolescent, when everyone agrees that the adolescent has demonstrated that she is capable of eating well and gaining (or maintaining) weight on her own. For example, the adolescent might begin requesting or ordering her own food and portioning out appropriate-size servings. Sessions become less frequent (scheduled every 2–3 weeks) to demonstrate further separation from the therapist's coaching and greater independence of the family and, subsequently, the adolescent.

> [Patty has increasingly become less resistant to eating regularly and now does so without prompts from her parents. Her parents feel that she is ready to start controlling her own eating.]
>
> THERAPIST: So it sounds like you are both saying that you feel Patty has been eating consistently and maintaining a healthy weight, and you feel you are ready to start giving her more control.
>
> MARY: Yeah, it has been really great—she now helps portion out the food for everyone, and gives herself the same portion as the rest of us. And she eats it all, too!
>
> FRANK: We still watch and make sure she is giving herself an appropriate portion, but we don't even have to say anything anymore.
>
> THERAPIST: Patty, do you feel you are doing better with your eating?
>
> PATTY: Yeah—I now eat what everyone else is eating. I even ate a second piece of garlic bread yesterday—I was the only one.
>
> BRANDON: Yes—even I didn't eat two!
>
> THERAPIST: So, parents, does it really comes down to whether you are ready to let Patty take more control, and whether you feel she is really ready to move on? If she isn't quite ready, things might not go so well; however, the ultimate goal is for her to do it on her own, so at some point you will need to give her a chance.
>
> MARY: I think Patty has shown that she is ready. We haven't had to watch her like a hawk the past few weeks. We don't have to bug her to eat more.
>
> FRANK: It isn't like we will stop watching her altogether.

THERAPIST: Right—you don't want to turn over all of the responsibility at once. That could be very overwhelming. What do you think might be a good first step?

MARY: Well, usually, I have been packing lunch for her the night before. Brandon packs his own lunch and Patty used to, before this all happened. Maybe Patty can start packing her own lunch and we can make sure it is sufficient and only step in if we see she starts trying to take less food.

The therapist continues to help the family navigate this transition. Additionally, he or she should prompt the family to think about the relation between developmental issues and their adolescent's ED. This can be achieved by working to make sure the adolescent is reintegrating back into healthy social relationships and possibly even start dating, as well as making sure the adolescent remains engaged in school and other activities she used to enjoy. It remains important for the adolescent to realize successes out of the home. Because these situations will be reintegrated into her life, the focus can change to settings in which the adolescent will need to increasingly master regular eating and appropriate exercise.

THERAPIST: So, Patty, we spent a lot of time talking about your eating, and a lot of other things have taken a back seat. What are you most looking forward to about next quarter in school?

PATTY: Well, I had to stop playing soccer, so I am looking forward to starting that up again. Also, every year in the spring there is a big team sleepover. I haven't been allowed to spend a night away from home. I am hoping that I will be able to go and spend the night!

Phase III

Interventions in Phase III

1. Review typical adolescent development, focusing on issues that may need to be addressed.

2. Identify for the family specific issues that may be pertinent to the adolescent.

3. Explore specific issues and help family members problem-solve.

4. Explore how the parents are doing as a couple.

5. Discuss what issues may arise in the future and how to handle them.

6. Terminate therapy.

Readiness to progress to Phase III is marked by the patient maintaining a stable weight between 95 and 100% of expected weight (taking into account height, age, and gender), while having regained control over her eating and exercise. The family is able to discuss issues not related to the adolescent's eating, and the patient regains functioning relationships with peers. The main goals of Phase III are to establish that ED symptoms no longer have to be a central topic of conversation within the family (specifically, between the parents and the patient), evaluate and review adolescent issues with the family and problem-solve best practices for dealing with these issues, assist the parents to transition to focusing on their relationship as a couple, and conclude treatment (Lock & Le Grange, 2012). In Phase III, sessions occur every 4–6 weeks. Some families may only need a handful of sessions in Phase III, while others benefit from remaining longer in treatment. The limited frequency of sessions in Phase III forces therapy to focus on only a few themes, encouraging the family to prioritize issues in session and understand the need to work as a family on other issues outside of therapy. During Phase III, treatment should explore adolescent themes and patterns of behavior. The disorder likely has set the adolescent back, behind her peers, and it is important to educate family members about the stages of development so that they can determine where issues may arise. Then the family members identify and evaluate the issues and problem-solve. The therapist might keep a record throughout treatment of any issues mentioned and reintroduce them now that the focus can be turned to issues other than eating. The therapist should check in with the parents as a couple and acknowledge that their child's ED may have been the focal point of their relationship over the course of treatment. The therapist should discuss with parents how to transition their relationship focus back to each other instead of ameliorating their child's ED. The therapist should help the family members plan for future issues that might come up (e.g., relapse); finally, the therapist should summarize each session and formally terminate the treatment at the last session. As with the way treatment began, it is important for the therapist to recognize each family member's contribution and say good-bye to each member.

FBT for BN

Although FBT is not a well-established treatment for BN, research findings suggest that it should be considered a possibly efficacious treatment for adolescent BN (Keel & Haedt, 2008). FBT for adolescent BN (FBT-BN) is very similar to FBT for AN (FBT-AN); however, it differs in several important ways (Le Grange & Lock, 2007). First, Phase I emphasizes regulating eating and eliminating binge and purge behaviors in FBT-BN, whereas Part I of FBT-AN emphasizes weight restoration. To eliminate binge and purge behaviors, the parents restrict access to binge-type foods and may restrict and monitor bathroom access. Of note, if an adolescent undergoing FBT-BN has a relatively low body weight, weight restoration should be addressed. The second major difference between FBT-BN and FBT-AN is that control of eating is never put entirely in the parents' hands like it is in FBT-AN, but through a more collaborative effort between parents and the adolescent. The rationale for this difference between treatments is twofold. First, adolescents with BN are not extremely low weight and in a state of starvation; their cognitive abilities are not as impaired nor is their health as gravely threatened. Second, adolescents seeking treatment for BN tend to be older than adolescents being treated for AN. Additionally, most adolescents with BN are similar to their peers in terms of development and autonomy, therefore making collaboration between adolescent and parents more feasible in treatment (Le Grange & Lock, 2007).

Another way FBT-BN differs from FBT-AN is that it is often more challenging given the higher rate of comorbid psychiatric disorders associated with BN (Le Grange & Lock, 2007). This makes it more difficult to stay focused on ED symptoms in treatment, for example, when other important issues arise that need therapeutic intervention (e.g., drug use, academic problems, risky behaviors). With self-starvation being of upmost concern due to its lethal nature, it is easier in FBT-AN to maintain sole focus on weight restoration and put other issues aside until later. One more major difference between FBT-BN and FBT-AN is that individuals with BN often feel guilt, shame, and discomfort regarding their symptoms (e.g., bingeing and purging). This often makes adolescents with BN more motivated to engage in treatment in the hope of reducing symptoms. Another challenge to FBT-BN, compared to FBT-AN, is the secretive nature of BN—the guilt and shame associated with the bingeing and purging make it likely that the parents are not fully aware of the adolescent's symptom severity. When using FBT to treat adolescents with AN, it is quite easy to convince parents of the seriousness of the condition because the parents can visually see that their child is very ill. This task is much more difficult in FBT-BN because, as previously discussed, many adolescents with BN keep their symptoms secret and appear healthy (e.g., healthy body weight). In summary, there are many similarities between FBT-BN and FBT-AN; however, therapists should not ignore the important differences between these treatments (Le Grange & Lock, 2007).

CONCLUSION

Eating disorders are serious mental health disorders that can cause significant impairment in child and adolescent development, including their serious effect on physical health. Family involvement is typically recommended in the assessment and treatment of EDs for this population. To date, FBT-AN is the only "well-established" treatment for any child and adolescent ED. Most research on assessment and treatment of EDs has been conducted in adults. More research is crucial to identify potential differences and establish evidence-based guidelines for assessment and treatment of EDs in children and adolescents.

REFERENCES

Adan, R. A. H., & Kaye W. H. (Eds.). (2011). *Behavioral neurobiology of eating disorders*. Heidelberg, Germany: Springer.

Allen, K. L., Byrne, S. M., Oddy, W. H., & Crosby, R. D. (2013). DSM-IV-TR and DSM-5 eating disorders in adolescents: Prevalence, stability, and psychosocial correlates in a population-based sample of male and female adolescents. *Journal of Abnormal Psychology, 122,* 720–732.

American Psychiatric Association. (2013). *Diagnostic and statistical manual of mental disorders* (5th ed.). Arlington, VA: Author.

American Psychological Association Task Force on Promotion and Dissemination of Psychological Procedures. (1995). Training in and dissemination of empirically validated psychological treatments: Report and recommendations. *Clinical Psychologist, 48,* 3–23.

Baldock, E., & Tchanturia, K. (2007). Translating laboratory research into practice: Foundations, functions and future of cognitive remediation therapy for anorexia nervosa. *Future Medicine, 4*(3), 285–292.

Biederman, J., Ball, S. W., Monuteaux, M. C., Surman, C. B., Johnson, J. L., & Zeitlin, S. (2007). Are girls with ADHD at risk for eating disorders?: Results from a controlled, five-year prospective study. *Journal of Developmental and Behavioral Pediatrics, 28*(4), 302–307.

Bleck, J. R., DeBate, R. D., & Olivardia, R. (2015). The comorbidity of ADHD and eating disorders in a nationally representative sample. *Journal of Behavioral Health Services and Research, 42*(4), 437–451.

Bryant-Waugh, R. J., Cooper, P. J., Taylor, C. L., & Lask, B. D. (1996). The use of the eating disorder examination with children: A pilot study. *International Journal of Eating Disorders, 19*(4), 391–397.

Bühren, K., Schwarte, R., Fluck, F., Timmesfeld, N., Krei, M., Egberts, K., et al. (2014). Comorbid psychiatric disorders in female adolescents with first-onset anorexia nervosa. *European Eating Disorders Review, 22,* 39–44.

Chambless, D. L., & Ollendick, T. H. (2001). Empirically supported psychological interventions: Controversies and evidence. *Annual Review of Psychology, 52,* 685–716.

Couturier, J., Kimber, M., & Szatmari, P. (2013). Efficacy of family-based treatment for adolescents with eating disorders: A systematic review and meta-analysis. *International Journal of Eating Disorders, 46*(1), 3–11.

Couturier, J., & Lock, J. (2006). What is remission in adolescent anorexia nervosa?: A review of various conceptualizations and quantitative analysis. *International Journal of Eating Disorders, 39*(3), 175–183.

Couturier, J., & Lock, J. (2007). A review of medication use for children and adolescents with eating disorders. *Journal of the Canadian Academy of Child and Adolescent Psychiatry, 16*(4), 173–176.

Crow, S. J., Mitchell, J. E., Roerig, J. D., & Steffen, K. (2009). What potential role is there for medication treatment in anorexia nervosa? *International Journal of Eating Disorders, 42*(1), 1–8.

Dahlgren, C. L., Lask, B., Landrø, N. I., & Rø, Ø. (2013). Neuropsychological functioning in adolescents with anorexia nervosa before and after cognitive remediation therapy: A feasibility trial. *International Journal of Eating Disorders, 46*(6), 576–581.

Dalle Grave, R., Calugi, S., Doll, H. A., & Fairburn, C. G. (2013). Enhanced cognitive behaviour therapy for adolescents with anorexia nervosa: An alternative to family therapy? *Behaviour Research and Therapy, 51*(1), 9–12.

DeBar, L. L., Wilson, G. T., Yarborough, B. J., Burns, B., Oyler, B., Hildebrandt, T., et al. (2013). Cognitive behavioral treatment for recurrent binge eating in adolescent girls: A pilot trial. *Cognitive and Behavioral Practice, 20*(2), 147–161.

Eisler, I., Dare, C., Hodes, M., Russell, G., Dodge, E., & Le Grange, D. (2000). Family therapy for adolescent anorexia nervosa: The results of a controlled comparison of two family interventions. *Journal of Child Psychology and Psychiatry, 41*(6), 727–736.

Fairburn, C. G. (2008). *Cognitive behavior therapy and eating disorders.* New York: Guilford Press.

Fairburn, C. G., & Beglin, S. J. (1994). Assessment of eating disorders: Interview or self-report questionnaire? *International Journal of Eating Disorders, 16*(4), 363–370.

Fairburn, C. G., & Cooper, Z. (1993). The Eating Disorder Examination (12th ed.). In C. G. Fairburn & G. T. Wilson (Eds.), *Binge eating: Nature, assessment, and treatment* (pp. 317–360). New York: Guilford Press.

Fairburn, C. G., Cooper, Z., & Shafran, R. (2003). Cognitive behavior therapy for eating disorders: A "transdiagnostic" theory and treatment. *Behaviour Research and Therapy, 41,* 509–528.

Fairweather-Schmidt, A. K., & Wade, T. (2014). DSM-5 eating disorders and other specified eating and feeding disorders: Is there a meaningful differentiation? *International Journal of Eating Disorders, 47,* 524–533.

Fichter, M. M., Herpertz, S., Quadflieg, N., & Herpertz-Dahlmann, B. (1998). Structured interview for anorexic and bulimic disorders for DSM-IV and ICD-10: Updated (third) revision. *International Journal of Eating Disorders, 24*(3), 227–249.

Fitzpatrick, K. K., Moye, A., Hoste, R., Lock, J., & Le Grange, D. (2010). Adolescent focused psychotherapy for adolescents with anorexia nervosa. *Journal of Contemporary Psychotherapy, 40*(1), 31–39.

Garner, D. M. (1991). *The Eating Disorder Inventory–C*. Lutz, FL: Psychological Assessment Resources.

Godart, N. T., Flament, M. F., Lecrubier, Y., & Jeammet, P. (2000). Anxiety disorders in anorexia nervosa and bulimia nervosa: Co-morbidity and chronology of appearance. *European Psychiatry, 15*, 38–45.

Goldschmidt, A. B., Doyle, A. C., & Wilfley, D. E. (2007). Assessment of binge eating in overweight youth using a questionnaire version of the Child Eating Disorder Examination with instructions. *International Journal of Eating Disorders, 40*(5), 460–467.

Guerdjikova, A. I., McElroy, S. L., Winstanley, E. L., Nelson, E. B., Mori, N., McCoy, J., et al. (2012). Duloxetine in the treatment of binge eating disorder with depressive disorders: A placebo-controlled trial. *International Journal of Eating Disorders, 45*(2), 281–289.

Holtkamp, K., Konrad, K., Kaiser, N., Ploenes, Y., Heussen, N., Grzella, I., et al. (2005). A retrospective study of SSRI treatment in adolescent anorexia nervosa: Insufficient evidence for efficacy. *Journal of Psychiatric Research, 39*(3), 303–310.

Hoopes, S. P., Reimherr, F. W., Hedges, D. W., Rosenthal, N. R., Kamin, M., Karim, R., et al. (2003). Treatment of bulimia nervosa with topiramate in a randomized, double-blind, placebo-controlled trial: Part 1. Improvement in binge and purge measures. *Journal of Clinical Psychiatry, 64*(11), 1335–1341.

Kass, A. E., Kolko, R. P., & Wilfley, D. E. (2013). Psychological treatments for eating disorders. *Current Opinion in Psychiatry, 26*, 549–555.

Kaufman, J., Birmaher, B., Brent, D., & Rao, U. (1997). Schedule for Affective Disorders and Schizophrenia for School-Age Children–Present and Lifetime version (K-SADS-PL): Initial reliability and validity data. *Journal of the American Academy of Child and Adolescent Psychiatry, 36*(7), 980–988.

Kaye, W. (2008). Neurobiology of anorexia and bulimia nervosa. *Physiology and Behavior, 94*(1), 121–135.

Kaye, W. H., Bulik, C. M., Thornton, L., Barbarich, N., Masters, K., & Price Foundation Collaborative Group. (2004). Comorbidity of anxiety disorders with anorexia and bulimia nervosa. *American Journal of Psychiatry, 161*, 2215–2221.

Keel, P. K., & Haedt, A. (2008). Evidence-based psychosocial treatments for eating problems and eating disorders. *Journal of Clinical Child and Adolescent Psychology, 37*(1), 39–61.

Klump, K. L., Bulik, C. M., Kaye, W. H., Treasure J., & Tyson, E. (2009). Academy for Eating Disorders position paper: Eating disorders are serious mental illnesses. *International Journal of Eating Disorders, 42*, 97–103.

Kotler, L. A., Devlin, M. J., Davies, M., & Walsh, B. T. (2003). An open trial of fluoxetine for adolescents with bulimia nervosa. *Journal of Child and Adolescent Psychopharmacology, 13*(3), 329–335.

Le Grange, D., Crosby, R. D., & Lock, J. (2008). Predictors and moderators of outcome in family-based treatment for adolescent bulimia nervosa. *Journal of the American Academy of Child and Adolescent Psychiatry, 47*(4), 464–470.

Le Grange, D., Crosby, R. D., Rathouz, P. J., & Leventhal, B. L. (2007). A randomized controlled comparison of family-based treatment and supportive psychotherapy for adolescent bulimia nervosa. *Archives of General Psychiatry, 64*(9), 1049–1056.

Le Grange, D., Eisler, I., Dare, C., & Russell, G. F. (1992). Evaluation of family treatments in adolescent anorexia nervosa: A pilot study. *International Journal of Eating Disorders, 12*(4), 347–357.

Le Grange, D., Hoste, R. R., Lock, J., & Bryson, S. W. (2011). Parental expressed emotion of adolescents with anorexia nervosa: Outcome in family-based treatment. *International Journal of Eating Disorders, 44*(8), 731–734.

Le Grange, D., & Lock, J. (2007). *Treating bulimia in adolescents: A family-based approach*. New York: Guilford Press.

Le Grange, D., Lock, J., Agras, W. S., Moye, A., Bryson, S. W., Jo, B., et al. (2012). Moderators and mediators of remission in family-based treatment and adolescent focused therapy for anorexia nervosa. *Behaviour Research and Therapy, 50*(2), 85–92.

Lock, J. (2011). Evaluation of family treatment models for eating disorders. *Current Opinion in Psychiatry, 24*(4), 274–279.

Lock, J., Agras, W. S., Bryson, S., & Kraemer, H. C. (2005). A comparison of short and long term family therapy for adolescent anorexia nervosa. *Journal of the American Academy of Child and Adolescent Psychiatry, 44*(7), 632–639.

Lock, J., & Le Grange, D. (2012). *Treatment manual for anorexia nervosa: A family-based approach* (2nd ed.). New York: Guilford Press.

Lock, J., Le Grange, D., Agras, W. S., Moye, A., Bryson, S. W., & Jo, B. (2010). Randomized clinical trial comparing family-based treatment with adolescent-focused individual therapy for adolescents with anorexia nervosa. *Archives of General Psychiatry, 67*(10), 1025–1032.

Maloney, M. J., McGuire, J. B., & Daniels, S. R. (1988). Reliability testing of a children's version of the Eating Attitude Test. *Journal of the American Academy of Child and Adolescent Psychiatry, 27*(5), 541–543.

Mazure, C. M., Halmi, K. A., Sunday, S. R., Romano, S. J., & Einhorn, A. M. (1994). The Yale–Brown–Cornell Eating Disorder Scale: Development, use, reliability and validity. *Journal of Psychiatric Research, 28*(5), 425–445.

Micali, N., & House, J. (2011). Assessment measures for child and adolescent eating disorders: A review. *Child and Adolescent Mental Health, 16*(2), 122–127.

Nickel, C., Tritt, K., Muehlbacher, M., Gil, F. P., Mitterlehner, F. O., Kaplan, P., et al. (2005). Topiramate treatment in bulimia nervosa patients: A randomized, double blind, placebo-controlled trial. *International Journal of Eating Disorders, 38*(4), 295–300.

Polivy, J., & Herman, C. P. (2002). Causes of eating disorders. *Annual Review of Psychology, 53*, 187–213.

Powers, P. S., & Cloak, N. L. (2012). Psychopharmacologic treatment of obesity and eating disorders in children and adolescents. *Child and Adolescent Psychiatric Clinics of North America, 21*(4), 831–859.

Pretorius, N., Dimmer, M., Power, E., Eisler, I., Simic, M., & Tchanturia, K. (2012). Evaluation of a cognitive remediation therapy group for adolescents with anorexia nervosa: Pilot study. *European Eating Disorders Review, 20*(4), 321–325.

Robin, A. L., Siegel, P. T., Moye, A. W., Gilroy, M., Dennis, A. B., & Sikand, A. (1999). A controlled comparison of family versus individual therapy for adolescents with anorexia nervosa. *Journal of the American Academy of Child and Adolescent Psychiatry, 38*(12), 1482–1489.

Rohde, P., Stice, E., & Marti, C. N. (2015). Development and predictive effects of eating disorder risk factors during adolescence: Implications for prevention efforts. *International Journal of Eating Disorders, 48*(2), 187–198.

Root, T. L., Poyastro Pinheiro, A., Thornton, L., Strober, M., Fernandez-Aranda, F., Brandt, H., et al. (2010). Substance use disorders in women with anorexia nervosa. *International Journal of Eating Disorders, 43*, 14–21.

Russell, G. F., Szmukler, G. I., Dare, C., & Eisler, I. (1987). An evaluation of family therapy in anorexia nervosa and bulimia nervosa. *Archives of General Psychiatry, 44*(12), 1047–1056.

Schmidt, U., Lee, S., Beecham, J., Perkins, S., Treasure, J., Yi, I., et al. (2007). A randomized controlled trial of family therapy and cognitive behavior therapy guided self-care for adolescents with bulimia nervosa and related disorders. *American Journal of Psychiatry, 164*(4), 591–598.

Schmidt, U., & Treasure, J. (1997). *Clinician's guide to getting better bit(e) by bit(e): A survival kit for sufferers of bulimia nervosa and binge eating disorders*. Hove, UK: Psychology Press.

Smink, F. R. E., van Hoeken, D., Oldehinkel, A. J., & Hoek, H. W. (2014). Prevalence and severity of DSM-5 eating disorders in a community cohort of adolescents. *International Journal of Eating Disorders, 47,* 610–619.

Stice, E., Marti, C., & Rohde, P. (2013). Prevalence, incidence, impairment, and course of the proposed DSM-5 eating disorder diagnoses in an 8-year prospective community study of young women. *Journal of Abnormal Psychology, 122,* 445–457.

Stiles-Shields, C., Hoste, R. R., Doyle, P., & Le Grange, D. (2012). A review of family-based treatment for adolescents with eating disorders. *Reviews on Recent Clinical Trials, 7,* 133–140.

Swanson, S. A., Crow, S. J., Le Grange, D., Swendsen, J., & Merikangas, K. R. (2011). Prevalence and correlates of eating disorders in adolescents. *Archives of General Pscyhiatry, 68,* 714–723.

Szmukler, G. I., Eisler, I., Russell, G. F., & Dare, C. (1985). Anorexia nervosa, parental "expressed emotion" and dropping out of treatment. *British Journal of Psychiatry, 147,* 265–271.

Tanofsky-Kraff, M., Shomaker, L. B., Olsen, C., Roza, C. A., Wolkoff, L. E., Columbo, K. M., et al. (2011). A prospective study of pediatric loss of control eating and psychological outcomes. *Journal of Abnormal Psychology, 120,* 108–118.

Tanofsky-Kraff, M., Wilfley, D. E., Young, J. F., Mufson, L., Yanovski, S. Z., Glasofer, D. R., et al. (2010). A pilot study of interpersonal psychotherapy for preventing excess weight gain in adolescent girls at-risk for obesity. *International Journal of Eating Disorders, 43(8),* 701–706.

Whitney, J., Easter, A., & Tchanturia, K. (2008). Service users' feedback on cognitive training in the treatment of anorexia nervosa: A qualitative study. *International Journal of Eating Disorders, 41(6),* 542–550.

Wilfley, D. E., Agras, W. S., Telch, C. F., Rossiter, E. M., Schneider, J. A., Cole, A. G., et al. (1993). Group cognitive-behavioral therapy and group interpersonal psychotherapy for the nonpurging bulimic individual: A controlled comparison. *Journal of Consulting and Clinical Psychology, 61(2),* 296–305.

Wilfley, D. E., Kolko, R. P., & Kass, A. E. (2011). Cognitive-behavioral therapy for weight management and eating disorders in children and adolescents. *Child and Adolescent Psychiatric Clinics of North America, 20(2),* 271–285.

Wilfley, D. E., MacKenzie, R. K., Welch, R. R., Ayres, V. E., & Weissman, M. M. (2000). *Interpersonal psychotherapy for group.* New York: Basic Books.

Wilfley, D. E., Welch, R. R., Stein, R. I., Spurrell, E. B., Cohen, L. R., Saelens, B. E., et al. (2002). A randomized comparison of group cognitive-behavioral therapy and group interpersonal psychotherapy for the treatment of overweight individuals with binge-eating disorder. *Archives of General Psychiatry, 59(8),* 713–721.

Wood, L., Al-Khairulla, H., & Lask, B. (2011). Group cognitive remediation therapy for adolescents with anorexia nervosa. *Clinical Child Psychology and Psychiatry, 16(2),* 225–231.

Young, J. F., & Mufson, L. (2003). *Manual for Interpersonal Psychotherapy Adolescent Skills Training (IPT-AST).* New York: Columbia University.

Zucker, N., Merwin, R., Elliott, C., Lacy, J., & Eichen, D. (2009). Assessment of eating disorder symptoms in children and adolescents. In J. L. Matson, F. Andrasik, & M. L. Matson (Eds.), *Assessing childhood psychopathology and developmental disabilities* (pp. 401–443). New York: Springer Science + Business Media.

CHAPTER 14

Substance Use Disorders

Eric F. Wagner, Ken Winters,
Tammy Chung, and Tracey Garcia

There are numerous features that characterize an adolescent's drug use: the age at which he or she initiates use; the pattern of use in terms of frequency, quantity, and duration; which drug or drugs the adolescent uses; the functional value of drug use for the adolescent (e.g., social benefits; psychological benefits); and the resulting personal and social consequences of use. We focus on this latter feature as it represents the most salient feature for how a substance use disorder (SUD) is defined.

THE DSM-5 DEFINITION OF SUDs

When drug use goes beyond occasional use (sometimes referred to as "recreational" or "experimental" use), it is common for the person to begin to experience symptoms of a drug use disorder. These symptoms are formally delineated by various nomenclatures, with the primary one used in the United States being the fifth edition of the *Diagnostic and Statistical Manual of Mental Disorders* (DSM-5; American Psychiatric Association, 2013). The 11 symptoms of an SUD reflect the salient problem behaviors that occur when an individual exhibits compulsive-like use of a drug: hazardous and harmful consequences; loss of control of one's use; and the narrowing of one's choices on a daily basis in order to accommodate drug-seeking and drug-using behaviors. Individuals are assigned an SUD diagnosis based on how many symptoms on that list they meet: no disorder (0–1), moderate (2–3), or severe (4 or more).

DSM-5 does not have distinct SUD criteria for adolescent and adults, and this issue has led to concerns about the applicability of the criteria to adolescents (Martin, Chung, & Langenbucher, 2008; Winters, Martin, & Chung, 2011). On the positive side, a sizable literature supports the validity of most of the 11 criteria when applied to adolescent populations (Chung & Martin, 2011). In addition, the elimination of the "legal problems" symptom in DSM-5 makes sense because this symptom tends to be less relevant for female and younger teenagers, and is significantly related to comorbid conduct disorder (Martin, Chung, Kirisci, & Langenbucher, 2006).

PREVALENCE AND COURSE

Peak risk for experimentation with, and escalation in consumption of, commonly used substances such as alcohol, marijuana, and other illicit drugs occurs during adolescence (Johnston, O'Malley, Miech, Bachman, & Schulenberg, 2014) National survey data of 12- to 17-year-olds indicated that prevalence rates of the prior 30 days' use of alcohol, marijuana, and other illicit drugs were 11.3, 7.1, and 3.0%, respectively (Substance Abuse and Mental Health Services Administration, 2014). Although only a minority of users become addicted, late adolescence (ages 17–18) marks a period of high risk for the onset of alcohol or marijuana dependence disorder (Kandel, Schaffran, Griesler, Samuolis, Davies, & Galanti, 2005; Wagner & Anthony, 2002). National data indicate that among 12- to 17-year-olds, 2.8% had alcohol dependence use disorder, 3.5% had an illicit dependence use disorder, and 5.2% had either an alcohol or illicit drug dependence use disorder in the previous year (Substance Abuse and Mental Health Services Administration, 2014).

For most substances, early onset of use (under age 17) is associated with greater risk for progression to dependence (Chen, Storr, & Anthony, 2009; Winters & Lee, 2008). Etiological models of SUD course propose that individual vulnerabilities (e.g., deviance proneness, history of trauma) interact with environmental context (e.g., substance-using peers) in determining SUD onset, duration, severity, and response to treatment (Brown et al., 2008). Also, because many teenagers meet criteria for more than one SUD (and often this occurs within 2 years of first use of a substance, to the point of developing an SUD symptom; Winters & Lee, 2008), there is likely a concentration of SUDs within a relatively small proportion of adolescents (Kaminer & Bukstein, 2008).

Adolescent-onset SUD is typically associated with a persistent course into young adulthood, such that among youth with an alcohol use disorder (AUD), a majority (55–62%) continued to have an alcohol diagnosis in young adulthood (Clark, De Bellis, Lynch, Cornelius, & Martin, 2003). Similarly, adolescent-onset of regular marijuana use has been associated with a chronic marijuana use disorder in young adulthood (Swift, Coffey, Carlin, Degenhardt, & Patton, 2008). Importantly, heavy substance use trajectories have been associated with co-occurring psychopathology (e.g., conduct problems) and other health risks (e.g., risky sexual behavior), suggesting a clustering of substance use problems with other problem behaviors and health risks that warrant attention in a high-risk subgroup of youth (Mustanski et al., 2013).

For alcohol and other drugs, early emerging SUD symptoms typically include substance-related interpersonal problems, difficulties in fulfilling major role obligations, and tolerance to drug effects (Chung & Martin, 2005; Wagner, Lloyd, & Gil, 2002). For marijuana and cigarettes, symptoms indicating impaired control over use (i.e., using more than intended) have been found to emerge within a year of regular use (DiFranza et al., 2002; Rosenberg & Anthony, 2001). Withdrawal is rarely endorsed by adolescents for most substances (Chung & Martin, 2005; Wagner et al., 2002), and emerges relatively late, in the context of chronic heavy use. However, some novice smokers report withdrawal at low levels of cigarette use (DiFranza et al., 2002), suggesting cross-drug differences in symptom development.

Posttreatment Trajectories of Substance Involvement and Psychosocial Outcomes

Studies of posttreatment SUD course have identified several prototypical trajectories of substance involvement, with the majority of youth showing stable remission or low levels of use, and a minority returning to regular or heavy substance use (Anderson, Ramo, Schulte, Cummins, & Brown, 2007; Chung & Maisto, 2006). Treated youth who are in remission or who demonstrate low substance use trajectories over follow-up had better emotional and social functioning than those who returned to heavy, chronic substance use (Brown, D'Amico, McCarthy, & Tapert, 2001). While improvements in some domains, such as school functioning, may occur within a year after treatment, improvements in other domains, such as family functioning, emerge more gradually over 2 years following treatment (Brown et al., 2001). Despite posttreatment improvements in multiple areas of functioning, treated youth continue to have lower levels of functioning compared to youth in the community (Winters, Stinchfield, Latimer, & Stone, 2008).

Studies of long-term adolescent treatment outcome reveal how developmental milestones (e.g., becoming a parent) and the transition to independent living are associated with change points in substance use trajectories. Long-term (e.g., up to 10-year) follow-up indicates that most youth maintain a low level of substance involvement posttreatment, a trajectory that is associated with better adult outcomes (e.g., employment; Anderson et al., 2007) and better neuropsychological functioning (Hanson, Cummins, Tapert, & Brown, 2011). More persistent and severe substance involvement trajectories are typically associated with concurrent psychopathology (e.g., conduct problems, depression), which can complicate SUD course and recovery (Tomlinson, Brown, & Abrantes, 2004).

Predictors of Outcome

Co-occurring psychopathology has been consistently associated with worse outcomes among adolescents with SUD (Chung & Maisto, 2006; Winters et al., 2008). Brain-based markers, such as greater white-matter integrity in prefrontal regions, show promise as predictors of better treatment outcome (Chung, Pajtek, & Clark, 2013). During treatment, factors associated with better outcomes include longer treatment duration, higher motivation to change substance use behavior, and family participation in treatment (Chung & Maisto, 2006; Waldron & Turner, 2008). Posttreatment factors associated with better outcomes include engagement in continuing care (e.g., Sterling, Chi, Campbell, & Weisner, 2009), and continued motivation to abstain from substance use (King, Chung, & Maisto, 2009). Although treatment can facilitate SUD remission, environmental factors (i.e., family, peers, neighborhood) that operate outside of treatment account for a large proportion of variance in outcome (Hsieh, Hoffmann, & Hollister,

1998; Kelly, Brown, Abrantes, Kahler, & Myers, 2008; Latimer, Newcomb, Winters, & Stinchfield, 2000).

ETIOLOGICAL/CONCEPTUAL MODELS OF SUDs

Multidimensional Perspective

A phenomenon as complex as adolescent SUDs requires an etiological model that is multifactorial. Such models have been developmental in nature (e.g., Tarter et al., 1999; Zucker, Fitzgerald, & Moses, 1995) and have focused on the multiple genetic and environment factors that influence the phenotypes of interest, such as age of onset of drug use, maintenance of this use, and the emergence of signs and symptoms of an SUD (Clark & Winters, 2002). At their core, these models posit that a youth's liability to development of an SUD is the sum of risk and protective factors, with genetic and environmental origins (Tarter et al., 1999). Moreover, these models emphasize the contrast between normal and atypical development, and the importance of considering qualitative change over time (Cicchetti & Cohen, 1995), consistent with the developmental psychopathology perspective.

Isolating SUD-related genetic factors at a molecular level is still an ongoing scientific challenge (Ducci & Goldman, 2008). This body of knowledge has led to the nomination of a wide range of candidate genetic variants, typically associated with functioning of neurotransmitters linked to brain reward pathways. The pursuit of such models will likely continue given that family, adoption, and twin studies offer support for the view that SUD etiology includes a genetic component (Rutter & Silberg, 2002).

Self-Regulation, Brain Development, and Risk for Drug Involvement

Self-regulation refers to the ability to control and to plan one's behaviors and to resist impulses to engage in behaviors that result in negative consequences. The ability to self-regulate behavioral impulses is critical for successfully dealing with the increased exposure to risk that typically occurs during adolescence, including drug use. Indicators of poor self-regulation during childhood have been linked to increased risk for initiating drug use and developing an SUD (Kirisci, Tarter, Vanyukov, Reynolds, & Habeych, 2004).

The brain continues to develop throughout adolescence and into young adulthood (Giedd, 2004). Longitudinal research demonstrates that higher-order association cortices develop later than do primary sensorimotor cortices, with the dorsolateral prefrontal cortex developing through the latest stages of adolescence. This different trajectory in maturational processes is believed to contribute to a greater tendency for risk taking (and poorer self-regulation) during adolescence. However, adolescent risk-taking behavior may be additionally influenced by the way youth process social and emotional cues (Steinberg, 2004).

Adolescent brain development raises concerns about the unique vulnerability to neurotoxicity attributable to drug use among teenagers. Animal studies have shown, for example, that prenatal or adolescent exposure to tetrahydrocannabinol (THC), the active ingredient in marijuana, can heighten sensitivity of the reward system to other drugs (Dinieri & Hurd, 2012); a heighted brain sensitivity to drugs may contribute to greater drug involvement and accelerated progression to drug-related problems. Also, human studies suggest impairment in memory brain structures (e.g., the hippocampus) and in memory tasks linked to heavy alcohol use and heavy marijuana use (Brown, Tapert, Granholm, & Delis, 2000; Filbey & Yezhuvath, 2013; Zalesky et al., 2012).

EVIDENCE-BASED TREATMENTS FOR SUDs IN ADOLESCENTS

According to the National Institute on Drug Abuse's (2014) "Principles of Adolescent Substance Use Disorder Treatment: A Research-Based Guide," adolescent substance abuse treatment is most commonly offered in outpatient settings. As a result, this section focuses on effective, well-established (as per Chambless & Ollendick, 2001) outpatient treatments. Becker and Curry (2008) conducted a quality of evidence review of randomized clinical trials (RCTs) of outpatient treatments for adolescent SUDs, and found strong research evidence in support of three well-established approaches: (1) ecological family therapy (EFT), (2) brief motivational interventions (BMI or motivational enhancement therapy [MET]), and (3) cognitive-behavioral therapy (CBT). EFT models consider adolescent substance use problems in the context of multiple interrelated, nested systems and provide interventions based on the particular client's social ecology (e.g., brief strategic family therapy [Robbins et al., 2011], contingency management with family engagement strategies [Henggeler, McCart, Cunningham, & Chapman, 2012], ecologically based family therapy [Slesnick, Erdem, Bartle-Haring, & Brigham, 2013], multidimensional family therapy [Liddle, Rowe, Daykof, Henderson, & Greenbaum, 2009], and multisystemic therapy [Borduin, Schaeffer, & Heiblum, 2009]).

BMI and MET models are designed to increase a client's motivation to reduce substance use, whereas CBT models work to modify dysfunctional (i.e., pathology-promoting) beliefs and cognitive processes, change specific behaviors in order to meet specific goals (e.g., reduction or cessation of substance use), and address social/environmental contexts that influence cognition and behavior (Becker & Curry, 2008). Both BMI and CBT models appear to be generally as effective in the short-term to midterm as EFTs (Dennis et al., 2004; Henderson, Dakof, Greenbaum, & Liddle, 2010; Slesnick et al., 2013). Treatments that combine BMI and CBT approaches also exist (e.g., MET/CBT [Dennis et al., 2004]; guided self-change [GSC; Wagner, Hospital, Graziano, Morris, & Gil, 2014]), and a growing empirical literature provides strong support for these hybrid approaches.

Pharmacotherapy

Continuing advances regarding the neurobiological basis of drug addiction have supported the potential role of various medications to treat substance use problems. But the bulk of this research literature pertains to adults, perhaps due to concerns that medications are not safe for youth and are a form of "chemical restraint" (Kaminer & Marsch, 2011). Moreover, adolescents are exceptionally skilled at spotting adult-generated hypocrisies, and the idea of prescribing a drug to treat a drug problem may be perceived as hypocritical by teenagers. Nonetheless, there exists a tiny but growing literature on pharmacotherapy for adolescent SUDs; the current literature consists mostly of case reports and small open-label studies, and is characterized by minimal, inconsistent findings and medication adherence issues.

Predictors (Moderators/Mediators) of Treatment Response

Gender

In terms of symptomatology and drug problem severity, Oplund, Winters, and Stinchfield (1995) found that males, compared to females, exhibited greater symptomatology; however, other studies have found that girls entering treatment had significantly higher scores on substance-use frequency and substance-use-related problems (Becker, Stein, Curry, & Hersh, 2012; Stevens, Estrada, Murphy, McKnight, & Tims, 2004). Furthermore, males have also been found to have worse treatment outcomes, to use more drugs after treatment, and to be less likely than females to attend aftercare (Catalano, Hawkins, Wells, Miller, & Brewer, 1990; Chung & Martin, 2001; Grella, Joshi, & Hser, 2004; Hsieh & Hollister, 2004; Latimer, Winters, Stinchfield, & Traver, 2000); however, Springer, Rivaux, Bohman, and Yeung (2006) found that in day treatment, females were more likely than males to leave treatment. Finally, several studies have found no gender differences in treatment outcomes in several studies (e.g., Anderson et al., 2007; Fickenscher, Novins, & Beals, 2006; Wagner et al., 2014; Winters, Lee, Botzet, Fahnhorst, & Nicholson, 2014).

Race/Ethnicity

Research findings have been mixed in regard to whether race/ethnicity affects treatment outcomes, and if so, the mechanisms through which it does so. Several researchers found that ethnicity did not moderate or predict treatment outcome variables (e.g., Becker et al., 2012; Latimer, Winters, et al., 2000; Wagner et al., 2014; Winters et al., 2014:). Conversely, Clair and colleagues (2013) found that among substance- abusing adolescents, ethnicity (defined as Hispanic, white, and African American) moderated the relationship between treatment modality (i.e., motivational interviewing or relaxation therapy) and alcohol use outcomes (i.e., number and percentage of heavy drinking days); however, ethnicity did not moderate the relationship between treatment modality and marijuana use outcomes. Using survival analysis, Springer and colleagues (2006) found that Mexican American adolescents in treatment were more likely than African American and European American adolescents. Additionally, Grella and colleagues (2004) found that European American adolescent patients were less likely to be abstinent at follow-up than were African American adolescents. Jainchill, Hawke, De Leon, and Yagelka (2000) found that at 1 year posttreatment, Hispanics' drug use was almost three times as likely to decline (i.e., marijuana, alcohol, illegal drugs) as African Americans or whites.

Age and Developmental Level

Research has consistently demonstrated that substance use is higher among older adolescents (Becker et al., 2012; Wallace et al., 2003); however, whether and how age affects substance use treatment outcomes remain unclear. For example, Winters and colleagues (2014) found that age did not moderate the relationship between treatment condition and treatment outcomes. Additionally, Latimer, Winters, and colleagues (2000) found that age did not predict variations in treatment outcome.

At the same time, several studies have demonstrated that age does modify treatment outcomes. Rivaux, Springer, Bohman, Wagner, and Gil (2006) found that older adolescents were less likely to have successful treatment outcomes; however, Gonzales, Ang, Murphy, Glik, and Anglin (2014) found that younger adolescents were more likely than older adolescents to relapse at discharge and at 90-day follow-up. Among Native American adolescents, Fickenscher and colleagues (2006) found that more older adolescent completed treatment than did younger adolescents, consistent with Godley, Godley, Funk, Dennis, and Loveland's (2001) finding that adolescents who were unplanned discharges (i.e., against staff advice or at staff request) from treatment were younger. However, Anderson and colleagues (2007) found that younger adolescents were more likely to be minor relapsers (i.e., using substance for less than 3 consecutive days on one occasion and not returning to intake level of use) than to be major relapsers. Further complicating the examination of the effects of age on substance use treatment outcomes is the reliance on chronological age as an explanatory variable, which is somewhat problematic because age is not always a proxy for developmental level (Achenbach & Rescorla, 2006). Even now, little is known about how developmental issues may affect treatment outcome, despite the array of changes brought about by the adolescent period (Wagner, 2009).

Psychiatric Comorbidity

Both internalizing (e.g., major depressive disorder [MDD], anxiety) and externalizing disorders (e.g., attention-deficit/hyperactivity disorder [ADHD], conduct disorder [CD]) often are comorbid with adolescent SUDs (Branson, Clemmey, Harrell, Subramaniam, & Fishman, 2012; Chan, Dennis, & Funk, 2008; Grella et al., 2004; Godley et al., 2001; Latimer, Ernst, Hennessey, Stinchfield, & Winters, 2004; Rowe, Liddle, Greenbaum, & Henderson, 2004; Tomlinson et al., 2004). Many adolescents with an SUD have multiple disorders, often simultaneously demonstrating both an internalizing and externalizing disorder (Chan et al., 2008; Rowe et al., 2004). In terms of prognosis, adolescents who are in treatment for substance use and have additional comorbid mental health diagnoses demonstrate worse treatment outcomes (Anderson et al., 2007; Chung & Martin, 2001; Tomlinson et al., 2004). Interestingly, adolescents with an SUD and comorbid internalizing disorders fare better in terms of treatment outcomes when compared to adolescents with a comorbid externalizing disorder (Winters et al., 2008). Furthermore, adolescents who present with both internalizing and externalizing symptoms typically have the highest relapse rates (McCarthy, Tomlinson, Anderson, Marlatt, & Brown, 2005; Rowe et al., 2004; Shane, Jasiukaitis, & Green, 2003; Tomlinson et al., 2004; Warden et al., 2012).

Drug Use Severity at Intake and Polysubstance Use

The severity of the drug use at intake and/or the presence of polysubstance use have been linked to relapse. Williams, Chang, and the Addiction Centre Research Group (2000) concluded that the most consistent relation to positive treatment outcome is lower pretreatment substance use. Indeed, several studies have demonstrated that higher pretreatment substance use negatively affects treatment outcomes in terms of drug use during treatment, treatment completion, and relapse (e.g., Anderson et al., 2007; Rawson, Gonzales, Obert, McCann, & Brethen, 2005; Schell, Orlando, & Morral, 2005; Tamm et al., 2013).

Family Variables

Adolescents from families that are cohesive and demonstrate high levels of positive family functioning demonstrate greater improvements in response to drug treatment (Brown, Myers, Mott, & Vik, 1994; Goldstein et al., 2013; Winters et al., 2008). Additionally, family participation in treatment has a positive impact on treatment outcomes (Smith, Sells, Rodman, & Reynolds, 2006; Winters et al., 2008, 2014). Furthermore, a familial environment that encourages or supports substance use, or a family environment with problematic family functioning, has deleterious effects on successful treatment outcomes (Dakof, Tejeda, & Liddle, 2001; Galaif, Hser, Grella, & Joshi, 2001; Grella et al., 2004). That said, several studies found that family factors did not affect treatment outcome, either directly or as a potential mediator (Anderson et al., 2007; Hsieh et al., 1998; Winters, Fahnhorst, Botzet, Lee, Lalone, 2012)

Peers

Associating with a deviant peer group has been consistently linked to growth in adolescent problem behaviors (Dishion, Bullock, & Granic, 2002; Dishion & Medici Skaggs, 2000). Furthermore, there is some evidence that aggregating peers in treatment groups might lead to iatrogenic effects on problem behavior (Dishion, McCord, & Poulin, 1999); however, when examining peer relationships outside of treatment groups, the association of peers relative to treatment outcomes is complex. In general, having less deviant peers, or a greater proportion of non-substance-using peers, increases the likelihood of better treatment outcomes (Anderson et al., 2007; Battjes, Gordon, O'Grady, & Kinlock, 2004; Winters et al., 2008). Conversely, association with negative peers appears to have a negative effect on treatment outcomes (i.e., relapse) (Ciesla, 2010; Jainchill et al., 2000; Latimer, Newcomb, et al., 2000). When examining the predictive power of peers on reduction in substance use, Latimer, Winters, and colleagues (2000) found that among a clinical sample of adolescents, having abstinent friends had greater predictive power than having drug-using friends.

ASSESSMENT

Developmental Issues

As noted earlier in this chapter, DSM-5 does not have distinct SUD criteria for adolescent versus adults. This is an important issue because symptoms of SUD may manifest differently in adolescent and adults, or may be interpreted differently by adolescents than by adults. For example, the DSM-5 symptom "spending much time trying to obtain alcohol, drinking, or getting over its effects" may be endorsed by an adolescent as a result of difficulties in obtaining alcohol related to his or her status as a minor, rather than because the teenager is exhibiting compulsive-like alcohol use, which is the intended meaning of the symptom (Harford, Grant, Yi, & Chiung, 2005). Another example is the tolerance symptom. Variability of developmental sensitivity to drugs can be affected by neurodevelopmental changes during adolescence (Giedd, 2004); thus, what might appear to be a sign of tolerance may be a result of developmental changes rather than metabolic tolerance (Chung, Martin, Winters, & Langenbucher, 2001). These examples highlight the importance of developmentally informed assessment measures.

Screening and Comprehensive Assessment Tools

The field uses numerous developmentally informed assessment tools. We distinguish two general types: screening and comprehensive assessment (Allen, 2003). The goal of screening is to identify accurately the youth who may have a problem and, if suggestive, merit detailed assessment. An ideal screening should take no longer than 30 minutes and should cover recent drug use quantity and frequency (e.g., "How often did you use drugs in the past 6 months?"), the presence of adverse consequences of use (e.g., "Has your drug use led to problems with your parents?"), and contextual factors (e.g., "Do your friends use alcohol or other drugs?"). If the screening reveals positive indications of a substance use problem, a comprehensive assessment should follow.

A comprehensive assessment seeks to evaluate whether a diagnosis is present and determines the extent and nature of treatment needs. Common topics for a comprehensive assessment include the age of onset and progression of use for specific substances, diagnostic symptoms, contexts of use (e.g., the usual times and places of drug use), typical behavioral and social antecedents associated with drug use, peer and family influences, and personal consequences of use (e.g., school, social, family, psychological functioning, and physical functioning).

Clinical Interview

The initial interview with the adolescent sets the tone for the entire assessment and treatment process; in this case, first impressions do very much matter. In order to maximize clinical participation and engagement from teenagers, it is advisable to follow these principles:

- Begin with the teenager alone, then follow with the parent portion of the interview.

- Do not sit behind a desk; avoid too much note taking, as this takes away from maintaining eye contact with the youth.

- Build rapport throughout by using a motivational interviewing approach; the early part of the interview should focus on the present situation; more historical issues can be addressed later in the interview. Avoid pontificating, lecturing, and admonishing.

- Be honest with the teenager that your task is to understand his or her situation; emphasize that the subsequent course of action will be negotiated based on the specifics of the teenager's situation.

- Without approving, acknowledge that drug use has a functional, purposeful value for the teenager.
- Serve as the teenager's advocate within appropriate limits; emphasize the adolescent's strengths and assets; when offering challenges or criticism, focus on the activity, not the person.

Self-Report

Clinical assessment relies heavily on the self-report method due to its convenience, efficiency, and value in obtaining information from the most knowledgeable source (Martin & Winters, 1998). Self-report tools generally fall into one of three types: self-administered questionnaire (SAQ), standard interview, or computer-assisted interview (CAI). There are several lines of evidence supporting the validity of self-report (e.g., Brown et al., 1998; Johnston, & O'Malley, 1997; Maisto, Connors, & Allen, 1995): (1) Youth in clinical settings self-report much higher rates of drug involvement and accompanying problems compared to nonclinical samples; (2) youth self-report low rates of faking tendencies (typically measured by lying and social desirability items embedded in self-report assessments); and (3) there is a general pattern of convergence when self-report is compared to the reports of other informants (e.g., parents and teachers) and archival records. But as with adults, there are several sources that can compromise the validity of self-report, including lack of insight, inattentiveness, or misunderstanding of the question, intent to distort, and concerns about the consequences of admitting to drug use (Maisto et al., 1995; Winters et al., 2011).

Parent Reports

Parents can provide detailed and accurate information regarding many mental health problems experienced by their son or daughter, particularly externalizing disorders such as ADHD and conduct problems (Ivens & Rehm, 1988; Rey, Schrader, & Morris-Yates, 1992). Yet clinical experience and research indicate that parents generally do not provide meaningful details about their child's drug use and related consequences. Diagnostic agreement between mothers' and children's reports of SUDs has shown a considerable range (Edelbrock, Costello, Dulcan, Calabro, & Kala, 1986; Weissman et al., 1987; Winters, Anderson, Bengston, Stinchfield, & Latimer, 2000). Peers are probably a more accurate source regarding a teenager's drug use, but it is not realistic to expect an adolescent's friend to participate in an assessment.

OVERVIEW AND DESCRIPTION
OF KEY COMPONENTS OF EFFECTIVE TREATMENTS

As we noted earlier in this chapter, there is strong research evidence in support of the following well-established outpatient approaches to treating substance use problems among adolescents: EFT, (BMI or MET, CBT, and hybrid BMI/CBT therapies, such as GSC (Sobell & Sobell, 2005). The following sections provide an overview and description of the key treatment strategies and related considerations for each of these treatment approaches.

Generally speaking, EFTs conceptualize adolescent substance use problems as family problems, and as a result focus on engaging family members, improving interactions and communication within the family, enhancing the family's problem solving, and capitalizing on supports from the wider social and education system (National Institute for Health and Care Excellence [NICE], 2014). Necessarily, EFTs are delivered to families (vs. individuals or larger groups); improvement in family functioning is viewed as the fundamental mechanism of change in EFTs. Unfortunately, family involvement can be a barrier to receiving treatment. Enrollment and retention problems in EFTs are not uncommon (Hooven, Pike, & Walsh, 2013), and these problems become more pronounced (1) with teenagers who have more severe substance use problems (Alexander, Robbins, & Sexton, 2000; Biglan & Metzler, 1999; Hogue, Liddle, Becker, & Johnson-Leckrone, 2002; Nock & Kazdin, 2001; Tolan & McKay, 1996), (2) when intervention is delivered over multiple sessions (McCollister, Freitas, Prado, & Pantin, 2013), and (3) with racial/ethnic minority adolescents (Hooven et al., 2013). Moreover, EFT approaches are more expensive and less cost-effective than BMI, CBT, or hybrid BMI/CBT approaches, especially with teenagers with low to moderate levels of substance use problems (Dennis et al., 2004; French et al., 2002, 2008). Also, compared with BMIs and CBTs, EFTs are more vulnerable to diminished effectiveness due to variations across therapists, clients, and settings in the therapeutic alliance (Hogue, Dauber, Stambaugh, Cecero, & Liddle, 2006; Huey, Henggeler, Brondino, & Pickrel, 2000).

BMIs (and METs) share in common the use of a client-centered, collaborative, goal-oriented conversation style designed to strengthen intrinsic motivation for, and commitment to, substance use reduction or cessation; this style derives from the spirit, principles, and practices of motivational interviewing (MI; Miller & Rollnick, 2013). Miller and Rollnick (2013) characterize MI as "a person-centered counseling style for addressing the common problem of ambivalence about change" (p. 24). Four key elements characterize the spirit of MI: partnership, acceptance, compassion, and evocation. In principal, MI-based interventions increase the likelihood of changes in problematic substance use behaviors by helping clients (1) recognize that problems exist in their lives, and (2) overcome ambivalence about changing their substance use. Ambivalence, which is considered a normal (i.e., not pathological) human process, is expressed through clients' in-session change talk (pro-change arguments) and sustain talk (anti-change arguments). MI practices are directed toward magnifying discrepancies between client goals and current behavior (which increases ambivalence), and are represented by the acronym OARS: asking Open-ended questions, Affirming, Reflecting, and Summarizing. In clinical practice, MI can be used in individual, face-to-face consultation or with couples, families, or groups. Moreover, there is empirical support for MI's delivery via telephone, televideo, computer, and print across a variety of cultures and special populations. While sharing an MI core, BMIs and METs differ in regard to contact time and appropriateness for different levels of SUD severity. BMIs typically take place over one or two sessions and target clients in the early stages of substance use problems. METs extend contact to five or more sessions and target clients with mild to moderate substance use problems.

CBTs derive directly from behavioral and social learning perspectives on behavior, and conceptualize substance use problems as learned behaviors that are initiated and maintained in the context of environmental factors (Waldron & Kaminer, 2004). Cognitive processes (e.g., an individual's perception and appraisal of the environment) that can promote substance use also are incorporated into CBT conceptualizations. From the CBT perspective, processes that can lead to substance use problems include the direct experience of drug effects as rewarding or punishing, the observation and imitation of substance-using models (e.g., parents, siblings, peers), social reinforcement for substance use, and cognitive phenomena that include the anticipated effects of substances (i.e., expectancies) and self-efficacy beliefs about the ability to resist use. While CBT-based interventions for substance use problems are many and varied, typical components of treatment include identifying the circumstances ("triggers") associated with substance use (e.g., the setting, time, or place), and developing strategies to manage urges and cravings (e.g., self-control, reinforcement for competing behaviors, coping skills training). In addition, CBT approaches often include skills-focused interventions (e.g., training in drug and alcohol refusal, communication skills, problem solving, and/or assertiveness), mood regulation interventions (e.g., relaxation training, anger management, modifying cognitive distortions), and relapse prevention. CBT sessions typically are delivered in individual or group formats, and often involve modeling, behavior rehearsal, feedback about behavior, and homework assignments.

Hybrid BMI/CBT therapies integrate motivational and cognitive-behavioral approaches for treating substance use problems. BMI/CBTs typically address motivation to change, build skills necessary to increase social support, promote participation in non-drug-related activities, and bolster substance use avoidance and non-substance-involved stress coping skills. GSC (Sobell & Sobell, 2005) is an integrated BMI/CBT treatment with several published RCTs supporting its efficacy for addressing alcohol and other drug (AOD) problems, as well as a growing literature supporting its efficacy with English- and Spanish-speaking teenagers (Breslin, Li, Sdao-Jarvie, Tupker, & Ittig-Deland, 2002; Gil, Wagner, & Tubman, 2004; Martínez Martínez, Pedroza Cabrera, de los Ángeles-Vacío Muro, Jiménez Pérez, & Salazar Garza, 2008; Martínez Martínez, Salazar Garza, Pedroza Cabrera, Ruiz Torres, & Ayala Velázquez, 2008; Wagner et al., 2014). Another popular hybrid BMI/CBT therapy is MET/CBT (Riley, Rieckmann, & McCarty, 2008), developed for the Cannabis Youth Treatment (CYT; see Dennis et al., 2004) study. While originally cast in both five- and 12-session versions, MET/CBT-5 has proven just as effective, and significantly less costly, than MET/CBT-12. MET/CBT-5 involves two individual sessions of MI followed by three group sessions of CBT.

An important consideration in the treatment of adolescent SUDs is where and with whom they take place. In regard to *where,* effective adolescent substance use treatment can take place in schools, homes, outpatient clinics, partial or inpatient hospitals, and residential facilities (e.g., a juvenile detention center). In regard to *with whom,* effective treatment can involve individual adolescents, adolescents and their families, groups of teens with substance use problems, and/or groups of parents of teens with substance use problems. As we noted earlier in this chapter, adolescent drug abuse treatment is most commonly offered in outpatient settings, which are best suited for adolescents with less severe substance use problems, few co-occurring mental health problems, and supportive living environments (NIDA, 2014). Adolescents who have more severe substance use problems, yet can still be safely managed while living at home, may be referred to partial hospitalization or "day treatment." Adolescents with the most severe substance use problems, which typically include complex psychiatric and/or medical problems and/or family issues, may be referred to residential treatment, which provides a 24-hour structured environment to facilitate amenability and response to treatment.

EVIDENCE-BASED TREATMENTS IN PRACTICE: THE EXAMPLE OF GSC

An extensive international literature has shown that GSC, when used with individuals, couples, or groups, has "consistently resulted in substantial and significant gains over the course of treatment that are maintained in follow-up" (Sobell & Sobell, 2005). GSC employs (1) a motivational client–therapist interactional style (see Miller & Rollnick, 2013), (2) a cognitive-behavioral approach to planning, implementing, and maintaining changes in AOD behaviors (see Kaminer & Waldron, 2006; Magill & Ray, 2009), and (3) a harm-reduction perspective for the treatment of addictive behaviors (see Monti et al., 1999; Ritter & Cameron, 2006). GSC's major treatment components include (1) weekly self-monitoring of behaviors targeted for change; (2) treatment goal advice, with clients selecting their own goal; (3) brief readings and homework assignments exploring high-risk situations, options, and action plans; (4) motivational strategies to increase clients' commitment to change; and (5) cognitive relapse prevention procedures. As noted earlier, a growing literature supports GSC's efficacy with English- and Spanish-speaking teenagers; a session-by-session outline of GSC, based on a recent RCT by Wagner and colleagues (2014), is provided in Table 14.1.

Case Example

The following fictional case example demonstrates the core and prototypical components of GSC treatment for adolescents with SUDs. The client, Carlos, a 16-year-old Hispanic male, had recently been expelled from the 11th grade. He was court-mandated to treatment after he was arrested and charged with possession of marijuana. In anticipation of GSC treatment, he completed a comprehensive assessment that covered substance use, negative consequences related to substance use, psychiatric symptomatology, juvenile justice system involvement, family dynamics, peer relations, and social support.

Session 1

Carlos was brought to the first therapy session by his mother, who agreed to be responsible for his transportation to and from session. After a brief introduction, the therapist asked Carlos to describe the details of his involvement in the legal system and his subsequent referral to GSC. Carlos recalled his arrest, stating that he was charged with "intent to sell" because of the amount of marijuana with which he was caught. He also pointed out that his personal preferences among substances were alcohol and cigarettes, not marijuana.

The therapist remarked while treatment would focus on substance use, she wanted to know more about who Carlos was before talking about his use. The GSC written exercise, "Things That Are Important to Me," which is designed to do just that, was completed by Carlos at this point. The exercise revealed that friends and faithfulness were important to the client, as well as setting and achieving goals, industry (working hard),

TABLE 14.1. GSC Intervention: Content of Sessions

Session 1

Explanation of the rationale behind GSC treatment, provision of personalized feedback on substance use patterns based on the assessment findings, review of a decisional balance exercise, setting goals for treatment, and completing self-monitoring exercises

Session 2

Review of past week substance use, examining personal antecedents ("triggers") and consequences of substance use and violence, discussing the management of occasional "slips" in attempts to change behavior, homework assignments, provision of feedback on drug use situation profiles based on the information obtained from baseline assessment, and evaluation of the client's perceptions of their substance use problems

Session 3

Review of past week substance use, examination of feelings and experiences that may contribute to a range of adolescent problem behaviors, refusal skills and social skills training, development of an options and actions plan for managing substance use and violence "trigger" situations, review of personal priorities, and development of a change plan

Session 4

Review of past week substance use, a second assessment of drug use situation profiles, and discussion of general causes of stress, coping with stress, and stress prevention

Session 5

Rereview and discussion of goals for change, review of past week substance use, development of a list of short- and long-term life goals, a reevaluation of the client's perceptions of their substance use problems, and a discussion of positive social supports for maintaining changes

Sessions 6 and 7

Optional sessions, as requested by client, to review any of the material covered in previous sessions

---

simplicity, and knowledge. After a brief discussion, next came the "Decision to Change" written exercise, which addresses the pros and cons of making substance use changes. Carlos completed it, and his pros for using alcohol were, "I don't have to deal with my problems or pay attention" and "It helps me calm down and relax;" his con for alcohol use was "I will have money problems." He elaborated:

"I don't go out of my way for school. I just don't care about it. But, in my house, like let's say I get mad at my dad, and we end up fighting or something, and my friends are there, or I just call them up and say, 'Hey, come pick me up.' And we hang out at his house and just drink or smoke something and I don't pay attention. I just start talking to my friends."

Following the pros and cons of use, the client completed "Goals for Change" Questionnaire. On a scale of 0 to 100, the level of importance for Carlos to change his alcohol use was 25 ("less important than most of the other things I would like to achieve now"), and his confidence to change was 100 ("I think I will definitely achieve my goal").

CARLOS: I care but I really don't care that much.

THERAPIST: So it's something that you want to work toward but there are other things that you want to do right now.

CARLOS: Yes, that sounds right.

THERAPIST: And it seems like when you make a decision and you set a goal for yourself, you are confident in your ability to achieve that goal. You are 100% confident.

CARLOS: Yes, I'm sure when I'm sure.

Next Carlos completed the "Session Check-In," on which past week substance use is recorded and reviewed. Carlos reported only 1 day of use over the past week, which was Saturday.

THERAPIST: Was drinking something you planned to do that day?

CARLOS: I was at the gas station to buy cigarettes and I decided to get some beer. I just felt like it. I just wanted to drink.

When asked what happened on the other 6 days, Carlos was not able to recall much. His goal for the next session was to use drugs fewer days of the week. When asked to rate his week on a scale of 0 ("lousy") to 10 ("fantastic"), the Carlos rated it as a 2.

Next, Carlos and therapist reviewed a personalized feedback summary derived from the client's comprehensive assessment. Carlos reported that he had had 10 or more drinks in the last month; it was noted that only 2.8% (i.e., 3 out of every 100) of students his age and gender drank as much or more than Carlos. He also reported having used cocaine at some point in his life; it was noted that only 4% of adolescents his age and gender report ever using cocaine.

To wrap up the session, the therapist asked Carlos what stood out for him in the day's material. He immediately stated that the personalized feedback summaries were the most meaningful to him because "It made me realize. I know I drink a lot, but I didn't realize it was that much."

Session 2

The session began with a brief review of Session 1. On his "Session Check-In," Carlos reported that he thought about using only once (on Sunday), but that he did not use that day. However, he used on 3 days (Thursday, Friday, and Saturday) without thinking about it first. He said he drank because he "felt the need to cope" and because he was "thirsty." The therapist also inquired about the days that Carlos avoided using, to which Carlos responded, "Someone could have given me money to buy it but I just didn't feel like drinking." His new goal was to use fewer days, and he rated his week at a 3.5, which was a bit higher than the previous week.

The "Session Check-In" was followed by a review if the Brief Situational Confidence Questionnaire (BSCQ), which addressed Carlos's confidence in his ability to resist using utilizing a 0- to 100-point scale. Carlos's confidence to resist using across different situations was as follows: Unpleasant Emotions (20), Physical Discomfort (100), Pleasant

Emotions (100), Testing Control over My Use of Alcohol or Drugs (100), Urges and Temptations (70), Conflict with Others (100), Social Problems at School (100), and Pleasant Times with Others (30). After identification of Carlos's low-confidence, high-risk situations, discussion flowed to the topic of *triggers*, defined as situations, behaviors, thoughts, or feelings, commonly associated with using alcohol or drugs, so that the trigger might make you want to use substances. Carlos identified his personal triggers as highly emotional situations, both negative and positive, especially "conflict with parents." He described his second trigger as "People in school telling me what to do."

Next, Carlos was asked to consider non-substance-use strategies for coping with triggers, and to complete a written "Options and Actions Plan" for each trigger. For the first trigger, "Parents getting mad at me," Carlos's options were (1) to smoke and drink with a friend, (2) to talk with a friend, and (3) to look at a magazine. His actions were to "have a friend pick me up" and "look at a magazine." For consequences, he stated that there were "no bad consequences" and that he would have more money (positive). For the second trigger, "School problems," Carlos's options were (1) listening to the teacher or (2) not paying attention. His actions were to "pay attention" or "find someone to talk to." His only consequence was that he "wouldn't get in trouble." In order to help Carlos prepare to put his action plan into effect, he and the therapist discussed facilitators and barriers to implementation.

The therapist then asked Carlos to consider the results from the "Where Are You Now Scale?" completed during his initial assessment. At that time, he rated himself at 8 ("not a huge problem, but somewhat"); now that he had begun GSC, he rated himself at a 7, indicating an increase in problem severity. When asked about this increase, Carlos replied that he now recognized that he drank too much, citing the personalized feedback from Session 1 as evidence. At the conclusion of the session, when asked to identify what stood out for him in that day, the Carlos reported, "I have been drinking a little bit more."

Session 3

The session began with a brief review of Session 2, with an emphasis on "Options and Actions." Carlos reported using his plan, noting, "I tried the one with my dad. . . . It went all right. I didn't drink." He also noted that he could not follow through on all of his actions because his friend showed up with his girlfriend, which meant that Carlos and his friend were unable to talk things through.

Carlos's goal for the next week was to "stay the same." The therapist noted that drinking one day a week seemed workable, and commented that this was a big change from previous sessions. Carlos's rating of his past week was a 4.5, an increase from 3.5 the week before. When asked what made this week better, Carlos noted, "That my dad actually trusted me." The therapist related this incident back to Carlos's triggers.

Next, the therapist introduced the *slip back effect*, which results from a brief return (i.e., lapse) to previous patterns of substance use. Discussion focused on how bad people may feel if they slip (i.e., the slip back effect), and how to prevent a slip from becoming a full-blown fall (i.e., relapse) to problematic substance use. The therapist presented ways to prevent a lapse from becoming a relapse. In response, to demonstrate his understanding of the slip back effect, Carlos related a story about how he had improved his grades, but when he received a poor grade ended up not caring and giving up. The therapist concluded discussion of the slip back effect by noting that acknowledging the effect did not equate with giving permission to have a slip.

Subsequently, the therapist moved on to discuss communication skills, the major focus of Session 3. This began with a discussion of alcohol- and drug-refusal skills. The therapist asked Carlos to think back to a recent occasion when he did not drink, even though he had the chance. Carlos related that he was not prone to giving in to peer pressure. The therapist referred back to Carlos's triggers, stating that possibly if Carlos could communicate better, he also could avoid drinking in other high-risk situations.

The therapist next defined communication skills and assertiveness, emphasizing that good communication involves both expressing oneself and listening to others. In addition, some time was spent discussing getting and showing respect when interacting with others. Next, Carlos read through a list of communication "rights," and completed "Steps Toward Better Communication," an exercise designed to strengthen effective communication skills by considering different approaches to social interaction. The therapist role-played with Carlos how best to respond to his trigger of having difficulty with his teachers. With practice and repetition, Carlos came see how he could control the tone and direction of the conversation by choosing his words carefully, and remaining calm.

To demonstrate the social skill of "avoid interrupting," the therapist asked Carlos to tell her about a magazine he had brought with him, then proceeded to continually interrupt him while he spoke. Eventually, they laughed, and she acknowledged that she was being rude and annoying by interrupting and not letting him speak. In the "Practicing Better Communication" exercise, Carlos chose to role-play with the therapist "a teacher blames you for something you didn't do." The therapist and Carlos conducted the role play, focusing on newly learned communication skills, with Carlos taking both the student and teacher roles. Finally, Carlos completed a "Change Plan Worksheet," which asks respondents to identify something relating to substance use that they want to change. Carlos's desired changes were to "cut down on my drinking and stop smoking cigarettes." The most important reason he wanted to make those changes was "I can't run half a block because of my smoking, which is embarrassing and the alcohol costs too much." The steps identified to implement his plan were "Don't buy any cigarettes or vodka and make good decisions." Carlos was able to name one friend who would be able to help by not drinking in front of him. Finally, when asked about things that could interfere with his plans, Carlos mentioned "school and parents getting mad at me"; in response, Carlos and the therapist briefly reviewed previously identified options and actions.

Session 4

The session began with Carlos completing another BSCQ in order to gauge his current situational confidence, followed by a review of communication skills from the previous session, during which Carlos offered the following example:

> CARLOS: My friend picked me up and we went to a party, not a keg party but a dancing party. Then it got boring so my friends said, "Let's go drink." They got money and went on a beer run, and I said, "I'm not going to drink today because I am sick and I don't really feel like drinking." I didn't want to smoke either but I ended up having a cigarette.

THERAPIST: It sounds like you did a great job avoiding drinking. You decided not to drink, and stuck to that decision and followed through on it. That was a real success, and you made it happen.

Carlos next reported that he did not think about or use any substances in the previous week, and that he accomplished this by avoiding using. His goals for the next week were to not use at all. His weekly rating was a 7.5, which he attributed to "finally getting some of my dad's trust back."

Carlos next completed "General Causes of Stress" written exercise, and reported the following sources of stress: "parents expecting me to be perfect," "parents expecting me to have perfect friends," "parents who fight," "having too much to do," and "teachers expecting too much."

THERAPIST: That's a lot of stress. How might your stress be related to your alcohol use?

CARLOS: Sometimes, when parents expect too much and expect me to be perfect, I would drink. It might happen too with other kinds of stress, but for sure for me when they got up in my face I would drink.

THERAPIST: So there seems for sure to be an association between stress from your parents and drinking. How about dealing with stress without drinking? What could you do instead?

CARLOS: Hmm . . . talking with friends. Maybe with my brother, since he knows about my parents fighting about the bills, the only reason they usually talk. And maybe exercise, though I doubt it because I don't have anyone to go to the gym with.

The therapist elaborated that stress could not be completely eliminated, but Carlos could control the number of things that stress him out, reduce the impact of that stress, and shorten the duration of the stress. Next, she asked Carlos to consider "Future Goals," and identify 1-month, 1-year, and 5-year goals for substance use and other areas of his life. In 1 month, Carlos's goal was to "stop or don't drink as much"; in other areas of his life, his goals were going to school and getting a job. In 1-year, his AOD use goal was to "just use on special occasions"; he also wanted to "have a job, go to school, and have a car." Finally, his 5-year AOD use goal remained "just use on special occasions"; his 5-year life goals included "finish high school and go to some type of college." Finally, the therapist asked Carlos to consider how the goals in the two columns (substance use and other areas of life) related to each other.

"I know if I go to school and drink, I won't do good. I won't be able to think about working. So I have to work really hard to achieve the substance use goals to achieve the other goals."

At the end of session, Carlos stated that he enjoyed discussing stress and how it could be a trigger, the awareness of which would make him more likely to choose non-substance-use options in order to deal with stress.

Session 5

Carlos opened the final GSC session by noting that the activities and discussion from the previous session "really got me thinking." Apparently, Carlos had encountered a friend who used crack cocaine, and whose life appeared bleak and aimless. This reminded Carlos of his future goals and the connection between substance use and other things he wanted to achieve. On the "Session Check-In," Carlos reported that he only thought about using on 1 day, but he did not use at all. He reported that he wanted to drink due to "thirst," but when he thought about using, he did something else. His goal for the upcoming week, "taking into consideration the holiday weekend," included "drink, but not as much." The therapist asked him to be more specific, to which Carlos replied, "Just drink on holidays and stop smoking (cigarettes)." He rated his past week as a 4.5, and commented that (1) his friends were still using around him and (2) his parents had decided to get a divorce, so he had been staying home more lately to stay out of trouble.

The majority of the remainder of the session involved comparing where Carlos was now to where he was when he began treatment. Referring back to the "Decision to Change Exercise" from Session 1, the therapist asked Carlos to review his original pros and cons and consider whether any of his reasons had changed since then. Carlos noted, "They are all the same," and added "having fewer problems at work and school" as another reason for changing. Next, the intake and Session 4 BSCQ profiles were compares. Session 4 confidence ratings were as follows: Unpleasant Emotions (70), Physical Discomfort (100), Pleasant Emotions (100), Testing Control over My Use of Alcohol or Drugs (100), Urges and Temptations (70), Conflict with Others (80), Social Problems at School (60), Pleasant Times with Others (100). The therapist asked Carlos what had increased his confidence, to which Carlos responded, "Gains in knowledge of triggers, options for responding to triggers, effective stress coping, and communication. Now I know that if someone, like my mom, gets me mad, now I know I have a different way." The therapist then asked Carlos to complete a "Goals for Change Questionnaire," and he gave an importance rating of 75 (compared to a Session 1 rating of 25) and a confidence rating of 100 (same score as Session 1). The therapist asked Carlos what he believed accounted for his change in importance and stability in confidence, to which he responded, "When I first came in I really didn't care about my drinking. Now I'm at 75 because I know I have a problem with drinking because other people drink to get drunk but they do it at a party once in a while. And when I look at myself I think I used to do it every weekend. When other people wanted to drink and didn't want to buy it, I wasted my money."

Carlos next completed his final "Where Are You Now?" scale. Carlos's rating was 9 because even though he was not drinking, he remained aware that high-risk situations could lead to drinking. Subsequently, the therapist asked Carlos to review the "Future Goals" form that he had completed the previous week; Carlos commented that his goals were still the same, but the therapist suggested that Carlos add goals for reducing his cigarette smoking. Carlos's resulting goals were to reduce the number of cigarettes in 1 month, and stop smoking in 1 year. Carlos reported that he particularly enjoyed reflecting back to the beginning of treatment and attributed his progress to tracking his use and thinking about it: "It's a whole different mentality."

The therapist then explained to Carlos that getting support is critical for maintaining changes and for continuing to make additional changes. To this end, Carlos was asked to generate a list of people who would be able to offer him support. Carlos listed three friends and talked about each one. The therapist also gave him a list of support numbers he could use.

Before saying good-bye, the therapist reviewed the positive changes Carlos has made, reinforcing his efforts, and discussed what Carlos would need to do to maintain his changes in alcohol use and to reduce his cigarette smoking. The therapist told him she enjoyed working with him and was impressed with how well he had made use of the material. She reminded Carlos that booster sessions would be available to him if he ever needed them. When asked if he had any final questions, Carlos talked about a friend whose substance use concerned him, and how he might help that friend. Carlos and the therapist discussed the importance of peer support, and the therapist gave him a GSC brochure to pass along to his friend. Finally, Carlos was provided a GSC certificate of completion, and the therapist shook Carlos's hand and wished him well.

REFERENCES

Achenbach, T. M., & Rescorla, L. A. (2006). Developmental issues in assessment, taxonomy, and diagnosis of psychopathology: Life span and multicultural perspectives. In D. Cicchetti & D. J. Cohen (Eds.), *Developmental psychopathology, theory and method* (pp. 139–180). Hoboken, NJ: Wiley.

Alexander, J. F., Robbins, M. S., & Sexton, T. L. (2000). Family-based interventions with older, at-risk youth: From promise to proof to practice. *Journal of Primary Prevention, 21*(2), 185–205.

Allen, J. P. (2003). Assessment of alcohol problems: An overview. In J. P. Allen & V. B. Wilson (Eds.), *Assessing alcohol problems: A guide for clinicians and researchers* (2nd ed., pp. 1–11). Rockville, MD: National Institute on Alcohol Abuse and Alcoholism.

American Psychiatric Association. (2013). *Diagnostic and statistical manual of mental disorders* (5th ed.). Arlington, VA: Author.

Anderson, K. G., Ramo, D. E., Schulte, M. T., Cummins, K. & Brown, S. A. (2007). Substance use treatment outcomes for youth: Integrating personal and environmental predictors. *Drug and Alcohol Dependence, 88,* 42–48.

Battjes, R. J., Gordon, M. S., O'Grady, K. E., & Kinlock, T. W. (2004). Predicting retention of adolescents in substance abuse treatment. *Addictive Behaviors, 29,* 1021–1027.

Becker, S. J., & Curry, J. F. (2008). Outpatient interventions for adolescent substance abuse: A quality of evidence review. *Journal of Consulting and Clinical Psychology, 76*(4), 531–543.

Becker, S. J., Stein, G. L., Curry, J. F., & Hersh, J. (2012). Ethnic differences among substance-abusing adolescents in a treatment dissemination project. *Journal of Substance Abuse Treatment, 42,* 328–336.

Biglan, A., & Metzler, C. (1999). A public health perspective for research on family-focused interventions. In R. Ashery, E. Robertson, & K. Kumpfer (Eds.), *Drug abuse prevention through family-focused interventions* (NIDA Research Monograph, pp. 430–458). Rockville, MD: National Institute on Drug Abuse.

Borduin, C. M., Schaeffer, C. M., & Heiblum, N. (2009). A randomized clinical trial of multisystemic therapy with juvenile sexual offenders: Effects on youth social ecology and criminal activity. *Journal of Consulting and Clinical Psychology, 77,* 26–37.

Branson, C. E., Clemmey, P., Harrell, P., Subramaniam, G., & Fishman, M. (2012). Polysubstance use and heroin relapse among adolescents following residential treatment. *Journal of Child and Adolescent Substance Abuse, 21,* 204–221.

Breslin, F. C., Li, S., Sdao-Jarvie, K., Tupker, E., & Ittig-Deland, V. (2002). Brief treatment for young substance abusers: A pilot study in an addiction treatment setting. *Psychology of Addictive Behaviors, 16*(1), 10–16.

Brown, S. A., D'Amico, E. J., McCarthy, D. M., & Tapert, S. F. (2001). Four-year outcomes from adolescent alcohol and drug treatment. *Journal of Studies on Alcohol, 62*(3), 381–388.

Brown, S. A., McGue, M., Maggs, J., Schulenberg, J., Hingson, R., Swartzwelder, S., et al. (2008). A developmental perspective on alcohol and youths 16 to 20 years of age. *Pediatrics, 121*(Suppl. 4), S290–S310.

Brown, S. A., Myers, M. G., Lippke, L., Tapert, S. F., Stewart, D. G., & Vik, P. W. (1998). Psychometric evaluation of the Customary Drinking and Drug Use Record (CDDR): A measure of adolescent alcohol and drug involvement. *Journal of Studies on Alcohol, 59,* 427–438.

Brown, S. A., Myers, M. G., Mott, M. A., & Vik, P. W. (1994). Correlates of success following treatment for adolescent substance abuse. *Applied and Preventive Psychology, 3,* 61–73.

Brown, S. A., Tapert, S. F., Granholm, E., & Delis, D. C. (2000). Neurocognitive functioning of adolescents: Effects of protracted alcohol use. *Alcohol Clinical and Experimental Research, 24,* 164–171.

Catalano, R. F., Hawkins, J. D., Wells, E. A., Miller, J., & Brewer, D. (1990). Evaluation of the effectiveness of adolescent drug abuse treatment, assessment of risks for relapse, and promising approaches for relapse prevention. *International Journal of the Addictions, 25,* 1085–1140.

Chambless, D. L., & Ollendick, T. H. (2001). Empirically supported psychological interventions: Controversies and evidence. *Annual Review of Psychology, 52,* 685–716.

Chan, Y. F., Dennis, M. L., & Funk, R. R. (2008). Prevalence and comorbidity of major internalizing and externalizing problems among adolescents and adults presenting to substance abuse treatment. *Journal of Substance Abuse Treatment, 34,* 14–24.

Chen, C. Y., Storr, C. L., & Anthony, J. C. (2009). Early-onset drug use and risk for drug dependence problems. *Addictive Behaviors, 34*(3), 319–322.

Chung, T., & Maisto, S. A. (2006). Relapse to alcohol and other drug use in treated adolescents: review and reconsideration of relapse as a change point in clinical course. *Clinical Psychology Review, 26,* 149–161.

Chung, T., & Martin, C. S. (2001). Classification and course of alcohol problems among adolescents in addictions treatment programs. *Alcoholism: Clinical and Experimental Research, 25,* 1734–1742.

Chung, T., & Martin, C. S. (2005). Classification and short-term course of DSM-IV cannabis, hallucinogen, cocaine, and opioid disorders in treated adolescents. *Journal of Consulting and Clinical Psychology, 73,* 995–1004.

Chung, T., & Martin, C. S. (2011). Prevalence and clinical course of adolescent substance use and substance use disorders. In Y. Kaminer & K. C. Winters (Eds.), *Clinical manual of adolescent substance abuse treatment* (pp. 1–24). Washington, DC: American Psychiatric Publishing.

Chung, T., Martin, C. S., Winters, K. C., & Langenbucher, J. W. (2001). Assessment of alcohol tolerance in adolescents. *Journal of Studies on Alcohol, 62,* 687–695.

Chung, T., Pajtek, S., & Clark, D. B. (2013). White matter integrity as a link in the association between motivation to abstain and treatment outcome in adolescent substance users. *Psychology of Addictive Behaviors, 27,* 533–542.

Cicchetti, D., & Cohen, D. J. (1995). Perspectives on developmental psychopathology. In D. Cicchetti & D. J. Cohen (Eds.), *Developmental psychopathology: Theory and methods* (pp. 3–20). New York: Wiley.

Ciesla, J. R. (2010). Evaluating the risk of relapse for adolescents treated for substance abuse. *Addictive Disorders and Their Treatment, 9,* 87–92.

Clair, M., Stein, L. A. R., Soenksen, S., Martin, R. A., Lebeau, R., & Golembseke, C. (2013). Ethnicity as a moderator of motivational interviewing for incarcerated adolescents after release. *Journal of Substance Abuse Treatment, 45,* 370–375.

Clark, D., & Winters, K. C. (2002). Measuring risks and outcomes in substance use disorders prevention research. *Journal of Consulting and Clinical Psychology, 70*, 1207–1223.

Clark, D. B., De Bellis, M. D., Lynch, K. G., Cornelius, J. R., & Martin, C. S. (2003). Physical and sexual abuse, depression and alcohol use disorders in adolescents: Onsets and outcomes. *Drug and Alcohol Dependence, 69*, 51–60.

Dakof, G. A., Tejeda, M., & Liddle, H. A. (2001). Predictor of engagement in adolescent drug abuse treatment. *Journal of the American Academy of Child and Adolescent Psychiatry, 40*, 274–281.

Dennis, M. L., Godley, S. H., Diamond, G., Tims, F. M., Babor, T., Donaldson, J., et al. (2004). The Cannabis Youth Treatment (CYT) study: Main findings from two randomized trials. *Journal of Substance Abuse Treatment, 27*(3), 197–213.

DiFranza, J. R., Savageau, J. A., Rigotti, N. A., Fletcher, K., Ockene, J. K., McNeill, A. D., et al. (2002). Development of symptoms of tobacco dependence in youths: 30 month follow up data from the DANDY study. *Tobacco Control, 11*, 228–235.

Dinieri, J. A., & Hurd, Y. L. (2012). Rat models of prenatal and adolescent cannabis exposure. *Methods of Molecular Biology, 829*, 231–242.

Dishion, T. J., Bullock, B. M., & Granic, I. (2002). Pragmatism in modeling peer influence: Dynamics, outcomes, and change processes. *Development and Psychopathology, 14*, 969–981.

Dishion, T. J., McCord, J., & Poulin, F. (1999). When interventions harm: Peer groups and problem behaviors. *American Psychologist, 54*, 755–764.

Dishion, T. J., & Medici Skaggs, N. (2000). An ecological analysis of monthly "bursts" in early adolescent substance use. *Applied Developmental Science, 4*, 89–97.

Ducci, F., & Goldman, D. (2008). Genetic approaches to addiction: Genes and alcohol. *Addiction, 9*, 1414–1428.

Edelbrock, C., Costello, A. J., Dulcan, M. K., Calabro, C. N., & Kala, R. (1986). Parent–child agreement on child psychiatric symptoms assessed via structured interview. *Journal of Child and Adolescent Psychiatry, 27*, 181–190.

Fickenscher, A. Novins, D. K., & Beals, J. (2006). A pilot study of motivation and treatment completion among American Indian adolescents in substance abuse treatment. *Addictive Behaviors, 31*, 1402–1414.

Filbey, F., & Yezhuvath, U. (2013). Functional connectivity in inhibitory control networks and severity of cannabis use disorder. *American Journal of Drug and Alcohol Abuse, 39*, 382–391.

French, M. T., Roebuck, M. C., Dennis, M. L., Diamond, G., Godley, S. H., Tims, F., et al. (2002). The economic cost of outpatient marijuana treatment for adolescents: Findings from a multi-site field experiment. *Addiction, 97*(Suppl. 1), 84–97.

French, M. T., Zavala, S. K., McCollister, K. E., Waldron, H. B., Turner, C. W., & Ozechowski, T. J. (2008). Cost-effectiveness analysis of four interventions for adolescents with a substance use disorder. *Journal of Substance Abuse Treatment, 34*(3), 272–281.

Galaif, E. R., Hser, Y., Grella, C. E., & Joshi, V. (2001). Prospective risk factors and treatment outcomes among adolescent drug users in DATOS-A. *Journal of Adolescent Research, 16*, 661–678.

Giedd, J. N. (2004). Structural magnetic resonance imaging of the adolescent brain. *Annuals of New York Academy of Sciences, 1021*, 77–85.

Gil, A. G., Wagner, E. F., & Tubman, J. G. (2004). Culturally sensitive substance abuse intervention for Hispanic and African American adolescents: Empirical examples from the Alcohol Treatment Targeting Adolescents in Need (ATTAIN) project. *Addiction, 99*, 140–150.

Godley, M. D., Godley, S. H., Dennis, M. L., Funk, R. R., & Passetti, L. L. (2006). The effect of assertive continuing care on continuing care linkage, adherence, and abstinence following residential treatment for adolescents with substance use disorders. *Addiction, 102*, 81–93.

Godley, M. D., Godley, S. H., Funk, R. R., Dennis, M. L., & Loveland, D. (2001). Discharge

status as a performance indicator: Can it predict adolescent substance abuse treatment outcome? *Journal of Child and Adolescent Substance Abuse, 11,* 91–109.

Goldstein, B. I., Strober, M., Axelson, D., Goldstein, T. R., Gill, M. K., Hower, H. et al. (2013).
Predictors of first-onset substance use disorders during the prospective course of bipolar
spectrum disorders in adolescents. *Journal of the American Academy of Child and Adolescent Psychiatry, 52,* 1026–1037.

Gonzales, R., Ang, A., Murphy, D. A., Glik, D. C., & Anglin, M. D. (2014). Substance use recovery outcomes among a cohort of youth participating in a mobile-based texting aftercare pilot
program. *Journal of Substance Abuse Treatment, 47,* 20–26.

Grella, C. E., Joshi, V., & Hser, Y. I. (2004). Effects of comorbidity on treatment processes outcomes among adolescents in drug treatment programs. *Journal of Child and Adolescent Substance Abuse, 13,* 13–31.

Hanson, K. L., Cummins, K., Tapert, S. F., & Brown, S. A. (2011). Changes in neuropsychological functioning over 10 years following adolescent substance abuse treatment. *Psychology of
Addictive Behaviors, 25,* 127–142.

Harford, T. C., Grant, B., Yi, H. Y., & Chiung, M. C. (2005). Patterns of DSM-IV alcohol abuse
and dependence criteria among adolescents and adults: Results from the 2001 National
Household Survey on Drug Abuse. *Alcohol Clinical and Experimental Research, 29,* 810–
828.

Henggeler, S. W., McCart, M. R., Cunningham, P. B., & Chapman, J. E. (2012). Enhancing the
effectiveness of juvenile drug courts by integrating evidence-based practices. *Journal of Consulting and Clinical Psychology, 80*(2), 264–275.

Hogue, A., Dauber, S., Stambaugh, L. F., Cecero, J. J., & Liddle, H. A. (2006). Early therapeutic
alliance and treatment outcome in individual and family therapy for adolescent behavior
problems. *Journal of Consulting and Clinical Psychology, 74*(1), 121–129.

Hogue, A., Liddle, H. A., Becker, D., & Johnson-Leckrone, J. (2002). Family-based prevention
counseling for high-risk young adolescents: Immediate outcomes. *Journal of Community
Psychology, 30*(1), 1–22.

Hooven, C., Pike, K., & Walsh, E. (2013). Parents of older at-risk youth: A retention challenge for
preventive intervention. *Journal of Primary Prevention, 34*(6), 423–438.

Hsieh, S., Hoffman, N. G., & Hollister, C. D. (1998). The relationship between pre-, during-,
post-treatment factors, and adolescent substance abuse behaviors. *Addictive Behaviors, 23,*
477–488.

Hsieh, S., & Hollister, C. D. (2004). Examining gender differences in adolescent substance abuse
behavior: Comparisons and implications for treatment. *Journal of Child and Adolescent
Substance Abuse, 13,* 53–70.

Huey, S. J., Jr., Henggeler, S. W., Brondino, M. J., & Pickrel, S. G. (2000). Mechanisms of change
in multisystemic therapy: Reducing delinquent behavior through therapist adherence and
improved family and peer functioning. *Journal of Consulting and Clinical Psychology, 68*(3),
451–467.

Ivens, C., & Rehm, L. P. (1988). Assessment of childhood depression: Correspondence between
reports by child, mother, and father. *Journal of the American Academy of Child and Adolescent Psychiatry, 27,* 738–747.

Jainchill, N., Hawke, J., De Leon, G., & Yagelka, J. (2000). Adolescents in therapeutic communi-
ties: One-year posttreatment outcomes. *Journal of Psychoactive Drugs, 32,* 81–94.

Johnston, L. D., & O'Malley, P. M. (1997). The recanting of earlier reported drug use by young
adults. *NIDA Research Monograph, 167,* 59–80.

Johnston, L. D., O'Malley, P. M., Miech, R. A., Bachman, J. G., & Schulenberg, J. (2014). *Monitoring the Future national results on drug use: 1975–2013: Overview, key findings on adolescent drug use.* Ann Arbor: Institute for Social Research, University of Michigan.

Kaminer, Y., & Bukstein, O. (Eds.). (2008). *Adolescent substance abuse: Psychiatric comorbidity
and high-risk behaviors.* New York: Routledge.

Kaminer, Y., & Marsch, L. A. (2011). Pharmacotherapy of adolescent substance use disorders. In Y. Kaminer & K. C. Winters (Eds.), *Clinical manual of adolescent substance abuse treatment* (pp. 163–186). Washington, DC: American Psychiatric Association.

Kaminer, Y., & Waldron, H. B. (2006). Evidence-based cognitive-behavioral therapies for adolescent substance use disorders: Applications and challenges. In H. A. Liddle & C. L. Rowe (Eds.), *Adolescent substance abuse: Research and clinical advances* (pp. 396–419). New York: Cambridge University Press.

Kelly, J. F., Brown, S. A., Abrantes, A., Kahler, C. W., & Myers, M. (2008). Social recovery model: An 8-year investigation of adolescent 12-step group involvement following inpatient treatment. *Alcoholism: Clinical and Experimental Research, 32,* 1468–1478.

King, K. M., Chung, T., & Maisto, S. A. (2009). Adolescents' thoughts about abstinence curb the return of marijuana use during and after treatment. *Journal of Consulting and Clinical Psychology, 77,* 554–565.

Kirisci, L., Tarter, R. E., Vanyukov, M., Reynolds, M., & Habeych, M. (2004). Relation between cognitive distortions and neurobehavior disinhibition on the development of substance use during adolescence and substance use disorder by young adulthood: A prospective study. *Drug and Alcohol Dependence, 76,* 125–133.

Latimer, W. W., Ernst, J., Hennessey, J., Stinchfield, R. D., & Winters, K. C. (2004). Relapse among adolescent drug abusers following treatment: The role of probable ADHD status. *Journal of Child and Adolescent Substance Abuse, 13,* 1–16.

Latimer, W. W., Newcomb, M., Winters, K. C., & Stinchfield, R. D. (2000). Adolescent substance abuse treatment outcome: The role of substance use problem severity, psychosocial, and treatment factors. *Journal of Consulting and Clinical Psychology, 68,* 684–696.

Latimer, W. W., Winters, K. C., Stinchfield, R., & Traver, R. E. (2000). Demographic, individual, and interpersonal predictors of adolescent alcohol and marijuana use following treatment. *Psychology of Addictive Behaviors, 14,* 162–173.

Liddle, H. A., Rowe, C. L., Dakof, G. A., Henderson, C. E., & Greenbaum, P. E. (2009). Multidimensional family therapy for young adolescent substance abuse: Twelve-month outcomes of a randomized controlled trial. *Journal of Consulting and Clinical Psychology, 77*(1), 12–25.

Magill, M., & Ray, L. A. (2009). Cognitive-behavioral treatment with adult alcohol and illicit drug users: A meta-analysis of randomized controlled trials. *Journal of Studies on Alcohol and Drugs, 70*(4), 516–527.

Maisto, S. A., Connors, G. J., & Allen, J. P. (1995). Contrasting self-report screens for alcohol problems: A review. *Alcoholism: Clinical and Experimental Research, 19,* 1510–1516.

Martin, C., & Winters, K. C. (1998). Diagnostic criteria for adolescent alcohol use disorders. *Alcohol Health and Research World, 22,* 95–106.

Martin, C. S., Chung, T., Kirisci, L., & Langenbucher, J. W. (2006). Item response theory analysis of diagnostic criteria for alcohol and cannabis use disorders in adolescents: Implications for DSM-V. *Journal of Abnormal Psychology, 115,* 807–814.

Martin, C. S., Chung, T., & Langenbucher, J. W. (2008). How should we revise diagnostic criteria for substance use disorders in the DSM-V? *Journal of Abnormal Psychology, 117,* 561–575.

Martínez Martínez, K. I., Pedroza Cabrera, F. J., de los Ángeles Vacío Muro, M., Jiménez Pérez, A. L., & Salazar Garza, L. (2008). Consejo breve para adolescentes escolares que abusan del alcohol [School-based brief intervention for adolescent alcohol abusers]. *Revista Mexicana De Análisis De La Conducta, 34*(2), 247–264.

Martínez Martínez, K. I., Salazar Garza, M. L., Pedroza Cabrera, F. J., Ruiz Torres, G. M., & Ayala Velázquez, H. E. (2008). Resultados preliminares del programa de intervención breve para adolescentes que inician el consumo de alcohol y otras drogas [Preliminary results of a brief intervention program for adolescents who have started using alcohol and other drugs]. *Salud Mental, 31*(2), 119–127.

McCarthy, D. M., Tomlinson, K. L., Anderson, K. G., Marlatt, G. A., & Brown, S. A. (2005).

Relapse in alcohol- and drug-disordered adolescents with comorbid psychopathology: Changes in psychiatric symptoms. *Psychology of Addicitve Behaviors, 19,* 28–34.

McCollister, K. E., Freitas, D. M., Prado, G., & Pantin, H. (2013). Opportunity costs and financial incentives for Hispanic youth participating in a family-based HIV and substance use preventive intervention. *Journal of Primary Prevention, 35,* 13–20.

Miller, W. R., & Rollnick, S. (2013). *Motivational interviewing: Helping people change* (3rd ed.). New York: Guilford Press.

Monti, P. M., Colby, S. M., Barnett, N. P., Spirito, A., Rohsenow, D. J., Myers, M., et al. (1999). Brief intervention for harm reduction with alcohol-positive older adolescents in a hospital emergency department. *Journal of Consulting and Clinical Psychology, 67*(6), 989–994.

Mustanski, B., Byck, G. R., Dymnicki, A., Sterrett, E., Henry, D., & Bolland, J. (2013). Trajectories of multiple adolescent health risk behaviors in a low-income African American population. *Development and Psychopathology, 25,* 1155–1169.

National Institute for Health and Care Excellence (NICE). (2014). *Special considerations for children and young people with alcohol-use disorders.* London: Author. Retrieved from *www.nice.org.uk/Guidance/PH24.*

National Institute on Drug Abuse (NIDA). (2014). *Principles of adolescent substance use disorder treatment: A research-based guide.* Bethesda, MD: Author.

Nock, M. K., & Kazdin, A. E. (2001). Parent expectancies for child therapy: Assessment and relation to participation in treatment. *Journal of Child and Family Studies, 10*(2), 155–180.

Oplund, E. A., Winters, K. C., & Stinchfield, R. D. (1995). Examining gender differences in drug-abusing adolescents. *Psychology of Addictive Behaviors, 19,* 167–175.

Rawson, R. A., Gonzales, R., Obert, J. L., McCann, M. J., & Brethen, P. (2005). Methamphetamine use among treatment-seeking adolescents in southern California: Participant characteristics and treatment response. *Journal of Substance Abuse Treatment, 29,* 67–74.

Rey, J. M., Schrader, E., & Morris-Yates, A. (1992). Parent–child agreement on children's behaviours reported by the Child Behaviour Checklist (CBCL). *Journal of Adolescence, 15,* 219–230.

Riley, K. J., Rieckmann, T., & McCarty, D. (2008). Implementation of MET/CBT 5 for Adolescents. *Journal of Behavioral Health Services and Research, 35*(3), 304–314.

Ritter, A., & Cameron, J. (2006). A review of the efficacy and effectiveness of harm reduction strategies for alcohol, tobacco and illicit drugs. *Drug and Alcohol Review, 25*(6), 611–624.

Rivaux, S. L., Springer, D. W., Bohman, T. Wagner, E. F., & Gil, A. G. (2006). Differences among substance abusing Latino, Anglo, and African-American juvenile offenders in predictors of recidivism and treatment outcome. *Journal of Social Work Practice in the Addictions, 6,* 5–29.

Robbins, M. S., Feaster, D. J., Horigian, V. E., Rohrbaugh, M., Shoham, V., Bachrach, K., et al. (2011). Brief strategic family therapy versus treatment as usual: Results of a multisite randomized trial for substance using adolescents. *Journal of Consulting and Clinical Psychology, 79*(6), 713–727.

Rosenberg, M. F., & Anthony, J. C. (2001). Early clinical manifestations of cannabis dependence in a community sample. *Drug and Alcohol Dependence, 64,* 123–131.

Rowe, C. L., Liddle, H. A., Greenbaum, P. E., & Henderson, C. E. (2004). Impact of psychiatric comorbidity on treatment of adolescent drug abusers. *Journal of Substance Abuse Treatment, 26,* 129–140.

Rutter, M., & Silberg, J. (2002). Gene–environment interplay in relation to emotional and behavioral disturbance. *Annual Review of Psychology, 53,* 463–490.

Schell, T. L., Orlando, M., & Morral, A. R. (2005). Dynamic effects among patients' treatment needs, beliefs, and utilization: A prospective study of adolescents in drug treatment. *Health Research and Educational Trust, 40,* 1128–1147.

Shane, P. A., Jasiukaitis, P., & Green, R. S. (2003). Treatment outcomes among adolescents with substance abuse problems: The relationship between comorbidities and post-treatment substance involvement. *Evaluation and Program Planning, 26,* 393–402.

Slesnick, N., Erdem, G., Bartle-Haring, S., & Brigham, G. S. (2013). Intervention with substance-abusing runaway adolescents and their families: Results of a randomized clinical trial. *Journal of Consulting and Clinical Psychology, 81*(4), 600–614.

Smith, T. E., Sells, S. P., Rodman, J., & Reynolds, L. R. (2006). Reducing adolescent substance abuse and delinquency: Pilot research of a family-oriented psychoeducation curriculum. *Journal of Child and Adolescent Substance Abuse, 15*, 105–115.

Sobell, M. B., & Sobell, L. C. (2005). Guided self-change model of treatment for substance use disorders. *Journal of Cognitive Psychotherapy, 19*(3), 199–210.

Springer, D. W., Rivaux, S. L., Bohman, T., & Yeung, A. (2006). Predicting retention in three substance abuse treatment modalities among Anglo, African American, and Mexican American juvenile offenders. *Journal of Social Service Research, 32*, 135–155.

Steinberg, L. (2004). Risk taking in adolescence: What changes, and why? *Annuals of the New York Academy of Sciences, 1021*, 51–58.

Sterling, S., Chi, F., Campbell, C., & Weisner, C. (2009). Three-year chemical dependency and mental health treatment outcomes among adolescents: The role of continuing care. *Alcoholism: Clinical and Experimental Research, 33*, 1417–1429.

Stevens, S. J., Estrada, B., Murphy, B. S., McKnight, K. M., & Tims, F. (2004). Gender differences in substance use, mental health, and criminal justice involvement of adolescents at treatment entry and at three, six, twelve, and thirty-six month follow-up. *Journal of Psychoactive Drugs, 36*, 13–25.

Substance Abuse and Mental Health Services Administration. (2014). *Results from the 2013 National Survey on Drug Use and Health: Summary of national findings* (NSDUH Series H-48, HHS Publication No. SMA 14-4863). Rockville, MD: Author.

Swift, W., Coffey, C., Carlin, J. B., Degenhardt, L., & Patton, G. C. (2008). Adolescent cannabis users at 24 years: Trajectories to regular weekly use and dependence in young adulthood. *Addiction, 103*, 1361–1370.

Tamm, L., Trello-Rishel, Riggs, P., Nakonezny, P. A., Acosta, M., Bailey, G., et al. (2013). Predictors of treatment response in adolescents with comorbid substance use disorder and attention-deficit/hyperactivity disorder. *Journal of Substance Abuse Treatment, 44*, 224–230.

Tarter, R. E., Vanyukov, M., Giancola, P., Dawes, M., Blackson, T., Mezzich, A., et al. (1999). Epigenetic model of substance use disorder etiology. *Development and Psychopathology, 11*, 657–683.

Tolan, P. H., & McKay, M. (1996). Preventing serious antisocial behavior in inner-city children: An empirically based family intervention program. *Family Relations, 45*(2), 148–155.

Tomlinson, K. L., Brown, S. A., & Abrantes, A. (2004). Psychiatric comorbidity and substance use treatment outcomes of adolescents. *Psychology of Addictive Behaviors, 18*, 160–169.

Wagner, E. F. (2009). Improving treatment through research: Directing attention to the role of development in adolescent treatment success. *Alcohol Research and Health, 32*, 67–75.

Wagner, E. F., Hospital, M. M., Graziano, J. N., Morris, S. L., & Gil, A. G. (2014). A randomized controlled trial of guided self-change with minority adolescents. *Journal of Consulting and Clinical Psychology, 82*, 1128–1139.

Wagner, E. F., Lloyd, D. A., & Gil, A. G. (2002). Racial/ethnic and gender differences in the incidence and onset age of DSM-IV alcohol use disorder symptoms among adolescents. *Journal of Studies on Alcohol, 63*, 609–619.

Waldron, H. B., & Kaminer, Y. (2004). On the learning curve: The emerging evidence supporting cognitive-behavioral therapies for adolescent substance abuse. *Addiction, 99*(Suppl. 2), 93–105.

Waldron, H. B., & Turner, C. W. (2008). Evidence-based psychosocial treatments for adolescent substance abuse. *Journal of Clinical Child and Adolescent Psychology, 37*, 238–261.

Wallace, J., Bachman, J., O'Malley, P., Schulenberg, J., Cooper, S., & Johnston, L. (2003). Gender and ethnic differences in smoking, drinking and illicit drug use among American 8th, 10th and 12th grade students, 1976–2000. *Addiction, 98*, 225–234.

Warden, D., Riggs, P. D., Min, S., Mikulich-Gilbertson, S. K., Tamm, L., Trello-Rishel, K., et al. (2012). Major depression and treatment response in adolescents with ADHD and substance use disorder. *Drug and Alcohol Dependence, 120,* 214–219.

Weissman, M. M., Wickramaratne, P., Warner, V., John, K., Prusoff, B. A., Merikangas, K. R., et al. (1987). Assessing psychiatric disorders in children: Discrepancies between mothers' and children's reports. *Archives of General Psychiatry, 44,* 747–753.

Williams, R. J., Chang, S. Y., & the Addiction Center Research Group. (2000). A comprehensive and comparative review of adolescent substance abuse treatment outcome. *Clinical Psychology: Science and Practice, 7,* 138–166.

Winters, K. C., Anderson, N., Bengston, P., Stinchfield, R. D., & Latimer, W. W. (2000). Development of a parent questionnaire for the assessment of adolescent drug abuse. *Journal of Psychoactive Drugs, 32,* 3–13.

Winters, K. C., Fahnhorst, T., Botzet, A., Lee, S., & Lalone, B. (2012). Brief intervention for drug-abusing adolescents in a school setting: Outcomes and mediating factors. *Journal of Substance Abuse Treatment, 42,* 279–288.

Winters, K. C., & Henly, G. A. (1994). *Personal Experience Inventory and manual.* Los Angeles: Western Psychological Services.

Winters, K. C., & Lee, S. (2008). Likelihood of developing an alcohol and cannabis use disorder during youth: Association with recent use and age. *Drug and Alcohol Dependence, 92,* 239–247.

Winters, K. C., Lee, S., Botzet, A., Fahnhorst, T., & Nicholson, A. (2014). One-year outcomes and mediators of a brief intervention for drug abusing adolescents. *Psychology of Addictive Behaviors, 28,* 464–474.

Winters, K. C., Martin, C. S., & Chung, T. (2011). Commentary on O'Brien: Substance use disorders in DSM-5 when applied to adolescents. *Addiction, 106,* 882–884.

Winters, K. C., Stinchfield, R. D., Latimer, W. W., & Stone, A. (2008). Internalizing and externalizing behaviors and their association with the treatment of adolescents with substance use disorder. *Journal of Substance Abuse Treatment, 35,* 269–278.

Zalesky, A., Solowij, N., Yücel, M., Lubman, D. I., Takagi, M., Harding, I. H., et al. (2012). Effect of long-term cannabis use on axonal fibre connectivity. *Brain, 135,* 2245–2255.

Zucker, R. A., Fitzgerald, H. E., & Moses, H. D. (1995). Emergence of alcohol problems and the several alcoholisms: A developmental perspective on etiologic theory and life course trajectory. In D. Cicchetti & D. J. Cohen (Eds.), *Developmental psychopathology: Risk, disorder and adaptation* (pp. 677–711). New York: Wiley.

CHAPTER 15

Tic Disorders
and Trichotillomania

David C. Houghton, Jennifer R. Alexander,
and Douglas W. Woods

Although they appear under different diagnostic categories in DSM-5 (American Psychiatric Association, 2013), tic disorders, such as Tourette's disorder (TD), and body-focused repetitive behaviors, such as trichotillomania (TTM; hair-pulling disorder), share common properties and respond to similar treatments. Both groups of disorders are defined by overt, repetitive behaviors that are largely driven by internal stimuli and strongly influenced by contextual variables. In addition, evidence suggests these disorders respond to habit reversal training, a form of behavioral therapy designed to manage symptoms by interrupting associations between repetitive behaviors and maintaining contextual variables. We provide in this chapter an overview of TD and TTM and discuss habit reversal training for both disorders.

TOURETTE'S DISORDER

The DSM-5 Definition of TD

TD is a childhood-onset neurodevelopmental disorder characterized by tics (i.e., involuntary and repetitive muscle movements [motor tics]) and vocalizations (vocal tics) that are not the result of a substance or an alternative mental or medical disorder (American Psychiatric Association, 2013). Unlike other tic disorders, diagnosis of TD requires the presence of at least two motor tics and one vocal tic. In addition, diagnosis of TD requires that tics persist for at least 1 year, though the tics need not occur concomitantly or consistently in terms of frequency, severity, or anatomical location. Other tic disorders can also be diagnosed. *Persistent (chronic) motor or vocal tic disorder* is defined as the presence of motor *or* vocal tics for at least 1 year, and *provisional tic disorder* is defined as the presence of motor and/or vocal tics for less than 1 year.

Prevalence and Course

Tics are relatively common, with some researchers suggesting that between 16.9 and 19.7% of children show tics at some point during development (e.g., Kurlan, McDermott, Deeley, & Como, 2001). Prevalence rates for tic disorders in children are much lower. Researchers suggest that tic disorders occur in 1.4–1.8% of children (Kraft et al., 2012; Scharf, Miller, Mathews, & Ben-Shlomo, 2012), and that TD occurs in between 0.3 and 1.0% of children (Khalifa & von Knorring, 2003; Robertson, 2008).

TD is two to nine times more common in males (Khalifa & von Knorring, 2003) and may be more prevalent in white children than in black and Hispanic children (Robertson, 2008). Recent evidence suggests that children from lower socioeconomic status (SES) backgrounds may be at a greater risk for a TD diagnosis (Miller, Scharf, Mathews, & Ben-Shlomo, 2014), but other studies have failed to demonstrate an association between SES and TD (Chao, Hu, & Pringsheim, 2014; Khalifa & von Knorring, 2005).

Tics, typically, simple motor tics, often emerge by age 6. Simple motor tics employ just one muscle group (e.g., eye blinking and eye rolling; Leckman et al., 1998). Simple vocal (phonic) tics, which consist of inarticulate sounds (e.g., coughing and throat clearing), typically emerge several years after the onset of simple motor tics (Leckman et al., 1998). Generally, both types of tics may increase in complexity over time; evolving into complex motor and vocal tics (Bloch & Leckman, 2009). Complex motor tics employ multiple muscle groups (i.e., jumping in the air while arching the back). There are two types of complex motor tics: strings of simple tics and more multifaceted, purposeful-looking movements. Complex vocal tics consist of strings of syllables, as well as words, phrases, repeating others' words or sounds, coprolalia (i.e., obscene words), and blocking (i.e., being unable to get a sound out).

Throughout the course of the disorder, tics tend to vary in terms of severity. Between the ages of 6 and 15, tic severity either progressively increases or is stable but high (Leckman et al., 1998). During late adolescence and early adulthood (i.e., 18–19 years of age), tics may significantly decrease in severity and frequency (Bloch & Leckman, 2009).

Common Comorbid Conditions

TD frequently co-occurs with other psychiatric conditions, as demonstrated by comorbidity rates ranging from 64 to 86% (Hirschtritt et al., 2015; Specht et al., 2011). Attention-deficit/hyperactivity disorder (ADHD) and obsessive–compulsive disorder (OCD) are the most commonly observed comorbid disorders. Although estimates vary, between 17 and 54% of those with TD have comorbid ADHD, and between 19 and 66% have comorbid OCD (Hirschtritt et al., 2015; Scharf et al., 2012; Specht et al., 2011). Other common comorbidities include anxiety, mood, and disruptive behavior disorders (Hirschtritt et al., 2015).

Etiological/Conceptual Models of TD

Biological Factors

The etiological origin of TD encompasses both environmental and genetic factors (Dietrich et al., 2015). Though genetic studies have yet to identify definitively any TD-producing genetic mutations, several candidate genes have been proposed (Albin & Mink, 2006; Lawson-Yuen, Saldivar, Sommer, & Picker, 2008; Nag et al., 2013; Scharf et al., 2013; Verkerk et al., 2003), and some studies suggest that certain pre- and perinatal variables (e.g., parental stress and mood, legal and illegal drug use during pregnancy, and the child's birthweight) may interact with the child's genetic composition to influence subsequent TD severity (Ben-Shlomo, Scharf, Miller, & Mathews, 2016; Mathews et al., 2006). Overall, the neurobiology of TD is complex, but the most well-supported biological model of TD involves dysfunction in corticostriatal–thalamocortical (CSTC) circuits (Albin & Mink, 2006; Felling & Singer, 2011; Leckman, Bloch, Smith, Larabi, & Hampson, 2010; Lerner et al., 2012). CSTC circuits link several regions of the frontal cortex, which are involved in executive functions, to subcortical structures that are involved in motor control and reinforcement learning. Several regions within the basal ganglia are responsible for performing action selection processes, whereby desired movements are facilitated and undesired (or competing) movements are inhibited (Mink, 2001). Researchers have suggested that tics are the result of deficient inhibition of competing motor programs that leads to excitatory cortical output and a proliferation of undesired movements (Albin & Mink, 2006). Within the CSTC model of TD, multiple structural and functional abnormalities are thought to contribute (Felling & Singer, 2011), as well as certain neurotransmitters (dopamine, glutamate, gamma-aminobutyric acid [GABA], and serotonin; Albin & Mink, 2006; Draper et al., 2014; Lerner et al., 2012; Puts et al., 2015).

Behavioral Factors

Most persons with TD report that they voluntarily perform tics in order to alleviate premonitory urges (PMUs), which are uncomfortable somatic sensations (e.g., feelings of tension or "energy surges") experienced immediately prior to tic onset (Leckman, Walker, Goodman, Pauls, & Cohen, 1994). This apparent relationship between tics and PMUs constitutes the basis of a negative reinforcement model, whereby the elimination of the aversive PMU reinforces tic expression (Evers & van de Wetering, 1994). Of note, younger children (i.e., < 10 years old) are less likely than older children to endorse the presence of PMUs, and PMUs tend to develop several years after tic onset (Banaschewski, Woerner, & Rothenberger, 2003; Leckman, Walker, & Cohen, 1993). Studies have also shown that (1) contextual variables impact tic occurrence, frequency, and severity (Conelea & Woods, 2008), (2) contingently reinforcing tic suppression leads to lengthier tic absences (Himle & Woods, 2005), and (3) some types of behavior therapy can be used to effectively manage tics (McGuire, Piacentini, et al., 2014).

Evidence-Based Treatments for TD

Various psychosocial and pharmacological treatments are available for TD. The following section provides a broad overview of psychosocial treatments for TD. See Gilbert and Jankovic (2014) for a review of pharmacological treatments for TD.

Psychosocial Interventions

Although not yet widely practiced due to lack of both awareness and availability (Marcks, Woods, Teng, & Twohig, 2004; Woods, Conelea, & Himle, 2010), behavior therapy is an effective means of treating TD. In fact, behavior therapy targets associations between tics and contextual variables, and is considered a first-line treatment for TD according to Canadian, European, and U.S. clinical guidelines (Murphy, Lewin, Storch, & Stock, 2013; Verdellen, van de Griendt, Hartmann, Murphy, & ESSTS Guidelines Group, 2011). The following section describes the evidence base for two empirically supported behavioral treatments for TD (i.e., habit reversal training/comprehensive behavioral intervention for tics, and exposure and response prevention) as well as several other promising psychosocial treatment options that have been tested primarily in adults with tic disorders (i.e., mindfulness-based stress reduction and cognitive psychophysiological treatment).

WELL-ESTABLISHED TREATMENTS

Habit Reversal Training (HRT) is a well-established treatment for TD, as evidenced by 35 studies showing significant results (Cook & Blacher, 2007; Himle, Woods, Piacentini, & Walkup, 2006) and a large average effect size ($d = 0.8$; Bate, Malouff, Thorsteinsson, & Bhullar, 2011). HRT is superior to other behavioral or psychosocial treatments, such as massed negative practice (Azrin & Peterson, 1990) and supportive psychotherapy (Deckersbach, Rauch, Buhlmann, & Wilhelm, 2006). However, in one trial, HRT was equivalent to exposure and response prevention (Verdellen, Keijsers, Cath, & Hoogduin, 2004).

Comprehensive behavioral intervention for tics (CBIT; Woods et al., 2008), which includes both HRT and several adjunctive components (described later), is another widely used and effective form of therapy for TD. Randomized controlled trials have demonstrated that CBIT results in greater tic reductions than psychoeducation and supportive therapy for both children (Piacentini et al., 2010) and adults (Wilhelm et al., 2012) with TD. CBIT also results in significantly improved long-term outcomes for tics, as well as anxiety, disruptive behavior, family strain, and social functioning (Woods et al., 2011). Notably, recent evidence suggests that CBIT administered via videoconference technology may be as effective as in-person CBIT (Himle et al., 2012; Himle, Olufs, Himle, Tucker, & Woods, 2010; Ricketts et al., 2016), suggesting that the dissemination potential for CBIT may be high.

PROBABLY EFFICACIOUS TREATMENT

Exposure and response prevention (ERP), based on the well-validated treatment for OCD (Abramowitz, 1997), is another form of behavioral treatment available for TD (Verdellen et al., 2004). Several case studies have documented ERP-produced tic reduction (Hoogduin, Verdellen, & Cath, 1997). To date, however, only one randomized controlled trial has been employed to examine ERP's effectiveness (Verdellen et al., 2004). Using a sample that included both children and adults, the authors found no significant differences between ERP and HRT in terms of treatment outcome. They suggested that ERP may be able to manage tics as well as HRT. However, it should be noted that ERP participants received twice as much treatment time as those who received HRT, which potentially confounded study results. See Table 15.1 for a comparison of HRT and ERP treatment components.

POSSIBLY EFFICACIOUS TREATMENTS

Several other behaviorally based treatments for TD appear to be efficacious but have been evaluated primarily in adults. Mindfulness-based stress reduction (MBSR) has been shown to be efficacious for chronic tic disorders in one study (Reese et al., 2015). In this small open trial with 18 participants ages 16–67, MBSR resulted in significant improvement in tic severity and tic-related impairment. Another behavioral treatment that has modest evidentiary support is based on a cognitive-behavioral psychophysiological model of tics (O'Connor, 2002). In this treatment model, the sensory phenomena and PMUs that are believed to instigate tics are directly targeted, and therapy aims to improve overall motor inhibition and motor planning. In an open trial of cognitive-behavioral psychophysiological treatment of 102 adults with chronic TDs, there were significant differences between pre- and posttreatment scores on measures of tic severity (O'Connor, Lavoie, Blanchet, & St-Pierre-Delorme, 2016).

TABLE 15.1. Comparisons between HRT/CBIT and ERP

	HRT/CBIT	ERP
Number of tics targeted:	Targets one tic at a time.	Targets all tics at once.
Components:	*Awareness training*: Increase client awareness of PMUs and tics. *Competing response training*: Teach client to perform a different action when PMU appears rather than performing the tic. *Social support*: Family members prompt and praise use of competing response.	*Exposure*: Expose client to PMUs. *Response prevention*: Teach client to suppress tics for extended periods of time despite feeling PMUs.
Sessions:	Eight sessions lasting 60–90 minutes each.	12 sessions lasting 120 minutes each.
Most recent manual:	*Managing Tourette Syndrome: A Behavioral Intervention for Children and Adults Therapist Guide* (Woods et al., 2008)	*Tics—Therapist Manual & Workbook for Children* (Verdellen, van de Griendt, Kriens, van Oostrum, & Chang, 2011)

Predictors of Treatment Response

Comorbid psychiatric conditions, particularly ADHD, tend to negatively impact TD treatment outcomes (McGuire, Piacentini, et al., 2014). This appears to be more of an issue with behavioral treatment than with pharmacological treatments. In fact, some pharmacological treatments, such as [a] 2 adrenergic agonists, successfully target both TD and ADHD symptomatology (Weisman, Qureshi, Leckman, Scahill, & Bloch, 2013). Other pharmacological treatments, such as stimulants, can significantly decrease ADHD symptomology without significantly increasing tic severity (Robertson, 2006).

McGuire, Piacentini, and colleagues (2014) also found that client age and the number of treatment sessions are positive predictors of treatment outcomes. Verdellen and colleagues (2004) suggested that a predictor of ERP treatment outcome is a client's ability to suppress tics successfully during therapy sessions. However, while Verdellen and colleagues considered tic suppression ability to be a motivational issue, it may also be a product of symptom severity or ability to facilitate behavioral inhibition.

Evidence-Based Assessment

Differential Diagnosis

It is important to differentiate between TD and other movement disorders, such as chorea, myoclonus, and dystonia (American Psychiatric Association, 2013). Several unique features differentiate between TD and other conditions. For instance, tics (1) are often immediately preceded by PMUs (Jankovic & Kurlan, 2011), (2) can typically be voluntarily suppressed for relatively small periods of time (Cohen, Leckman, & Bloch, 2013), and (3) often wax and wane in response to contextual variables.

Tics may also be difficult to differentiate from stereotypic movement disorders and compulsions associated with OCD. Stereotypies are repetitive and involuntary movements (American Psychiatric Association, 2013) that, unlike the majority of tics, are not associated with PMUs and can be immediately and dramatically reduced upon distraction (Singer, 2013). Moreover, stereotypies typically have an earlier age of onset than tics and tend be longer in duration (American Psychiatric Association, 2013; Singer, 2013). Compulsions in OCD can appear to be similar to complex tics, and differential diagnosis can be complicated by the high comorbidity rate between OCD and TD. Compulsions tend to have uniquely cognitive components and are associated with physiological arousal, such that compulsions are typically performed in an attempt to nullify obsessions, thoughts, or fears. In contrast, tics are typically performed in an attempt to alleviate aversive sensations (i.e., PMUs), which are somatic rather than cognitive. Furthermore, compulsions are typically more consciously and carefully executed than tics (American Psychiatric Association, 2013). Via clinical interview, detailed characteristics and psychosocial histories are often required in order to elucidate whether presenting symptoms should be classified as tics, compulsions, or stereotypies.

Clinical Interview

There are structured or semistructured interviews to aid in clinical interviews for TD, such as the Diagnostic Interview Schedule for Children (Lucas et al., 2001) and the

Anxiety Disorders Interview Schedule (Silverman & Albano, 1996). However, a detailed clinical intake should include a summary of the child's and family's medical and mental history, as well as the child's substance use history. In addition, an intake should include information regarding the emergence of the suspected TD symptomatology. Of particular interest is the timing of symptom emergence, a description of early symptoms, and any major events that occurred immediately prior to symptom emergence. Although direct observation of the child's tics by a clinician or physician is preferred, indirect reports (i.e., reports from parents) may be sufficient to make a diagnosis in certain cases, particularly because children may not exhibit tics initially in the presence of health care providers.

Assessment Tools

Tic severity may be assessed using a variety of techniques, but common measures do exist (see the review by McGuire, Kugler, Park, & Horng, 2012).

Several experts continue to use observational methods of tic severity, such as video observation (Chappell et al., 1994) and client self-monitoring estimates. Himle, Chang, and colleagues (2006) determined that independent observations of tic frequency tends to generalize across settings; tic frequency counts based on recordings of the individual at home significantly correlate with tic frequency counts from recordings of the individual in a clinical setting. Moreover, the authors demonstrated that partial-interval coding, a quick, efficient coding technique, was just as accurate and reliable in assessing tic frequency as an event frequency coding technique. Goetz, Tanner, Wilson, and Shannon (1987) also demonstrated the reliability and validity of a rating scale for the observational coding of tics that measures (1) number of body areas affected, (2) frequency of tics, and (3) severity of tics. Self-monitoring and observational measures have several advantages, such as external validity and ease of implementation, but objective measures of tic severity are also commonly used.

The *Yale Global Tic Severity Scale* (YGTSS; Leckman et al., 1989), the most commonly used tic severity measure (Cohen et al., 2013), is a clinician-rated measure in which the client's tic performance over the preceding week is rated on five indicators: number of tics, tic frequency, tic noticeability, tic complexity, and impairment due to tics. The YGTSS provides separate indices for motor and vocal tics, as well as global composites. The total tic severity score is calculated by adding the motor and vocal tic indices, resulting in total scores that range from 0 to 50. Research suggests that the YGTSS has high concurrent validity (Leckman et al., 1989; Walkup, Rosenberg, Brown, & Singer, 1992), high interrater reliability (Walkup et al., 1992), and strong internal consistency (Storch et al., 2005).

The *Premonitory Urge for Tics Scale* (PUTS; Woods, Piacentini, Himle, & Chang, 2005) is a nine-item self-report measure of the PMUs endorsed by the client and their relationship with the client's tics. PUTS items are rated on a 1- ("not at all true") to 4-point ("very much true") scale, resulting in total scores ranging from 9 to 36. Analysis of the scale suggests that the PUTS has high internal consistency and concurrent validity (Reese et al., 2014; Woods et al., 2005).

The *Parent Tic Questionnaire* (PTQ; Chang, Himle, Tucker, Woods, & Piacentini, 2009) assesses clients' motor and vocal tic severity via parental ratings on 14 commonly reported motor tics and 14 commonly reported vocal tics. Parents are asked to indicate whether each of these tics is present or absent in the client. Subsequently, parents rate the frequency and intensity of all present tics, both of which are measured on a 4-point scale. For each present tic, frequency and intensity ratings are added together to form severity scores. In turn, the severity scores for all motor tics are added together to form a motor tic severity score, and the severity scores for all vocal tics are added together to form a vocal tic severity score. Higher scores indicate greater severity. Chang and colleagues (2009) found that the PTQ demonstrates high internal consistency, high temporal stability, and strong convergent validity.

The *Hopkins Motor and Vocal Tic Scale* (HMVTS; Walkup et al., 1992) assesses tic severity over the preceding week by means of clinician and parental ratings of each tic. Both parties individually rate each tic's severity, in terms of tic frequency, intensity, interference, and impairment, along a 10 cm rank visual scale. These rankings are then converted into three final scores: parent-rated assessment, clinician-rated assessment, and overall assessment. Final scores range from 0 ("no tics") to 5 ("severe tics"). Walkup and colleagues (1992) determined that the scale has good interrater reliability and high concurrent validity.

Summary

TD is an etiologically complex neurobehavioral disorder, characterized by tics that typically emerge in early childhood but decrease in severity upon adulthood. Several behavioral (and pharmacological) interventions are effective in reducing TD symptoms. Efficacy of behavioral treatment tends to be influenced by factors such as age, ADHD comorbidity, and therapeutic contact. Despite these acknowledged impediments, behavior therapy (i.e., HRT/CBIT) is recognized as a well-established treatment for the disorder. After discussion of a related condition, TTM, we present an overview of HRT.

TRICHOTILLOMANIA

The DSM-5 Definition of TTM

TTM is an obsessive–compulsive-related disorder that affects both adult and pediatric populations (American Psychiatric Association, 2013). Individuals with TTM have hair loss as a result of repeatedly pulling out their hair, despite repeated attempts to decrease or stop pulling. For a TTM diagnosis, hair pulling must cause clinically significant distress or impairment and cannot be attributed to a medical condition or another mental disorder.

Prevalence and Course

Most epidemiological research on TTM has focused on adults. Prevalence estimates show that subclinical hair pulling occurs in 6.8–22% of adults (Duke, Bodzin, Tavares, Geffken, & Storch, 2009; Hajcak, Franklin, Simons, & Keuthen, 2006; Hansen, Tishelman, Hawkins, & Doepke, 1990; Woods, Miltenberger, & Flach, 1996) and TTM occurs in 0.6–1% of adults (Christenson, Pyle, & Mitchell, 1991; Rothbaum, Shaw, Morris, & Ninan, 1993). Some have suggested that TTM prevalence in children and adolescents is comparable to that in adults (e.g., King, Scahill, & Vitulano, 1995), but others have argued that hair pulling in very young children might occur in rates as high as 9.25% (e.g., Wright & Holmes, 2003).

Research supports the notion of a bimodal age of onset, whereby some individuals begin pulling during early childhood (<5 years old; Walther et al., 2014) and others tend to start during early adolescence (ages 11–14 years; Snorrason, Belleau, & Woods, 2012). Those in the early-onset subgroup are believed to have a higher likelihood of spontaneous remission than those in the late-onset subgroup (Swedo, Leonard, Lenane, & Rettew, 1992). However, other reports suggest that a significant number of adults with chronic hair pulling began pulling during early childhood (Snorrason et al., 2012), thus calling into question whether age of onset is a useful predictor of prognosis. Nevertheless, TTM typically shows a chronic but fluctuating course that rarely remits completely (Diefenbach, Reitman, & Williamson, 2000), and symptoms can be interspersed between weeks or months of pulling-free periods (Bohne, Keuthen, & Wilhelm, 2005).

Common Comorbid Conditions

Research indicates that 38% of treatment-seeking children and adolescents with TTM have at least one comorbid diagnosis (Tolin, Franklin, Diefenbach, Anderson, & Meunier, 2007). The most common comorbidity in children appears to be anxiety disorders (30%), but up to 11% may have a comorbid externalizing disorder (primarily ADHD). Studies also indicate elevated rates of anxiety and depressive symptoms in pediatric populations with TTM (Franklin et al., 2008; Lewin et al., 2009). Unfortunately, there has been little research on comorbidity in child/adolescent TTM samples; much more research has been conducted on adult samples. Research on adult samples has shown that adult comorbidity rates may be higher than those in children (40–50%; Lochner et al., 2012; Odlaug, Kim, & Grant, 2010; Tolin et al., 2007). The most frequent comorbidities in adults are mood (14–60%) and anxiety (2.3–57%) disorders (Christenson, Mackenzie, & Mitchell, 1991; Christenson & Mansueto, 1999; Odlaug et al., 2010; van Minnen, Hoogduin, Keijsers, Hellenbrand, & Hendriks, 2003), addictive disorders (2.6–22%; Christenson, 1995; Christenson, Mackenzie, Mitchell, & Callies, 1991; Grant & Odlaug, 2008; Keuthen et al., 2012; Odlaug & Grant, 2008; Schlosser, Black, Blum, & Goldstein, 1994), and OCD (5–27%; Christenson, 1995; Christenson, Mackenzie, Mitchell, et al., 1991; Lochner, Seedat, & Stein, 2010; Odlaug & Grant, 2008; Schlosser et al., 1994).

It has been suggested that TTM belongs to a larger category of related conditions called body-focused repetitive behavior disorders (BFRBDs; Teng, Woods, Twohig, & Marcks, 2002), which include chronic skin picking, nail biting, cheek/lip biting, thumb sucking, teeth grinding, and other similar behaviors. Indeed, a growing body of evidence suggests that TTM and other BFRBDs co-occur at high rates, share many phenomenological characteristics, and might have similar risk factors (Snorrason et al., 2012; Stein et al., 2008; Teng et al., 2002).

Beyond specific psychiatric comorbidities, the global impact of TTM on psychosocial functioning is substantial. Feelings of physical unattractiveness, shame, and worthlessness are experienced in a majority of TTM sufferers (Stemberger, Thomas, Mansueto, & Carter, 2000). In particular, TTM appears to have a negative impact on the social lives of sufferers. Peers tend to view hair pulling negatively (Marcks, Woods, &

Ridosko, 2005; Woods, Fuqua, & Outman, 1999), and children with TTM have reported that their social lives and relationships have been damaged by the disorder (Franklin et al., 2008). The effects of TTM also penetrate the academic environment, wherein students report absences due to TTM symptoms and difficulties performing schoolwork and studying (Franklin et al., 2008). Of note, very young children (<5 years old) appear to be less negatively affected (Walther et al., 2014), perhaps due to (1) the possibility that early-onset TTM has a better prognosis and less severity than late-onset TTM, (2) the fact that young children have fewer opportunities to receive negative social reactions to their hair pulling/loss, or (3) that hair pulling in very young children is viewed as benign and therefore receives less stigmatization.

Etiological/Conceptual Models of TTM

Biological Factors

There is little available research on the neurobiology of TTM, especially when compared with research on TD, but existing evidence implicates the same CSTC circuits as underlying pathological hair pulling. Moreover, some evidence has supported the notion of a genetic vulnerability to TTM (Hemmings et al., 2006; King et al., 1995; Novak, Keuthen, Stewart, & Pauls, 2009; Zuchner et al., 2006). Structural imaging research has detected abnormal volumes in prefrontal cortical regions (Chamberlain et al., 2008; Odlaug, Chamberlain, Derbyshire, Leppink, & Grant, 2014; Roos, Grant, Fouche, Stein, & Lochner, 2015; White et al., 2013) and the basal ganglia (O'Sullivan et al., 1997; Roos et al., 2015), and there is evidence for disorganized functional connectivity between the cortex and basal ganglia (Chamberlain et al., 2010; Roos, Fouche, Stein, & Lochner, 2013). This converging evidence suggests that, similar to TD, individuals with TTM have impaired top-down control over their actions and that motor programs supporting hair pulling behavior are disinhibited and overactive. Moreover, research suggests that serotonergic, dopaminergic, and glutamatergic neurotransmission might facilitate aforementioned pathophysiology of TTM (Grant, Odlaug, & Kim, 2009; Martin, Scahill, Vitulano, & King, 1998; Swedo et al., 1989; Van Ameringen, Mancini, Oakman, & Farvolden, 1999), mirroring findings in TD. It should be noted that much of the research on the neurobiology of TTM was conducted with adults and may not necessarily apply in children. For instance, although N-acetylcysteine, a glutamate modulator, has shown evidence for efficacy in adults with TTM (Grant et al., 2009), it has shown null results in children (Bloch, Panza, Grant, Pittenger, & Leckman, 2013).

Behavior

Hair pulling may serve to decrease or distract one from aversive cognitive and affective states. Several studies have found that hair pulling is frequently triggered by stress, boredom, and tension (Christenson, Ristvedt, & Mackenzie, 1993; Diefenbach, Mouton-Odum, & Stanley, 2002; Diefenbach, Tolin, Meunier, & Worhunsky, 2008; Teng, Woods, Marcks, & Twohig, 2004), but this feature might be absent in very young children (Walther et al., 2014). Paradoxically, hair pulling might temporarily alleviate these aversive internal states, but episodes of pulling tend to be followed by feelings of guilt, sadness, and anger (Diefenbach, Mouton-Odum, & Stanley, 2002). Some have suspected that hair pulling is associated with a process known as *experiential avoidance* (Begotka, Woods, & Wetterneck, 2004; Norberg, Wetterneck, Woods, & Conelea, 2007), which is defined as a tendency to avoid aversive thoughts and emotions at the expense of valued behavior. In fact, Houghton and colleagues (2014) found that this process mediated the relationship between emotional variables (e.g., anxiety, depression) and hair pulling.

Finally, phenomenological accounts of hair pulling have led researchers to offer two distinct styles of pulling, known as "automatic" and "focused." Automatic pulling is believed to involve pulling that is performed with little or no conscious intent, and that might be reinforced by tactile stimulation (Flessner et al., 2007). Focused pulling, performed actively and with conscious intent, has been associated with higher depression and anxiety (Begotka et al., 2004) and experiential avoidance (Houghton et al., 2014).

Evidence-Based Treatments for TTM

Behavioral Interventions

In contrast to the range of evidence-based psychosocial treatments for TD, no treatment can be considered well established for pediatric TTM (Woods & Houghton, 2016). However, in this section, we discuss treatments with some levels of empirical support and their components. See McGuire, Ung, and colleagues (2014) for a meta-analysis that includes pharmacological treatments for TTM.

The treatment with the highest level of support for pediatric TTM is HRT, which has been tested in three different studies. Azrin, Nunn, and Frantz (1980) compared HRT to massed negative practice (an ineffective therapy) in 34 persons, four of whom were children. Using self-reported frequency of hair pulling as the primary outcome measure, results showed a significant advantage for HRT as evidenced by all children and 91% of total participants, showing significant reductions in hair pulling, and gains were maintained in 87% of participants at 22-month follow-up. However, because neither a psychometrically valid assessment measure was used nor were the child results reported separately, the results of this study must be interpreted with caution. HRT was also tested with three adolescents in a multiple baseline design using direct observation of behavior with reliability checks as the primary outcome measures (Rapp, Miltenberger, Long, Elliot, & Lumley, 1998). Results showed substantial reductions in time spent pulling hair and significant improvements in hair appearance; gains were maintained at 27 weeks posttreatment by two of the three participants. More recently, Franklin, Edson, Ledley, and Cahill (2011) tested HRT versus a minimal attention control condition in a randomized trial with 24 children and adolescents. The HRT group saw significant improvement, whereas the control group did not. Moreover, the HRT group did not experience significant relapse at 8-week follow-up.

The evidence base suggests HRT is well established in adults but only probably efficacious in children. Other assorted behavioral techniques also have been tested for pediatric TTM, but only possess experimental status. These experimental behavioral techniques include response prevention (Massong, Edwards, Sitton, & Hailey, 2002), differential reinforcement (Altman, Grahs, & Friman, 1982), and a combination of these techniques (Blum, Barone, & Friman, 1993); all studies showed positive effects.

Novel Psychosocial Treatments

Although behavioral treatments have shown promise for TTM, researchers have proposed that strategies aimed at regulating negative cognition/affect might boost the efficacy of these interventions. As such, several trials of mood-enhanced habit reversal therapies have been conducted for adult TTM. Cognitive-behavioral therapy (CBT) plus HRT has been tested in two studies, one for adults and another for children. CBT for TTM includes HRT along with coping strategies for cognitive, affective, and somatic variables that might trigger hair pulling. An uncontrolled pediatric trial tested CBT + HRT in 22 children (Tolin et al., 2007). Results showed that 77% of children were treatment responders at posttreatment, and 64% were still responding at 6-month follow-up. The adult trial (Ninan, Rothbaum, Marsteller, Knight, & Eccard, 2000) tested CBT + HRT versus clomipramine (a selective serotonin reuptake inhibitor [SSRI]) and wait-list placebo in 23 persons and found that CBT + HRT outperformed both other conditions.

Two other treatments similar to CBT have also been combined with HRT and tested in adults: acceptance and commitment therapy (Woods, Wetterneck, & Flessner, 2006) and dialectical behavior therapy (DBT; Keuthen et al., 2012). Both showed positive results. However, these treatments have only been tested in controlled studies with adults, and only in a recent case study of a 15-year-old female has DBT + HRT substantially reduced hair pulling (Welch & Kim, 2012).

Predictors of Treatment Response

Consistent with the lack of quality treatment studies of pediatric TTM, literature on treatment outcome moderators and mediators is limited. Franklin, Edson, and Freeman (2010) found no age effects associated with behavior therapy for pediatric TTM. McGuire, Ung, and colleagues (2014) found no moderating effects of comorbid anxiety and depression in their meta-analysis of treatment for TTM, but they did find that increased therapeutic contact hours and mood-enhanced forms of behavior therapy did moderate successful outcomes.

With respect to potential mechanisms of change, evidence from recent trials of mood-enhanced behavior therapy suggests that improvements in emotion regulation skills mediate therapeutic outcome, but this notion has only been tested with CBT for adults (Keuthen et al., 2012; Woods, Wetterneck, et al., 2006).

Evidence-Based Assessment

Differential Diagnosis

The first step in assessment involves differentiating between TTM and dermatological disorders, similar obsessive–compulsive conditions, substance use disorders, and psychotic disorders.

Several medical and dermatological conditions can cause hair loss (Stefanato, 2010). Typically, these conditions can be diagnosed via skin biopsy and/or dermoscopy (Abraham, Torres, & Azulay-Abulafia, 2010). Examples include alopecia areata, male or female pattern alopecia, and telogen effluvium (Mostaghimi, 2012). Additionally, there are several characteristics that differentiate TTM from alternative causes of alopecia. For instance, hair loss resulting from TTM generally results in irregularly shaped patches of baldness and/or broken hairs. Also, the remaining hairs of persons with TTM remain firmly affixed to the dermis and are not easily removed by slight tugs, which would suggest weakened hair roots or follicles. For a more detailed discussion of the differentiation of dermatological conditions and TTM, see Mostaghimi (2012).

OCD and TTM can be difficult to distinguish, but there are several key differences. First, hair pulling in TTM tends to be pleasurable and "ego-syntonic," whereas compulsions in OCD tend to be somewhat aversive and "ego-dystonic." Second, OCD is generally characterized by unwanted, intrusive, and repetitive thoughts, which are less common in TTM. Third, persons with OCD tend to have multiple compulsions that express themselves across several behavioral domains, whereas persons with TTM focus on hair pulling. Finally, OCD tends to respond positively to SSRIs, which tend to be less effective for TTM. Of note, TTM and OCD co-occur frequently (see the earlier section on comorbidity), and the presence of obsessions and compulsions unrelated to hair pulling does not preclude a TTM diagnosis.

Body dysmorphic disorder (BDD) can also be difficult to differentiate from TTM. BDD involves preoccupation with a real or imagined defect in physical appearance and repeated attempts to alter or "fix" that defect. This concern over physical appearance has parallels to cognitive aspects of TTM, in that persons with TTM often report desires to pull hairs that are "out of place" or that have certain physical properties (i.e., rough texture, non-parsimonious color, bent shape). Also, persons with BDD often display repeated checking behavior and repetitive attempts to conceal or directly alter their physical appearance, which can mirror the compulsive aspects of TTM (e.g., spending time in front of mirrors pulling hairs or concealing the effects of pulling). However, there are several features that clearly differentiate TTM from BDD. First, the obsessional concerns about appearance inherent to BDD are often far more excessive than the hair-related cognitions in TTM. Likewise, persons with TTM frequently experience guilt and regret following pulling episodes, and shame and embarrassment regarding their hair loss, whereas persons with BDD continually desire and rarely feel remorse over extreme attempts to alter their appearance (American Psychiatric Association, 2013).

Substance abuse, particularly with psychostimulants, should also be carefully screened for when considering a TTM diagnosis. Numerous case reports have suggested that hair pulling can onset or be exacerbated after exposure to stimulants (e.g., Adderall and cocaine), and that pulling quickly remits after cessation of stimulants (George & Moselhy, 2005; Hamalian & Citrome, 2010; Martin et al., 1998; Narine, Sarwar, & Rais, 2013). As such, clinicians should ask whether hair pulling frequently occurs while under the influence of substances. If it is determined that the use of a substance overlaps or contributes to hair pulling, it is wise to delay TTM diagnosis until the client has stopped using substances for at least 6 weeks, whereupon reassessment should be undertaken to determine if hair pulling is a stand-alone problem (Flessner, 2012).

Finally, hair pulling can occur in the context of a psychotic disorder (American Psychiatric Association, 2013). In these cases, delusions or hallucinations compel the psychotic individual to pull out his or her hair, but this does not qualify for a diagnosis of TTM.

Clinical Interview

There is no existing structured or semistructured interview that includes current DSM-5 criteria for TTM. Nevertheless, the clinician should ask the child where the pulling takes place (e.g., scalp, eyebrows, or eyelashes), and, if the child is postpubescent, should ask whether the child also pulls hair on other sites on the body (e.g., axillary, pubic, chest). The clinician should also explore where and how often hair pulling occurs, the methods used to pull (e.g., tweezers, fingernails), how aware the child is of pulling during episodes, whether any postpulling behavior occurs (e.g., ingesting pulled hairs), and the impact hair pulling has on the child's functionality. Depending on the child's maturity, insight, and willingness to disclose personal information, secondary reports from parents might be useful. Separate interviews may also be warranted if the child is nervous or refuses to speak openly about hair pulling around his or her parents.

Assessment Tools

There are several methods for assessing TTM, including direct methods that take physical samples or video recordings and indirect self-, parent-, and clinician-rated measures. We discuss in this section several tools for determining symptom severity, pulling subtype, and overall impairment.

Several direct methods of assessing TTM typically involves having clients monitor hair pulling in a diary or save pulled hairs. Utilizing self-monitoring methods is advantageous in that it may potentially be more accurate and lead to increased client awareness of pulling, but compliance is difficult to verify and practical limitations (i.e., client misplacing the form) are numerous (Rothbaum & Ninan, 1994). If choosing to collect pulled hairs, therapists should instruct clients to place pulled hairs inside an envelope or plastic bag, so that the therapist may attain an accurate count of pulled hairs. Although this method may provide an accurate means to identify the exact number of pulled hairs, it suffers from the same disadvantages regarding compliance and practicality, as does self-monitoring by diary (Rothbaum & Ninan, 1994).

Other direct methods of assessing TTM include videotaping clients, directly observing clients, and taking photographs of pulling and/or pulling sites. Videotaping or other means of direct observation allow the clinician to accurately assess the frequency, duration, and other characteristics of hair pulling in a naturalistic sense, but is also limited by practical concerns (e.g., time, observational effects) and client reactivity (Mackenzie, Ristvedt, Christenson, Lebow, & Mitchell, 1995; Rapp, Miltenberger, Galensky, Ellingson, & Long, 1999). Perhaps the most widely used direct measure of hair pulling involves photographing affected areas. Photographing pulling areas is a valid and naturalistic measure of hair pulling severity and treatment response (Houghton et al., 2016; Rosenbaum & Ayllon, 1981; Rothbaum & Ninan, 1994). However, there are no standardized guidelines for performing photographic assessment, and some clients may object to the use of photographs for monitoring treatment progress, particularly in private body areas.

Because each direct measure of TTM severity described earlier has disadvantages, only some are suitable for everyday clinical practice. The method that is perhaps best suited for normal clinical application is having the client create daily diaries on the frequency of hair pulling. This method has few disadvantages, in that it is not highly invasive and does not require much effort, and it can serve a secondary purpose of helping the child pay attention to how much and in which contexts he or she pulls on a daily basis. By comparison, having the child save pulled hairs can often create resistance and should only be used when the child has significant difficulties in making accurate judgments about pulling frequency (i.e., cannot remember how much he or she pulled earlier that day when filling out a diary). Direct observational methods such as videotaping and observation are rarely employed in normal clinical practice unless there is doubt as to whether the child is actually pulling hair, and photographs are best suited for research contexts and program evaluation rather than normal clinical practice. Indeed, a better tolerated and similarly valid method to assess hair pulling severity at single and multiple time points is to use standardized self-report instruments, which are described below.

The *Trichotillomania Scale for Children* (TSC; Tolin et al., 2008), a 12-item self-report measure with both parent and child versions, consists of two components: severity and distress/impairment. Each item consists of three sentences that reflect varying degrees of hair-pulling severity. Items are scaled from 0 to 2, with higher scores indicating more severe symptoms. The TSC total score and both subscales possess adequate reliability, but mixed convergent validity (Tolin et al., 2008). Furthermore, the parent version has shown questionable validity (Tolin et al., 2008).

The *National Institutes of Health Trichotillomania Scale* (Swedo et al., 1989) is a two-part, clinician-rated scale measuring both TTM severity and impairment. The severity index, the NIMH Trichotillomania Severity Scale, consists of five items that measure pulling frequency in the previous week and day, resistance to urges, pulling-related distress, and functional impairment. Items are scored from 0 to 5, resulting in a total score ranging from 0 to 25. The impairment index, the NIMH Trichotillomania Impairment Scale, consists of a single item with a 0- to 10-point Likert scale, with higher scores reflecting greater impairment. The NIMH Trichotillomania scale has shown adequate psychometric properties in both adults and children (Diefenbach, Tolin, Crocetto, Maltby, & Hannan, 2005; Franklin et al., 2011; Swedo et al., 1989).

The *Milwaukee Inventory for Styles of Trichotillomania—Child Version* (MIST-C; Flessner et al., 2007) is a 25-item self-report measure of automatic and focused pulling styles. A two-factor solution has been identified that correspond to each pulling style: a 21-item focused factor and a 4-item automatic factor. The scale showed acceptable internal consistency, as well as good convergent and discriminant validity (Flessner et al., 2007).

Several other self-report measures exist for TTM but have only been evaluated in adults (Diefenbach et al., 2005), such as the *Massachusetts General Hospital Hairpulling Scale* (O'Sullivan et al., 1995) and the *Psychiatric Institute Trichotillomania Scale* (Winchel et al., 1992), and should only be used with caution in older adolescents.

TREATMENT OF TD AND TTM IN CHILDREN AND ADOLESCENTS

Overview and Theoretical Framework

HRT-based treatments have the largest evidence base of any psychosocial treatment for pediatric TD and TTM. Although there are several nuances in the presentation of behavior therapy for either condition, the core principles of HRT remain the same. The behavioral model on which HRT is based recognizes the role of neurobiological factors (particularly for TD) but posits that the expression of tics and hair pulling are heavily influenced by contextual factors. For instance, several antecedents that often occur prior to tic and hair-pulling symptoms include PMUs, tension, anxiety, and boredom. Several consequences that often follow tics and hair pulling include relief of antecedent feelings and/or pleasurable somatic sensations (e.g., feeling a hair follicle pop out of the scalp). This process tends to reinforce TD and TTM symptoms when those particular antecedents are present. HRT interrupts that reinforcement process by blocking engagement in tics or hair pulling. In addition, functional assessment/intervention and stimulus control procedures are used to reduce the influence of other problematic contextual variables (e.g., tic-contingent caregiver attention, access to tweezers). The subsequent sections provide a detailed description of each of these techniques, and Table 15.2 presents a breakdown of how the components of treatment are often presented.

However, we mention two cautions prior to our discussion of therapy components. First, behavior therapy for TD and TTM should always begin with the presentation of basic psychoeducation. This educational information can be drawn from research presented herein, as well as a more detailed reading of the literature. How psychoeducation is performed can vary according to time demands, clinician preferences, and detail requested by the caregivers and child. Thus, we do not present a formal guideline for how psychoeducation should be conducted. Second, one major difference in the implementation of HRT for these conditions is that HRT for TD focuses on one tic at a time. This is done because tics are heterogeneous, and HRT procedures for one tic can easily be ineffective for another. Before beginning the active components of HRT for TD, the clinician should obtain a "tic hierarchy," in which each tic receives a rating from 1 to 10 describing the level of distress or impairment. The most bothersome tic on the hierarchy is targeted first. Each session thereafter typically focuses on incrementally less bothersome tics. For TTM, hair pulling in all locations can be targeted simultaneously.

Habit Reversal Training

Awareness Training

The goal of awareness training is to teach clients to recognize the occurrence of tics or hair pulling and the triggers, or "warning signs," that precede them. Many children with

TABLE 15.2. Components of Behavior Therapy for TD and TTM

TD	TTM
• Assessment	• Assessment
• Psychoeducation	• Psychoeducation
• Function-based intervention	• Function-based intervention and stimulus control
• HRT for Tic 1, Tic 2, . . .	• HRT
• Relaxation training	• Optional relaxation training or other additional components

TD and TTM are not fully aware of every instance of their repetitive behavior, so this exercise sets the precedent for future exercises aimed at symptom suppression.

Typically, awareness training begins with the client providing a very detailed description of his or her tics or hair pulling, otherwise known as a *response description* (Himle, Woods, et al., 2006). This description needs to be highly detailed. For response description in TD, the clinician should direct the client to describe the ways in which specific muscles are used in creating the targeted tic. In addition, the child should be asked to describe any sensations that precede that tic (i.e., premonitory urges). Response description in TTM should involve describing how the hand is used to pull, the posture enacted during pulling, and any prepulling ritualistic behaviors (e.g., stroking the hair). Similar to awareness training in TD, the child is directed to describe any sensations or behaviors that precede hair pulling.

In the response detection phase of awareness training, the clinician tests the child's ability to detect the presence of his or her tics or hair pulling. To do so, the clinician instructs the child to signal (e.g., raise a finger) when a symptom has occurred or is about to occur (i.e., when he or she experiences an urge). In the therapy session, the clinician and child engage in conversation or play while the child is asked to acknowledge the tic/ hair pulling. When the child correctly raises his or her finger (e.g., a tic occurs and child immediately raises his or her finger), the therapist praises the child. When the child forgets to raise a finger following a tic or hair-pulling behavior, the therapist briefly stops the conversation/play and reminds the child to raise a finger when the target behavior occurs. This continues until the child is aware of approximately 80% of tics/hair pulling as it happens in the session. For behavior therapy to be effective, awareness of symptoms is a prerequisite, and this exercise primes the child for implementation of future therapeutic exercises aimed at interrupting symptom performance.

TD Case Example

CLINICIAN: So, Kyle, what tics have been going on during the previous week?

KYLE: I do this one a lot (*Displays a head-jerking tic.*): lifting my head and jutting out my jaw. (*Describes a few other tics.*)

CLINICIAN: Let's get an idea of how bothersome or annoying each tic is, so that we can figure out which one to go after first. On a scale from 0 to 10, with 10 being most bothersome and 0 being not bothersome at all, how would you rate each of your tics?

KYLE: The head jerking tic is definitely very annoying. It's probably a 9. (*Describes lower ratings for several other tics.*)

CLINICIAN: What we typically do in this treatment is first target the tic that is bothering you the most, which sounds like the head-jerking tic. Right?

KYLE: Yes, definitely.

CLINICIAN: OK. One of the first things we want to do is to get you to know every time the tic happens. You may already know exactly how many times your tic happens, so this might go really quick, but you might only know when it happens sometimes, so this may help.

KYLE: Sure.

CLINICIAN: When we get to know when something is happening, we first need to really think about what it is we are talking about. Let's start by having you give me a very detailed description of your tic. Please tell me everything about your tic. What muscles are you using when you do the head-jerking tic?

KYLE: Well, I kind of tense the back of my neck and pull my head up. Then, I tense my jaw and push my chin out while pulling my shoulders back.

CLINICIAN: OK. That's a great description. What happens to you before the head-jerking tic happens? Do you feel anything weird going on?

KYLE: It's kind of like a knife or a toothpick that's poking me in the back of the neck, and it's really annoying. When I do this (*Raises his head and juts out jaw.*], it feels a little better and the poking sensation goes away. I also have some tension or force in my neck that makes me want to do it.

CLINICIAN: Once you feel this tension and poking feeling and start doing the tic, I also noticed that your eyes start looking upward. Did you know that?

KYLE: No, but I guess I do that as well.

CLINICIAN: There is sometimes more going on with a tic than we notice. Your eyes go up, your eyebrows go up, and you probably feel a stretching feeling in your neck muscles. Do a couple more head jerking tics so that we can see what's going on. Do you feel anything in your chest?

KYLE: I guess so, because my shoulders start to move back a bit and I feel it in my chest.

CLINICIAN: Let's pull this all together. You feel a tension or force in your neck as well as a poking sensation. Then, the muscles in the back of your neck start tensing, you start looking up, the front of your neck tightens, your shoulders push back, your chest tightens, and you push your jaw out. Is that right?

KYLE: Yes.

CLINICIAN: What happens to those tense and poking feelings after you do the tic?

KYLE: They go away, but then come right back.

CLINICIAN: OK. Now what I would like to do, Kyle, is a little practice exercise. For the next few minutes I want to sit here and talk, but I don't want to talk about your tics. Let's talk about something else. During our talk, I want you to do something for me. Every time you have that feeling in the back of your neck or you start to do the head jerking tic, I want you to raise a finger and let me know that you caught it. If you catch it, I'm going to say, "Good job." If you miss it, I'm going to say, "Oh, there was one. Don't forget." Make sense?

KYLE: Sure.

CLINICIAN: So what's your favorite sport?

KYLE: Baseball. (*Raises finger but doesn't tic.*)

CLINICIAN: Did you just have an urge to tic there?

KYLE: Yes.

CLINICIAN: Good job. Do you play baseball? Which position?

KYLE: Shortstop. (*Raises finger and performs tic.*)

CLINICIAN: Good job. So you're responsible for catching all the ground balls and throwing out the runner?

KYLE: I try to.

CLINICIAN: Are you a big hitter as well?

KYLE: Sure. I always try to knock it out of the park. (*Performs head-jerking tic.*)

CLINICIAN: Did you catch that one? Make sure you tell me when you have that tic. What other kinds of things do you do for fun?

KYLE: I play piano.

CLINICIAN: Great. How long have you been playing piano?

KYLE: I started taking lessons several years ago, but I played long before that, when I was very young. (*Raises finger and performs tic.*)

CLINICIAN: Good job. You must be pretty good at the piano by now.

KYLE: Sure, I can play a lot of songs.

CLINICIAN: You know what I noticed here, Kyle? I noticed that you can identify just about every tic before it happens, which means you have a big advantage over your tics. You know when tics are going to happen each time, so that means you can start to take control of them. Let's do a different exercise where we figure out how to do that.

Competing Response Training

Inhibiting tics or pulling is not simple, and many clients can become rightly skeptical when they are told that HRT involves managing symptoms through behavioral efforts alone. However, the potency of HRT is due primarily to the use of a competing behavior that provides the child with an active alternative to ticcing or pulling.

Using data obtained during response description, a competing response (CR) for ticcing or pulling is generated. Three rules need to be followed when selecting a competing response. First, the behavior must be physically incompatible with ticcing or pulling, so that the child cannot engage in the behavior while the CR is engaged. Second, the CR must be a behavior that can be done anywhere for at least a few minutes; that is, the CR must not require external equipment or intense effort that cannot be sustained for an extended period of time. Third, the CR should be less noticeable to others than the ticcing or hair pulling.

CRs for TD often involve the antagonistic use of muscles involved in the targeted tic (Azrin & Nunn, 1973), such as gently tensing the neck muscles in response to a head-jerking tic. However, research has shown that noncompeting CRs may also be effective (Evers & van de Wetering, 1994). While the CR for tics must be formulated on an individual basis for each specific tic (see Table 15.3 for examples), CRs for hair pulling are more uniform. The most common CR for TTM is placing the arm that is used to pull down by the sides and gently clenching the fists. Other examples of CRs for TTM include folding the arms together or clasping the hands together. For both TD and TTM, selecting a competing response should be a collaborative process that affords the child autonomy over his or her actions and promotes self-efficacy.

In introducing the CR training component, the clinician starts by stating that the next step of treatment involves choosing an "exercise" that will help the child stop the ticcing or hair pulling. This exercise should be performed whenever the child feels the urge to tic or pull or after ticcing or pulling is already occurring. Before allowing the child to select a CR, the clinician states the three rules to selecting CRs, and when the child offers an option, it should be checked against these rules. For instance, if a child suggests sitting on his or her hands for hair pulling, the clinician might respond with, "That's a pretty good option. Sitting on your hands might work most of the time, but I don't think it follows rule 2. You can't sit on your hands everywhere because you're not always sitting down." This process continues until a good CR is agreed on, whereupon the child should receive instructions for CR implementation.

In implementing the CR, the child is told to engage in his or her "exercise" for 1 minute or until the urge to do the behavior diminishes (based on findings by Twohig & Woods, 2001) whenever he or she feels the urge to tic/pull or finds him- or herself ticcing/pulling. The therapist should model the use of the CR, showing how the CR looks and how it is possible to continue behaving normally while engaging in the CR. Next, the child is told to engage in the CR during session whenever an urge appears or when the child finds him- or herself ticcing/pulling. The therapist provides praise for correct use of the CR, and gentle reminders are provided after omissions. At the end of the session, the clinician instructs the child to begin using the CR outside of session every time a symptom or urge occurs.

Any concerns over implementation should be problem-solved collaboratively. For instance, a child might be resistant to using a diaphragmatic breathing CR when chatting with friends. A solution may be to teach the client how to communicate in a controlled way on the exhale of the CR. Clinicians should also remember that CRs do not always result in immediate symptom reductions and are not always effective. Clinicians should address these problems by encouraging the child to keep trying or by implementing simple alterations, such as selecting a new CR. Many children can become frustrated that performing the CR takes significant effort and/or that their urges are still occurring despite implementation of the CR. In these cases, the clinician should advise the child that performing the CR tends to get easier over time and ticcing/pulling generally declines after at least a few days of using the CR.

TTM Case Example

CLINICIAN: We are now going to learn how to do something called the competing response. For now, let's call this your "exercise." The reason I am asking you to do this exercise is to give you something to prevent your hair pulling from happening. After you do the exercise long enough, it will become very natural and the pulling will decrease. I will ask you to do this exercise for 1 minute each time you pull or notice one of your signals or urges we talked about earlier.

KARA: OK. I guess I can try it.

CLINICIAN: The first rule for picking a good exercise is that is has to be something that makes pulling impossible. You can't be able to do the exercise and pull at

TABLE 15.3. Examples of Common Tics and Their Corresponding Competing Responses

Tic	Competing response
Eye blinking	Controlled blinking
Head jerking	Tensing of the neck and shoulders
Shoulder shrugging	Pushing shoulder downward and clenching back and chest muscles
Mouth movements	Slight clenching of the jaw and pursing of the lips
Abdominal tensing	Controlled, diaphragmatic breathing
Squeaking	Controlled breathing in through the mouth and out through the nose
Nose blowing	Controlled breathing in through the nose and out through the mouth

the same time. The second rule is that the exercise needs to be something you could do anywhere without it being very difficult to do, so you can't have any tools or props to do it. Finally, the exercise has to be less noticeable than hair pulling because we don't want to make you do something silly.

KARA: OK.

CLINICIAN: When you pull from your scalp, you bring your right hand up to the right side of your head and comb through the hair with your fingers until you find a hair to pull. Right?

KARA: Yes. I pretty much always do it that way.

CLINICIAN: Based on the rules I have given you, what kind of exercise could you do to prevent pulling from happening?

KARA: I could put my hand in my pocket when I feel the urge to pull.

CLINICIAN: That's a pretty good option. However, I'm worried that you might not always wear clothes with pockets, meaning that it violates rule 2.

KARA: Oh, you're right.

CLINICIAN: So what could you do that doesn't require pockets?

KARA: Maybe I could make my hand into a fist and hold it down away from my head. That way, I could never pull and do the exercise at the same time.

CLINICIAN: Yes! I think that works. Watch me demonstrate how you would do that exercise, and you can try it after me. (*Demonstrates.*) Now I want you to try doing the exercise. You might not want to pull in room right now with me, but for the sake of practice, I want you to pretend to start pulling and then use the exercise just like you would in real life. While you're doing this, let's talk about something other than hair pulling. What's your favorite subject in school?

KARA: I like Spanish class. It's fun to learn another language and practice it with others. (*Hand starts to move toward head but drops down and forms a fist.*)

CLINICIAN: Good job. Are you fluent in Spanish?

KARA: I can read a few words at a time, but sometimes the verb tenses mix me up. (*Combs hand through hair.*)

CLINICIAN: Was that just a signal that hair pulling might start to happen? Remember, your hand going to your head is a signal, and whenever you do a signal you should use the exercise. Also, remember to hold the exercise for 1 minute.

KARA: Oh, yeah. Sometimes I just comb through my hair without thinking.

CLINICIAN: I understand, but let's try to remember to use the exercise whenever we start the process that often leads to pulling. Also, let's remember to hold the exercise for 1 minute.

[At the end of the session]

CLINICIAN: Now you have seen the exercise that you will be expected to do. Remember, you should do this exercise for 1 minute each time you pull or notice a signal or urge to pull. Before we end today, I want to make sure that you're willing to do the exercise. I know that the exercise probably doesn't feel natural and it might be a little annoying, but you will get better at it and it will begin to feel normal. Are there any situations where you think the exercise will be harder or where you won't be willing to do it?

Social Support

Because the procedures described earlier undoubtedly require significant effort to implement, motivation can be a critical factor in the success of HRT. In the social support component, an adult (typically a parent) is asked to support the child's engagement in treatment. The support person should verbally reinforce the child when he or she engages in the CR at the appropriate time. A simple comment such as "Good job using your exercise" or "Way to go!" is sufficient. Likewise, when ticcing or hair pulling is observed but no competing response is used, the support person should remind the child to use the CR in a supportive and nonjudgmental tone. For instance, when a child starts ticcing repeatedly without using the exercise, the parent might say, "Remember to use your exercise." Children should never be reprimanded upon the occurrence of ticcing or hair pulling. Likewise, support should not be contingent on the presence or absence of symptoms, but rather on treatment engagement. Instead of focusing on tics by saying, "You're having a lot of tics right now," the emphasis should be placed on using the CR. The goal of social support is for the child to receive reinforcement for effort alone, regardless of the effectiveness.

Behavioral Reward Program

To increase and maintain participant motivation for treatment, Woods and colleagues (2008) suggest that parents implement a behavioral reward program to reinforce their child's treatment compliance. Should parents decide to implement such a program, the rules of the program, as well as the possible rewards, should be outlined at the beginning of treatment in consultation with the clinician. Importantly, clinicians should stress that rewards be contingent on treatment compliance rather than on symptom reduction.

Compliance can be objectively measured, for example, by homework completion and session attendance.

Function-Based Intervention and Stimulus Control

Because tics are impacted by contextual influences (Conelea & Woods, 2008) and hair pulling is typically performed in specific situations or with certain tools, function-based interventions and stimulus control procedures have been implemented in behavior therapy to prevent harmful bouts of ticcing or pulling.

Function-based interventions are intended to disrupt relationships between symptom performance and identifiable antecedent and consequent variables that impact symptom severity. Such relationships are often described during a functional assessment interview. These symptom-exacerbating variables can occur prior to symptoms and make the target behaviors more likely to occur (i.e., antecedents), or they can occur after symptoms and temporarily attenuate symptoms but ultimately impact their performance (i.e., consequences). For instance, some children report that riding in cars makes tics worse. In this case, both the parent and child would be encouraged to be mindful of car rides and prepare to use CRs when getting on the road. If a certain situation that is avoidable tends to exacerbate symptoms, such as playing video games or spending time in front of the mirror, this situation might be avoided during the acute stages of treatment (i.e., limiting the time that the child is allowed to play video games or use of the bathroom mirror).

An example of a relevant consequence variable is getting to leave dinner and eat in front of the television because of ticcing. Such a scenario may reinforce the occurrence of tics, and as a result, the child may continue to have severe ticcing bouts at dinner as long as the reward of being excused is available. An appropriate function-based intervention in this case would be to recommend that the parents refrain from directing any sort of special attention toward ticcing (at dinner time or during any other circumstance), ideally creating a tic-neutral environment (Woods et al., 2008). As with competing responses, determine appropriate function-based interventions based on input from the clinician, the child, the child's parents, and even teachers, if necessary.

TD Case Example

CLINICIAN: Kyle, would I be right to say that your tics tend to get worse sometimes and at other times are not that bad?

KYLE: Sure! Sometimes they just come one after the other and it's like they won't stop. Other times, I barely have any at all.

CLINICIAN: You know what? I figured that was the case because that is what most kids with tics say. Tics can happen at any time, but I bet there are some situations in which you know that your tics will get worse.

KYLE: Oh, yeah! When I'm in gym class at school my tics tend to go crazy. They just won't stop and it's really embarrassing.

CLINICIAN: Is there anything about gym class that bothers you?

KYLE: Not really. It's just really loud and there are a lot of things going on. Somehow, my tics must think it's time to all come out.

CLINICIAN: What happens when you're in gym and all of these tics start happening?

KYLE: My gym coach, Mr. Griffin, lets me go hang out on the sidelines until my tics calm down. He is really nice and knows that I cannot help it.

CLINICIAN: Mr. Griffin sounds like a cool guy. But, how does it make you feel when you're not getting to play sports in gym with your friends?

KYLE: I guess it makes me feel bad sometimes. I don't mind playing dodgeball and some of the other games. However, I do hate having to do any exercises or running because I'm not very good at it.

CLINICIAN: I see. Do the tics get really bad when you have to run or do exercises?

KYLE: That's when they are the worst. I get really anxious about having to do those things and my tics go crazy.

CLINICIAN: I think I understand. Tics can do that sort of thing. I think we should have a chat with Mr. Griffin and see if we can figure out how to take care of this. It's great that he understands your tics, but I bet we can help your tics without having to miss gym class.

Stimulus control for TTM follows a similar path, whereby the clinician elucidates environmental cues that tend to make pulling more likely to happen or more severe. Common examples of cues for pulling are presented in Table 15.4. Here, we further illustrate the example relating to pulling while doing homework. Many children find that they pull with their unoccupied hand while studying, writing, or drawing with their dominant hand. During these times, it is helpful to occupy the free hand with a toy or ball that can be squeezed or mindlessly manipulated, as pulling cannot be performed while the object is in the hand. Related stimulus control procedures can involve setting limits on certain activities (e.g., limiting time in the bathroom) or removing pulling-related objects from the child's possession (e.g., tweezers). Several consequences to hair pulling should also be monitored, such as playing with the hair, running the hair along the lips, or biting or chewing on the hair. These rituals should be targeted because they also tend to reinforce pulling behavior. During treatment, these procedures should be continually monitored and adjusted to meet the needs of the client and ensure proper implementation and effect.

TTM Case Example

CLINICIAN: You know, Kara, I bet there are some times when you pull a whole lot and others where you don't pull so much. Is that true?

KARA: Of course. If I pulled all the time, I would be completely bald!

CLINICIAN: That's true. But when is your pulling the worst or when do you do it the most?

KARA: I guess I pull the most when I'm sitting on my bed and when I'm in the bathroom.

CLINICIAN: OK. What happens on the bed when you're pulling?

TABLE 15.4. Examples of Common Cues for Hair Pulling and Related Stimulus Control Procedures

Cue	Stimulus control procedure
Pulling with tweezers	Remove tweezers from the home or give them to parents.
Pulling in front of the bathroom mirror	Limit time in bathroom using egg timer; remove several bright lights from vanity to make hair examination more difficult; cover mirrors with blankets.
Pulling while doing homework	Place a small stress ball in free hand so that it is occupied and not pulling.
Pulling while on the couch watching television	Sit in the center of the couch so that the arm is not propped up against the arm rest and next to the scalp; use stress ball to occupy hands.
Pulling at night while in bed	Place gloves or mittens on the hands.
Pulling in the car	If the child is old enough, have him or her sit in the front seat, where he or she can be observed and reminded to use CR.

KARA: I have a little pocket mirror that I use to look at my eyebrows, and I pick up my tweezers and start pulling.

CLINICIAN: So, you're using the mirror to look at the hairs and you use the tweezers to pull. What about the bathroom?

KARA: Well, it's kind of the same. I look in the mirror and use the tweezers to pull?

CLINICIAN: Do you ever pull without the tweezers?

KARA: Yes, but not very much because it's kind of difficult, especially since I keep my nails short. The tweezers make it really easy.

CLINICIAN: I see. I think that we should consider giving up the pocket mirror and the tweezers for now. You can still do your makeup in the bathroom mirror, but I want you to also set a timer so that you're not spending a lot of time in the bathroom. Would 5 minutes be good?

KARA: Well, that's not a lot of time to do my hair and makeup.

CLINICIAN: How about this? Set the timer when you start doing your hair and makeup. If the timer goes off before you're finished, you can set another minute or two. But, if the timer goes off and you're done or you are finding yourself pulling or wanting to pull, you get out of the bathroom. The point is to remind yourself to only stay in the bathroom for as long as you have to, and not linger there when pulling is more likely to happen. Also, do you ever do anything with your hairs after you pull them?

KARA: Yes. I like to roll the hairs in between my fingers and play with them.

CLINICIAN: OK. When you find yourself doing that, I want you to throw the hair away and use your exercise. Playing with the hair tends to lead to more pulling.

Relaxation Training

Because tics and hair pulling are often exacerbated when children experience increased stress or anxiety, it can be useful to implement basic relaxation training alongside HRT procedures. Although relaxation training is helpful for many clients, it is not effective as a monotherapy (Bergin, Waranch, Brown, Carson, & Singer, 1998) and can be downplayed or abandoned if the child does not tolerate it or becomes disengaged.

There are two basic procedures involved in relaxation training: progressive muscle relaxation and diaphragmatic breathing. Progressive muscle relaxation involves breaking the body down into smaller muscle groups (e.g., feet and calves, thighs and hips, abdominal section and lower back, hands and arms, shoulders and chest) and slowly tensing and relaxing these regions. Each region should be held tense for 5–7 seconds and relaxed for 10–20 seconds. Progressive muscle relaxation generally produces a soothing feeling. Diaphragmatic breathing focuses on achieving a relaxed state by regulating breathing behavior. Participants are encouraged to breathe deeply and slowly, using their diaphragm to push air out and draw air in for 5-second intervals. This procedure generally slows the heart rate and prevents hyperventilation, thus producing a calming sensation and attenuating stress.

CONCLUSION

TD and TTM are similar behavior disorders characterized by repetitive and problematic behaviors. Both disorders can create significant problems for children and adolescents. It is likely that neurobiological factors have a large role in TD and TTM, but behavioral research has led to well-supported models based on behavioral principles. Indeed, while some medications may be effective (particularly for TD), they rarely result in complete symptom remission and may lead to unwanted side effects. Behavioral interventions are evidence-based for both conditions, especially when they contain HRT.

Although the prevalence rates of TD and TTM are low, the number of clinicians who are educated about these conditions and corresponding evidence-based treatments are perhaps too low (Woods, Conelea, & Walther, 2007; Woods, Flessner, et al., 2006). Making a larger impact on these conditions requires not only conducting future research but also disseminating evidence-based practices to behavior therapists, counselors, social workers, physicians, and education specialists.

REFERENCES

Abraham, L. S., Torres, F. N., & Azulay-Abulafia, L. (2010). Dermoscopic clues to distinguish trichotillomania from patchy alopecia areata. *Anais Brasileiros de Dermatologia, 85*(5), 723–726.

Abramowitz, J. S. (1997). Effectiveness of psychological and pharmacological treatments for obsessive–compulsive disorder: A quantitative review. *Journal of Consulting and Clinical Psychology, 65*(1), 44–52.

Albin, R. L., & Mink, J. W. (2006). Recent advances in Tourette syndrome research. *Trends in Neurosciences, 29*(3), 175–182.

Altman, K., Grahs, C., & Friman, P. C. (1982). Treatment of unobserved trichotillomania by attention-reflection and punishment of an apparent covariation. *Journal of Behavior Therapy Experimental Psychiatry, 13*(4), 337–340.

American Psychiatric Association. (2013). *Diagnostic and statistical manual of mental disorders* (5th ed.). Arlington, VA: Author.

Azrin, N. H., & Nunn, R. G. (1973). Habit-reversal: A method of eliminating nervous habits and tics. *Behaviour Research and Therapy, 11*(4), 619–628.

Azrin, N. H., Nunn, R. G., & Frantz, S. E. (1980). Treatment of hairpulling (trichotillomania): A comparative study of habit reversal and negative practice training. *Journal of Behavior Therapy and Experimental Psychiatry, 11*(1), 13–20.

Azrin, N. H., & Peterson, A. L. (1990). Treatment of Tourette's syndrome by habit reversal: A waiting-list control group comparison. *Behavior Therapy, 21*(3), 305–318.

Banaschewski, T., Woerner, W., & Rothenberger, A. (2003). Premonitory sensory phenomena and suppressibility of tics in Tourette syndrome: Developmental aspects in children and adolescents. *Developmental Medicine and Child Neurology, 45*(10), 700–703.

Bate, K. S., Malouff, J. M., Thorsteinsson, E. T., & Bhullar, N. (2011). The efficacy of habit reversal therapy for tics, habit disorders, and stuttering: A meta-analytic review. *Clinical Psychology Review, 31*(5), 865–871.

Begotka, A. M., Woods, D. W., & Wetterneck, C. T. (2004). The relationship between experiential avoidance and the severity of trichotillomania in a nonreferred sample. *Journal of Behavior Therapy and Experimental Psychiatry, 35*(1), 17–24.

Ben-Shlomo, Y., Scharf, J. M., Miller, L. L., & Mathews, C. A. (2016). Parental mood during pregnancy and post-natally is associated with offspring risk of Tourette syndrome or chronic tics: Prospective data from the Avon Longitudinal Study of Parents and Children (ALSPAC). *European Child and Adolescent Psychiatry, 25*(4), 373–381.

Bergin, A., Waranch, H. R., Brown, J., Carson, K., & Singer, H. S. (1998). Relaxation therapy in Tourette syndrome: A pilot study. *Pediatric Neurology, 18*(2), 136–142.

Bloch, M. H., Landeros-Weisenberger, A., Dombrowski, P., Kelmendi, B., Wegner, R., Nudel, J., et al. (2007). Systematic review: Pharmacological and behavioral treatment for trichotillomania. *Biological Psychiatry, 62*(8), 839–846.

Bloch, M. H., & Leckman, J. F. (2009). Clinical course of Tourette syndrome. *Journal of Psychosomatic Research, 67*(6), 497–501.

Bloch, M. H., Panza, K. E., Grant, J. E., Pittenger, C., & Leckman, J. F. (2013). Acetylcysteine in the treatment of pediatric trichotillomania: A randomized, double-blind, placebo-controlled add-on trial. *Journal of the American Academy of Child and Adolescent Psychiatry, 52*(3), 231–240.

Blum, N. J., Barone, V. J., & Friman, P. C. (1993). A simplified behavioral treatment for trichotillomania: Report of two cases. *Pediatrics, 91*(5), 1–4.

Bohne, A., Keuthen, N., & Wilhelm, S. (2005). Pathologic hairpulling, skin picking, and nail biting. *Annals of Clinical Psychiatry, 17*(4), 227–232.

Chamberlain, S. R., Hampshire, A., Menzies, L. A., Garyfallidis, E., Grant, J. E., Odlaug, B. L., et al. (2010). Reduced brain white matter integrity in trichotillomania: A diffusion tensor imaging study. *Archives of General Psychiatry, 67*(9), 965–971.

Chamberlain, S. R., Menzies, L. A., Fineberg, N. A., Del Campo, N., Suckling, J., Craig, K., et al. (2008). Grey matter abnormalities in trichotillomania: Morphometric magnetic resonance imaging study. *British Journal of Psychiatry, 193*(3), 216–221.

Chang, S., Himle, M. B., Tucker, B. T. P., Woods, D. W., & Piacentini, J. (2009). Initial psychometric properties of a brief parent-report instrument for assessing tic severity in children with chronic tic disorders. *Child and Family Behavior Therapy, 31*(3), 181–191.

Chao, T. K., Hu, J., & Pringsheim, T. (2014). Prenatal risk factors for Tourette syndrome: A systematic review. *BMC Pregnancy and Childbirth, 14*(1), 53.

Chappell, P. B., McSwiggan-Hardin, M. T., Scahill, L., Rubenstein, M., Walker, D. E., Cohen, D. J., et al. (1994). Videotape tic counts in the assessment of Tourette's syndrome: Stability, reliability, and validity. *Journal of the American Academy of Child and Adolescent Psychiatry, 33*(3), 386–393.

Christenson, G. A. (1995). Trichotillomania-from prevalence to comorbidity. *Psychiatric Times, 12*(9), 44–48.

Christenson, G. A., Mackenzie, T. B., & Mitchell, J. E. (1991). Characteristics of 60 adult hair pullers. *American Journal of Psychiatry, 148*(3), 365–370.

Christenson, G. A., Mackenzie, T. B., Mitchell, J. E., & Callies, A. L. (1991). A placebo-controlled, double-blind crossover study of fluoxetine in trichotillomania. *American Journal of Psychiatry, 148*(11), 1566–1571.

Christenson, G. A., & Mansueto, C. S. (1999). Trichotillomania: Descriptive characteristics and phenomenology. In D. J. Stein, G. A. Christenson, & E. Hollander (Eds.), *Trichotillomania* (pp. 1–42). Washington, DC: American Psychiatric Press.

Christenson, G. A., Pyle, R. L., & Mitchell, J. E. (1991). Estimated lifetime prevalence of trichotillomania in college students. *Journal of Clinical Psychiatry, 54*(2), 72–73.

Christenson, G. A., Ristvedt, S. L., & Mackenzie, T. B. (1993). Identification of trichotillomania cue profiles. *Behaviour Research and Therapy, 31*(3), 315–320.

Cohen, S. C., Leckman, J. F., & Bloch, M. H. (2013). Clinical assessment of Tourette syndrome and tic disorders. *Neuroscience and Biobehavioral Reviews, 37*(6), 997–1007.

Conelea, C. A., & Woods, D. W. (2008). The influence of contextual factors on tic expression in Tourette's syndrome: A review. *Journal of Psychosomatic Research, 65*(5), 487–496.

Cook, C. R., & Blacher, J. (2007). Evidence-based psychosocial treatments for tic disorders. *Clinical Psychology Science and Practice, 14*, 252–267.

Deckersbach, T., Rauch, S., Buhlmann, U., & Wilhelm, S. (2006). Habit reversal versus supportive psychotherapy in Tourette's disorder: A randomized controlled trial and predictors of treatment response. *Behaviour Research and Therapy, 44*(8), 1079–1090.

Diefenbach, G. J., Mouton-Odum, S., & Stanley, M. A. (2002). Affective correlates of trichotillomania. *Behaviour Research and Therapy, 40*(11), 1305–1315.

Diefenbach, G. J., Reitman, D., & Williamson, D. A. (2000). Trichotillomania: A challenge to research and practice. *Clinical Psychology Review, 20*(3), 289–309.

Diefenbach, G. J., Tolin, D. F., Crocetto, J., Maltby, N., & Hannan, S. (2005). Assessment of trichotillomania: A psychometric evaluation of hair-pulling scales. *Journal of Psychopathology and Behavioral Assessment, 27*(3), 169–178.

Diefenbach, G. J., Tolin, D. F., Meunier, S., & Worhunsky, P. (2008). Emotion regulation and trichotillomania: A comparison of clinical and nonclinical hair pulling. *Journal of Behavior Therapy and Experimental Psychiatry, 39*(1), 32–41.

Dietrich, A., Fernandez, T. V., King, R. A., State, M. W., Tischfield, J. A., Hoekstra, P. J., et al. (2015). The Tourette International Collaborative Genetics (TIC Genetics) study, finding the genes causing Tourette syndrome: Objectives and methods. *European Child and Adolescent Psychiatry, 24*(2), 141–151.

Draper, A., Stephenson, M. C., Jackson, G. M., Pépés, S., Morgan, P. S., Morris, P. G., & Jackson, S. R. (2014). Increased GABA contributes to enhanced control over motor excitability in Tourette syndrome. *Current Biology, 24*(19), 2343–2347.

Duke, D. C., Bodzin, D. K., Tavares, P., Geffken, G. R., & Storch, E. A. (2009). The phenomenology of hairpulling in a community sample. *Journal of Anxiety Disorders, 23*(8), 1118–1125.

Evers, R. A., & van de Wetering, B. J. (1994). A treatment model for motor tics based on a specific tension-reduction technique. *Journal of Behavior Therapy and Experimental Psychiatry, 25*(3), 255–260.

Felling, R. J., & Singer, H. S. (2011). Neurobiology of Tourette syndrome: Current status and need for further investigation. *Journal of Neuroscience, 31*(35), 12387–12395.

Flessner, C. A. (2012). Diagnosis and comorbidity. In J. E. Grant, D. J. Stein, D. W. Woods, & N. J. Keuthen (Eds.), *Trichotillomania, skin picking, and other body-focused repetitive behaviors* (pp. 83–96). Washington, DC: American Psychiatry Publishing.

Flessner, C. A., Woods, D. W., Franklin, M. E., Keuthen, N. J., Piacentini, J., Cashin, S. E., et al. (2007). The Milwaukee Inventory for Styles of Trichotillomania—Child Version (MIST-C): Initial development and psychometric properties. *Behavior Modification, 31*(6), 896–918.

Franklin, M. E., Edson, A. L., & Freeman, J. B. (2010). Behavior therapy for pediatric trichotillomania: Exploring the effects of age on treatment outcome. *Child and Adolescent Psychiatry and Mental Health, 4*(1), 18.

Franklin, M. E., Edson, A. L., Ledley, D. A., & Cahill, S. P. (2011). Behavior therapy for pediatric trichotillomania: A randomized controlled trial. *Journal of the American Academy of Child and Adolescent Psychiatry, 50*(8), 763–771.

Franklin, M. E., Flessner, C. A., Woods, D. W., Keuthen, N. J., Piacentini, J. C., Moore, P., et al. (2008). The child and adolescent trichotillomania impact project: Descriptive psychopathology, comorbidity, functional impairment, and treatment utilization. *Journal of Developmental and Behavioral Pediatrics, 29*(6), 493–500.

George, S., & Moselhy, H. (2005). Cocaine-induced trichotillomania. *Addiction, 100*(2), 255–256.

Gilbert, D. L., & Jankovic, J. (2014). Pharmacological treatment of Tourette syndrome. *Journal of Obsessive–Compulsive and Related Disorders, 3*, 407–414.

Goetz, C. G., Tanner, C. M., Wilson, R. S., & Shannon, K. M. (1987). A rating scale for Gilles de la Tourette's syndrome: Description, reliability, and validity data. *Neurology, 37*(9), 1542–1544.

Grant, J. E., & Odlaug, B. L. (2008). Clinical characteristics of trichotillomania with trichophagia. *Comprehensive Psychiatry, 49*(6), 579–584.

Grant, J. E., Odlaug, B. L., & Kim, S. W. (2009). N-Acetylcysteine, a glutamate modulator, in the treatment of trichotillomania. *Archives of General Psychiatry, 66*(7), 756–763.

Hajcak, G., Franklin, M. E., Simons, R. F., & Keuthen, N. J. (2006). Hairpulling and skin picking in relation to affective distress and obsessive–compulsive symptoms. *Journal of Psychopathology and Behavioral Assessment, 28*(3), 177–185.

Hamalian, G., & Citrome, L. (2010). Stimulant-induced trichotillomania. *Substance Abuse, 31*(1), 68–70.

Hansen, D. J., Tishelman, A. C., Hawkins, R. P., & Doepke, K. J. (1990). Habits with potential as disorders: Prevalence, severity, and other characteristics among college students. *Behavior Modification, 14*(1), 66–80.

Hemmings, S. M. J., Kinnear, C. J., Lochner, C., Seedat, S., Corfield, V. A., Moolman-Smook, J. C., et al. (2006). Genetic correlates in trichotillomania—a case–control association study in the South African Caucasian population. *Israel Journal of Psychiatry and Related Sciences, 43*(2), 93–101.

Himle, M. B., Chang, S., Woods, D. W., Pearlman, A., Buzzella, B., Bunaciu, L., et al. (2006). Establishing the feasibility of direct observation in the assessment of tics in children with chronic tic disorders. *Journal of Applied Behavior Analysis, 39*(4), 429–440.

Himle, M. B., Freitag, M., Walther, M., Franklin, S. A., Ely, L., & Woods, D. W. (2012). A randomized pilot trial comparing videoconference versus face-to-face delivery of behavior therapy for childhood tic disorders. *Behaviour Research and Therapy, 50*(9), 565–570.

Himle, M. B., Olufs, E., Himle, J., Tucker, B. T. P., & Woods, D. W. (2010). Behavior therapy for tics via videoconference delivery. *Cognitive and Behavioral Practice, 17*, 359–337.

Himle, M. B., & Woods, D. W. (2005). An experimental evaluation of tic suppression and the tic rebound effect. *Behaviour Research and Therapy, 43*(11), 1443–1451.

Himle, M. B., Woods, D. W., Piacentini, J. C., & Walkup, J. T. (2006). Brief review of habit reversal training for tourette syndrome. *Journal of Child Neurology, 21*(8), 719–725.

Hirschtritt, M. E., Lee, P. C., Pauls, D. L., Dion, Y., Grados, M. A., Illmann, C., et al. (2015). Lifetime prevalence, age of risk, and genetic relationships of comorbid psychiatric disorders in tourette syndrome. *JAMA Psychiatry, 72*(4), 325–333.

Hoogduin, K., Verdellen, C., & Cath, D. (1997). Exposure and response prevention in the treatment of Gilles de la Tourette's syndrome: Four case studies. *Clinical Psychology and Psychotherapy, 4*(2), 125–135.

Houghton, D. C., Compton, S. N., Twohig, M. P., Saunders, S. M., Frankli, M. E., Neal-Barnett, A. M., et al. (2014). Measuring the role of psychological inflexibility in trichotillomania. *Psychiatry Research, 220*(1), 356–361.

Houghton, D. C., Franklin, M. R., Twohig, M. P., Franklin, M. E., Compton, S. N., Neal-Barnett, A. M., et al. (2016). Photographic assessment of change in trichotillomania: Psychometric properties and variables influencing interpretation. *Journal of Psychopathology and Behavioral Assessment, 38*(3), 505–513.

Jankovic, J., & Kurlan, R. (2011). Tourette syndrome: evolving concepts. *Movement Disorders, 26*(6), 1149–1156.

Keuthen, N. J., Rothbaum, B. O., Fama, J., Altenburger, E., Falkenstein, M. J., Sprich, S. E., et al. (2012). DBT-enhanced cognitive-behavioral treatment for trichotillomania: A randomized controlled trial. *Journal of Behavioral Addictions, 1*(3), 106–114.

Khalifa, N., & von Knorring, A.-L. (2003). Prevalence of tic disorders and Tourette syndrome in a Swedish school population. *Developmental Medicine and Child Neurology, 45*(5), 315–319.

Khalifa, N., & von Knorring, A.-L. (2005). Tourette syndrome and other tic disorders in a total population of children: Clinical assessment and background. *Acta Paediatrica, 94*(11), 1608–1614.

King, R. A., Scahill, L., & Vitulano, L. A. (1995). Childhood trichotillomania: Clinical phenomenology, comorbidity, and family genetics. *Journal of the American Academy of Child and Adolescent Psychiatry, 34*(11), 1451–1459.

Kraft, J. T., Dalsgaard, S., Obel, C., Thomsen, P. H., Henriksen, T. B., & Scahill, L. (2012). Prevalence and clinical correlates of tic disorders in a community sample of school-age children. *European Child and Adolescent Psychiatry, 21*(1), 5–13.

Kurlan, R., McDermott, M. P., Deeley, C., & Como, P. G. (2001). Prevalence of tics in schoolchildren and association with placement in special education. *Neurology, 59*(3), 414–420.

Lawson-Yuen, A., Saldivar, J. S., Sommer, S., & Picker, J. (2008). Familial deletion within NLGN4 associated with autism and Tourette syndrome. *European Journal of Human Genetics, 16*(5), 614–618.

Leckman, J. F., Bloch, M. H., Smith, M. E., Larabi, D., & Hampson, M. (2010). Neurobiological substrates of Tourette's disorder. *Journal of Child and Adolescent Psychopharmacology, 20*(4), 237–247.

Leckman, J. F., Riddle, M. A., Hardin, M. T., Ort, S. I., Swartz, K. L., Stevenson, J., et al. (1989). The Yale Global Tic Severity Scale: Initial testing of a clinician-rated scale of tic severity. *Journal of the American Academy of Child and Adolescent Psychiatry, 28*(4), 566–573.

Leckman, J. F., Walker, D. E., & Cohen, D. J. (1993). Premonitory urges in Tourette's syndrome. *American Journal of Psychiatry, 150*(1), 98–102.

Leckman, J. F., Walker, D. E., Goodman, W. K., Pauls, D. L., & Cohen, D. J. (1994). "Just right" perceptions associated with compulsive behavior in Tourette's syndrome. *American Journal of Psychiatry, 151*(5), 675–680.

Leckman, J. F., Zhang, H., Vitale, A., Lahnin, F., Lynch, K., Bondi, C., et al. (1998). Course of tic severity in Tourette syndrome: The first two decades. *Pediatrics, 102*(1, Pt. 1), 14–19.

Lerner, A., Bagic, A., Simmons, J. M., Mari, Z., Bonne, O., Xu, B., et al. (2012). Widespread abnormality of the [γ]-aminobutyric acid-ergic system in Tourette syndrome. *Brain: A Journal of Neurology, 135*(Pt. 6), 1926–1936.

Lewin, A. B., Piacentini, J., Flessner, C. A., Woods, D. W., Franklin, M. E., Keuthen, N. J., et al. (2009). Depression, anxiety, and functional impairment in children with trichotillomania. *Depression and Anxiety, 26*(6), 521–527.

Lochner, C., Grant, J. E., Odlaug, B. L., Woods, D. W., Keuthen, N. J., & Stein, D. J. (2012). DSM-5 Field Survey: Hair-pulling disorder (trichotillomania). *Depression and Anxiety, 29*(12), 1025–1031.

Lochner, C., Seedat, S., & Stein, D. J. (2010). Chronic hair-pulling: Phenomenology-based sub-types. *Journal of Anxiety Disorders, 24*(2), 196–202.

Lucas, C. P., Zhang, H., Fisher, P. W., Shaffer, D., Regier, D. A., Narrow, W. E., et al. (2001). The DISC Predictive Scales (DPS): Efficiently screening for diagnoses. *Journal of the American Academy of Child and Adolescent Psychiatry, 40*(4), 443–449.

Mackenzie, T. B., Ristvedt, S. L., Christenson, G. A., Lebow, A. S., & Mitchell, J. E. (1995). Iden-tification of cues associated with compulsive, bulimic, and hair-pulling symptoms. *Journal of Behavior Therapy and Experimental Psychiatry, 26*(1), 9–16.

Marcks, B. A., Woods, D. W., & Ridosko, J. L. (2005). The effects of trichotillomania disclosure on peer perceptions and social acceptability. *Body Image, 2*(3), 299–306.

Marcks, B. A., Woods, D. W., Teng, E. J., & Twohig, M. P. (2004). What do those who know, know?: Investigating providers' knowledge about Tourette's syndrome and its treatment. *Cognitive and Behavioral Practice, 11,* 298–305.

Martin, A., Scahill, L., Vitulano, L., & King, R. A. (1998). Stimulant use and trichotillomania. *Journal of the American Academy of Child and Adolescent Psychiatry, 37*(4), 349–350.

Massong, S. R., Edwards, R. P., Sitton, L. R., & Hailey, B. J. (2002). A case of trichotillomania in a three year old treated by response prevention. *Journal of Behavior Therapy and Experi-mental Psychiatry, 11,* 223–225.

Mathews, C. A., Bimson, B., Lowe, T. L., Herrera, L. D., Budman, C. L., Erenberg, G., et al. (2006). Association between maternal smoking and increased symptom severity in Tourette's syndrome. *American Journal of Psychiatry, 163*(6), 1066–1073.

McGuire, J. F., Kugler, B. B., Park, J. M., & Horng, B. (2012). Evidence-based assessment of com-pulsive skin picking, chronic tic disorders and trichotillomania in children. *Child Psychiatry and Human Development, 43*(6), 855–883.

McGuire, J. F., Piacentini, J., Brennan, E. A., Lewin, A. B., Murphy, T. K., Small, B. J., et al. (2014). A meta-analysis of behavior therapy for Tourette syndrome. *Journal of Psychiatric Research, 50,* 106–112.

McGuire, J. F., Ung, D., Selles, R. R., Rahman, O., Lewin, A. B., Murphy, T. K., et al. (2014). Treating trichotillomania: A meta-analysis of treatment effects and moderators for behavior therapy and serotonin reuptake inhibitors. *Journal of Psychiatric Research, 58,* 76–83.

Miller, L. L., Scharf, J. M., Mathews, C. A., & Ben-Shlomo, Y. (2014). Tourette syndrome and chronic tic disorder are associated with lower socio-economic status: Findings from the Avon Longitudinal Study of Parents and Children cohort. *Developmental Medicine and Child Neurology, 56*(2), 157–163.

Mink, J. W. (2001). Basal ganglia dysfunction in Tourette's syndrome: A new hypothesis. *Pediatric Neurology, 25,* 190–198.

Mostaghimi, L. (2012). Dermatological assessment of hair pulling, skin picking, and nail biting. In J. E. Grant, D. J. Stein, D. W. Woods, & N. J. Keuthen (Eds.), *Trichotillomania, skin pick-ing, and other body-focused repetitive behaviors* (pp. 97–112). Washington, DC: American Psychiatric Association.

Murphy, T. K., Lewin, A. B., Storch, E. A., & Stock, S. (2013). Practice parameter for the assess-ment and treatment of children and adolescents with tic disorders. *Journal of the American Academy of Child and Adolescent Psychiatry, 52*(12), 1341–1359.

Nag, A., Bochukova, E. G., Kremeyer, B., Campbell, D. D., Muller, H., Valencia-Duarte, A. V., et al. (2013). CNV analysis in Tourette syndrome implicates large genomic rearrangements in COL8A1 and NRXN1. *PLoS ONE, 8*(3), e59061.

Narine, C., Sarwar, S. R., & Rais, T. B. (2013). Adderall-induced trichotillomania: A case report. *Innovations in Clinical Neuroscience, 10*(7–8), 13–14.

Ninan, P. T., Rothbaum, B. O., Marsteller, F. A., Knight, B. T., & Eccard, M. B. (2000). A pla-cebo-controlled trial of cognitive-behavioral therapy and clomipramine in trichotillomania. *Journal of Clinical Psychiatry, 61*(1), 47–50.

Norberg, M. M., Wetterneck, C. T., Woods, D. W., & Conelea, C. A. (2007). Experiential avoidance as a mediator of relationships between cognitions and hair-pulling severity. *Behavior Modification, 31*(4), 367–381.

Novak, C. E., Keuthen, N. J., Stewart, S. E., & Pauls, D. L. (2009). A twin concordance study of trichotillomania. *American Journal of Medical Genetics, 150B*(7), 944–949.

O'Connor, K. (2002). A cognitive-behavioral/psychophysiological model of tic disorders. *Behaviour Research and Therapy, 40*(10), 1113–1142.

O'Connor, K., Lavoie, M., Blanchet, P., & St-Pierre-Delorme, M.-È. (2016). Evaluation of a cognitive psychophysiological model for management of tic disorders: An open trial. *British Journal of Psychiatry, 209*(1), 76–83.

Odlaug, B. L., Chamberlain, S. R., Derbyshire, K. L., Leppink, E. W., & Grant, J. E. (2014). Impaired response inhibition and excess cortical thickness as candidate endophenotypes for trichotillomania. *Journal of Psychiatric Research, 59*, 167–173.

Odlaug, B. L., & Grant, J. E. (2008). Trichotillomania and pathologic skin picking: Clinical comparison with an examination of comorbidity. *Annals of Clinical Psychiatry, 20*(2), 57–63.

Odlaug, B. L., Kim, S. W., & Grant, J. E. (2010). Quality of life and clinical severity in pathological skin picking and trichotillomania. *Journal of Anxiety Disorders, 24*(8), 823–829.

O'Sullivan, R. L., Keuthen, N. J., Hayday, C. F., Ricciardi, J. N., Buttolph, M. L., Jenike, M. A., et al. (1995). The Massachusetts General Hospital (MGH) Hairpulling Scale: 2. Reliability and validity. *Psychotherapy and Psychosomatics, 64*(3–4), 146–148.

O'Sullivan, R. L., Rauch, S. L., Breiter, H. C., Grachev, I. D., Baer, L., Kennedy, D. N., et al. (1997). Reduced basal ganglia volumes in trichotillomania measured via morphometric magnetic resonance imaging. *Biological Psychiatry, 42*(1), 39–45.

Piacentini, J., Woods, D. W., Scahill, L., Wilhelm, S., Peterson, A. L., Chang, S., et al. (2010). Behavior therapy for children with Tourette disorder. *Journal of the American Medical Association, 303*(19), 1929–1937.

Puts, N. A., Harris, A. D., Crocetti, D., Nettles, C., Singer, H. S., Tommerdahl, M., et al. (2015). Reduced GABAergic inhibition and abnormal sensory processing in children with Tourette syndrome. *Journal of Neurophysiology, 114*(2), 808–817.

Rapp, J. T., Miltenberger, R. G., Galensky, T. L., Ellingson, S. A., & Long, E. S. (1999). A functional analysis of hair pulling. *Journal of Applied Behavior Analysis, 32*(3), 329–337.

Rapp, J. T., Miltenberger, R. G., Long, E. S., Elliot, A. J., & Lumley, V. A. (1998). Simplified habit reversal treatment for chronic hair pulling in three adolescents: A clinical replication with direct observation. *Journal of Applied Behavior Analysis, 31*(2), 299–302.

Reese, H. E., Vallejo, Z., Rasmussen, J., Crowe, K., Rosenfield, E., & Wilhelm, S. (2015). Mindfulness-based stress reduction for Tourette syndrome and chronic tic disorder: A pilot study. *Journal of Psychosomatic Research, 78*(3), 293–298.

Ricketts, E. J., Goetz, A. R., Capriotti, M. R., Bauer, C. C., Brei, N. G., Himle, M. B., et al. (2016). A randomized waitlist-controlled pilot trial of voice over Internet protocol-delivered behavior therapy for youth with chronic tic disorders. *Journal of Telemedicine and Telecare, 22*(3), 153–162.

Robertson, M. M. (2006). Attention deficit hyperactivity disorder, tics and Tourette's syndrome: The relationship and treatment implications: A commentary. *European Child and Adolescent Psychiatry, 15*(1), 1–11.

Robertson, M. M. (2008). The prevalence and epidemiology of Gilles de la Tourette syndrome: Part 1. The epidemiological and prevalence studies. *Journal of Psychosomatic Research, 65*(5), 461–472.

Roos, A., Grant, J. E., Fouche, J. P., Stein, D. J., & Lochner, C. (2015). A comparison of brain volume and cortical thickness in excoriation (skin picking) disorder and trichotillomania (hair pulling disorder) in women. *Behavioural Brain Research, 279*, 255–258.

Rosenbaum, M. S., & Ayllon, T. (1981). The behavioral treatment of neurodermatitis through habit reversal. *Behaviour Research and Therapy, 19*, 313–318.

Rothbaum, B. O., & Ninan, P. T. (1994). The assessment of trichotillomania. *Behaviour Research and Therapy, 32*(6), 651–662.

Rothbaum, B. O., Shaw, L., Morris, R., & Ninan, P. T. (1993). Prevalence of trichotillomania in a college freshman population. *Journal of Clinical Psychiatry, 54*(2), 72–73.

Scharf, J. M., Miller, L. L., Mathews, C. A., & Ben-Shlomo, Y. (2012). Prevalence of Tourette syndrome and chronic tics in the population-based Avon Longitudinal Study of Parents and Children Cohort. *Journal of the American Academy of Child and Adolescent Psychiatry, 51*(2), 192–201.

Scharf, J. M., Yu, D., Mathews, C. A., Neale, B. M., Stewart, S. E., Fagerness, J. A., et al. (2013). Genome-wide association study of Tourette's syndrome. *Molecular Psychiatry, 18*(6), 721–728.

Schlosser, S., Black, D. W., Blum, N., & Goldstein, R. B. (1994). The demography, phenomenology, and family history of 22 persons with compulsive hair pulling. *Annals of Clinical Psychiatry, 6*(3), 147–152.

Silverman, W. K., & Albano, A. M. (1996). *Anxiety Disorders Interview Schedule for DSM-IV: Child Interview Schedule.* Boulder, CO: Graywind.

Singer, H. S. (2013). Motor control, habits, complex motor stereotypies, and Tourette syndrome. *Annals of the New York Academy of Sciences, 1304*(1), 22–31.

Snorrason, I., Belleau, E. L., & Woods, D. W. (2012). How related are hair pulling disorder (trichotillomania) and skin picking disorder?: A review of evidence for comorbidity, similarities and shared etiology. *Clinical Psychology Review, 32*(7), 618–629.

Specht, M. W., Woods, D. W., Piacentini, J., Scahill, L., Wilhelm, S., Peterson, A. L., et al. (2011). Clinical characteristics of children and adolescents with a primary tic disorder. *Journal of Developmental and Physical Disabilities, 23*(1), 15–31.

Stefanato, C. M. (2010). Histopathology of alopecia: A clinicopathological approach to diagnosis. *Histopathology, 56*(1), 24–38.

Stein, D. J., Flessner, C. A., Franklin, M., Keuthen, N. J., Lochner, C., & Woods, D. W. (2008). Is trichotillomania a stereotypic movement disorder?: An analysis of body-focused repetitive behaviors in people with hair-pulling. *Annals of Clinical Psychiatry, 20*(4), 194–198.

Stemberger, R. M. T., Thomas, A. M., Mansueto, C. S., & Carter, J. G. (2000). Personal toll of trichotillomania: Behavioral and interpersonal sequelae. *Journal of Anxiety Disorders, 14*(1), 97–104.

Storch, E. A., Murphy, T. K., Geffken, G. R., Sajid, M., Allen, P., Roberti, J. W., et al. (2005). Reliability and validity of the Yale Global Tic Severity Scale. *Psychological Assessment, 17*(4), 486–491.

Swedo, S. E., Leonard, H. L., Lenane, M. C., & Rettew, D. C. (1992). Trichotillomania: A profile of the disorder from infancy through adulthood. *International Pediatrics, 7*, 144–150.

Swedo, S. E., Leonard, H. L., Rapoport, J. L., Lenane, M. C., Goldberger, E. L., & Cheslow, D. L. (1989). A double-blind comparison of clomipramine and desipramine in the treatment of trichotillomania (hair pulling). *New England Journal of Medicine, 321*(8), 497–501.

Teng, E. J., Woods, D. W., Marcks, B. A., & Twohig, M. P. (2004). Body-focused repetitive behaviors: The proximal and distal effects of affective variables on behavioral expression. *Journal of Psychopathology and Behavioral Assessment, 26*(1), 55–64.

Teng, E. J., Woods, D. W., Twohig, M. P., & Marcks, B. A. (2002). Body-focused repetitive behavior problems: Prevalence in a nonreferred population and differences in perceived somatic activity. *Behavior Modification, 26*(3), 340–360.

Tolin, D. F., Diefenbach, G. J., Flessner, C. A., Franklin, M. E., Keuthen, N. J., Moore, P., et al. (2008). The Trichotillomania Scale for Children: Development and validation. *Child Psychiatry and Human Development, 39*(3), 331–349.

Tolin, D. F., Franklin, M. E., Diefenbach, G. J., Anderson, E., & Meunier, S. A. (2007). Pediatric trichotillomania: Descriptive psychopathology and an open trial of cognitive behavioral therapy. *Cognitive Behaviour Therapy, 36*(3), 129–144.

Twohig, M. P., & Woods, D. W. (2001). Evaluating the duration of the competing response in habit reversal: A parametric analysis. *Journal of Applied Behavior Analysis, 34*(4), 517–520.

Van Ameringen, M., Mancini, C., Oakman, J. M., & Farvolden, P. (1999). The potential role of haloperidol in the treatment of trichotillomania. *Journal of Affective Disorders, 56*(2–3), 219–226.

van Minnen, A., Hoogduin, K. A., Keijsers, G. P., Hellenbrand, I., & Hendriks, G. J. (2003). Treatment of trichotillomania with behavioral therapy or fluoxetine: A randomized, waiting-list controlled study. *Archives of General Psychiatry, 60*(5), 517–522.

Verdellen, C. W. J., Keijsers, G. P. J., Cath, D. C., & Hoogduin, C. A. L. (2004). Exposure with response prevention versus habit reversal in Tourette's syndrome: A controlled study. *Behaviour Research and Therapy, 42*(5), 501–511.

Verdellen, C., van de Griendt, J., Hartmann, A., Murphy, T., & ESSTS Guidelines Group. (2011). European clinical guidelines for Tourette syndrome and other tic disorders: Part III. Behavioural and psychosocial interventions. *European Child and Adolescent Psychiatry, 20*(4), 197–207.

Verdellen, C., van de Griendt, J., Kriens, S., van Oostrum, I., & Chang, I. (2011). *Tics—Therapist manual and workbook for children.* Amsterdam, The Netherlands: Boom uitgevers.

Verkerk, A. J. M. H., Mathews, C. A., Joosse, M., Eussen, B. H. J., Heutink, P., Oostra, B. A., et al. (2003). CNTNAP2 is disrupted in a family with Gilles de la Tourette syndrome and obsessive compulsive disorder. *Genomics, 82*(1), 1–9.

Walkup, J. T., Rosenberg, L. A., Brown, J., & Singer, H. S. (1992). The validity of instruments measuring tic severity in Tourette's syndrome. *Journal of the American Academy of Child and Adolescent Psychiatry, 31*(3), 472–477.

Walther, M. R., Snorrason, I., Flessner, C. A., Franklin, M. E., Burkel, R., & Woods, D. W. (2014). The Trichotillomania Impact Project in Young Children (TIP-YC): Clinical characteristics, comorbidity, functional impairment and treatment utilization. *Child Psychiatry and Human Development, 45*(1), 24–31.

Weisman, H., Qureshi, I. A., Leckman, J. F., Scahill, L., & Bloch, M. H. (2013). Systematic review: Pharmacological treatment of tic disorders—efficacy of antipsychotic and alpha-2 adrenergic agonist agents. *Neuroscience and Biobehavioral Reviews, 37*(6), 1162–1171.

Welch, S. S., & Kim, J. (2012). DBT-enhanced cognitive behavioral therapy for adolescent trichotillomania: An adolescent case study. *Cognitive and Behavioral Practice, 19*(3), 483–493.

White, M. P., Shirer, W. R., Molfino, M. J., Tenison, C., Damoiseaux, J. S., & Greicius, M. D. (2013). Disordered reward processing and functional connectivity in trichotillomania: A pilot study. *Journal of Psychiatric Research, 47*(9), 1264–1272.

Wilhelm, S., Peterson, A. L., Piacentini, J., Woods, D. W., Deckersbach, T., Sukhodolsky, D. G., et al. (2012). Randomized trial of behavior therapy for adults with Tourette syndrome. *Archives of General Psychiatry, 69*(8), 795–803.

Winchel, R. M., Jones, J. S., Molcho, A., Parsons, B., Stanley, B., & Stanley, M. (1992). The Psychiatric Institute Trichotillomania Scale (PITS). *Psychopharmacology Bulletin, 28*(4), 463–476.

Woods, D. W., Conelea, C. A., & Himle, M. B. (2010). Behavior therapy for Tourette's disorder: Utilization in a community sample and an emerging area of practice for psychologists. *Professional Psychology: Research and Practice, 41*(6), 518–525.

Woods, D. W., Conelea, C. A., & Walther, M. R. (2007). Barriers to dissemination: Exploring the criticisms of behavior therapy for tics. *Clinical Psychology Science and Practice, 14*(3), 279–282.

Woods, D. W., Flessner, C. A., Franklin, M. E., Keuthen, N. J., Goodwin, R. D., Stein, D. J., et al. (2006a). The Trichotillomania Impact Project (TIP): Exploring phenomenology, functional impairment, and treatment utilization. *Journal of Clinical Psychiatry, 67*(12), 1877–1888.

Woods, D. W., Fuqua, R. W., & Outman, R. C. (1999). Evaluating the social acceptability of persons with habit disorders: The effects of topography, frequency, and gender manipulation. *Journal of Psychopathology and Behavioral Assessment, 21*(1), 1–18.

Woods, D. W., & Houghton, D. C. (2016). Evidence-based psychosocial treatments for pediatric body-focused repetitive behavior disorders. *Journal of Clinical Child and Adolescent Psychology, 45*(3), 227–240.

Woods, D. W., Miltenberger, R. G., & Flach, A. D. (1996). Habits, tics, and stuttering. Prevalence and relation to anxiety and somatic awareness. *Behavior Modification, 20*(2), 216–225.

Woods, D. W., Piacentini, J., Chang, S., Deckersbach, T., Ginsburg, G., Peterson, A., et al. (2008). *Managing Tourette syndrome: A behavioral intervention for children and adults therapist guide*. New York: Oxford University Press.

Woods, D. W., Piacentini, J., Himle, M. B., & Chang, S. (2005). Premonitory Urge for Tics Scale (PUTS): Initial psychometric results and examination of the premonitory urge phenomenon in youths with tic disorders. *Journal of Developmental and Behavioral Pediatrics, 26*(6), 397–403.

Woods, D. W., Piacentini, J. C., Scahill, L., Peterson, A. L., Wilhelm, S., Chang, S., et al. (2011). Behavior therapy for tics in children: Acute and long-term effects on psychiatric and psychosocial functioning. *Journal of Child Neurology, 26*(7), 858–865.

Woods, D. W., Wetterneck, C. T., & Flessner, C. A. (2006). A controlled evaluation of acceptance and commitment therapy plus habit reversal for trichotillomania. *Behaviour Research and Therapy, 44*(5), 639–656.

Wright, H. H., & Holmes, G. R. (2003). Trichotillomania (hair pulling) in toddlers. *Psychological Reports, 92*(1), 228–230.

Zuchner, S., Cuccaro, M. L., Tran-Viet, K. N., Cope, H., Krishnan, R. R., Pericak-Vance, M. A., et al. (2006). SLITRK1 mutations in trichotillomania. *Molecular Psychiatry, 11*(10), 888–889.

PART III

SPECIAL POPULATIONS AND APPLICATIONS

CHAPTER 16

Cognitive-Behavioral Treatment for Children with Autism Spectrum Disorder

Angela Scarpa, Tyler A. Hassenfeldt,
and Tony Attwood

We describe in this chapter the potential use of caregiver-assisted cognitive-behavioral therapy (CBT) to treat difficulties with emotional competence and dysregulation in youth with autism spectrum disorder (ASD). Our focus is primarily on school-age children* (preschool and beyond) with ASD who do not have language or cognitive impairment and can therefore benefit most readily from CBT. After an overview on ASD symptoms, assessment and treatments, we discuss how CBT can be successfully modified for use with the ASD population and developmental considerations that need to be addressed. We then review specific CBTs designed to treat anxiety, anger, and emotion regulation in children with ASD, ending with a case example of a specific CBT modification and developmental adaptation for young children with ASD, called the Stress and Anger Management Program (STAMP; Scarpa, Wells, & Attwood, 2013).

THE DSM-5 DEFINITION OF ASD

ASD is a lifelong neurodevelopmental condition characterized by a continuum of difficulties in social communication and interaction, as well as behavioral differences, such as repetitive body mannerisms, interests that are unique in topic or severity, compulsions,

---

*Unless otherwise indicated, the word "children" is used flexibly in this chapter to refer to both children and adolescents.

and sensory sensitivities or preferences (Volkmar, Reichow, Westphal, & Mandell, 2014). Classic autism was first identified by Leo Kanner (1943) and originally was thought to be a relatively rare disorder that affected approximately 3 in 10,000 children. Around the same time, Hans Asperger described a group of children with similar characteristics, but no language or cognitive delay, formerly referred to as Asperger syndrome upon its characterization by Lorna Wing (1981). Autism was not included in the Diagnostic and Statistical Manual of Mental Disorders (DSM) until 1980, and Asperger's disorder in 1994, within the category of pervasive developmental disorders. Most recently, the fifth edition (DSM-5) groups all of these categories into one unified construct of ASD (American Psychiatric Association, 2013).

The spectrum of ASD refers to the notion that symptoms may vary in severity and may change over time in development. For example, some individuals with ASD may have language or intellectual impairments, while others may not. Although abilities vary, the symptoms of ASD do cause adaptive behavior difficulties, such as psychological disorders or problems in daily living skills, occupational functioning, or peer relationships.

PREVALENCE AND COURSE

A recent report by the Centers for Disease Control and Prevention (CDC) estimates that 1 in 68 children (1.47%) in the United States meets diagnostic criteria for ASD, representing an increase of 123% in prevalence since the first surveillance study in 2002 (Baio, 2014). Similarly, the National Survey of Children's Health estimated parent-reported prevalence to be 2% among children ages 6–17 years in 2011–2012, representing an increase of 67% since 2007 (Blumberg et al., 2013). Taken together, these findings suggest that the prevalence range of ASD is one out of every 50–68 children in the United States, or approximately 1–1.5 million children ages 0–17 years. Cost analyses suggest that the economic burden of pediatric ASD is substantial due to the costs associated with increased use of health services, school supports, ASD-related therapy, family services, and caregiver time. In one study, the total societal cost in the United States for children with parent-reported ASD was estimated at $11.5 billion in 2011, at an individual cost of at least $17,000 more per year to care for a child with versus without ASD (Lavelle, 2014).

Symptoms of ASD appear early in development, although they are typically not reported until around age 2 years, when communication difficulties and lack of other skills become increasingly noticeable. Even at 12–18 months, children who are later diagnosed with ASD may show signs of the disorder, such as lack of pointing, showing emotion, orienting to their spoken name, or looking at faces. Despite greater knowledge about early signs, the ASD diagnosis is often not made until age 4 years or older according to the last CDC report (Baio, 2014). ASD is a chronic condition, and although there are often gradual improvements with age, most children with ASD are likely to continue to experience problems throughout their lifetime (Howlin, 2014). Intellectual ability, language development, and severity of ASD symptoms are the strongest childhood predictors of adult outcomes. Still, due to social impairments and comorbid conditions, adults with ASD continue to have low rates of positive outcomes such as living independently or maintaining employment.

COMMON COMORBID CONDITIONS

In addition to the chronic course of ASD symptoms, ASD has been associated with a host of comorbid psychiatric conditions that occur at a greater than expected rate compared to the general populations (Leyfer et al., 2006; Moseley, Tonge, Brereton, & Einfeld, 2011; Simonoff et al., 2008). Ghaziuddin, Weidmer-Mikhail, and Ghaziuddin (1998) found that two-thirds of people with ASD met criteria for a comorbid psychiatric disorder, such as attention-deficit/hyperactivity disorder (ADHD), anxiety disorders, mood problems, and self-injurious behavior. Emotional difficulties may be most notable in children with ASD who do not have co-occurring cognitive or language impairments, possibly because more typical assessments can be used to capture problems in this population (Volkmar et al., 2014). It is also possible that more capable children with ASD are more aware of their differences, leading to greater difficulties with adjustment, anxiety, or depression.

Children with ASD also often have deficits in emotional competence (Bauminger-Zviely, 2013; Begeer, Koot, Rieffe, Meerum Terwogt, & Stegge, 2008) due to alexithymia and theory of mind deficits coupled with brain-based connectivity differences and compromised brainstem regulation (Mazefsky et al., 2013). As such, children with ASD may find it difficult to recognize and label emotions in themselves and in others (Downs & Smith, 2004; Sofronoff, Attwood, Hinton, & Levin, 2007), and to express their emotions (Shalom et al., 2006). Moreover, children with ASD tend to demonstrate more negative emotional reactions than their typically developing peers (Capps, Kasari, Yirmiya, & Sigman, 1993; Joseph & Tager-Flusberg, 1997), and are often described by their parents as more likely to experience tantrums and meltdowns (Myles & Southwick, 2005). These difficulties in turn may lead to some of the heightened psychiatric comorbidities we noted earlier, including increased rates of anxiety, mood, and behavioral disorders. Mazefsky and colleagues (2013) argue that the overarching concept of emotion dysregulation in children with ASD helps to explain their difficulty with emotional competence, as well as resultant mood and behavioral comorbidity.

EVIDENCE-BASED TREATMENTS FOR ASD

Evolving Conceptualization and Treatment

Early psychoanalytic views in the 1950s and 1960s described autism as a form of childhood schizophrenia, characterized by "autistic aloneness" or rejection of reality, and caused by cold and distant parenting (Baker, 2013). This psychogenic view of autism was popularized by Bettleheim (1967) in *Empty Fortress,* and at that time led to long-term institutionalization of patients. A paradigm shift occurred in the late 1960s and 1970s, when the psychogenic perspective was replaced by findings supporting a biological origin for autism (Rimland, 1964), and behavioral approaches to treatment became more acceptable, which paved the way for research on behavioral interventions or applied behavior analysis. Lovaas (1987) demonstrated significant improvements in intellectual functioning and school placement in the first randomized controlled trial of intensive behavioral treatment, often referred to as applied behavior analysis (ABA), applied to children with autism, which was later replicated by McEachin, Smith, and Lovaas (1993). Interventions based on ABA are now considered to be well-established forms of treatment for young children with ASD (Smith & Iadarola, 2015). Multiple reviews have outlined effective components and/or guidelines for behavioral interventions (e.g., National Academy of Sciences & National Research Council, 2001; Reichow, 2012; Rogers & Vismara, 2008) that are considered at least moderately effective in the treatment of autism (Maglione, Gans, Das, Timbie, & Kasari, 2012). More recently, cognitive-behavioral interventions have emerged as promising evidence-based approaches for the treatment of anxiety, depression, and social deficits in children with ASD (Attwood & Garnett, 2016; National Autism Center, 2015; Scarpa, White, & Attwood, 2013; Wong et al., 2013), and are most applicable for those without intellectual or language impairment, formerly referred to as "high-functioning ASD" or Asperger's disorder.

Current Established, Emerging, and Unestablished Treatments

Many ASD programs are pseudoscientific, and are marketed toward parents, who are provided anecdotal evidence that appears convincing. As such, efforts to help discriminate between interventions that are and are not evidence-based and effective are worthwhile and helpful. A panel of experts in the field of autism reviewed 361 psychosocial studies of treatment for children with ASD (through age 22) that were published from 2007 to 2011 (National Autism Center, 2015). Ratings of studies were based on their methodological rigor, leading to the assignment of efficacy ratings to the interventions.

Fourteen interventions fell into the "Established" evidence group, which means that there is sufficient evidence to confidently state that they are effective (National Autism Center, 2015). These interventions include behavioral interventions, cognitive-behavioral intervention packages, comprehensive behavioral treatment for young children, such as early intensive behavioral intervention, ABA, language training (production), modeling, natural teaching strategies, parent training, peer training package, pivotal response training (PRT), schedules, scripting, self-management, social skills package, and story-based intervention. The STAMP treatment, which is described herein, and its predecessor, the Exploring Feelings program, are examples of cognitive-behavioral intervention packages.

Eighteen interventions fell into the "Emerging" evidence group, which indicates that at least one study supported the effectiveness of this treatment, but that additional high-quality studies are needed to better cement the intervention's actual effectiveness. These interventions included augmentative and alternative communication (AAC) devices, developmental relationship-based treatment, exercise, exposure, functional communication training, imitation-based intervention, initiation training, language training (production and understanding), massage therapy, a multicomponent package, music therapy, a picture exchange communication system (PECS), a reductive package, sign instruction, a social communication intervention, structured teaching, a technology-based intervention, and theory of mind training.

Finally, 13 interventions fell in the "Unestablished" evidence group, which means that they were not supported by research (i.e., panelists could not rule out the possibility that these interventions might be ineffective and/or harmful). These interventions were animal-assisted therapy, auditory integration training, concept mapping, developmental individual-difference, relationship-based (DIR)/floortime therapy, facilitated communication, gluten-free/casein-free diet, movement-based intervention, the Social Emotional Neuroscience and Endocrinology (SENSE) Theatre intervention, a sensory integration package, shock therapy, a social-behavioral learning strategy, a social cognition intervention, and a social thinking intervention.

Psychopharmacology in ASD

Only two drugs are approved by the U.S. Food and Drug Administration for the treatment of irritability in ASD (risperidone and aripiprazole; Spencer et al., 2013). However, other drugs are sometimes prescribed in other capacities (e.g., "off-label" use) to help treat other symptoms of ASD. In a study of 33,565 children with ASD (ages 0–20 years), Spencer and colleagues found that 64% used at least one psychotropic medication. Thirty-five percent had been prescribed multiple psychotropic drugs. Children who were more likely to be prescribed psychotropic drugs included those who were older, those who had seen a psychiatrist, and those who had comorbid diagnoses (e.g., seizure disorder, ADHD, anxiety, unipolar or bipolar depression). The preponderance of children taking one or more psychotropic medications, despite the lack of evidence on the effectiveness of "off-label" usages, indicates the need for better standards of care in this area.

EVIDENCE-BASED ASSESSMENT AND TREATMENT IN PRACTICE

Assessment

Diagnostic Screening and Evaluation

The current "gold standard" of ASD assessment for children is multi-modal and interdisciplinary (Mazefsky & White, 2013). Children first are usually screened for ASD to establish whether a more in-depth diagnostic evaluation is indicated. Some common screening measures completed by parents or teachers include the Modified Checklist for Autism in Toddlers—Revised with Follow-Up (M-CHAT-R/F; Robins et al., 2014), the Social Responsiveness Scale—Second Edition (SRS-2; Constantino & Gruber, 2012), Social Communication Questionnaire (SCQ; Rutter, Bailey, & Lord, 2003), and Autism-Spectrum Quotient (Baron-Cohen, Wheelwright, Skinner, Martin, & Clubley, 2001). These may be supplemented by more traditional behavioral/social–emotional rating scales, such as the Child Behavior Checklist (CBCL; Achenbach, Dumenci, & Rescorla, 2001; Achenbach & Rescorla, 2000) or the Behavior Assessment System for Children, Second Edition (BASC-2; Reynolds & Kamphaus, 2004), which may also help to rule out comorbid diagnoses.

If a diagnostic evaluation is indicated, recommended components include a review of school, medical, and/or previous testing records, parent interview, developmental and cognitive testing, a play-based observation, and a measure of adaptive behavior skills. The Autism Diagnostic Interview—Revised (ADI-R; Rutter, Le Couteur, & Lord, 2003) and the Autism Diagnostic Observation Schedule, Second Edition (ADOS-2; Lord et al., 2012), are considered to be "gold standard" assessment tools for obtaining a complete developmental history and observing symptoms of ASD during standardized tasks, though other interviews and observational measures exist. Current levels of adaptive functioning can be assessed with the Vineland Adaptive Behavior Scales (VABS), the Adaptive Behavior Assessment System (ABAS), or the Developmental Profile, Third

Edition (DP-3). Traditional intellectual testing or screening may be conducted with tools such as the Wechsler Scales (e.g., Wechsler Intelligence Scale for Children, Fifth Edition [WISC-V]; Wechsler Adult Intelligence Scale, Fourth Edition [WAIS-IV]) or the Kaufman Assessment Battery for Children, Second Edition (KABC-II; Kaufman Brief Intelligence Test, Second Edition [KBIT-2]), though it is cautioned that other tools are warranted for nonverbal children or with severe language impairment. Additional recommended components include a medical evaluation and teacher consultation when possible.

Most importantly, it is critical that a developmental history be taken into account (in addition to current functioning) in order to gain information from multiple reporters, and to compare testing results and presence of symptoms to the published diagnostic criteria. Clinicians should also have training and experience specific to ASD and related disorders. Readers are referred to Saulnier and Ventola (2012) for a more thorough understanding of how to conduct a detailed, accurate evaluation of ASD symptoms.

Assessment of Comorbid Psychiatric Conditions and Treatment Outcome

The assessment of psychiatric comorbidity and its change after treatment is complicated. Few measures have been validated to assess for comorbidity in children with ASD. Some interviews that have been used are the Kiddie Schedule for Affective Disorders and Schizophrenia (Kaufman, Birmaher, Brent, Rao, & Ryan, 1996), the Anxiety Disorders Interview Schedule (Silverman & Albano, 1996), and the Autism Comorbidity Interview (Lainhart, Leyfer, & Folstein, 2003), among others. Whichever measure is used, it is important to consider baseline functioning of the child and how/whether current symptoms are different or worse than usual. It is also important to note that some symptoms (e.g., rituals) may be part of the ASD syndrome, and do not necessarily indicate a comorbid disorder (e.g., obsessive–compulsive disorder [OCD]). Understanding the temporal ordering of symptoms may help clarify whether there are two discrete disorders or whether the symptoms instead represent different expressions within the autism spectrum.

In any CBT program, it is important that assessments be conducted to monitor treatment readiness and outcome. Unfortunately, few, if any, outcome measures have been explicitly developed and normed for use in the ASD population. The most extensive work has been completed on measures of anxiety in ASD. Some anxiety self-report instruments have been found to have good psychometric properties in children with ASD (i.e., the Multidimensional Anxiety Scale for Children [MASC], the Spence Children's Anxiety Scale [SCAS], the Revised Children's Anxiety and Depression Scale [RCADS], and the Screen for Child Anxiety-Related Emotional Disorders [SCARED]), but only the MASC has shown sensitivity to change, and age 6 is the youngest age studied (Lecavalier et al., 2014; Wigham & McConachie, 2014). There is also some initial indication that the SCAS may show good agreement between child and parent report, indicating that some children with ASD may be able to self-report on symptoms of anxiety (Ozsivadjian, Hibberd, & Hollocks, 2014), but this work needs replication. The Anxiety Disorders Interview Schedule (ADIS) and the Pediatric Anxiety Rating Scale (PARS) are clinician interviews that have also shown limited to good reliability and validity, and sensitivity to change, but these require clinician training and are time-intensive (Lecavalier et al., 2014). Even these measures, however, may not tap into symptoms of anxiety as they are uniquely experienced and expressed by children with ASD (e.g., in response to transitions, changes in routine, loud noises, unpredictable situations), or they may rely on a caregiver noticing changes in emotion expression or a child verbalizing his or her experience (both of which may be minimized in children with ASD). As such, further research is needed on appropriate ways to measure emotions and their sensitivity to change in children with ASD, and these studies need to extend beyond measures of anxiety. The Aberrant Behavior Checklist (ABC; Aman & Singh, 1986) is one measure that taps into other ASD characteristics (e.g., irritability, hyperactivity), with good psychometric support for use within a sample of children with ASD and is sensitive to parent training treatment outcome. Meanwhile, clinicians should continue to use careful multimethod assessment of their clients with ASD by self-report, other report, and observation to obtain the most comprehensive picture of abilities and change, and incorporate evidence-based ASD measures as they become available.

Parent Considerations During Assessment and Treatment

It is important to consider that parents of children who are referred for ASD asessment are likely to be under considerable strain in relation to their children's behaviors and diagnostic ambiguity, and are suffering from a lack of support from family members, their children's school, and elsewhere. In addition to the direct impact of ASD on children, the strain of caregiving for a child with ASD can affect the parents, child, and siblings. Caregivers of children with ASD experience greater levels of parenting stress (Estes et al., 2013); moreover, increased levels of stress in parents of children with ASD are highly correlated to child problem behavior (Davis & Carter, 2008). The relationship between parenting stress and child behavior is thought to be bidirectional, such that child problem behavior decreases parenting efficacy and increases parental depression/anxiety, which in turn can exacerbate the problem behavior (Rezendes & Scarpa, 2011). As a result, this stress can affect family relationships, psychological well-being, and the child's treatment success. In summary, clinicians do well to recognize that parents may be depleted when they present for assessment; joining with parents, validating their experiences, and being empathetic are likely to go a long way in helping parents feel understood and supported.

Treatment

Overview and Description of Key Treatment Components

CBT is an approach that merges behavior therapy with cognitive therapy, using short-term, problem-focused cognitive and behavioral strategies based on empirical data and theory from the fields of learning and cognition. The cognitive components of CBT primarily focus on helping clients identify and change maladaptive attitudes and beliefs, which subsequently change cognitive processing, emotional experiences, and problem behaviors, but CBT may also include techniques to change behavior by modifying associated responses and/or antecedents and consequences in the situation (Craske, 2010). The therapeutic process involves teaching and guiding the client toward more adaptive ways of thinking and behaving, making use of both cognitive and behavioral strategies to varying degrees, generally including the following components: (1) psychoeducation, (2) somatic management, (3) cognitive restructuring, (4) problem solving, (5) exposure, and (6) relapse prevention (Velting, Setzer, & Albano, 2004).

Although this approach was historically developed for the treatment of adults, there is a general consensus that CBT approaches have empirical support for treating psychological disorders of childhood (e.g., Weisz & Kazdin, 2010). CBT approaches for children, however, must consider developmental issues related to the fact that children are dependent on larger systems within which they are embedded, and that they also display a wide range of cognitive maturation or abilities (Ollendick, Grills, & King, 2001; Scarpa & Lorenzi, 2013). To be sensitive to these issues, the CBT approach may be modified to include parents or other key caregivers in the treatment process. To address cognitive challenges, therapists are well advised to incorporate concrete and tangible examples, to use methods that match the child's cognitive abilities, and to incorporate lessons into developmentally appropriate play routines.

Given that children are inherently dependent on caregivers, they rarely refer themselves to treatment. Therefore, it is important for therapists to assess the child's motivation and modify CBT to include enjoyable activities appropriate for the child's age or developmental level. Parents are often critical to treatment success by helping children complete homework assignments and generalize skills to outside settings, and monitoring whether their own behaviors are directly or indirectly impacting the child. Children may also enter treatment with varying levels of cognitive abilities or maturation, so treatment needs to be tailored to their developmental level. For example, games, songs, and favorite characters might be included, pictures may be used to illustrate concepts, interactive and experiential learning activities can keep children interested and show them concepts in a more concrete way, puppet shows can relay key lessons, and specific words may be modified to the child's level of comprehension. Studies have shown the success of using developmentally modified CBT for use with children as young as 3 years old (Scarpa & Lorenzi, 2013).

The National Standards Project (National Autism Center, 2015) broke intervention opportunities into 10 developmental skills that should be *increased* in children with ASD: academics, communication, problem solving, social, learning readiness, motor skills, personal responsibility, placement (i.e., working toward placement in a less restrictive environment), play, and self-regulation. Additionally, four types of behaviors that are often targeted to be *decreased* include "general symptoms" of ASD, disruptive behaviors, repetitive behaviors or thoughts, and sensory or emotional dysregulation (e.g., anxiety/depression, sleep difficulties).

Moderators to Consider

Other cognitive factors and abilities may need to be considered when applying CBT to a child with ASD. Current estimates indicate that almost 50% of school-age children with ASD have IQ within the normal range (Baio, 2014). Nonetheless, because the cognitive profile on an IQ test may be very uneven, an evaluation of children's cognitive and processing strengths and weaknesses can be helpful in adapting CBT to their abilities. For example, a child with advanced reading comprehension may benefit from reading text about CBT concepts. A child with advanced visual reasoning skills, on the other hand, may benefit from having concepts represented by computer programs, imagery, and demonstration. Those with slower information processing may need additional time to cognitively process and respond to information, and it is helpful to add reminders and written instructions to minimize the need to rely on memory.

Children with ASD may also have comorbid ADHD, which can cause significant functional impairment of sustained attention and increase hyperactivity/impulsivity. In these cases, targeted behavioral interventions with frequent schedules of reinforcement (e.g., token economies) can be incorporated into the sessions to aid with following rules and completing activities (Carlson & Tamm, 2000). Consistent with educational modifications that have been found to be helpful for children with ADHD (DuPaul & Stoner, 2003), children with ASD are more responsive to programs that are highly structured, with short, discrete activities and assignments broken down into smaller units, in keeping with the children's attention span. Other helpful educational modifications that can be adapted for use in CBT include highlighting relevant information, using graphics or visual aids, clearly posting rules, repeating instructions, providing a visual schedule. The clinician should regularly monitor and give feedback to maintain attention, and the amount of environmental distractions should be reduced. Stimulant and atypical antipsychotic medication may also help manage symptoms in some children with comorbid ASD and ADHD (Hazell, 2007; Reiersen & Todd, 2008), though results of many medication studies are still equivocal.

CBT Modifications for Treatment of ASD

Modifications can make CBT more suitable and accessible for children with ASD and must take into account needs that are both similar to those of other children and unique to ASD (Attwood & Scarpa, 2013; Moree & Davis, 2010; Rotheram-Fuller & MacMullen, 2011). As noted earlier, all children (especially at younger ages) generally may benefit from the inclusion of parents/caregivers, concrete examples, developmentally appropriate play routines, and techniques that are matched to their cognitive abilities. For all children, issues involving sexuality may increase as they approach their teenage and young adult years, and the increased cognitive and social demands in middle school and high school may trigger difficulties leading them to seek or to be referred for treatment at this time.

Children with ASD, however, may have unique characteristics that require further modification or consideration when attempting CBT. In particular, the CBT therapist needs to assess and consider the following ASD-specific factors: language/communication abilities, interpersonal/social abilities, cognitive and behavioral inflexibility, and sensory sensitivities. In addition, children with ASD may be affected by other cognitive factors that can impact CBT, as noted earlier. As such, it is important to assess these cognitive, social, and emotional skills prior to implementing CBT. In addition, children with ASD are known to have difficulties with generalization to new contexts and often respond well to immediate reinforcement, both of which also have implications for techniques to incorporate within a CBT approach. See Table 16.1 for a list of ASD-related characteristics or issues and possible corresponding CBT modifications.

TABLE 16.1. ASD-Related Factors and Corresponding CBT Modifications

ASD-related factors	CBT modifications
Language/ communication abilities (including pragmatics)	• Use visual aids, pictures, written worksheets • Simplify words • Break lessons into smaller chunks • Use concrete examples • Hands-on activities, role plays, in vivo rehearsal • Provide reminders of topic or questions • Double-check comprehension • Signal when to initiate or stop talking • Teach conversational skills • Provide scripts or vocabulary for unknown words (e.g., for emotions; asking for help) • Explore nonverbal options for expression (e.g., through music, rating scales, drawing)
Interpersonal/ social abilities	• Teach "mind-reading" • Attend to actions that reflect therapeutic alliance • Provide many opportunities for practice both in and out of session • Use role plays, in vivo or video modeling, and rehearsals • Use group activities and cooperative games • Use special interests to encourage rapport
Cognitive/ behavioral inflexibility	• Use questions and multiple-choice options to encourage thinking of new strategies • Treat all comments with positivity and model how to handle mistakes (e.g., through self-talk) • Incorporate written or visual schedules • Include breaks between activities • Teach anxiety reduction techniques to cope with changes • Use special interests as motivators and self-regulatory strategies
Sensory issues	• Change therapy environment according to what can be tolerated by client (e.g., dim lighting, no perfumes) • Ask client before engaging in any physical contact, such as handshakes • Play calming music or white noise if client is overstimulated by sounds • Teach client how to recognize and communicate harmful sensations such as pain or discomfort • Find appropriate ways to satisfy sensory needs as self-regulation (e.g., chewing gum)
Other cognitive factors and comorbid ADHD	• Present CBT concepts according to cognitive strengths (e.g., visually or in text) • Provide frequent reminders • Repeat material to aid processing • Use token economies or reinforcement system • Use short, discrete activities • Break assignments into smaller units • Clearly post rules • Provide frequent feedback • Minimize distractions
Generalization	• Include parents/caregivers • Provide homework or practice assignments • Use video modeling or coaching of behaviors in nonclinical settings • Incorporate group work for social skills

LANGUAGE/COMMUNICATION ABILITIES

Because CBT makes frequent use of Socratic questioning and psychoeducation, it is important to consider the child's ability to understand and use language. To our knowledge, no controlled studies have examined CBT in nonverbal or intellectually disabled children with ASD; therefore, the effectiveness of CBT in this population remains unknown. It seems plausible, however, that CBT can be used with nonverbal people with ASD if they have the cognitive capability and a functional communication system that the therapist can use. Nonetheless, many children with ASD do not experience a language delay or deficits in verbal speech, but they vary widely on this dimension. For children with poorer verbal skills, it can be helpful to present materials visually (e.g., a picture of a person smiling to represent happiness), to break material down into smaller chunks that they can understand, to use words that are less complex, and to provide concrete examples of abstract concepts (e.g., a toolbox to fix feelings).

Research on theory of mind (Baron-Cohen, 2001) and alexithymia (Hill, 2004; Tani et al., 2004) suggests that some children with ASD have difficulty understanding the emotions and intentions of others and/or cannot label their own emotional states. They may have difficulty putting their own emotional experiences and thoughts into words. However, they may use other brain mechanisms that permit more deliberate analytical processing to compensate for the lack of automatic emotion recognition. In these cases, it is helpful in CBT to teach analytical strategies for processing social and emotional situations, to provide a vocabulary of emotion words in affective education, to use scripts (as in social stories or comic strips) to teach appropriate expression, and to provide other means of expressing internal emotional states. For example, the CBT therapist can suggest that the child rate his or her experience on a number scale, express him- or herself in music or drawing, or send an e-mail that allows more analytical processing.

Children with ASD often have difficulties with the pragmatics or use of language in social contexts (Twachtman-Cullen, 2000). In ASD, some problems with pragmatics may be seen in inappropriate initiations and stereotyped speech (e.g., talking repetitively about things that may not interest others; turning the conversation to a favorite theme), poor use of context (e.g., being overliteral; not understanding metaphor), and difficulty with social reciprocity (e.g., ignoring conversation initiated by others). Regarding use of context, youth with ASD may not perceive how intonation and emphasis affect meaning, and they may struggle with literal interpretations of idioms, metaphor, and sarcasm. Therefore, it is important that the CBT therapist provide very concrete examples of constructs (i.e., visual supports, simplified metaphors, hands-on learning, role plays) and double-check that the child with ASD has understood the information correctly.

Due to problems with initiations, providing too much information, or lack of coherence, the CBT therapist may find that the child with ASD seems to get off-topic or go on tangents. In these cases, it is helpful to remind the client with ASD about the initial topic or question and provide cues either to cut off tangents or help the client expand on his or her specific points. Finally, difficulty with social reciprocity can impair the "art" of conversation. The child or adolescent with ASD may not engage in social chitchat or the give-and-take of conversation, making it harder for the CBT therapist to sustain the interaction. Shorter sessions or training on conversational skills may be helpful.

INTERPERSONAL/SOCIAL ABILITIES

Social difficulties represent a primary form of impairment in ASD, as reflected in the diagnostic criteria (American Psychiatric Association, 2013). Specifically, children with ASD may have difficulty with social reciprocity (as we noted earlier when discussing pragmatics), reading and using nonverbal cues (e.g., gestures, facial expressions, intonation) to understand the feelings and intentions of others or the meaning of a situation, establishing appropriate peer relationships, and adjusting their behavior to match social contexts (e.g., acting differently at home than at school). Social competence may therefore refer both to the ability to understand social situations (i.e., social cognition) and to behave appropriately (i.e., social interactions) (Bauminger-Zviely, 2013).

To assist clients with deficits in social cognition, it is helpful to teach them "mind-reading" skills; that is, the client is taught how to use nonverbal cues to read the emotions or intentions of others, and also how to use gestures and facial expressions to express his or her own emotions. It is important to note that a limited range of affective display can lead others to the impression that children with ASD do not experience emotions; however, research indicates that they do experience emotions but may not know how to express themselves, or may have limited facial expressions (Ben Shalom et al., 2006). While the therapist can model, role-play, and behaviorally rehearse these competencies with the child, several computer-assisted programs are also available to help children learn to read facial expressions in others (e.g., Beaumont & Sofronoff, 2013; Tanaka, 2010).

Regarding the development of relationships and appropriate social skills, some individuals with ASD may appear aloof or disinterested due to lack of range of facial expressivity, flat affect, and poor intonation or communication. Thus, it is important for CBT therapists to attend to other cues of their therapeutic alliance (e.g., words, behaviors) and to teach the client words and nonverbal cues that convey interest in others. Moreover, multiple interventions now exist to promote appropriate social skills in the ASD population (Scarpa, White, et al., 2013).

COGNITIVE/BEHAVIORAL INFLEXIBILITY

Part of the diagnostic picture of ASD includes repetitive/stereotyped behaviors and fixated interests, which can be thought of as behavioral or cognitive rigidity. Such inflexibility can lead to a great deal of functional impairment, as emotional outbursts often result when the child is interrupted or prevented from engaging in the interests/behaviors, or the time spent in these activities may preclude participation in more appropriate undertakings. Inflexibility may be a result of problems with shifting attention, an executive cognitive function (Hill, 2008; Ozonoff et al., 2004), leading to perseveration or a "one-track mind" that can interfere with learning from mistakes or conceptualizing new alternative responses (Attwood & Scarpa, 2013). To encourage flexible thinking and behaviors in the context of CBT, the therapist can ask the child to think of additional strategies (e.g., "What else can you try?") and use multiple-choice options to offer possible solutions rather than expecting the child to generate them spontaneously. To address fear of making mistakes, it is helpful for the clinician to accept every comment positively and without criticism, then model how to handle mistakes calmly. For example, the clinician can model self-talk (e.g., "If I stay calm, I can solve the problem more quickly").

Behavioral inflexibility can also make transitions more difficult for the child with ASD or present as a need for sameness, which was first described by Kanner (1943). Because of this desire to maintain sameness, the child may need help with transitions and preparation for unexpected change. It can be helpful to include breaks between activities if time is needed to transition from one task to the next. A written or visual schedule of activities for the session may also help the child understand the expected session routine (Dalrymple, 1995). By the same token, improving flexibility may be one of the targets of treatment, and the therapist may wish to build-in opportunities to practice veering from rituals and routines through mild exposures and anxiety reduction techniques (e.g., progressive muscle relaxation, deep breathing).

Last, as another example of cognitive inflexibility (also discussed earlier in the section on pragmatics), children with ASD may perseverate on topics of interest to them. In these cases, the therapist may need to signal when to stop a conversation and move on to a new topic. However, it may also be helpful to use special interests as a motivating tool or a proactive method of improving mood. Therefore, it is important to teach children with ASD the difference between passively responding to cognitions and actively using their interests as a coping tool (i.e., as a method of self-regulation).

SENSORY ISSUES

There is a need to consider the sensory profile of the person with ASD, especially in terms of auditory, olfactory, and tactile sensory sensitivity (Attwood & Scarpa, 2013). Both over- and underresponsivity, along with low sensory seeking, has been associated with higher levels of negative emotionality in children with ASD (Ben-Sasson et al., 2008), possibly due to having overwhelming sensations and not being able to identify them due to alexithymia (Liss, Mailloux, & Erchull, 2008). Therefore, it is helpful to assess for sensory issues and arrange the therapy environment to promote the client's tolerability and comfort. For example, the lighting may need to be dimmed or changed to nonfluorescent. Smells, such as perfumes or deodorants, may need to be minimized. If snacks are provided, texture and taste need to be considered. Therapists may need to ask the client first, before engaging in any physical gestures, such as patting him or her on the back for praise, handshakes, tapping his or her arm to gain attention, or hugs for comfort. Calming music or sounds may be played for clients who are very oversensitive to auditory stimulation. Other clients may be underresponsive to some sensations (e.g., pain) that are important to notice, and the clinician may need to help clients identify and express those experiences (e.g., help-seeking behaviors). The clinician may also help clients identify appropriate ways to satisfy their sensory needs that will not be disruptive or stigmatizing, yet may have a powerful effect in regulating their stress or anxiety. For example, the client may chew gum or manipulate a small object in his or her pocket to receive sensory input.

GENERALIZATION

One often-noted limitation of ASD treatments is the lack of generalization to other people and settings (Schreibman, 2000). Therefore, it is important to incorporate ways to promote generalization within any CBT program. As noted earlier, including parents is an important developmental modification for CBT with children in general, and this seems especially pronounced for children with ASD (Reaven & Blakeley-Smith, 2013; Sofronoff, Attwood, & Hinton, 2005). Including parents in CBT seems especially helpful in facilitating at-home practice and greater involvement for youth with ASD (Puleo & Kendall, 2011).

By the same token, homework and practice assignments are important CBT components that promote real-life application outside of the session. A project that may be completed between each CBT session needs to be discussed at the start of the next session. It is important that parents and teachers outside of the CBT program are aware of the assignments so they can help with implementation at home and/or school. Because many children with ASD have had negative experiences with homework, the CBT therapist may need to spend extra time to explain the importance of completing the assignments and incorporate appropriate reinforcements.

Last, other strategies can be used to facilitate out-of-session generalization, such as video modeling of behaviors in other settings. The clinician or a caregiver may also accompany children to other settings (e.g., a bowling alley or pizzeria) to coach and practice skills *in vivo*. For social skills, incorporating group work into the CBT sessions is especially useful to practice new behaviors.

Application of CBT Used for Emotion Regulation Treatment in ASD

The last decade has seen the emergence of multiple studies on the efficacy of modified CBT for treating children with ASD, especially for anxiety and social competence (see Danial & Wood, 2013; Lang, Regester, Lauderdale, Ashbaugh, & Haring, 2010; Scarpa, White, et al., 2013; Sukhodolsky, Bloch, Panza, & Reichow, 2013). Most of these studies provide promising evidence for the benefits of CBT, with small effects that are at least comparable, if not better, than psychopharmacological management of emotional and behavioral symptoms (Selles & Storch, 2013). In particular, because of its heightened comorbidity and interaction with social deficits in ASD, anxiety has been most extensively studied.

Several gaps remain in this treatment literature. First, although there has been a predominance of CBT studies of anxiety, few studies have examined the use of CBT for treating anger problems or challenging behaviors, despite the fact that aggression and irritability are often prime symptoms for clinical referral (Myles & Southwick, 2005). Behavioral interventions and medication are often first lines of treatment for these problems in children with ASD (Dawson & Burner, 2011; McCracken et al., 2002), but we maintain that modified CBT would provide useful contributions by addressing cognitive mediators of anger/irritability, adding affective education, capitalizing on analytic capabilities, and improving self-efficacy and self-regulation. Second, there is a lack of research on CBT efficacy for treatment of young children with ASD (the youngest age noted in recent reviews is 7 years). However, it is clear from the larger literature on CBT that this approach can be developmentally adapted for children as young as age 3 years. Since early intervention is widely recommended for the best prognosis in ASD, it is worthwhile to apply and test developmental modifications for CBT efficacy in young children with ASD.

Mazefsky and colleagues (2013) propose that emotion dysregulation is inherent in ASD and provides a transdiagnostic explanation for many of clhildren's emotional and social difficulties and comorbid disorders. As such, treatment of emotion regulation problems in young children with ASD may have widespread benefits in both preventing later mood, anxiety, and externalizing behavior problems and promoting positive social development.

Based on the Exploring Feelings CBT program for anxiety and anger in 9- to 12-year-old children with ASD, STAMP, a manualized caregiver-assisted group CBT for the treatment of emotion dysregulation, has been developmentally adapted for 5- to 7-year-old children and modified to be suitable for ASD (Scarpa, Wells, et al., 2013). The focus of STAMP is on affective education and skills building for emotion regulation, including physical (i.e., energy-releasing), relaxation (i.e., soothing), social (i.e., seeking help from others), thinking (i.e., cognitive restructuring), and special interest (i.e., enjoyable) tools—thereby incorporating both cognitive and behavioral interventions throughout the 9-week program (Scarpa, Reyes, & Attwood, 2013). See Table 16.2 for topics covered in each of the nine 1-hour sessions.

Developmental modifications include the use of stories, games, and singing geared toward preschool or kindergarten maturity levels (e.g., Duck, Duck, Goose; Musical Chairs), which are used to provide instruction and rehearsal of CBT concepts, as well as to facilitate cognitive restructuring. During the child group session, parents/caregivers meet with a separate therapist in another room to discuss the material being taught to the children and to observe the child session through a monitor. Parents/caregivers are included as a critical component to promote generalization of skills to settings outside of the clinic and to facilitate home practice assignments. STAMP also is modified for children with ASD to include a routine schedule (i.e., *Welcome Time, Singing, Story Time, Activity/Lesson Time, Snack,* and *Goodbyes*), visual supports, both nonverbal and verbal ways to express feelings and thoughts, and concrete examples of abstract concepts (e.g., a physical toolbox to illustrate coping skills). Stickers are used as part of a token economy to reinforce following rules. A group format is used to promote the use of skills in a social setting. Breaks and a snack are also built into the routine. In a small randomized controlled trial, STAMP was found to benefit young children with ASD by decreasing parent-reported negativity/lability, increasing parent-reported emotion regulation, increasing child knowledge of emotion regulation strategies, and shortening duration of observed child outbursts (Scarpa & Reyes, 2011).

TABLE 16.2. Topics covered in STAMP

- Session 1. Affective Education: Understanding Positive Emotions (Happiness)
- Session 2. Affective Education: Understanding Positive Emotions (Relaxation) and Negative Emotions (Anger, Anxiety); Introduction of the Emotional Toolbox
- Session 3. Emotional Toolbox 1: Physical and Relaxation Tools
- Session 4. Emotional Toolbox 2: Social Tools
- Session 5. Emotional Toolbox 3: Thinking Tools
- Session 6. Emotional Toolbox 4: Special Interest Tools
- Session 7. Emotional Toolbox 5: Identifying Appropriate and Inappropriate Tools
- Session 8. Review Session: Create a Production (similar to a commercial) to Highlight Tools to Remember
- Session 9. Wrap-Up: Farewell and Party

It is important to note that STAMP was developed and tested for use with young children with ASD using a group format. However, the components of STAMP (i.e., affective education, cognitive restructuring, and the emotional toolbox) have been tested and used successfully with older children and young adults (e.g., Attwood & Garnett, 2016; Sofronoff et al., 2005, 2007). STAMP can also be adapted to work with individual clients and families when a group format is not available or feasible. In these cases, it may be helpful to bring in other family members, siblings, family friends, or colleagues into the session for games and activities, if possible.

In STAMP, cognitive interventions are included through the use of stories, comic strips with thinking bubbles, and thinking tools introduced in the emotional toolbox. For example, in Session 5 on thinking tools, the children are read a story about a dog that is unable to fall asleep until he thinks about all the things he likes to do during the day. Through this story, the children are taught the concept of thoughts (i.e., words or pictures in your head), and how sometimes they can use thoughts to feel better, just like the dog in the story. Parents are also taught how to use comic strip stories with thought bubbles as a nonverbal method to illustrate a conflict the child may have experienced, and the parent is asked to practice with the child during the week, so that the child can see how his or her thoughts may have affected his or her feelings. During the session, children play games and draw pictures that illustrate thoughts that can make them "feel better" or "feel worse." In these very concrete and child-friendly ways, the children are taught how to modify thoughts to feel better.

Behavioral interventions in STAMP include the use of contingencies, especially in the forms of points, stickers, and praise. From the very beginning in Session 1, we explain to the children that they can earn points for "following the rules and using their tools." The rules include listening to the speaker, keeping their hands to themselves, and using calm voices. Children earn points that are tracked throughout the session, then turn in those points for stickers at the end of the session. After the children together earn a predetermined number of stickers, the entire group is rewarded with a party. In this way, the program uses both individual and group contingencies to encourage appropriate behavior and use of the skills learned in the toolbox.

Specific skills in the emotional toolbox are taught through modeling and rehearsal. Therapists model the skills, present the skills in a story and lesson, and the children then can rehearse the skills through games. For example, in Session 8 on social tools, a story is presented about a dog that is lonely and searches for a friend to feel better. The children are taught that sometimes they can seek out other people or even animals to feel better. The therapists provide and model several scripts (e.g., "I feel angry. Can you help me?"), which the children then practice through a puppet show. To facilitate recall of the tools, the children are taught a song (to the tune of "If You're Happy and You Know It"), with each verse devoted to a specific tool. The song is repeated each week, with the addition of a new tool that corresponds to that week's lesson. In Session 8, for example, they sing, "If I'm angry and I know it—ask for help." The song provides another method, besides behavioral rehearsal and visual aids, to promote memory in the children, and it is also something they can easily practice with their parents at home.

It is always important to consider how physiology contributes to emotions and emotion regulation. Heart rate, respiration, and muscle tension, for example, tend to increase with intense anxiety or anger. Therefore, in Session 2 on physical and relaxation tools, we teach children to recognize these physical changes in their own bodies. Using a portable heart rate monitor that is placed on the child, the children can observe how heart rate increases when they become tense and decreases when they use paced breathing or some other form of relaxation. In this way, the children learn in a very concrete manner how to use physical and relaxation tools to help with physiological hyperreactivity.

In addition, STAMP considers other environmental and systemic contributions by including parents/caregivers in the treatment and incorporating home practice assignments after each session. As noted earlier, any CBT for children must consider the role of parents as part of the larger system within which children are embedded. This is especially important for children with ASD, who need extra assistance with involvement and practice outside of session. We have found that parent participation improves the parents' own sense of confidence in helping their child, thus empowering them by giving them skills and tools as well. The parents are then better equipped to serve as coaches who can help their children practice the skills at home and elsewhere, and complete homework assignments.

Case Example

Assessment of History and Emotion Regulation Problems

Lucas* was a European American male enrolled in the STAMP program. He was 4 years, 11 months old at intake and turned 5 during the 9-week program. He presented with a Full Scale IQ of 92, as measured by the KBIT-2 (Kaufman & Kaufman, 2004), suggesting appropriate cognitive and language ability for this program. Lucas was accompanied to sessions by both of his biological parents, Sally (age 35 years) and Jim (age 36 years), both of whom had graduate-level educations.

Lucas did not have a notable developmental history. He spoke his first word around age 12 months but did not speak much until 18 months. At the time he entered STAMP, Lucas attended a private preschool 5 days a week. He did not receive any special school services at the time, and had only recently been diagnosed with ASD. While he reportedly loved going to school, he received warnings or negative behavior ratings approximately half the time. Lucas had also been attending behavioral therapy sessions at another clinic for 3–4 months.

Sally, a stay-at-home mother, reported that Lucas hit and pushed other children when he was angry, and that he was very shy and anxious when meeting new adults. Lucas was reportedly difficult to discipline, and his mother found it hard to anticipate what would trigger his tantrums. Lucas had "little tolerance for delayed gratification" and became very upset if his requests were not honored immediately. While the family found time-outs to be effective in the short term, they had not been helpful in shaping behavior as a long-term solution. Sally found that Lucas had difficulty learning from natural consequences. As an example, Sally stated that Lucas never received what he wanted after screaming or hitting, but he continued to use these behaviors to try to access the activity or object he desired. While Lucas was generally described as happy, his parents also characterized him as "easily upset/frustrated." He was also sometimes aggressive, including hitting, kicking, head butting, and pushing.

At intake, we administered several measures to assess Lucas's current levels of anxiety and/or anger. As noted earlier, few measures have been normed for young children

---

*Clients' real names have been changed for the purpose of this case example.

or for children with ASD. Therefore, we adapted some measures from other studies that have used them with ASD samples. These measures are described here.

WHAT MAKES MY CHILD ANGRY/ANXIOUS?

When Sally and Jim were questioned about Lucas's anxiety using the What Makes my Child Angry/Anxious Questionnaire (adapted from Attwood, 2004a, 2004b), they reported that Lucas became moderately to very anxious in the following situations, in ascending order: being teased at school; playing on the playground, thinking about what other children thought of him; ghosts; making a mistake on his schoolwork; crying; looking funny in front of other people; being alone; vomiting; and not being able to breathe. In an open-ended question on the same measure, Sally and Jim reported that Lucas also worried about meeting new people, especially adults, and grooming habits, such as having his toenails trimmed, taking medicine, and brushing his teeth.

Regarding anger, Lucas's parents reported that he became angry in a variety of situations. A number of these scenarios were reported to make him "very angry," including when people interfered with his games, when people stopped him from doing what he wanted to do, when someone pushed him, when things got broken, when someone took his things, when he had to do something he did not want to do, when people did not listen to him, and when people did not understand him. Other situations that were rated as high in intensity included getting his work wrong, when someone shouted at him, and when he was interrupted. In each of these situations, Lucas was reported to become angry often to very often (3's and 4's on a Likert scale ranging from 1 to 4, with 1 meaning "hardly ever" and 4 meaning "very often").

SPENCE PRESCHOOL ANXIETY SCALE

The Spence Preschool Anxiety Scale (SPAS; Spence, Rapee, McDonald, & Ingram, 2001) asks parents to rate anxiety on 28 items on a scale of 0 ("not true at all") to 4 ("very often true"). Prior to treatment, Lucas had high levels of social anxiety (total = 17 out of 24) and physical injury fears (total = 13 out of 28). His parents reported lower scores for him on the Generalized Anxiety (total = 7 out of 20), Obsessive–Compulsive Disorder (total = 1 out of 20), and Separation Anxiety (total = 7 out of 20) scales. Overall, Lucas received a Total Score of 45 on the SPAS.

ABC—COMMUNITY VERSION

The ABC (Aman & Singh, 1986) is a 58-item checklist of problem behaviors often associated with ASD, including irritability, hyperactivity, lethargy, stereotypy, and inappropriate speech, rated by parents on a scale of 0 ("not at all a problem") to 3 ("the problem is severe in degree"). At intake, Lucas's parents endorsed high scores on the Irritability (total = 29 out of 45) and Hyperactivity (total = 21 out of 48) subscales. He earned low scores on the Lethargy (total = 3 out of 48), Stereotypy (total = 0 out of 21), and Inappropriate Speech (total = 2 out of 12) scales. Overall, Lucas scored a total of 55 points on the ABC.

BEHAVIORAL MONITORING

Lucas's parents were also asked to monitor the intensity and frequency of their child's emotional outbursts that were a result of anger or anxiety over 7 consecutive days. Prior to STAMP, Lucas had 53 tantrums in 7 days, with an average intensity of 7.22 (rated on a Likert scale of 1 to 10, with 1 meaning "not intense" and 10 meaning "extremely intense"). Each tantrum was an average of 3 minutes in duration.

PROFILE OF ANGER/ANXIETY COPING SKILLS

Due to STAMP's heavy emphasis on teaching coping skills, Lucas's parents were asked to complete the Profile of Anger/Anxiety Coping Skills—Parent Interview (adapted from Willner, Brace, & Phillips, 2005), which asks them to recall and rate the use of coping skills for situations that typically made Lucas angry and anxious. Sally and Jim identified three situations in which Lucas had difficulty managing his anger (e.g., when Lucas did not get to do something he wanted to do immediately, when he was told "no," or during transitions such as going to school or bedtime). Lucas was reported to use a total of eight coping skills across these situations (e.g., walking away, doing something else, asking for help, or using humor), but no particular skill was used more than "occasionally." Regarding anxiety, Sally and Jim reported that Lucas became anxious about grooming habits, when meeting new people, and when performing in front of other people (e.g., answering questions in class). Lucas was reported to use a total of 11 coping skills to manage his anxiety in these situations, such as doing something else, asking someone for help, rethinking the situation, being assertive, and using humor. Each coping skill was reported to be used "occasionally."

In summary, Lucas was described as a generally happy boy who had a tendency to overreact to situations that involved transitions, delay of gratification, and being around or being evaluated by unfamiliar people. His parents reported that he experienced high levels of social anxiety and physical injury anxiety, as well as hyperactivity and irritability. He had multiple emotional outbursts of moderate to high intensity and short duration (about 3 minutes each) daily. Although he had the ability to use a variety of coping strategies, he used them infrequently.

Treatment and Outcome Monitoring

Lucas was the youngest participant ever to complete STAMP, as he turned 5 years old within a few weeks after the start of treatment. Therefore, clinicians paid close attention to the developmental appropriateness of the STAMP curriculum for a younger child. Lucas responded well to modified treatment, especially the use of visual aids (e.g., Schedule Poster, Sticker Board, weekly activities) and concrete examples during the teaching of coping skills (e.g., making his toolbox from a shoebox). Lucas put his favorite cat toy into his Emotional Toolbox, which he brought to the second session with him. This toy became one of his preferred coping tools, representing both a special interest tool (i.e., his interest in animals) and a social tool (i.e., his ability to use his pet cat for comfort at home). His excitement to share this toy with the therapists and other group members also allowed him an age-appropriate way to socialize and begin to "come out of his shell."

At times, Lucas was distracted by the outbursts and impulsivity of an older child, who was having difficulty engaging with the material. However, the introduction of a structured behavioral management component and scheduled breaks within the group sessions (i.e., token economy for following rules) helped to decrease these disruptions, which allowed Lucas to better focus on the curriculum. Lucas also seemed to have an auditory sensitivity to singing and did not like to participate in this activity during the group session. As such, the therapists modified this aspect for Lucas, so that he could recite his portions or simply sit back and listen to the others at a distance that was comfortable for him.

In qualitative feedback, Sally and Jim reported that they found learning the tools to be the most helpful part of the program, and that their favorite aspect was being able to observe their child live during parent sessions. Lucas did not like to sing the "If I'm angry" song, so his parents turned it into a poem to read to him. Similarly, they were able to modify homework assignments to Lucas's interests and ability level. For example, during the affective education component, children were asked to cut out faces from magazines and label the emotions. Since Lucas enjoyed working with numbers, his mother had him rate the faces on a number scale from "a little happy" to "very very happy" (i.e., ecstatic), and taught him the feeling words as part of the activity. In these ways, it was crucial to the success of the therapy to include Lucas's parents because they facilitated his participation in the program and his ability to engage in and understand assignments.

Because no measures currently exist to assess change in emotion regulation in young children with ASD, we used a multimethod approach to monitor outcome. The following outcomes were noted for Lucas.

PROFILE OF ANGER/ANXIETY COPING SKILLS

After treatment, Sally and Jim indicated that Lucas became angry when he was told "no," when his activity was interrupted, or when he was told to wait. He was reported to use 16 coping skills, including relaxing, counting to 10, being assertive, and rethinking the situation, in addition to the skills he used prior to treatment. While he still did not use any specific skill more than "occasionally," he did double the number of skills that he used overall. This may show that introducing the Emotional Toolbox to Lucas enhanced the diversity of coping tools he was able to employ.

Regarding anxiety, after treatment, Lucas was reported to be anxious about taking medicine, being presented with a new situation, and being asked to perform in front of others. He used a total of 12 coping skills, one more than he had used prior to treatment. He also used one new coping skill (walking away) after treatment, which he had not previously used to cope with his anxiety.

SPENCE PRESCHOOL ANXIETY SCALE

After completing STAMP, Lucas's overall score on the SPAS decreased by 12 points, from 45 to 33. Lucas had lower scores on all scales except the Generalized Anxiety scale, which increased from 7 to 8. Previously, Lucas's highest scores had been on the Social Anxiety scale, which decreased from 17 to 15, and on the Physical Injury Fears scale, which decreased from 13 to 8. Additionally, Lucas's score on the Separation Anxiety scale decreased from 7 to 2, and his Obsessive–Compulsive Disorder score decreased from 1 to 0. His experience in a group setting with non-school peers may have helped him practice separating from his parents in a new setting. Moreover, he appeared to learn skills to reduce physiological arousal and to cope with social fears in a group.

ABERRANT BEHAVIOR CHECKLIST

Posttreatment, Lucas's overall score on the ABC decreased from 55 to 40. Decreases were seen on every scale (except for Stereotypy, for which Lucas earned 0 at both time points). Lucas's highest scores were on the Irritability and Hyperactivity subscales. His Irritability score decreased from 29 to 23, and his Hyperactivity score decreased from 21 to 15. It is likely that Lucas's ability to monitor and manage his affective states improved through the STAMP curriculum, as seen through his parents' perception of decreased irritability. While hyperactivity is not specifically targeted through STAMP, Lucas entered the program as a child without siblings and with little exposure to a formal classroom setting. The structured STAMP setting included behavior management by two trained clinicians and an intensive clinician:child ratio of 3:2. These unique properties may have shaped the impulsivity and high energy levels that his parents had previously seen in the home. Finally, Lucas's Lethargy score decreased slightly from 3 to 2, and his Inappropriate Speech score decreased from 2 to 0.

BEHAVIORAL MONITORING

After STAMP, Lucas's observed outbursts decreased from 53 to 25 over a 7-day period, a reduction of more than half as compared to his pretreatment frequency. The intensity of Lucas's outbursts stayed the same (7.22 on a scale of 1 to 10), and the average length increased from 3 minutes to 5.32 minutes. However, the total duration of Lucas's tantrums decreased from 159.5 minutes to 133 minutes posttreatment. This may indicate more variability in the length of Lucas's outbursts. It is possible that Lucas was using more skills from his Emotional Toolbox to deal with minor upsets but still needed practice with higher-level anxiety situations in which his tantrums lasted longer.

In summary, 5-year-old Lucas was able to successfully complete this modified group CBT. Especially helpful modifications included parent participation, home practice assignments, visual aids, concrete examples, and the use of a group setting. Capitalizing on his special interests also made the treatment more enjoyable and accessible for this young boy with ASD. His repertoire of coping skills increased after treatment, along with reductions in anxiety, irritability, and frequency of emotional outbursts. The structure of treatment also seemed to help with reduction of hyperactive/impulsive behaviors.

SUMMARY AND RECOMMENDATIONS

Although CBT has been an established form of treatment for adults for some time, recent studies suggest that it may be useful for children as young as age 3 years if developmental modifications are made. To promote success in children, CBT therapists should consider the incorporation of parents/caregivers, inclusion of concrete examples, matching treatment to the child's cognitive abilities, and using play or other age-appropriate interests to teach CBT concepts and skills. In addition to these developmental adaptations, CBT can be modified to meet the unique social, communication, and behavioral needs of children with ASD (e.g., use of visual aids, schedules, nonverbal methods of expression, group settings, behavioral management), and multiple studies have now noted benefits of modified CBT for treating anxiety and social skills in youth with ASD. Such modifications are often minor and may reflect overall good practice for CBT in children, regardless of diagnosis, but the logical and structured approach of CBT often makes it generally a good fit for the analytic nature of people with ASD, who may benefit from addressing cognitive biases, affective knowledge deficits, and social and behavioral skills. Further research is needed to refine CBT for this population, including the extent of parental/family involvement, adaptation for children who are nonverbal and/or have intellectual impairments, use in early intervention (i.e., preschool and young children), extension for difficulties beyond anxiety and social competence, and development of appropriate treatment outcome measures.

REFERENCES

Achenbach, T. M., Dumenci, L., & Rescorla, L. A. (2001). Ratings of relations between DSM-IV diagnostic categories and items of the CBCL/6–18, TRF, and YSR. Burlington: University of Vermont.

Achenbach, T. M., & Rescorla, L. A. (2000). *Manual for the ASEBA preschool forms & profiles: An integrated system of multi-informant assessment; Child behavior checklist for ages 1½–5; Language development survey; Caregiver–teacher report form.* Burlington: University of Vermont.

Aman, M., & Singh, N. (1986). *Aberrant Behavior Checklist: Manual.* East Aurora, NY: Slosson Educational.

American Psychiatric Association. (2013). *Diagnostic and statistical manual of mental disorders* (5th ed.). Arlington, VA: Author.

Attwood, T. (2004a). *Exploring Feelings (anger): Cognitive behavior therapy to manage anger.* Arlington, TX: Future Horizons.

Attwood, T. (2004b). *Exploring Feelings (anxiety): Cognitive behavior therapy to manage anxiety.* Arlington, TX: Future Horizons.

Attwood, T., & Garnett, M. (2016). *Exploring depression and beating the blues: A CBT guide to understanding and coping with depression in Asperger's syndrome [ASD-Level 1].* London: Jessica Kingsley.

Attwood, T., & Scarpa, A. (2013). Modifications of CBT for use with children and adolescents with high functioning ASD and their common difficulties. In A. Scarpa, S. W. White, & T. Attwood (Eds.), *CBT for children and adolescents with high-functioning autism spectrum disorders* (pp. 27–44). New York: Guilford Press.

Baio, J. (2014). Prevalence of autism spectrum disorders among children aged 8 years: Autism and Developmental Disabilities Monitoring Network, 11 Sites, United States, 2010. *Morbidity and Mortality Weekly Report Surveillance Summaries, 63*(SS02), 1–21.

Baker, J. P. (2013). Autism at 70—redrawing the boundaries. *New England Journal of Medicine, 369*(12), 1089–1091.

Baron-Cohen, S. (2001). Theory of mind and autism: A review. In L. M. Glidden (Ed.), *International Review of Research in Mental Retardation: Autism* (pp.169–184). San Diego, CA: Academic Press.

Baron-Cohen, S., Wheelwright, S., Skinner, R., Martin, J., & Clubley, E. (2001). The Autism-Spectrum Quotient (AQ): Evidence from Asperger syndrome/high-functioning autism, males and females, scientists and mathematicians. *Journal of Autism and Developmental Disorders, 31*(1), 5–17.

Bauminger-Zviely, N. (2013). Cognitive-behavioral–ecological intervention to facilitate social-emotional understanding and social interaction in youth with high-functioning ASD. In A. Scarpa, S. W. White, & T. Attwood (Eds.), *CBT for children and adolescents with high-functioning autism spectrum disorders* (pp. 226–258). New York; Guilford Press.

Beaumont, R., & Sofronoff, K. (2013). Multimodal intervention for social skills training in students with high-functioning ASD: The Secret Agent Society. In A. Scarpa, S. W. White, & T. Attwood (Eds.), *CBT for children and adolescents with high-functioning autism spectrum disorders* (pp. 173–198). New York: Guilford Press.

Begeer, S., Koot, H. M., Rieffe, C., Meerum Terwogt, M., & Stegge, H. (2008). Emotional competence in children with autism: Diagnostic criteria and empirical evidence. *Developmental Review, 28*(3), 342–369.

Ben-Sasson, A., Cermak, S. A., Orsmond, G. I., Tager-Flusberg, H., Kadlec, M. B., & Carter, A. S. (2008). Sensory clusters of toddlers with autism spectrum disorders: Differences in affective symptoms. *Journal of Child Psychology and Psychiatry, 49*(8), 817–825.

Ben Shalom, D., Mostofsky, S. H., Hazlett, R. L., Goldberg, M. C., Landa, R. J., Faran, Y., et al. (2006). Normal physiological emotions but differences in expression of conscious feelings in children with high-functioning autism. *Journal of Autism and Developmental Disorders, 36*, 395–400.

Bettelheim, B. (1967). *Empty fortress.* New York: Simon & Schuster.

Blumberg, S. J., Bramlett, M. D., Kogan, M. D., Schieve, L. A., Jones, J. R., & Lu, M. C. (2013). Changes in prevalence of parent-reported autism spectrum disorder in school-aged US children: 2007 to 2011–2012. *National Health Statistics Reports, 65*, 1–11.

Capps, L., Kasari, C., Yirmiya, N., & Sigman, M. (1993). Parental perception of emotional expressiveness in children with autism. *Journal of Consulting and Clinical Psychology, 61*(3), 475–484.

Carlson, C. L., & Tamm, L. (2000). Responsiveness of children with attention deficit–hyperactivity disorder to reward and response cost: Differential impact on performance and motivation. *Journal of Consulting and Clinical Psychology, 68*(1), 73.

Constantino, J. N., & Gruber, C. P. (2012). *Social Responsiveness Scale, second edition (SRS-2).* Los Angeles: Western Psychological Services.

Craske, M. G. (2010). *Cognitive-behavioral therapy.* Washington, DC: American Psychological Association.

Dalrymple, N. J. (1995). Environmental supports to develop flexibility and independence. In K. A. Quill (Ed.), *Teaching children with autism: Strategies to enhance communication and socialization* (pp. 243–264). New York: Delmar.

Danial, J. T., & Wood, J. J. (2013). Cognitive behavioral therapy for children with autism: Review and considerations for future research. *Journal of Developmental and Behavioral Pediatrics, 34*(9), 702–715.

Davis, N. O., & Carter, A. S. (2008). Parenting stress in mothers and fathers of toddlers with autism spectrum disorders: Associations with child characteristics. *Journal of Autism and Developmental Disorders, 38*(7), 1278–1291.

Dawson, G., & Burner, K. (2011). Behavioral interventions in children and adolescents with autism spectrum disorder: A review of recent findings. *Current Opinion in Pediatrics, 23*(6), 616–620.

Downs, A., & Smith, T. (2004). Emotional understanding, cooperation, and social behavior in high-functioning children with autism. *Journal of Autism and Developmental Disorders, 34*(6), 625–635.

DuPaul, G. J., & Stoner, G. (2003). *ADHD in the schools* (2nd ed.). New York: Guilford Press.

Estes, A., Olson, E., Sullivan, K., Greenson, J., Winter, J., Dawson, G., et al. (2013). Parenting-related stress and psychological distress in mothers of toddlers with autism spectrum disorders. *Brain and Development, 35*(2), 133–138.

Ghaziuddin, M., Weidmer-Mikhail, E., & Ghaziuddin, N. (1998). Comorbidity of Asperger syndrome: A preliminary report. *Journal of Intellectual Disability Research, 42,* 279–283.

Hazell, P. (2007). Drug therapy for attention-deficit/hyperactivity disorder-like symptoms in autistic disorder. *Journal of Peadiatrics and Child Health, 43,* 19–24.

Hill, E. L. (2004). Executive dysfunction in autism. *Trends in Cognitive Sciences, 8,* 26–32.

Hill, E. L. (2008). Executive functioning in autism spectrum disorder: Where it fits in the causal model. In E. McGregor, M. Nunez, K. Cebula, & J. C. Gomez (Eds.), *Autism: An integrated view from neurocognitive, clinical, and intervention research* (pp. 145–166). Malden, MA: Blackwell.

Howlin, P. (2014). Outcomes in adults with autism spectrum disorders. In F. R. Volkmar, S. Rogers, R. Paul, & K. A. Pelphrey (Eds.), *Handbook of autism and pervasive developmental disorders* (pp. 97–116). Hoboken, NJ: Wiley.

Joseph, R. M., & Tager-Flusberg, H. (1997). An investigation of attention and affect in children with autism and Down syndrome. *Journal of Autism and Developmental Disorders, 27*(4), 385–396.

Kanner, L. (1943). Autistic disturbances of affective contact. *Nervous Child, 2*(3), 217–250.

Kaufman, A. S., & Kaufman, N. L. (2004). *Kaufman Brief Intelligence Test* (2nd ed.). Bloomington, MN: Pearson.

Kaufman, J., Birmaher, B., Brent, D., Rao, U., & Ryan, N. (1996). *Diagnostic Interview: Kiddie SADS—Present and Lifetime Version (K-SADS-PL).* Pittsburgh, PA: University of Pittsburgh Medical Center.

Lainhart, J. E., Leyfer, O. T., & Folstein, S. E. (2003). *Autism Comorbidity Interview—Present and Lifetime Version (ACI-PL).* Salt Lake City: University of Utah.

Lang, R., Regester, A., Lauderdale, S., Ashbaugh, K., & Haring, A. (2010). Treatment of anxiety in autism spectrum disorders using cognitive behaviour therapy: A systematic review. *Developmental Neurorehabilitation, 13*(1), 53–63.

Lavelle, T. A. (2014). Economic burden of autism spectrum disorders in US. *PharmacoEconomics and Outcomes News, 697*(1), 5.

Lecavalier, L., Wood, J. J., Halladay, A. K., Jones, N. E., Aman, M. G., Cook, E. H., et al. (2014). Measuring anxiety as a treatment endpoint in youth with autism spectrum disorder. *Journal of Autism and Developmental Disorders, 44*(5), 1128–1143.

Leyfer, O. T., Folstein, S. E., Bacalman, S., Davis, N. O., Dinh, E., Morgan, J., et al. (2006). Comorbid psychiatric disorders in children with autism: Interview development and rates of disorders. *Journal of Autism and Developmental Disorders, 36*(7), 849–861.

Liss, M., Mailloux, J., & Erchull, M. J. (2008). The relationships between sensory processing sensitivity, alexithymia, autism, depression, and anxiety. *Personality and Individual Differences, 45,* 255–259.

Lord, C., Rutter, M., DiLavore, P., Risi, S., Gotham, K., & Bishop, S. (2012). *Autism Diagnostic Observation Schedule—2nd edition (ADOS-2).* Los Angeles: Western Psychological Corporation.

Lovaas, O. I. (1987). Behavioral treatment and normal educational and intellectual functioning in young autistic children. *Journal of Consulting and Clinical Psychology, 55*(1), 3–9.

Maglione, M. A., Gans, D., Das, L., Timbie, J., & Kasari, C. (2012). Nonmedical interventions for children with ASD: Recommended guidelines and further research needs. *Pediatrics, 130*(Suppl. 2), S169–S178.

Mazefsky, C. A., Herrington, J., Siegel, M., Scarpa, A., Maddox, B. B., Scahill, L., et al. (2013). The role of emotion regulation in autism spectrum disorder. *Journal of the American Academy of Child and Adolescent Psychiatry, 52*(7), 679–688.

Mazefsky, C. A., & White, S. W. (2013). The role of assessment in guiding treatment planning for youth with ASD. In A. Scarpa, S. W. White, & T. Attwood (Eds.), *CBT for children and adolescents with high-functioning autism spectrum disorders* (pp. 45–72). New York: Guilford Press.

McCracken, J. T., McGough, J., Shah, B., Cronin, P., Hong, D., Aman, M. G., et al. (2002). Risperidone in children with autism and serious behavioral problems. *New England Journal of Medicine, 347*(5), 314–321.

McEachin, J. J., Smith, T., & Lovaas, O. I. (1993). Long-term outcome for children with autism who received early intensive behavioral treatment. *American Journal of Mental Retardation, 97*, 359–391.

Moree, B. N., & Davis, T. E., III. (2010). Cognitive-behavioral therapy for anxiety in children diagnosed with autism spectrum disorders: Modification trends. *Research in Autism Spectrum Disorders, 4*(3), 346–354.

Moseley, D. S., Tonge, B. J., Brereton, A. V., & Einfeld, S. L. (2011). Psychiatric comorbidity in adolescents and young adults with autism. *Journal of Mental Health Research in Intellectual Disabilities, 4*(4), 229–243.

Myles, B. S., & Southwick, J. (2005). *Asperger syndrome and difficult moments: Practical solutions for tantrums, rage, and meltdowns.* Lenexa, KS: AAPC.

National Academy of Sciences & National Research Council. (2001). *Educating children with autism.* Washington, DC: ERIC Clearinghouse.

National Autism Center. (2015). Findings and conclusions: National Standards Project, Phase 2. Retrieved from *www.nationalautismcenter.org/national-standards-project/phase-2*.

Ollendick, T. H., Grills, A. E., & King, N. (2001). Applying developmental theory to the assessment and treatment of childhood disorders: Does it make a difference? *Clinical Psychology and Psychotherapy, 8*, 304–314.

Ozonoff, S., Cook, I., Coon, H., Dawson, G., Joseph, R.M., Klin, A., et al. (2004). Performance on Cambridge Neuropsychological Test Automated Battery sub-tests sensitive to frontal lobe function in people with autistic disorder: Evidence from the Collaborative Programs of Excellence in Autism Network. *Journal of Autism and Developmental Disorders, 34*, 139–150.

Ozsivadjian, A., Hibberd, C., & Hollocks, M. J. (2014). Brief report: The use of self-report measures in young people with autism spectrum disorder to access symptoms of anxiety, depression, and negative thoughts. *Journal of Autism and Developmental Disorders, 44*, 969–974.

Puleo, C. M., & Kendall, P. C. (2011). Anxiety disorders in typically developing youth: Autism spectrum symptoms as a predictor of cognitive-behavioral treatment. *Journal of Autism and Developmental Disorders, 41*(3), 275–286.

Reaven, J., & Blakeley-Smith, A. (2013). Parental involvement in treating anxiety in youth with high-functioning ASD. In A. Scarpa, S. W. White, & T. Attwood (Eds.), *CBT for children and adolescents with high functioning autism spectrum disorders* (pp. 97–122). New York: Guilford Press.

Reichow, B. (2012). Overview of meta-analyses on early intensive behavioral intervention for young children with autism spectrum disorders. *Journal of Autism and Developmental Disorders, 42*(4), 512–520.

Reiersen, A. M., & Todd, R. D. (2008). Co-occurrence of ADHD and autism spectrum disorders: Phenomenology and treatment. *Expert Review of Neurotherapeutics, 8*(4), 657–669.

Reynolds, C. R., & Kamphaus, R. W. (2004). *BASC-2: Behavior Assessment System for Children.* San Antonio, TX: Pearson.

Rezendes, D. L., & Scarpa, A. (2011). Associations between parental anxiety/depression and child behavior problems related to autism spectrum disorders: The roles of parenting stress and parenting self-efficacy. *Autism Research and Treatment, 2011*, Article ID 395190.

Rimland, B. (1964). *Infantile autism: The syndrome and its implications for a neural theory of behavior.* New York: Appleton-Century-Crofts.

Robins, D. L., Casagrande, K., Barton, M., Chen, C. M. A., Dumont-Mathieu, T., & Fein, D. (2014). Validation of the Modified Checklist for Autism in Toddlers, Revised with Follow-Up (M-CHAT-R/F). *Pediatrics, 133*(1), 37–45.

Rogers, S. J., & Vismara, L. A. (2008). Evidence-based comprehensive treatments for early autism. *Journal of Clinical Child and Adolescent Psychology, 37*(1), 8–38.

Rotheram-Fuller, E., & MacMullen, L. (2011). Cognitive-behavioral therapy for children with autism spectrum disorders. *Psychology in the Schools, 48,* 263–271.

Rutter, M., Bailey, A., & Lord, C. (2003). *The Social Communication Questionnaire: Manual.* Los Angeles: Western Psychological Services.

Rutter, M., Le Couteur, A., & Lord, C. (2003). *Autism Diagnostic Interview—Revised.* Los Angeles: Western Psychological Services.

Saulnier, C. A., & Ventola, P. E. (2012). *Essentials of autism spectrum disorders evaluation and assessment.* Hoboken, NJ: Wiley.

Scarpa, A., & Lorenzi, J. (2013). Cognitive-behavioral therapy with children and adolescents: History and principles. In A. Scarpa, S. W. White, & T. Attwood (Eds.), *CBT for children and adolescents with high-functioning autism spectrum disorders* (pp. 3–26). New York: Guilford Press.

Scarpa, A., & Reyes, N. M. (2011). Improving emotion regulation with CBT in young children with high functioning autism spectrum disorders: A pilot study. *Behavioural and Cognitive Psychotherapy, 39*(4), 495–500.

Scarpa, A., Reyes, N., & Attwood, T. (2013). Cognitive behavioral treatment for stress and anger management in young children with ASD: The Exploring Feelings program. In A. Scarpa, S. W. White, & T. Attwood (Eds.), *CBT for children and adolescents with high functioning autism spectrum disorders* (pp. 147–172). New York: Guilford Press.

Scarpa, A., Wells, A. O., & Attwood, T. (2013). *Exploring Feelings for young children with high-functioning autism or Asperger's disorder: The STAMP treatment manual.* London: Jessica Kingsley.

Scarpa, A., White, S. W., & Attwood, T. (Eds.). (2013). *CBT for children and adolescents with high-functioning autism spectrum disorders.* New York: Guilford Press.

Schreibman, L. (2000). Intensive behavioral/psychoeducational treatments for autism: Research needs and future directions. *Journal of Autism and Developmental Disorders, 30*(5), 373–378.

Selles, R. R., & Storch, E. A. (2013). Translation of anxiety treatment to youth with autism spectrum disorders. *Journal of Child and Family Studies, 22*(3), 405–413.

Shalom, D. B., Mostofsky, S. H., Hazlett, R. L., Goldberg, M. C., Landa, R. J., Faran, Y., et al. (2006). Normal physiological emotions but differences in expression of conscious feelings in children with high-functioning autism. *Journal of Autism and Developmental Disorders, 36*(3), 395–400.

Silverman, W. K., & Albano, A. M. (1996). *Anxiety Disorders Interview Schedule for DSM-IV: Parent Interview Schedule.* San Antonio, TX: Psychological Corporation.

Simonoff, E., Pickles, A., Charman, T., Chandler, S., Loucas, T., & Baird, G. (2008). Psychiatric disorders in children with autism spectrum disorders: prevalence, comorbidity, and associated factors in a population-derived sample. *Journal of the American Academy of Child and Adolescent Psychiatry, 47*(8), 921–929.

Smith, T., & Iadarola, S. (2015). Evidence base update for autism spectrum disorder. *Journal of Clinical Child and Adolescent Psychology, 44*(6), 897–922.

Sofronoff, K., Attwood, T., & Hinton, S. (2005). A randomised controlled trial of a CBT intervention for anxiety in children with Asperger syndrome. *Journal of Child Psychology and Psychiatry, 46*(11), 1152–1160.

Sofronoff, K., Attwood, T., Hinton, S., & Levin, I. (2007). A randomized controlled trial of a cognitive behavioural intervention for anger management in children diagnosed with Asperger syndrome. *Journal of Autism and Developmental Disorders, 37,* 1203–1214.

Spence, S. H., Rapee, R., McDonald, C., & Ingram, M. (2001). The structure of anxiety symptoms among preschoolers. *Behaviour Research and Therapy, 39*(11), 1293–1316.

Spencer, D., Marshall, J., Post, B., Kulakodlu, M., Newschaffer, C., Dennen, T., et al. (2013).

Psychotropic medication use and polypharmacy in children with autism spectrum disorders. *Pediatrics, 132*(5), 833–840.

Sukhodolsky, D. G., Bloch, M. H., Panza, K. E., & Reichow, B. (2013). Cognitive-behavioral therapy for anxiety in children with high-functioning autism: A meta-analysis. *Pediatrics, 132*(5), e1341–e1350.

Tanaka, J. T. (2010). Using computerized games to teach face recognition skills to children with autism spectrum disorder: The Let's Face It! program. *Journal of Child Psychology and Psychiatry, 51*(8), 944–952.

Tani, P., Joukamaa, M., Lindberg, N., Nieminen-von Wendt, T., Virkkala, J., Appelberg, B., et al. (2004). Asperger syndrome, alexithymia and sleep. *Neuropsychobiology, 49*, 64–70.

Twachtman-Cullen, D. (2000). More able children with autism spectrum disorders: Sociocommunicative challenges and guidelines for enhancing abilities. In A. M. Wetherby & B. M. Prizant (Eds.), *Autism spectrum disorders: A transactional developmental perspective* (pp. 225–249). Baltimore: Brookes.

Velting, O., Setzer, N., & Albano, A. (2004). Update on and advances in assessment and cognitive-behavioral treatment of anxiety disorders in children and adolescents. *Professional Psychology: Research and Practice, 35*, 42–54.

Volkmar, F. R., Reichow, B., Westphal, A., & Mandell, D. S. (2014). Autism and the autism spectrum: Diagnostic concepts. In F. R. Volkmar, S. Rogers, R. Paul, & K. A. Pelphrey (Eds.), *Handbook of autism and pervasive developmental disorders* (pp. 3–27). Hoboken, NJ: Wiley.

Weisz, J. R., & Kazdin, A. E. (Eds.). (2010). *Evidence-based psychotherapies for children and adolescents* (2nd ed.). New York: Guilford Press.

Wigham, S., & McConachie, H. (2014). Systematic review of the properties of tools used to measure outcomes in anxiety intervention studies for children with autism spectrum disorders. *PLoS ONE, 9*(1), e85268.

Willner, P., Brace, N., & Phillips, J. (2005). Assessment of anger coping skills in individuals with intellectual disabilities. *Journal of Intellectual Disability Research, 49*, 329–339.

Wing, L. (1981). Asperger's syndrome: A clinical account. *Psychological Medicine, 11*(1), 115–129.

Wong, C., Odom, S. L., Hume, K., Cox, A. W., Fettig, A., Kucharczyk, S., et al. (2013). *Evidence-based practices for children, youth, and young adults with autism spectrum disorder.* Chapel Hill: University of North Carolina, Frank Porter Graham Child Development Institute, Autism Evidence-Based Practice Review Group.

CHAPTER 17

Anxiety and Related Problems in Early Childhood

Elyse Stewart and Jennifer Freeman

BACKGROUND

The fifth edition of the *Diagnostic and Statistical Manual for Mental Disorders* (DSM-5; American Psychiatric Association, 2013) specifically defines the criteria for anxiety disorders; however, these criteria encompass all age ranges. Developmental level is an important factor to consider while making a diagnosis, especially since anxiety in younger children may manifest differently than that of an older child. Younger children may not have the language or cognitive capabilities to verbalize their feelings and explain their anxious cognitions. This can certainly complicate assessments; therefore, clinicians should rely on multiple informants, including their own clinical impressions, before deciding on a diagnosis. Each of the anxiety disorders and related problems is detailed below in relation to how it may present in young children:

- *Separation anxiety disorder* is characterized by an extreme attachment to a parent or caregiver. Many younger children experience developmentally typical separation anxiety; however, it can become problematic if it persists. When a separation from that caregiver occurs, the child experiences great distress. In young children, this distress presents as crying and clinging to the caregiver. Caregivers often describe their young child as their "shadow" because the child follows them wherever they go. Symptoms may initially present in situations such as a transition to preschool. Older children may have more anticipatory anxiety about future separations because they have acquired more future planning skills, whereas younger children typically experience the most distress at the time of separation, which is reflective of younger children's developmental level.

- *Selective mutism* occurs when the child is unable to speak in certain situations. Caregivers may describe how their young child is talkative at home but extremely shy in other situations. Selective mutism can be misconstrued as shyness, especially by caregivers of younger children. This "shyness" is often tolerated and not viewed as serious because young children do not have as many social expectations; in turn, this may deter the young child's family from seeking treatment. Selective mutism can become most impairing when the young child transitions to preschool. This is a critical time when selective mutism can be impairing to both the social and academic development of the young child.

- *Social anxiety* is another disorder that may be misconstrued as "shyness" in young children. Older children can typically verbalize their fear of embarrassment or judgment by others, whereas younger children may not report this. A younger child may hide his or her face when meeting new people or tantrum in social situations. He or she may not play with the other children and may avoid social interactions.

- *Specific phobia* presents as an intense fear of a certain situation or thing. Again, younger children may not be able to verbalize what exactly they fear, but caregivers can use observational data to inform the clinician. Young children may tantrum in the presence of the source of their phobia, seek out their caregiver, and/or hide. Clinicians should be mindful that it is developmentally typical for young children to have fears and should assess for severity of interference and distress to inform the diagnosis of a specific phobia.

- *Panic disorder* may present as physical symptoms in young children. A young child may complain of dizziness, shortness of breath, or a stomachache. The child may not want to leave his or her house for fear of feeling that way again. This may result in tantruming if the caregiver pressures the child to leave.

- *Generalized anxiety disorder* in young children presents as worry about a variety of things. Caregivers often describe their young children as having an older soul because they worry about "adult" things. Overall these children are characterized as "worriers." Symptoms of generalized anxiety disorder in young children may present as seeking reassurance by asking a lot of questions. These questions can be about anything they perceive as scary in the moment, such as schedule changes, schoolwork, or the weather.

- *Posttraumatic stress disorder* may be characterized as intense fear and anxiety after experiencing a traumatic event. A young child may become generally irritable and/or emotionally unexpressive. The child may tantrum in the presence of triggers that remind him or her of the traumatic event.

- *Obsessive–compulsive disorder* (OCD) in young children can present in a variety of ways. Young children may not have the ability to express their obsessions or to link their obsessions with their compulsions. In this case, the clinician must again defer to the caregiver reports and any observational data. Caregivers may be able to observe the young child's compulsions and may even take part in some. For example, a young child may have a specific nightly ritual in which his or her caregiver must say a "script" before bedtime. A clinician can assess the distress and interference by asking the caregiver about how the child would react if he or she were unable to complete the compulsion or by asking about the degree to which the caregiver is accommodating the child's symptoms.

Anxiety in younger children is just as common, persistent, and impairing as anxiety experienced by older children (Hirshfeld-Becker, Micco, Mazursky, Bruett, & Henin, 2011; Mian, 2014). Anxiety disorders are among the most common and the earliest forms of psychopathology to emerge in childhood, with mean onset ranging from ages 6 to 12 years (Cartwright-Hatton, McNally, & White, 2005; Fox et al., 2012). Community samples of children and adolescents have found lifetime prevalence estimates of childhood anxiety disorders ranging from 14 to 25% (Costello, Egger, & Angold, 2004). Specifically, for young children, a prevalence rate of 9% is estimated (Comer et al., 2012; Egger & Angold, 2006).

In a longitudinal cohort study, Copeland, Angold, Shanahan, and Costello (2014) found that for a large proportion of children, anxiety symptoms persisted into adolescence and early adulthood. In one study, 82% of a control sample of 4- to 7-year-olds with an anxiety disorder diagnosis maintained that diagnosis 6 months later (Hirshfeld-Becker et al., 2010). Furthermore, in untreated behaviorally inhibited 3- to 5-year-olds, of which 91.5% met criteria for an anxiety disorder diagnosis, the anxiety disorder persisted 1 year later (Rapee, Kennedy, Ingram, Edwards, & Sweeney, 2005). In addition, Wichstrom, Belsky, and Berg-Nielsen (2013) found that behavioral inhibition (BI), parental anxiety, and peer victimization in children age 4 function as risk factors in developing an anxiety disorder by age 6. These studies, in addition to others, attest to the chronic and rather stable nature of untreated anxiety disorders across development (Karevold, Roysamb, Youngstrom, & Mathiesen, 2009).

There are long-term consequences of childhood anxiety disorders that indicate poor prognosis (Cartwright-Hatton et al., 2005). Young children with anxiety disorders are at greater risk for developing another psychiatric condition later in life, such as further anxiety, mood disorders, depression, increased levels of suicidality, emotional problems, and substance abuse (Cartwright-Hatton, 2013; Hirshfeld-Becker et al., 2011; Kendall et al., 2010). Significant anxiety symptoms in young children have been linked to greater functional impairment such as academic underperformance and difficulty with relationships (Cartwright-Hatton, 2013; Fox et al., 2012). Anxiety symptoms investigated in an epidemiological sample of first graders were predictive of anxiety symptoms and academic decline in fifth grade (Ialongo, Edelsohn, Werthamer-Larsson, Crockett, & Kellam, 1995). Clearly, anxiety disorders experienced by young children are a critical clinical issue.

Additionally, young children are often at risk for having more than one anxiety disorder because anxiety disorders are frequently comorbid with other anxiety disorders (Connolly & Bernstein, 2007). Anxiety disorders in children are also associated with depression (Angold & Costello, 1993; Lewinsohn, Zinbarg, Seeley, Lewinsohn, & Sack, 1997), attention-deficit/hyperactivity disorder (Kendall, Brady, & Verduin, 2001), and oppositional defiant disorder (Manassis & Monga, 2001).

The development of anxiety problems in youth is conceptualized as an interplay between biological and environmental risk factors (Connolly & Bernstein, 2007). Genetics and child temperament, specifically, BI, are biological factors that may be contributors (Biederman et al., 1993; Kagan & Snidman, 1999). Environmental factors may include parents' own anxiety and parent–child interactions, such as parenting style and attachment (Hirshfeld et al., 1997; Rapee, 1997; Warren, Huston, Egeland, & Sroufe, 1997).

Due to the high risks associated with anxiety, early intervention is essential. Research suggests that early intervention targets an advantageous developmental stage of increased neuroplasticity in younger children (Mian, 2014). Also, targeting anxiety symptoms early on can potentially offset the trajectory of the poor prognoses we mentioned previously. Despite the necessity of early intervention, younger children are less likely to get treatment (Egger & Angold, 2006). Parents are more likely to seek treatment for disruptive behavior problems than for anxiety (Pavuluri, Luk, & McGee, 1996). Consequently, it is estimated that over 80% of children with an anxiety disorder do not receive mental health services (Merikangas, 2011). Despite the high-risk factors associated with young childhood anxiety, early interventions that specifically focus on these risks are in the beginning stages of investigation (Rapee, Kennedy, Ingram, Edwards, & Sweeney, 2010).

The treatment of anxiety disorders with cognitive-behavioral therapy (CBT) has strong empirical support with regard to its efficacy with older children and adolescents (Hirshfeld-Becker et al., 2011). The vast majority of CBT for anxiety research, however, is limited to children age 7 and older (Hirshfeld-Becker et al., 2011). Typically when younger children have been included in studies, they were few in number, as evidenced by higher mean ages, and results are often not broken down to explore the differences in the youngest children (Hirshfeld-Becker et al., 2011; Puliafico, Comer, & Albano, 2013). Although CBT is a well-established treatment, a simple downward extension of this treatment to a younger population is insufficient (Comer et al., 2012; Puliafico et al., 2013). Young children may not yet have the necessary developmental skills to engage in this type of treatment effectively (Comer et al., 2012; Puliafico et al., 2013). In recent years, the greater push to investigate anxiety in young children has resulted in emerging support for the effectiveness of CBT for this population (Cartwright-Hatton et al., 2005, 2011; Comer et al., 2012; Donovan & March, 2014; Hirshfeld-Becker et al., 2008, 2010, 2011; Monga, Young, & Owens, 2009; van der Sluis, van der Bruggen, Brechman-Toussaint, Thissen, & Bogels, 2012; Waters, Ford, Wharton, & Cobham, 2009). Further investigation of particular mechanisms for change within these evidence-based treatment approaches is also warranted.

EVIDENCE-BASED TREATMENTS

As previously mentioned, there has long been a dearth of research in regard to empirically supported treatment for younger children with anxiety disorders (Comer et al., 2012). Recently, researchers have begun to address this need by developing developmentally sensitive CBT protocols. Select studies are highlighted below (for a more comprehensive listing of all researched-based approaches, see Table 17.1).

Preventive CBT

The preventive treatment of anxiety in young children has been investigated by several researchers and is a possibly efficacious treatment approach (Cartwright-Hatton et al., 2005; Fox et al., 2012; Kennedy, Rapee, & Edwards, 2009; Rapee, 2013; Rapee et al., 2005, 2010). Rapee and colleagues (2005) conducted a randomized controlled trial (RCT) with parent-focused group CBT. One hundred forty-six children ages 3–5 with high levels of BI were included in the study. Key treatment components included psychoeducation, parent management technique, hierarchy building, and exposure. Parents' anxieties were also addressed through the teaching of cognitive restructuring. Posttreatment, children's anxiety symptoms significantly decreased. These gains were maintained at a 3-year follow-up (Rapee et al., 2010). At an 11-year follow-up, Rapee (2013) found

TABLE 17.1. Evidence-Based Treatment Approaches for Young Children with Anxiety

Treatment approach	Type of study	Disorder/ criteria	Ages	N	Duration	Key treatment components	Results	Citation
Family-focused group CBT								
CBT "Strengthening Early Emotional Development" (SEED) with child and parent groups	Open trial	Impairing anxiety symptoms ranging from subthreshold to clinically severe	3–5	16	10 weeks	Parenting skills, hierarchies, exposure, social skills, relaxation, and emotion regulation	Reduced child and parental anxiety symptoms, increased child emotional understanding, and parental confidence. Gains were maintained at 3-month follow-up.	Fox et al. (2012)
					Prevention of anxiety disorders			
Parent-focused group CBT								
Parent-focused group CBT	Open trial, pilot study	Referred for anxiety; scored at or above clinical cutoff on Internalizing scale of CBCL	4–9	11	10 weeks	Parenting techniques with an emphasis on encouraging brave behaviors and discouraging anxious behaviors, and anxiety management skills including problem solving, distraction, hierarchy building, and exposure	CBCL Internalizing scores dropped significantly posttreatment. At 3-month follow-up, the mean Internalizing score was further reduced, which may indicate continued improvement.	Cartwright-Hatton et al. (2005)
Parent-focused group CBT vs. wait-list controls	RCT	High levels of BI, met criteria for one or more anxiety disorder, and a parent with a current anxiety disorder	3–4	71	8 sessions	Psychoeducation, parenting skills, exposure, cognitive restructuring, and coping skills for both child and parent anxieties	At 6-month follow-up 46.7% of children no longer met criteria for an anxiety disorder compared to 6.7% of wait-list controls	Kennedy et al. (2009)
Parent-focused group CBT vs. no intervention	RCT	High levels of BI	3–5	146	6 sessions	Psychoeducation, parent-management techniques, hierarchies, exposure, and cognitive restructuring for parent anxieties	Significantly reduced anxiety symptoms but not BI. At 12-month follow-up 50% had anxiety disorder diagnoses compared to 90% at pretreatment.	Rapee et al. (2005)

(continued)

	3-year follow-up		121		Significant reduction in number of diagnoses from pretreatment to 1-, 2-, and 3-year follow-ups, reduction in clinical severity of primary diagnosis from pretreatment to 2- and 3-year follow-ups, and reduction in anxiety symptoms from pretreatment to 3-year follow-up.	Rapee et al. (2010)
	11-year follow-up		103		Significant differences in number of internalizing disorders, maternal ratings of anxiety symptoms, and self-rated life interference for females who received treatment.	Rapee (2013)

School-based intervention

Intervention	Design	Age	N	Sessions	Outcomes	Reference
CBT "Fun FRIENDS" with an emphasis on social–emotional learning school-based intervention with parent and child group sessions	Open trial No specific criteria–universal prevention	4–6	70	10 sessions	Delivered by classroom teachers; social–emotional competence building such as developing sense of self, social skills, self-regulation, responsibility for self and others, and prosocial behavior; cognitive-behavioral skills such as problem solving, relaxation, cognitive restructuring, and exposure Anxiety symptoms significantly decreased for females.	Pahl & Barrett (2007)
	RCT	4–7	488		Reduced BI, behavioral difficulties, parenting distress, and improved social and emotional competence, and parent–child interactions.	Anticich, Barrett, Silverman, Lacherez, & Gillies (2013)

(continued)

497

TABLE 17.1. (continued)

Treatment approach	Type of study	Disorder/ criteria	Ages	N	Duration	Key treatment components	Results	Citation
SAD								
Disorder-specific programs								
PCIT	Case series, pilot study	SAD	4–8	3	6–7 sessions	CDI phase included positive attention for brave behaviors and planned ignoring for anxious or oppositional behaviors; PDI phase included skills for leading interactions with their child, such as directing their child and giving time-outs; parents received immediate feedback through "bug-in-ear" communication with the therapist, and parents were praised for using skills effectively	No longer met criteria for SAD posttreatment.	Choate, Pincus, Eyberg, & Barlow (2005)
	Preliminary case series	SAD	4–8	10	10 weeks	Modified PCIT- included CDI and PDI phases in addition to more anxiety-focused parenting skills such as selective attention and reinforcement for brave behaviors	Decrease in severity of symptoms but did not reach nonclinical levels at posttreatment.	Pincus et al. (2005, 2008)
	Preliminary RCT findings	SAD	4–8	34	9 sessions	Modified PCIT- included CDI and PDI phases in addition to a bravery-directed interaction (BDI) phase including exposure situations	Significant improvements compared to wait-list controls.	Pincus et al. (2008)
CBT with parent training vs. wait-list controls	RCT	SAD	5–7	43	16 sessions	Psychoeducation, hierarchy building, cognitive restructuring, exposure, and parent training	76.19% no longer met criteria for SAD compared to 13.64% of the wait-list controls. Improvements were maintained at 4-week follow-up.	Schneider et al. (2011)

(continued)

498

Specific phobia

Intervention	Design	Age	N	Duration	Components	Outcomes	Citation
Parent-applied play therapy: bibliotherapy and games vs. emotive performances vs. no treatment	RCT	Specific phobia–darkness	4–8	78	5 weeks	Parent training, modeling, role playing, positive reinforcement, feedback, and graded exposure; treatment delivered by parents	Reduction in phobia posttreatment and continued reduction at 12-month follow-up.	Santacruz, Méndez, & Sánchez-Meca (2006)

Anxiety-related disorders

Intervention	Design	Disorder	Age	N	Duration	Components	Outcomes	Citation
Internet-delivered family-based CBT	Preliminary case series	OCD	4–8	5	12 sessions	Parent training, address parental accommodation of symptoms, externalizing, hierarchy building, and exposure with response prevention; treatment delivered via Internet-based program and video teleconferencing	60% no longer met criteria for an OCD diagnosis posttreatment.	Comer et al. (2014)
Family-based CBT (FB-CBT) with exposure with response prevention vs. family-based relaxation therapy (FB-RT)	RCT, preliminary findings	OCD	5–8	42	12 sessions	Modified psychoeducation; parent-based skills; simplification of CBT skills; parent involvement; exposure with response prevention; and family context, specifically, parent's response to their child's anxieties	69% achieved clinical remission of OCD symptoms compared to 20% in the FB-RT control group.	Freeman et al. (2008)
	RCT	OCD	5–8	127	14 weeks		72% of children compared to 41% for FB-RT improved as rated by their clinician on the CGI-I Scale. There was also a significant decrease in CY-BOCS scores for FB-CBT compared to FB-RT.	Freeman, Sapyta, et al. (2014)
Family-based CBT vs. wait-list controls	RCT	OCD	M = 6	7		Psychoeducation, exposure with response prevention, contingency management, address parental accommodation of symptoms	33–66% reduction in OCD symptoms, and six of the seven children were rated as treatment responders.	Ginsburg, Burstein, Becker, & Drake (2011)

(continued)

499

TABLE 17.1. (continued)

Treatment approach	Type of study	Disorder/ criteria	Ages	N	Duration	Key treatment components	Results	Citation
Family-based CBT	Case example	OCD	4	1	12 sessions	Exposure with response prevention, differential reinforcement of other behaviors, behavioral parent training, and addressing family accommodation	Significant reduction in OCD symptoms posttreatment; gains were maintained at 3-month follow-up.	Labouliere, Arnold, Storch, & Lewin (2014)
Family-based CBT vs. treatment as usual (TAU)	RCT, pilot study	OCD	3–8	31	12 sessions	Psychoeducation, parent tools, differential reinforcement, and exposure with response prevention	65% were rated as treatment responders and 35.2% achieved symptom remission compared 7% treatment responders and 0% remission in the TAU group	Lewin et al. (2014)
Multimodal treatment	Case series	Selective mutism	3–5	7	14 weeks	Psychoeducation, defocused communication, stimulus fading/sliding-in techniques, games, and rewards	Speech significantly increased posttreatment.	Oerbeck, Johansen, Lundahl, & Kristensen (2012)

Transdiagnostic anxiety programs

Family-focused individual CBT

Treatment approach	Type of study	Disorder/ criteria	Ages	N	Duration	Key treatment components	Results	Citation
Individualized family-focused CBT "Being Brave"	Open trial, pilot study	BI, elevated symptoms on Withdrawn or Anxious/ Depressed scale of CBCL with a parent who has a lifetime history of an anxiety disorder and/or a current anxiety disorder diagnosis	4–7	9	20 weeks	Adapted from Kendall's Coping Cat treatment. Includes parent involvement, coping skills, problem solving, and graded exposure with reinforcement	Eight of nine children improved on number of anxiety diagnoses, anxiety symptoms, and ability to cope with feared situations.	Hirshfeld-Becker et al. (2008)

(continued)

		Age	N	Duration	Components	Results	
High-risk children with SAD, social phobia, GAD, or specific phobia	RCT	4–7	64	20 sessions	Parent involvement, coping skills, problem solving, and graded exposure with reinforcement	59% no longer met criteria for anxiety disorder diagnoses posttreatment and at 12-month follow-up.	Hirshfeld-Becker et al. (2010)

Family-focused group CBT

		Age	N	Duration	Components	Results	
Group CBT, both parent and child sessions vs. wait-list controls	Nonrandomized trial, pilot study	Social anxiety, SAD, GAD, and/or selective mutism	5–7	32	12 weeks	Labeling feelings, relaxation, cognitive strategies, psychoeducation, parent management and behavioral strategies, and desensitization strategies	71.9% decreased by at least one anxiety diagnosis and 43.8% no longer met criteria for any anxiety disorder diagnoses posttreatment.	Monga et al. (2009)
Parent-only group CBT "Take Action" vs. Parent–child group CBT "Take Action" vs. wait-list controls	RCT	Specific phobia, social phobia, GAD, and/or SAD	4–8	60	10 weeks	Psychoeducation, relaxation, coping skills, graded exposure, problem solving, and social skills training	84% of parent-only group and 74% of parent–child group no longer met criteria for their primary diagnosis compared to 18% of wait-list controls. No significant differences between treatment groups.	Waters et al. (2009)

Parent-focused group CBT

			Age	N	Duration	Components	Results	
Parent-focused group CBT "Parent Survival Course" (PSC)	Open trial; pilot study	Moderate to severe difficulties with behavior and low socioeconomic status	2–4	43	8 sessions	Parenting skills with emphasis on positive attention, planned ignoring, and rewards; this program was not specifically tailored to address internalizing problems	Both internalizing and externalizing scores dropped significantly posttreatment; 6-month follow-up indicated that posttreatment scores were maintained.	Cartwright-Hatton et al. (2005)

(continued)

TABLE 17.1. (continued)

Treatment approach	Type of study	Disorder/criteria	Ages	N	Duration	Key treatment components	Results	Citation
Parent-focused group CBT "Timid to Tiger" vs. wait-list controls	RCT	CBCL Internalizing score or Preschool Behavior Checklist Internalizing score at or above clinical cutoff	2–9	74	10 sessions	Parenting skills including attention, play, rewards, limit setting, and ignoring; psychoeducation on anxiety; and skills to manage worry, such as problem solving distraction, hierarchies, and exposure	57% of children no longer met criteria for their primary diagnosis in comparison to 15% of the wait-list controls. Also, 32% no longer had any anxiety diagnoses compared to 6% of the wait-list controls; 12-month follow-up indicated that posttreatment gains were maintained.	Cartwright-Hatton et al. (2011)
Parent-focused group CBT and individualized telephone sessions "Confident Kids"	Open trial, pilot study	Presenting with anxiety symptoms	4–7	26	8	Parenting skills and guided exposure	Reduced anxiety and BI and improved parenting practices.	van der Sluis et al. (2012)
PCIT								
PCIT "CALM Program" vs. wait-list controls	RCT	SAD, social anxiety disorder, GAD, and/or specific phobias	4–8	9	12 sessions	Behavioral parent training, therapist provides live coaching through "bug-in-ear" to promote brave child behaviors, and practice in-session exposures; follow DADS steps: Describe situation, Approach situation, give Direct command for child to join situation, provide Selective attention	85.7% no longer met criteria for any disorders posttreatment. 100% response rate for SAD, social anxiety disorder, GAD, selective mutism, and ODD.	Comer et al. (2012)
Technology-based parent-focused CBT								
Parent online CBT "BRAVE-Online" vs. wait-list control	RCT	Social phobia, SAD, specific phobia, or GAD	3–6	52	6 sessions with 2 booster sessions after 1 month and after 3 months	Psychoeducation; anxiety management strategies such as relaxation, self-talk, exposure, problem-solving; and reinforcement of brave behavior	39.1% no longer met criteria for an anxiety disorder compared to 25.9% of wait-list controls. At 6-month follow-up 70.6% of treated children no longer met criteria for their primary diagnosis.	Donovan & March (2014)

that females who completed their prevention program had less internalizing disorders and less self-rated life interference from symptoms.

Family-Focused Individual CBT

Family-focused individual CBT is also a possibly efficacious treatment (Hirshfeld-Becker et al., 2008, 2010). Hirshfeld-Becker and colleagues (2010) developed the Being Brave program, a 20-session manualized treatment protocol for high-risk children with separation anxiety disorder (SAD), social phobia, generalized anxiety disorder (GAD), and/or specific phobia. This manual is an adaptation of Kendall's Coping Cat treatment and focuses on parent involvement, coping skills, problem solving, and graded exposure with reinforcement (Kendall & Hedtke, 2006). The RCT included 64 children ages 4–7 and took place over 20 weekly sessions. Sessions 1–6 and 20 were for parents only, and Sessions 7–19 included both the child and parents (Hirshfeld-Becker et al., 2010). Upon completion of treatment, 59% of the children no longer met criteria for an anxiety disorder diagnosis. There was a 69% response rate on the Clinical Global Impressions Scale (CGI; Guy, 1976) for anxiety compared to a 32% response rate for waitlist controls. Posttreatment, children experienced a greater reduction in anxiety symptoms, and the parent group's coping increased more than did the wait list. Additionally, these gains were maintained at a follow-up 1 year later. Clinicians should refer to the Being Brave protocol as a solid framework example for treating young children with anxiety.

Family-Focused Group CBT

Group CBT with both parent and child sessions is a possibly efficacious treatment. Monga and colleagues (2009) investigated this treatment in a nonrandomized trial of children ages 5–7 with social anxiety, SAD, GAD, and/or selective mutism. Thirty-two children and their parents completed treatment across 12 weeks. Treatment focused on psychoeducation, parent management, and behavioral strategies. It also addressed labeling feelings, relaxation, cognitive strategies, and desensitization strategies. Posttreatment, 43.8% of the children no longer met criteria for any anxiety disorder diagnoses.

Waters and colleagues (2009) also investigated this treatment in an RCT along with parent-only group CBT in their Take Action program. This study included 60 children ages 4–8 and took place across 10 weeks. The program focused on psychoeducation, relaxation, coping skills, graded exposures, problem solving, and social skills training. No significant differences were found between parent-only group CBT and family-focused group CBT. Eighty-four percent of the parent-only group CBT and 74% of the parent–child group CBT no longer met criteria for their primary diagnosis compared to 18% of wait-list controls.

Parent-Focused Group CBT

Parent-only group CBT is a possibly efficacious treatment. Cartwright-Hatton and colleagues (2011) developed the Timid to Tiger program and conducted an RCT with 74 children ages 2–9. Children were at or above the clinical cutoff for their internalizing score on the Child Behavior Checklist (CBCL; Achenbach, 1991) or the Preschool

Behavior Questionnaire (Behar, 1977) for study inclusion. Treatment took place over 10 sessions and focused on psychoeducation, parenting skills, problem solving, and exposure. Posttreatment, 57% of children no longer met criteria for their primary diagnosis in comparison to 15% of the wait-list controls.

Technology-Based Parent-Focused CBT

Parent online CBT is a possibly efficacious treatment. The BRAVE-Online program was completed by parents of 52 children ages 3–6 with social phobia, SAD, specific phobia, or GAD in an RCT (Donovan & March, 2014). Treatment was across six sessions, with two booster sessions, after 1 month and after 3 months. Key components included psychoeducation and anxiety management strategies such as relaxation, exposure, problem solving, and reinforcement of brave behavior. Posttreatment, 39.1% of children no longer met criteria for an anxiety disorder diagnosis compared to 25.9% of wait-list controls.

Parent–Child Interaction Therapy

Parent–child interaction therapy (PCIT), a possibly efficacious treatment approach for young children with anxiety disorders, was originally developed to treat young children with disruptive behavior problems (McNeil & Hembree-Kigin, 2010). It is a directive, short-term treatment in which the clinician monitors parent–child interactions and gives immediate feedback through "bug-in-ear" communication. PCIT consists of two components: child-directed interaction (CDI) and parent-directed interaction (PDI). The CDI component includes training parents to give positive attention to appropriate behavior and actively ignore undesired behaviors. The PDI component includes training parents to use effective commands and follow through with consequences for misbehavior. This helps to shape the child to act more appropriately.

Pincus, Eyberg, and Choate (2005) modified the PCIT treatment model to apply to young children with separation anxiety. They used both components, PDI and CDI, but added a bravery-directed interaction (BDI) component as well. During this, parents were taught to encourage their child to approach the feared situation and to respond to their child positively for his or her efforts. The preliminary results from this treatment approach were successful (Pincus, Santucci, Ehrenreich, & Eyberg, 2008).

Given this success, Comer and colleagues (2012) extended this program for use in young children with social phobia, GAD, SAD, and/or specific phobia. They, too, were successful in their preliminary investigation. Of the nine children who completed treatment, all but one child no longer met criteria for an anxiety disorder diagnosis. Children also showed functional improvement at posttreatment. PCIT appears to be a promising treatment approach for young children with anxiety. Although further research is necessary, parent training can be a powerful tool for clinicians to disseminate.

CBT for Other Anxiety

Individual family-based CBT for children with OCD has been established as a probably efficacious treatment (Freeman, Garcia, et al., 2014). This treatment adapted to a younger population is a possibly efficacious treatment. The Pediatric OCD Treatment

Study for Young Children (POTS Jr) is an RCT of family-based CBT in comparison to family-based relaxation therapy (RT) across multiple sites (Freeman, Sapyta, et al., 2014). The study included 127 children ages 5 through 8 with an OCD diagnosis. The treatment included 12 sessions, and the protocol was a developmentally sensitive downward extension of the successful POTS I and POTS II trials (Pediatric OCD Treatment Study Team, 2004). The study highlights the importance of the clinician tailoring the treatment to a developmentally appropriate level that is unique based on the child's presentation and overall level of understanding. The clinicians in the POTS Jr studies modified psychoeducation, simplified CBT skills, and increased focus on parent-based skills (Freeman et al., 2012). The treatment rationale is often difficult for young children to process. In an effort to remedy this, the first two sessions were parent-only sessions that focused on psychoeducation and ensuring parents' comprehension of the rationale. Given the young age of the child, clinicians were mindful that this may be parents' first encounter with the mental health treatment for their child. In their child's absence, parents were allowed the opportunity to process any emotions and concerns regarding their child's illness. The clinician also helped parents to delineate between OCD impairing symptoms in relation to other behavior problems, rigidity, or normal developmental rituals. Parent involvement and behavioral parenting techniques were key. Clinicians externalized OCD, empowering children to "be the boss" and made the exposure into a game as much as possible. Freeman, Sapyta, and colleagues (2014) found their approach to be effective, as 69% of the children in the family-based CBT group achieved OCD remission in comparison to 20% of children in the family-based RT group.

Acceptance and Commitment Therapy

Acceptance and commitment therapy (ACT) is a novel psychosocial intervention that is in the early stages of investigation with anxious youth. This approach has been largely implemented with adults; however, there is an emerging literature on its application with children and adolescents (Coyne, McHugh, & Martinez, 2011). Currently there are no specific guidelines for implementing ACT with younger children. The ACT model works by encouraging patients to live consistently with their values despite the discomfort that may accompany anxious thoughts (Twohig et al., 2015). The therapeutic process in ACT relies on the patient's willingness to accept anxious thoughts and feelings, and not to allow those feelings to change the course of his or her behavior toward life values. Randomized trials of ACT that contained exposure showed this model is useful for treating anxiety disorders and OCD in adults (Arch et al., 2012; Craske et al., 2014). Other research indicates that ACT without in-session exposure also to be useful for OCD and related disorders (Twohig et al., 2015).

Pharmacological Interventions

There is a paucity of research on the use of psychotropic medication in young children with anxiety (Barterian & Rappuhn, 2014; Gleason et al., 2007). Consistent with the treatment of older children, selective serotonin reuptake inhibitors (SSRIs) were found to be the most widely prescribed medication for internalizing problems in young children (Barterian & Rappuhn, 2014; Gleason et al., 2007). In a review of the current research,

Barterian and Rappuhn found preliminary support for the medication's effectiveness in reducing anxiety symptoms; however, they strongly caution that this support was established primarily through case studies and therefore lacks the necessary methodological adherence. Gleason and colleagues (2007) advise that medication should not be the first line of treatment for young children with anxiety disorders. Clinicians should reevaluate the child's diagnosis, clinical picture, and adequacy of the psychotherapy the child received before considering medication (Gleason et al., 2007). Currently, pharmacological interventions have not yet been investigated in young children with anxiety disorders through an RCT. Further research is needed to establish pharmacological interventions as a safe and effective treatment practice for this population.

EVIDENCE-BASED ASSESSMENT AND TREATMENT IN PRACTICE

Assessment

Differential Diagnoses

When assessing for anxiety disorders in young children, it is necessary to consider differential diagnoses, specifically, pervasive developmental disorders (PDDs) and other behavioral problems should be considered. Symptoms of PDD or other behavioral problems may appear topographically, similar to symptoms of anxiety; therefore, it is important to assess for the function of the behavior in question. For instance, avoidance in anxiety may look similar to that in oppositional behavior. The anxious child avoids feeling uncomfortable and is having a fear response, whereas the oppositional child seeks some form of reinforcement, such as attention. Additionally, both children with anxiety and those with PDD experience rigidity and desire for predictability, and the clinician should examine the child's social functioning further. It is also sometimes important to consider the differences among mood disorders, eating disorders, tic and other obsessive–compulsive spectrum disorders, and between specific anxiety disorders themselves. This highlights the need to obtain a complete history of the child and pose questions in relation to the function of symptoms, the context in which the symptoms are occurring, and the course of symptoms (Freeman et al., 2012).

Clinical Interview

Versions of structured interviews such as the Schedule for Affective Disorders and Schizophrenia for School-Age Children—Present and Lifetime Versions (K-SADS-PL; Kaufman, Birmaher, Brent, & Rao, 1997) and the Anxiety Disorders Interview Scheduled for DSM-IV: Child and Parent Versions (ADIS-IV-C/P; Silverman & Albano, 1996) have been used effectively in RCTs of young children with anxiety and related problems (Cartwright-Hatton et al., 2011; Donovan & March, 2014; Freeman, Garcia, et al., 2014; Hirshfeld-Becker et al., 2010; Kennedy et al., 2009; Lewin et al., 2014; Waters et al., 2009). The K-SADS is often administered to assess psychiatric diagnoses in children as young as age 5 (Hirshfeld-Becker & Biederman, 2002; Youngstrom, Gracious, Danielson, Findling, & Calabrese, 2003). It is recommended that parents be the main contributors to the interview given that young children's ability to actively participate may vary (Freeman et al., 2012).

Developmental considerations must be made in the assessment process for young children. Interview questions should be tailored to the cognitive and developmental abilities of the presenting child (Freeman et al., 2012). It is challenging for younger children to understand questions that relate to their thoughts, and they have difficulty reflecting on concepts such as estimating, averaging, and duration in relation to their symptom expression (Grave & Blissett, 2004). Freeman and colleagues (2012) emphasize the importance of using concrete examples to obtain child-report information about symptoms and behavior. Parents can be helpful "translators" for their children during this process by providing recent examples and, if necessary, rewording clinicians' questions specific to their own child's understanding (Freeman et al., 2012). The accuracy of child reports is often unclear and clinical judgment must be used in determining how helpful the child's report will be during the assessment (Choudhury, Pimentel, & Kendall, 2003; Freeman et al., 2012; Safford, Kendall, Flannery-Schroeder, Webb, & Sommer, 2005). Clinicians must also be mindful of the shorter attention spans of younger children and maintain a balance between a thorough assessment and the child's cooperation with the assessment (Freeman et al., 2012). Given the young age of the child, the assessment may be families' first contact with the mental health system. Hence, special considerations should be made to ensure the comfort of the children and families (Freeman et al., 2012). This can be achieved through patience in explaining terminology to parents and having fun activities or snacks available for the children.

During assessment, it is important to gather information from multiple informants, so the clinician can obtain a complete picture of the child's symptoms (Kraemer et al., 2003). It is the clinician's role to gather and translate these views into the clinical setting. The method in which the clinician uncovers the child's symptoms through the assessment process will affect the available knowledge for tailoring treatment.

Parent-Report and Self-Report Measures

Parent-report measures such as the Screen for Anxiety Related Disorders—Revised (SCARED-R; Muris, Merckelbach, Van Brakel, & Mayer, 1999) and child-report measures such as the Multidimensional Anxiety Scale for Children (MASC; March, 1997) can provide valuable information to the clinician's assessment. The SCARED-R and MASC are well-established screens for anxiety disorders with children above age 8, yet they have been used in RCTs with younger children with anxiety and related problems (Cartwright-Hatton et al., 2011; Freeman, Garcia, et al., 2014). It is suggested that the MASC be read aloud, and it is most appropriate for children at least 6 years old (Cartwright-Hatton et al., 2011).

The selection and administration of measures to young children must be considered carefully. Children at this age may not be able to complete self-report forms and articulate answers (Freeman et al., 2012). Clinicians must use their judgment when considering child reports of symptoms. Assessment has widely relied on parent reports and clinician observation due to the developmental limitations of young children to reflect on their own mental status (Achenbach, McConaughy, & Howell, 1987; Freeman et al., 2012; Measelle, John, Ablow, Cowan, & Cowan, 2005).

Although limited in number, researchers have developed specific measures for assessing anxiety in a younger population. These measures can be found in Table 17.2.

TABLE 17.2. Assessment Measures for Anxiety in Young Children

Measure	Citation	Reporter	Recommended assessment age of patient	Purpose	Psychometrics
Berkeley Puppet Interview (BPI)	Ablow & Measelle (1993)	Child	Tested in ages 3–6	Screen for emotional and behavioral problems through the interactive use of puppets	Sufficient test–retest reliability, adequate congruent validity, and concurrent validity are supported more for externalizing problems than internalizing problems. It has demonstrated sensitivity to change and was tested in a Dutch community sample.
Child Behavior Checklist (CBCL)	Achenbach (1991)	Parent	Preschool version for ages 1.5–5	Screening for behavioral and emotional problems including subscales for Internalizing and Externalizing symptoms	Good reliability and validity. Very high sensitivity and specificity.
Children's Moods Fears and Worries Questionnaire (CMFWQ)	Broeren & Muris (2008)	Parent	Tested in ages 2–6	Screen for internalizing problems	Demonstrated convergent and discriminant validity in a Dutch community sample and Australian clinical sample.
Picture Anxiety Test (PAT)	Dubi, Lavallee, & Schneider (2012)	Child	Tested in ages 5–7	Assesses anxiety and avoidance	Moderate to high internal consistency, high convergent validity, and high discriminant validity. Researchers encourage its use in conjunction with diagnostic interviews, such as, the Anxiety Disorders Interview Schedule (ADIS). Tested in clinically anxious children and healthy controls.
Koala Fear Questionnaire (KFQ)	Muris et al. (2003)	Child	Tested in ages 4–12	Assesses fears and fearfulness	With older children researchers found support for convergent validity, good internal consistency, and test–retest reliability. Preliminary support for similar psychometrics was reported for younger children.
Preschool Anxiety Scale—Revised (PAS-R)	Edwards, Rapee, Kennedy, & Spence (2010)	Parent	Tested in ages 2–6	Screen for anxiety problems	Moderate to high internal consistency, good test–retest reliability, and established discriminative validity. Tested in a community sample.

508

Other Anxiety Measures

Freeman, Flessner, and Garcia (2011) investigated the use of the Children's Yale–Brown Obsessive Compulsive Scale (CY-BOCS; Scahill, Riddle, McSwiggin-Hardin, & Ort, 1997) with children ages 5–8. The CY-BOCS has been validated for ages 8–17 and assesses current OCD symptoms and severity (Scahill et al., 1997). For use with younger children in an RCT treatment outcome study, the CY-BOCS showed questionable reliability for the Obsessions subscale and good reliability for the Compulsions subscale and Total Scale (Freeman et al., 2011). The Total Scale showed mixed discriminant validity, strong convergent validity, and sensitivity to change. Overall, the preliminary use of the CY-BOCS in a younger population appears promising.

Tailoring Treatment

Key Treatment Components for Treating Anxiety in Young Children

PARENT INVOLVEMENT

Parent involvement is essential, especially while treating younger children (Freeman, Sapyta, et al., 2014; Hirshfeld-Becker & Biederman, 2002; Mian, 2014). Unlike older children, younger children may not have the developmental savvy to generalize treatment outside of therapy sessions. Given the greater dependence of younger children, it is the parents' role to disseminate treatment into the household and serve as their children's treatment "coach" (Ginsburg & Schlossberg, 2002). Parent "buy-in" is necessary for the treatment plan to be consistent, both in therapy sessions and, most importantly, at home. Ensuring that parents receive adequate psychoeducation and truly understand the treatment model further aids their children's treatment.

PSYCHOEDUCATION

Keeping in mind the developmental limitations of young children to understand treatment fully, it is essential that parents completely comprehend the treatment rationale and be capable of following through with it. Young children can better understand the treatment through watching their parents apply CBT principles at home (Freeman et al., 2012). The clinician should provide in detail the expectations of treatment and stress the importance of the parents' full participation in "coaching" their child to approach rather than avoid fearful situations. Unlike treatment for older children, it is recommended that parents attend their own psychoeducation session without their child present (Freeman et al., 2012). This gives the parents an opportunity to process any of their own emotions on the impact of their child's symptoms and also provides an open context for parents to explore the treatment rationale with the clinician (Freeman et al., 2012).

> "No one likes to feel anxious. So, it is only natural that your child avoids anxiety-provoking situations; however, this avoidance is not solving the problem and in fact is causing increased fear of that situation as he or she continues to avoid it. The thing about anxiety is that it always goes down over time—it's a temporary emotion. In treatment we are going to work to encourage approach and discourage avoidance. Meaning that you will encourage your child to be brave through approaching

anxiety-provoking situations and help him or her 'ride out' the anxious feelings without avoiding or escaping from them. Over time, your child's anxiety with that situation will decrease. You will be an important part of your child's treatment. I will guide you in coaching your child to be brave, and it will be your job to make sure that your child continues to practice bravery at home."

The use of examples, visual imagery, and analogies may help to explain more abstract treatment concepts. For instance, it may be useful to draw pictures, such as drawing out the habituation curve for parents. The following is another example of how the process of habituation can be explained through the use of an analogy:

"Have you ever jumped into a pool or the ocean and felt really cold? At first you feel very uncomfortable and you want to get out right away. But what happens if you stay in the water? You get used to it even though the temperature hasn't changed. The same thing happens when you feel nervous. In the same way that your body gets used to temperature, your body gets used to feeling nervous. . . . "

When providing psychoeduction to the child, the clinician should attempt to make it as hands-on, engaging, and simple as possible. The clinician can take advantage of developmentally appropriate materials such as big pieces of paper to draw on with markers or building blocks. At this time, the clinician should introduce to the child the concept of being brave. The clinician may inquire about a favorite athlete, role model, or superhero, explore with the child what challenges that person has overcome, and why it makes that person brave ("How is Superman brave? Do you think he felt scared before defeating the villain? Did he face his fear?"). The child can then reflect back on what makes the hero brave and how he or she can be brave in his or her own life ("How can you be brave like Superman? Do you think you could face [feared stimuli] just like Superman faced the villain?").

If the child engages with this, then the clinician can ask him or her to draw and name his or her anxiety as a supervillain. This externalizing technique has been shown to be especially useful in young children with OCD (March & Mulle, 1998).

FAMILY PROCESS COMPONENTS

Clinicians should be flexible in addressing family process components such as family accommodation, criticism, and blame (Freeman et al., 2012). Parents themselves may be anxious and consequently unaware of how their actions may influence their child's behavior (Last, Hersen, Kazdin, Orvaschel, & Perrin, 1991). Some parents may accommodate their child's anxious symptoms by enabling avoidance, restricting independence, and displaying overprotection (Rapee, Schniering, & Hudson, 2009). Parents often accommodate to protect their child from being distressed, angry, or hostile. This is a natural urge for parents; therefore, it is necessary for the clinician to outline how accommodation can hinder opportunities for their child to be brave on his or her own. It may be helpful for the clinician to address accommodation in a process-oriented rather than a didactic manner (Freeman et al., 2012). Parents should gradually allow their child to act autonomously in anxiety-provoking situations in order to help him or her to build anxiety management skills.

"It is certainly difficult to watch your child experience distress; however, if you continually rescue your child from distress, then he or she will never learn how to handle it on his or her own. The process of rescuing can also incorrectly reinforce your child's perception that the situation is indeed scary and that it warrants rescuing. Your child needs the opportunity to prove to him- or herself that he or she is capable of confronting fears. It will be an exposure for you as parents to tolerate being in the presence of your distressed child. Just as exposures get easier over time with practice for your child, it will get easier for you as parents to watch your child complete them."

The clinician should also work to reduce criticism and hostility related to the child's anxiety symptoms and promote positive family problem solving (Freeman et al., 2012).

"Parents often have a number of thoughts/worries about why their child has anxiety problems. Anxiety is a biological disorder. It is not your child's fault, or yours, that he or she has anxiety. There is nothing that you or your child has 'done' to make him or her have anxiety. It is important not to be critical or angry about these behaviors and to remind yourself that your child is not doing these behaviors on purpose or to upset you."

Barriers to treatment success, such as secondary gains for the child and/or the family, can be explored as well (Freeman et al., 2012).

PARENTING TOOLS

Parenting tools focus on effective management of the young child's anxiety (Freeman et al., 2012). Parents can help shape brave behavior through the use of parenting tools such as differential attention, modeling, and scaffolding (Freeman et al., 2012; Hirshfeld-Becker et al., 2011; Mian, 2014). *Differential attention,* that is, ignoring undesired behaviors and rewarding desired behaviors, should be consistent with an established reward program for the child. For children who are oppositional toward participating, contingency management techniques can be implemented (i.e., the child receives a preferred reward only after trying an exposure). Parents can also model brave behavior for their child. The philosophy of "facing our fears" can become incorporated into the household and foster a supportive family environment. Additionally, through scaffolding, the parents help their child build emotion regulation skills. Parents can guide their child's emotional regulation during anxious moments, helping the child ultimately to internalize his or her response as self-regulation (Freeman et al., 2012). The clinician can have parents reflect on their behavior and on how their child responds and learns from that. All parenting tools should be practiced at home and rehearsed in session.

"You mentioned that you have an important presentation coming up for work. This would be a great opportunity for you to model brave behavior for your child. Share with your child how you were brave in giving your presentation despite feeling anxiety. Children are very much aware of the behavior of others, and they can learn a lot through observation. Modeling treatment-consistent behavior for your child can be very powerful."

EXPOSURE

Exposure is a crucial component to the treatment of anxiety. It teaches the child that there are more options than just avoidance when encountering a scary situation (Freeman et al., 2012). While working with younger children, the clinician should move more slowly up the child's fear hierarchy and exposures should be shorter (Hirshfeld-Becker et al., 2011). The process of creating a fear hierarchy should involve an active collaboration between the parents and their child (Freeman et al., 2012). The child should gradually be exposed to the anxiety-provoking situations until fear decreases. Exposures with younger children should be modified to capture their attention. Whenever possible, exposures should be made into a fun and engaging process, like a game, but not distract them from the feared stimulus (Freeman et al., 2012).

Often during exposure children use a "fear thermometer" to rate their anxiety levels. This tool may be difficult for younger children to use. Adaptation of the thermometer can be based on the child's level of understanding (Freeman et al., 2012). Some children may benefit from more concrete examples, such as pictures of happy and sad faces; varying size cups to express small, medium, or large amounts of discomfort; or a traffic light to indicate that they're feeling green, yellow, or red. The clinician should always bear in mind the child's ability to accurately report on their distress level. Sometimes young children can have an "all-or-nothing" (0 to 10) experience in regard to their anxiety ratings during an exposure task (Freeman et al., 2012). In this case, the clinician should anticipate the pattern and break down the situation for the child while training the parents to identify their child's subtle behavior cues (Freeman et al., 2012). It is important that the clinician reads the child's behavior cues in order to properly titrate the child's exposure in the moment (Freeman et al., 2012). Sometimes the child may not be able to express his or her anxious feelings, in which case the clinician must use his or her own judgment to gauge the difficulty of exposures. Overall, the clinician should encourage a broad, approach-oriented behavioral model for parents to adhere to with their child and especially to practice at home (Freeman et al., 2012).

COGNITIVE TECHNIQUES

Cognitive techniques such as challenging thoughts may be effective with younger children. Studies have shown success with young children distinguishing between negative and positive cognitions, and also reframing thoughts on anxiety-provoking situations as no longer being a prompt to escape (Hirshfeld-Becker et al., 2008; Pahl & Barrett, 2007). Cognitive techniques should not serve as reassurance during an exposure, but rather as a postprocessing tool. Once the child's anxiety has decreased, the clinician can help to identify how the child previously overestimated the amount of danger and/or underestimated his or her own ability to face it.

> "Wow! You did a great job practicing [exposure]. Beforehand you were really worried about [feared consequence], and you thought that you wouldn't be able to face it. Did that bad thing happen? How do you think you did? I know it was scary for you at first, but I noticed that it got easier after a while. You were so brave for sticking with it."

ADDRESSING MOTIVATION

It is especially important that young children receive external motivators for their successes during treatment. Often young children lack intrinsic motivation because they may not have gained the appropriate insight into their symptoms and may not see how those symptoms negatively affect their environment. The clinician and parents can come up with a rewards system to address this need. The child should receive immediate rewards for brave behavior, such as attention through praise and a star on his or her chart that he or she can "cash-in" for a tangible prize.

> "A reward is a form of positive attention that is very effective in increasing behaviors you want to see more of. All of us need rewards to do things that are challenging—for example, most of us would not go to work every day unless we received a paycheck. We will be asking your child to change some behaviors that will likely be pretty challenging for him or her to do. A positive reward plan will be an important motivator to help your child face his or her fears. When talking about positive rewards, sometimes parents think it sounds like bribing their child to behave; however, positive rewards are actually very different from bribery. The major difference is that these types of rewards are planned and proactive. Rewards are connected to specific behaviors, both of which have been determined ahead of time. The rewards are set up ahead of time to help your child stay motivated to control his or her behavior and to make good behavioral choices. This is very different than pulling rewards out because of desperation (e.g., giving a child having a tantrum in a toy store a toy to get him or her to be quiet)."

Early in treatment, the clinician can inquire about how anxious symptoms get in the way of things that the child likes doing. Family members can be particularly helpful in identifying concrete examples of how the child's symptoms are impairing. Some reasons a child would want to beat anxiety may include the following: Symptoms take up time, they make the child feel uncomfortable, and they cause arguments between the child and parents. It may be useful to revisit these reasons throughout the course of treatment to boost motivation.

Treatment Protocols

Overall, the following treatment adaptations are crucial in treating younger children with anxiety: (1) Parents need to be involved in all phases of treatment; (2) clinicians should make special considerations for the individual child's developmental characteristics and tailor psychoeducation, exposures, and homework tasks, respectively; and (3) the family context (patterns of family accommodation, lack of familiarity with the mental health system, and parental psychopathology), particularly the parents' responses to their child's anxieties, should be understood by the clinician (Freeman et al., 2012).

This treatment is intentionally geared toward changing the parents' behavior and having the young child follow suit. Parents experience their own "exposure" throughout the course of treatment as they learn to tolerate their own anxiety in the face of supporting their distressed child through difficult tasks both at home and in session (Freeman et al., 2012).

TABLE 17.3. Outline of Treatment Protocol for Young Children with Anxiety Disorders

Duration	Focus/objective	Homework
Two sessions without the child present; should be revisited at last session on maintaining gains	Psychoeducation for parents • Provide education about anxiety • Differentiating between anxious and nonanxious behaviors • Describe treatment in detail • Stress the importance of family involvement • Address parents' own anxieties	Have parents be keen observers of their child's behavior and their reactions to it. Parents can relate the "ABC's" (Antecedents, Behavior, and Consequence) to situations in order to further their own understanding of the anxiety process.
Two sessions; dependent on child's level of understanding	Psychoeducation for child • Concrete and specific in explaining anxiety. Can use pictorial treatment aids or incorporate stories or cartoons • Provide rationale for being brave (introduction to exposures)	Explore brave role models with the child and have parents help the child to identify anxiety in the moment.
Two sessions; may be paired with parent psychoeducation but relevant throughout treatment	Family process issues • Reducing accommodation • Reducing criticism • Promoting positive family problem solving • Increasing parents own understanding of modeling anxiety	Have parents identify and change their behaviors that perpetuate the anxious cycle, such as excessive reassurance. The parents should prompt and assist their child in problem solving when anxious situations arise.
Eight or more sessions; throughout the remainder of treatment and concurrent with "Child Tools." At this point the clinician can revisit any previous treatment components as needed.	Parent tools • Parents are "coaches" for their child • Differential attention • Modeling • Scaffolding • Frequent and immediate reinforcement such as stickers or small prizes for desired behaviors • Hierarchy building (along with the clinician) • Reinforcement of brave behavior • Clinician models how to assist the child during exposure in session for parents • Parents practice exposure with their child at home • Problem solving	Parents should be modeling brave behavior. The child receives praise and rewards at home for brave behavior. The parents should make exposures a daily practice for homework and reinforce their child for trying.
	Child tools • Externalizing (optional) • Fear thermometer to rate anxiety • Learning about exposures • Making exposures playful, fun, and engaging but not distracting; when it can't be fun, make it rewarding through positive reinforcement • Cognitive techniques • Problem solving	Have the child with parent assistance regularly practice exposures and problem solving at home and in session.

A treatment protocol guideline largely based on Hirshfeld-Becker and colleagues' (2010) Being Brave program and Freeman and colleagues' (2012) POTS Jr may be found in Table 17.3.

CONCLUSION

Anxiety in young children is of clinical importance. It is clearly prevalent, yet there is only beginning research on effective assessment and treatment approaches. While treating younger children with anxiety, clinicians should be mindful of the individual child's ability to understand treatment and tailor his or her approach accordingly. Preliminary support exists for developmentally sensitive downward extensions of CBT treatment protocols, but further investigation is definitely warranted.

REFERENCES

Ablow, J., & Measelle, J. (1993). *The Berkeley Puppet Interview (BPI): Interviewing and coding system manuals*. Berkeley: University of California, Department of Psychology.

Achenbach, T. M. (1991). *Manual for the Child Behavior Checklist/4–18 and 1991 profile*. Burlington: University of Vermont, Department of Psychiatry.

Achenbach, T. M., McConaughy, S. H., & Howell, C. T. (1987). Child/adolescent behavioral and emotional problems: Implications of cross-informant correlations for situational specificity. *Psychological Bulletin, 101*(2), 213–232.

American Psychiatric Association. (2013). *Diagnostic and statistical manual of mental disorders* (5th ed.). Arlington, VA: Author.

Angold, A., & Costello, E. J. (1993). Depressive comorbidity in children and adolescents. *American Journal of Psychiatry, 150*(12), 1779–1791.

Anticich, S. A. J., Barrett, P. M., Silverman, W., Lacherez, P., & Gillies, R. (2013). The prevention of childhood anxiety and promotion of resilience among preschool-aged children: A universal school based trial. *Advances in School Mental Health Promotion, 6*(2), 93–121.

Arch, J. J., Eifert, G. H., Davies, C., Vilardaga, J. C. P., Rose, R. D., & Craske, M. G. (2012). Randomized clinical trial of cognitive behavioral therapy (CBT) versus acceptance and commitment therapy (ACT) for mixed anxiety disorders. *Journal of Consulting and Clinical Psychology, 80*(5), 750–765.

Barterian, J. A., & Rappuhn, E. (2014). Current state of evidence for medication treatment of preschool internalizing disorders. *Scientific World Journal, 2014*, Article 286085.

Behar, L. B. (1977). The Preschool Behavior Questionnaire. *Journal of Abnormal Child Psychology, 5*(3), 265–275.

Biederman, J., Rosenbaum, J. F., Bolduc-Murphy, E. A., Faraone, S. V., Chaloff, J., Hirshfeld, D. R., et al. (1993). A 3-year follow-up of children with and without behavioral inhibition. *Journal of the American Academy of Child and Adolescent Psychiatry, 32*(4), 814–821.

Broeren, S., & Muris, P. (2008). Psychometric evaluation of two new parent-rating scales for measuring anxiety symptoms in young Dutch children. *Journal of Anxiety Disorders, 22*(6), 949–958.

Cartwright-Hatton, S. (2013). Treating anxiety in early life. *British Journal of Psychiatry, 203*(6), 401–402.

Cartwright-Hatton, S., McNally, D., Field, A. P., Rust, S., Laskey, B., Dixon, C., et al. (2011). A new parenting-based group intervention for young anxious children: Results of a randomized controlled trial. *Journal of the American Academy of Child and Adolescent Psychiatry, 50*(3), 242–251.

Cartwright-Hatton, S., McNally, D., & White, C. (2005). A new cognitive behavioural parenting intervention for families of young anxious children: A pilot study. *Behavioural and Cognitive Psychotherapy, 33*(2), 243–247.

Choate, M. L., Pincus, D. B., Eyberg, S. M., & Barlow, D. H. (2005). Parent–child interaction therapy for treatment of separation anxiety disorder in young children: A pilot study. *Cognitive and Behavioral Practice, 12*(1), 126–135.

Choudhury, M. S., Pimentel, S. S., & Kendall, P. C. (2003). Childhood anxiety disorders: Parent–child (dis)agreement using a structured interview for the DSM-IV. *Journal of the American Academy of Child and Adolescent Psychiatry, 42*(8), 957–964.

Comer, J. S., Furr, J. M., Cooper-Vince, C. E., Kerns, C. E., Chan, P. T., Edson, A. L., et al. (2014). Internet-delivered, family-based treatment for early-onset OCD: A preliminary case series. *Journal of Clinical Child and Adolescent Psychology, 43*(1), 74–87.

Comer, J. S., Puliafico, A. C., Aschenbrand, S. G., McKnight, K., Robin, J. A., Goldfine, M. E., et al. (2012). A pilot feasibility evaluation of the CALM program for anxiety disorders in early childhood. *Journal of Anxiety Disorders, 26*(1), 40–49.

Connolly, S. D., & Bernstein, G. A. (2007). Practice parameter for the assessment and treatment of children and adolescents with anxiety disorders. *Journal of the American Academy of Child and Adolescent Psychiatry, 46*(2), 267–283.

Copeland, W. E., Angold, A., Shanahan, L., & Costello, E. J. (2014). Longitudinal patterns of anxiety from childhood to adulthood: The Great Smoky Mountains study. *Journal of the American Academy of Child and Adolescent Psychiatry, 53*(1), 21–33.

Costello, E. J., Egger, H. L., & Angold, A. (2004). Developmental epidemiology of anxiety disorders. In T. H. Ollendick & J. S. March (Eds.), *Phobic and anxiety disorders in children and adolescents: A clinician's guide to effective psychosocial and pharmacological interventions.* (pp. 61–91). New York: Oxford University Press.

Coyne, L. W., McHugh, L., & Martinez, E. R. (2011). Acceptance and commitment therapy (ACT): Advances and applications with children, adolescents, and families. *Child and Adolescent Psychiatric Clinics of North America, 20*(2), 379–399.

Craske, M. G., Niles, A. N., Burklund, L. J., Wolitzky-Taylor, K. B., Vilardaga, J. C. P., Arch, J. J., et al. (2014). Randomized controlled trial of cognitive behavioral therapy and acceptance and commitment therapy for social phobia: Outcomes and moderators. *Journal of Consulting and Clinical Psychology, 82*(6), 1034–1048.

Donovan, C. L., & March, S. (2014). Online CBT for preschool anxiety disorders: A randomised control trial. *Behaviour Research and Therapy, 58*, 24–35.

Dubi, K., Lavallee, K. L., & Schneider, S. (2012). The Picture Anxiety Test (PAT): Psychometric properties in a community sample of young children. *Swiss Journal of Psychology, 71*(2), 73–81.

Edwards, S. L., Rapee, R. M., Kennedy, S. J., & Spence, S. H. (2010). The assessment of anxiety symptoms in preschool-aged children: The revised Preschool Anxiety Scale. *Journal of Clinical Child and Adolescent Psychology, 39*(3), 400–409.

Egger, H. L., & Angold, A. (2006). Common emotional and behavioral disorders in preschool children: presentation, nosology, and epidemiology. *Journal of Child Psychology and Psychiatry, 47*(3–4), 313–337.

Fox, J. K., Warner, C. M., Lerner, A. B., Ludwig, K., Ryan, J. L., Colognori, D., et al. (2012). Preventive intervention for anxious preschoolers and their parents: Strengthening early emotional development. *Child Psychiatry and Human Development, 43*(4), 544–559.

Freeman, J., Flessner, C. A., & Garcia, A. (2011). The Children's Yale–Brown Obsessive Compulsive Scale: Reliability and validity for use among 5 to 8 year olds with obsessive–compulsive disorder. *Journal of Abnormal Child Psychology, 39*(6), 877–883.

Freeman, J., Garcia, A., Benito, K., Conelea, C., Sapyta, J., Khanna, M., et al. (2012). The Pediatric Obsessive Compulsive Disorder Treatment Study for Young Children (POTS Jr): Developmental considerations in the rationale, design, and methods. *Journal of Obsessive–Compulsive and Related Disorders, 1*(4), 294–300.

Freeman, J., Garcia, A. M., Coyne, L., Ale, C., Przeworski, A., Himle, M., et al. (2008). Early childhood OCD: Preliminary findings from a family-based cognitive-behavioral approach. *Journal of the American Academy of Child and Adolescent Psychiatry, 47*(5), 593–602.

Freeman, J., Garcia, A., Frank, H., Benito, K., Conelea, C., Walther, M., et al. (2014). Evidence base update for psychosocial treatments for pediatric obsessive–compulsive disorder. *Journal of Clinical Child and Adolescent Psychology, 43*(1), 7–26.

Freeman, J., Sapyta, J., Garcia, A., Compton, S., Khanna, M., Flessner, C., et al. (2014). Family-based treatment of early childhood obsessive–compulsive disorder: The Pediatric Obsessive–Compulsive Disorder Treatment Study for Young Children (POTS Jr)—a randomized clinical trial. *JAMA Psychiatry, 71*(6), 689–698.

Ginsburg, G. S., Burstein, M., Becker, K. D., & Drake, K. L. (2011). Treatment of obsessive compulsive disorder in young children: An intervention model and case series. *Child and Family Behavior Therapy, 33*(2), 97–122.

Ginsburg, G. S., & Schlossberg, M. C. (2002). Family-based treatment of childhood anxiety disorders. *International Review of Psychiatry, 14*(2), 143–154.

Gleason, M. M., Egger, H. L., Emslie, G. J., Greenhill, L. L., Kowatch, R. A., Lieberman, A. F., et al. (2007). Psychopharmacological treatment for very young children: Contexts and guidelines. *Journal of the American Academy of Child and Adolescent Psychiatry, 46*(12), 1532–1572.

Grave, J., & Blissett, J. (2004). Is cognitive behavior therapy developmentally appropriate for young children?: A critical review of the evidence. *Clinical Psychology Review, 24*(4), 399–420.

Guy, W. (1976). *Clinical global impressions ECDEU Asessment Manual for Psychopharmacology* (pp. 218–222). Rockville, MD: National Institute for Mental Health.

Hirshfeld, D. R., Biederman, J., Brody, L., Faraone, S. V., & Rosenbaum, J. F. (1997). Associations between expressed emotion and child behavioral inhibition and psychopathology: A pilot study. *Journal of the American Academy of Child and Adolescent Psychiatry, 36*(2), 205–213.

Hirshfeld-Becker, D. R., & Biederman, J. (2002). Rationale and principles for early intervention with young children at risk for anxiety disorders. *Clinical Child and Family Psychology Review, 5*(3), 161–172.

Hirshfeld-Becker, D. R., Masek, B., Henin, A., Blakely, L. R., Pollock-Wurman, R. A., McQuade, J., et al. (2010). Cognitive behavioral therapy for 4- to 7-year-old children with anxiety disorders: A randomized clinical trial. *Journal of Consulting and Clinical Psychology, 78*(4), 498–510.

Hirshfeld-Becker, D. R., Masek, B., Henin, A., Blakely, L. R., Rettew, D. C., Dufton, L., et al. (2008). Cognitive-behavioral intervention with young anxious children. *Harvard Review of Psychiatry, 16*(2), 113–125.

Hirshfeld-Becker, D. R., Micco, J. A., Mazursky, H., Bruett, L., & Henin, A. (2011). Applying cognitive-behavioral therapy for anxiety to the younger child. *Child and Adolescent Psychiatric Clinics of North America, 20*(2), 349–368.

Ialongo, N., Edelsohn, G., Werthamer-Larsson, L., Crockett, L., & Kellam, S. (1995). The significance of self-reported anxious symptoms in first grade children: Prediction to anxious symptoms and adaptive functioning in fifth grade. *Journal of Child Psychology and Psychiatry, 36*(3), 427–437.

Kagan, J., & Snidman, N. (1999). Early childhood predictors of adult anxiety disorders. *Biological Psychiatry, 46*(11), 1536–1541.

Karevold, E., Roysamb, E., Youngstrom, E., & Mathiesen, K. S. (2009). Predictors and pathways from infancy to symptoms of anxiety and depression in early adolescence. *Developmental Psychology, 45*(4), 1051–1060.

Kaufman, J., Birmaher, B., Brent, D., & Rao, U. (1997). Schedule for Affective Disorders and Schizophrenia for School-Age Children—Present and Lifetime version (K-SADS-PL): Initial reliability and validity data. *Journal of the American Academy of Child and Adolescent Psychiatry, 36*(7), 980–988.

Kendall, P. C., Brady, E. U., & Verduin, T. L. (2001). Comorbidity in childhood anxiety disorders and treatment outcome. *Journal of the American Academy of Child and Adolescent Psychiatry, 40*(7), 787–794.

Kendall, P. C., Compton, S. N., Walkup, J. T., Birmaher, B., Albano, A. M., Sherrill, J., et al. (2010). Clinical characteristics of anxiety disordered youth. *Journal of Anxiety Disorders, 24*(3), 360–365.

Kendall, P. C., & Hedtke, K. A. (2006). *The Coping Cat workbook.* Ardmore, PA: Workbook.

Kennedy, S. J., Rapee, R. M., & Edwards, S. L. (2009). A selective intervention program for inhibited preschool-aged children of parents with an anxiety disorder: Effects on current anxiety disorders and temperament. *Journal of the American Academy of Child and Adolescent Psychiatry, 48*(6), 602–609.

Kraemer, H. C., Measelle, J. R., Ablow, J. C., Essex, M. J., Boyce, W. T., & Kupfer, D. J. (2003). A new approach to integrating data from multiple informants in psychiatric assessment and research: Mixing and matching contexts and perspectives. *American Journal of Psychiatry, 160*(9), 1566–1577.

Labouliere, C. D., Arnold, E. B., Storch, E. A., & Lewin, A. B. (2014). Family-based cognitive-behavioral treatment for a preschooler with obsessive–compulsive disorder. *Clinical Case Studies, 13*(1), 37–51.

Last, C. G., Hersen, M., Kazdin, A., Orvaschel, H., & Perrin, S. (1991). Anxiety disorders in children and their families. *Archives of General Psychiatry, 48*(10), 928–934.

Lewin, A. B., Park, J. M., Jones, A. M., Crawford, E. A., De Nadai, A. S., Menzel, J., et al. (2014). Family-based exposure and response prevention therapy for preschool-aged children with obsessive–compulsive disorder: A pilot randomized controlled trial. *Behaviour Research and Therapy, 56*, 30–38.

Lewinsohn, P. M., Zinbarg, R., Seeley, J. R., Lewinsohn, M., & Sack, W. H. (1997). Lifetime comorbidity among anxiety disorders and between anxiety disorders and other mental disorders in adolescents. *Journal of Anxiety Disorders, 11*(4), 377–394.

Manassis, K., & Monga, S. (2001). A therapeutic approach to children and adolescents with anxiety disorders and associated comorbid conditions. *Journal of the American Academy of Child and Adolescent Psychiatry, 40*(1), 115–117.

March, J. S. (1997). *Multidimensional Anxiety Scale for Children.* North Tonawanda, NY: Multi-Health Systems.

March, J. S., & Mulle, K. (1998). *OCD in children and adolescents: A cognitive-behavioral treatment manual.* New York: Guilford Press.

McNeil, C., & Hembree-Kigin, T. (2010). *Parent–child interaction therapy.* New York: Springer-Verlag.

Measelle, J. R., John, O. P., Ablow, J. C., Cowan, P. A., & Cowan, C. P. (2005). Can children provide coherent, stable, and valid self-reports on the big five dimensions?: A longitudinal study from ages 5 to 7. *Journal of Personality and Social Psychology, 89*(1), 90–106.

Merikangas, K. R. (2011). What is a case?: New lessons from the Great Smoky Mountains Study. *Journal of the American Academy of Child and Adolescent Psychiatry, 50*(3), 213–215.

Mian, N. D. (2014). Little children with big worries: Addressing the needs of young, anxious children and the problem of parent engagement. *Clinical Child and Family Pscholology Review, 17*(1), 85–96.

Monga, S., Young, A., & Owens, M. (2009). Evaluating a cognitive behavioral therapy group program for anxious five to seven year old children: A pilot study. *Depression and Anxiety, 26*(3), 243–250.

Muris, P., Meesters, C., Mayer, B., Bogie, N., Luijten, M., Geebelen, E., et al. (2003). The Koala Fear Questionnaire: A standardized self-report scale for assessing fears and fearfulness in pre-school and primary school children. *Behaviour Research and Therapy, 41*(5), 597–617.

Muris, P., Merckelbach, H., Van Brakel, A., & Mayer, A. B. (1999). The revised version of the Screen for Child Anxiety Related Emotional Disorders (SCARED-R): Further evidence for its reliability and validity. *Anxiety Stress, and Coping, 12*(4), 411–425.

Oerbeck, B., Johansen, J., Lundahl, K., & Kristensen, H. (2012). Selective mutism: A home- and kindergarten-based intervention for children 3–5 years: A pilot study. *Clinical Child Psychology and Psychiatry, 17*(3), 370–383.

Pahl, K. M., & Barrett, P. M. (2007). The development of social–emotional competence in preschool-aged children: An introduction to the Fun FRIENDS Program. *Australian Journal of Guidance and Counselling, 17*(1), 81–90.

Pavuluri, M. N., Luk, S. L., & McGee, R. (1996). Help-seeking for behavior problems by parents of preschool children: A community study. *Journal of the American Academy of Child and Adolescent Psychiatry, 35*(2), 215–222.

Pediatric OCD Treatment Study Team. (2004). Cognitive-behavior therapy, sertraline, and their combination for children and adolescents with obsessive–compulsive disorder: The Pediatric OCD Treatment Study (POTS) randomized controlled trial. *Journal of the American Medical Association, 292*(16), 1969–1976.

Pincus, D. B., Eyberg, S. M., & Choate, M. L. (2005). Adapting parent–child interaction therapy for young children with separation anxiety disorder. *Education and Treatment of Children, 28*(2), 163–181.

Pincus, D. B., Santucci, L. C., Ehrenreich, J. T., & Eyberg, S. M. (2008). The implementation of modified parent–child interaction therapy for youth with separation anxiety disorder. *Cognitive and Behavioral Practice, 15*(2), 118–125.

Puliafico, A. C., Comer, J. S., & Albano, A. M. (2013). Coaching approach behavior and leading by modeling: Rationale, principles, and a session-by-session description of the CALM program for early childhood anxiety. *Cognitive and Behavioral Practice, 20*(4), 517–528.

Rapee, R. M. (1997). Potential role of childrearing practices in the development of anxiety and depression. *Clinical Psychology Review, 17*(1), 47–67.

Rapee, R. M. (2013). The preventative effects of a brief, early intervention for preschool-aged children at risk for internalising: Follow-up into middle adolescence. *Journal of Child Psychology and Psychiatry, 54*(7), 780–788.

Rapee, R. M., Kennedy, S., Ingram, M., Edwards, S., & Sweeney, L. (2005). Prevention and early intervention of anxiety disorders in inhibited preschool children. *Journal of Consulting and Clinical Psychology, 73*(3), 488–497.

Rapee, R. M., Kennedy, S. J., Ingram, M., Edwards, S. L., & Sweeney, L. (2010). Altering the trajectory of anxiety in at-risk young children. *American Journal of Psychiatry, 167*(12), 1518–1525.

Rapee, R. M., Schniering, C. A., & Hudson, J. L. (2009). Anxiety disorders during childhood and adolescence: Origins and treatment. *Annual Review of Clinical Psychology, 5*, 311–341.

Safford, S. M., Kendall, P. C., Flannery-Schroeder, E., Webb, A., & Sommer, H. (2005). A longitudinal look at parent–child diagnostic agreement in youth treated for anxiety disorders. *Journal of Clinical Child and Adolescent Psychology, 34*(4), 747–757.

Santacruz, I., Méndez, F. J., & Sánchez-Meca, J. (2006). Play therapy applied by parents for children with darkness phobia: Comparison of two programmes. *Child and Family Behavior Therapy, 28*(1), 19–35.

Scahill, L., Riddle, M. A., McSwiggin-Hardin, M., & Ort, S. I. (1997). Children's Yale–Brown Obsessive Compulsive Scale: Reliability and validity. *Journal of the American Academy of Child and Adolescent Psychiatry, 36*(6), 844–852.

Schneider, S., Blatter-Meunier, J., Herren, C., Adornetto, C., In-Albon, T., & Lavallee, K. (2011). Disorder-specific cognitive-behavioral therapy for separation anxiety disorder in young children: A randomized waiting-list-controlled trial. *Psychotherapy and Psychosomatics, 80*(4), 206–215.

Silverman, W. K., & Albano, A. M. (1996). *Anxiety Disorders Interview Schedule for DSMI-IV Child version: Clinical manual.* Albany, NY: Graywind.

Twohig, M. P., Abramowitz, J. S., Bluett, E. J., Fabricant, L. E., Jacoby, R. J., Morrison, K. L., et al. (2015). Exposure therapy for OCD from an acceptance and commitment therapy (ACT) framework. *Journal of Obsessive–Compulsive and Related Disorders, 6,* 167–173.

van der Sluis, C. M., van der Bruggen, C. O., Brechman-Toussaint, M. L., Thissen, M. A., & Bogels, S. M. (2012). Parent-directed cognitive behavioral therapy for young anxious children: A pilot study. *Behavior Therapy, 43*(3), 583–592.

Warren, S. L., Huston, L., Egeland, B., & Sroufe, L. A. (1997). Child and adolescent anxiety disorders and early attachment. *Journal of the American Academy of Child and Adolescent Psychiatry, 36*(5), 637–644.

Waters, A. M., Ford, L. A., Wharton, T. A., & Cobham, V. E. (2009). Cognitive-behavioural therapy for young children with anxiety disorders: Comparison of a Child + Parent condition versus a Parent Only condition. *Behaviour Research and Therapy, 47*(8), 654–662.

Wichstrom, L., Belsky, J., & Berg-Nielsen, T. S. (2013). Preschool predictors of childhood anxiety disorders: A prospective community study. *Journal of Child Psychology and Psychiatry, 54*(12), 1327–1336.

Youngstrom, E., Gracious, B., Danielson, C., Findling, R., & Calabrese, J. (2003). Toward an integration of parent and clinician report on the Young Mania Rating Scale. *Journal of Affective Disorders, 77*(2), 179–190.

CHAPTER 18

Transdiagnostic Approaches and Sleep Disturbance

Allison G. Harvey

While progress toward establishing evidence-based psychological treatments for most mental disorders has been excellent, much work remains. As summarized elsewhere (Harvey & Gumport, 2015), the effect sizes can be small to moderate, gains may not persist, and there are a small proportion of patients who derive little or no benefit. Hence, there is an ongoing need for innovation to develop new treatments and to continue to improve existing ones. This is a domain in which our field has been active and successful, yet there is great need for continued progress.

ARE THERE ADVANTAGES TO TRANSDIAGNOSTIC APPROACHES?

There are a range of rigorous review processes that have compiled lists of evidence-based psychological treatments (e.g., *www.psychologicaltreatments.org*; *www.nrepp.samhsa. gov*; National Institute for Health and Care Excellence [NICE]). It seems highly unlikely that any one therapist will be able to master them all. The problem that emerges is known as the "too many empirically supported treatments problem" (Weisz, Ng, & Bearman, 2014, p. 68). One relatively new treatment—the transdiagnostic approach—holds potential for contributing to a resolution of this problem.

The transdiagnostic approach involves targeting treatment at a *transdiagnostic process,* defined as a common process that occurs across more than one mental disorder (e.g., Barlow, Allen, & Choate, 2004; Fairburn, Cooper, & Shafran, 2003; Harvey, Watkins, Mansell, & Shafran, 2004; Kring & Sloan, 2009). This is in contrast to the approach that most groups tend to use, the *disorder-focused* approach, in which researchers tend to target a specific disorder and try to understand the etiology and maintenance of that one disorder so as to develop more effective strategies to treat that disorder. There is no doubt that the disorder-focused approach has greatly advanced our understanding of, and ability to treat, several mental disorders. However, it is suggested that there may be several advantages in having more research groups work transdiagnostically.

First, if a transdiagnostic process contributes to the maintenance of symptoms across multiple disorders, then one potentially powerful approach would be to focus treatment on that process rather than on the large number of discrete disorders currently listed in DSM-5. In this way, perhaps a transdiagnostic perspective would result in more effective and efficient treatments. This is an empirical question that has yet to be explored.

Second, *comorbidity,* or the coexistence of two or more disorders (Angold, Costello, & Erkanli, 1999; de Graaf, Bijl, Smit, Vollebergh, & Spijker, 2002) is a major challenge for clinicians. It is clear that comorbidity is the norm rather than the exception for mental illness. Indeed, a staggering 50% of people who meet diagnostic criteria for a mental disorder in a specific year meet criteria for more than one disorder (Kessler, Chiu, Demler, Merikangas, & Walters, 2005). Hence, a problem faced by clinicians is which disorder/s to prioritize when developing a treatment plan. Treating transdiagnostic processes, or processes common across the comorbidities, provides one path forward. It is noteworthy that the comorbidity picture is particularly complicated in youth. Garber and Weersing (2010) highlight that comorbidity varies by age and developmental stage. For example, anxiety is more prevalent in children, rates of depression increase in teens, and comorbid anxiety and depression tend to be more prevalent in older than in younger teens. Interestingly, anxiety and depression are not distinguishable in young children (third graders). However, after just a few more years of development, anxiety and depression have become distinguishable (Cole, Truglio, & Peeke, 1997). Indeed, Ehrenreich-May and Chu (2013, pp. 3–4) note that "in child and adolescent populations, the call for transdiagnostic approaches is even more relevant. High comorbidity rates, shifting symptom profiles, and complex family contexts all complicate the typical treatment approach." An empirical question for the future will be to delineate the transdiagnostic processes that are common across the fluctuating anxiety and depression symptoms observed in youth.

Finally, as already mentioned, a transdiagnostic approach may reduce the current heavy burden on clinicians, who must learn multiple disorder-focused protocols, often with common theoretical underpinnings and interventions. Moreover, a transdiagnostic approach might lead the field to be able to specify a single treatment or treatment components that are effective across a wide range of disorders (Harvey et al., 2004; Mansell, Harvey, Watkins, & Shafran, 2009). If this turned out to be possible it would certainly have an impact on the "too many empirically supported treatments problem" (Weisz, et al., 2014, p. 68).

A BRIEF STATUS UPDATE ON PROGRESS TOWARD ESTABLISHING TRANSDIAGNOSTIC EVIDENCE-BASED PSYCHOLOGICAL TREATMENTS

There continues to be very nice progress toward developing transdiagnostic treatments that target transdiagnostic processes. As summarized elsewhere (Harvey & Gumport, 2015), examples include treatments that focus across the anxiety disorders and depression in adults (Craske et al., 2011; Farchione et al., 2012; McManus, Shafran, & Cooper, 2010; Norton, 2012); across anxiety, depression, and conduct problems in youth (Bilek & Ehrenreich-May, 2012; Fraire & Ollendick, 2013; Weisz et al., 2012); across all of the eating disorders (Fairburn et al., 2009), as well as schizophrenia (Bentall et al., 2009), bipolar disorder (Ellard, Deckersbach, Sylvia, Nierenberg, & Barlow, 2012), and sleep problems (Harvey, 2008, 2009; Harvey, Murray, Chandler, & Soehner, 2011). Also, specific treatments targeting transdiagnostic processes, such as rumination (Nolen-Hoeksema & Watkins, 2011) and perfectionism (Egan, Wade, & Shafran, 2011), have been shown to be effective (Riley, Lee, Cooper, Fairburn, & Shafran, 2007; Watkins et al., 2011).

A particularly successful youth transdiagnostic treatment—the modular approach to therapy for children (MATCH)—provides an approach to treating anxiety, depression, and conduct problems (Weisz et al., 2012). In an evaluation of MATCH, a total of 84 community clinicians were randomly assigned to one of three conditions for the treatment of 174 clinically referred youth ages 7–13 years: usual care, standard manualized disorder-focused treatment (i.e., cognitive behavioral therapy for depression, cognitive behavioral therapy for anxiety, and behavioral parent training for conduct problems), or a modular treatment that integrates the procedures from the three separate treatments and includes detailed guides for therapists as to the conditions under which the various elements should be administered. The best outcome was observed for the modular treatment (MATCH), which produced significantly steeper trajectories of improvement relative to both usual care and to standard manualized disorder-focused treatment. Notably, outcomes from the disorder-focused manualized treatments did not differ significantly from the outcomes of usual care (Weisz et al., 2012). This study was conducted across outpatient settings (i.e., not in a university/medical school setting), and 40% of the therapists were social workers, 24% were psychologists, and 36% had various other qualifications. This is a much more representative sample of mental health providers than is typical in treatment research conducted in university settings. This research represents an encouraging "new wave" of research that is actually conducted in the settings for which it is intended and demonstrates the potential utility of transdiagnostic and modular treatments.

RESEARCH DOMAIN CRITERIA

Any discussion of transdiagnostic approaches would not be complete without mention of the Research Domain Criteria (RDoC), an important initiative of the National Institute of Mental Health in the United States. It is a massive effort that is decidedly transdiagnostic. The encouragement is to focus future research on determining the common processes and the specific processes by comparing *across* mental disorders. Instead, the mandate is to conduct research on genes, molecules, cells, physiology, behavior, and self-reports within one or more research domains *across disorders* (Insel et al., 2010). Sleep and circadian rhythms are one of the research domains specified within RDoC. The domains have been defined on the basis of their potential as *causal mechanisms in mental disorders*. In other words, this effort "uncouples research efforts from clinically familiar diagnostic categories to focus directly on fundamental mechanisms of psychopathology" in the hope of speeding progress toward discovering new and more effective treatments (Sanislow et al., 2010, p. 631)

IS THE TRANSDIAGNOSTIC PERSPECTIVE NEW?

There are ways in which the approach to psychopathology in youth has always been more "transdiagnostic" relative to the adult literature. For example, the Coping Cat (Kendall & Hedtke, 2006) is a treatment designed for children ages 8–13 who have generalized anxiety disorder, separation anxiety disorder, or social anxiety disorder. In other words, this treatment cuts across anxiety disorders. In adults, there tend to be different protocols for each anxiety disorder. Also, as we have previously highlighted (Harvey et al., 2004), the importance of cognitive and behavioral processes in mental disorders has long been recognized by clinicians and researchers. For example, research on behavioral processes, such as conditioning and reinforcement contingencies, led to a range of treatments and techniques that were largely transdiagnostic and came to be known collectively as behavior therapy (Pavlov, 1928; Skinner, 1959; Watson & Rayner, 1920; Wolpe, 1958). Also, A. T. Beck (1967) had a common proposal that he recognized as relevant across the disorders: that cognitive processes, including unhelpful beliefs, illogical thinking, and distorted perception, were crucial to understanding and treating mental disorders. These ideas led to the birth of cognitive therapy and cognitive-behavioral therapy.

THE DEVELOPMENT OF A
TRANSDIAGNOSTIC SLEEP AND CIRCADIAN INTERVENTION

For the remainder of this chapter I describe a transdiagnostic sleep and circadian treatment for youth (TranS-C-Youth) that is currently being tested. A fair question to ask is: Why develop such a transdiagnostic intervention for youth?

First, sleep problems in youth are complicated and tend to not fit into neat DSM-5 categories. A brief description of the common DSM-5 diagnoses during the teenage years are presented in Table 18.1. However, real-life sleep and circadian problems are not so neatly categorized. Indeed, there is evidence that, in youth, insomnia can overlap with hypersomnia (Breslau, Roth, Rosenthal, & Andreski, 1996; Liu et al., 2007), delayed sleep phase (Giglio et al., 2010), and irregular sleep–wake schedules. Although there is a need for longitudinal studies to verify this clinical impression, during assessments, many youth report changes to the specific type of sleep problem they experience over development. So while there are disorder-focused treatments for specific types of sleep disturbance, such as insomnia, in specific diagnostic groups such as depression (Clarke et al., 2015), a TranS-C-Youth—one that includes modules covering all of the sleep problems experienced by youth and whose selection is based on the specific sleep problems present—may be more helpful.

We illustrate this point more fully by describing the typical set of sleep-related vicious cycles experienced by youth. As we describe these, we invite the reader to notice the lack of fit between this clinical picture and DSM-5 categories in Table 18.1. As described elsewhere (Harvey, 2016), in youth, a biological shift in the circadian system at puberty

TABLE 18.1. DSM-5 Sleep–Wake Disorders that are Prevalent in Youth

Insomnia Disorder

A predominant complaint of dissatisfaction with sleep quantity or quality, associated with:
- Difficulty getting to sleep
- Difficulty maintaining sleep
- Waking up too early in the morning

The sleep difficulty occurs despite adequate opportunity for sleep and must be accompanied by significant daytime impairment. The sleep difficulty occurs at least three nights per week and must be present for at least 3 months.

Hypersomnolence Disorder

Excessive sleepiness (hypersomnolence) despite a main sleep period lasting at least 7 hours, with at least one of the following symptoms:
- Recurrent periods of sleep or lapses into sleep within the same day
- A prolonged main sleep episode of more than 9 hours per day that is nonrestorative (i.e., unrefreshing)
- Difficulty being fully awake after abrupt awakening

The sleep difficulty must be accompanied by significant daytime impairment. The sleep difficulty occurs at least three times per week and must be present for at least 3 months.

Circadian Rhythm Sleep–Wake Disorders
- *Delayed sleep phase type:* A pattern of delayed sleep onset and awakening times, with an inability to fall asleep and awaken at a desired or conventionally acceptable earlier time.
- *Irregular sleep–wake type:* A temporally disorganized sleep–wake pattern, such that the timing of sleep and wake periods is variable throughout the 24-hour period.

Note. Adapted from American Psychiatric Association (2013). Copyright © 2013 American Psychiatric Association. Adapted by permission.

in the direction of a delayed sleep phase (Carskadon, Acebo, & Jenni, 2004; Lee, Hummer, Jechura, & Mahoney, 2004) is compounded by social changes, such as less parental control, increased access to stimulating social activities (music, Internet, text messaging, etc.), and increased use of alcohol and substances that contribute to sleep disruption. Together, the social influences interact with the biological tendencies toward phase delay and can spiral quickly into a pattern of very delayed bedtimes. Yet school and work usually require a fixed, early wake-up time (Hansen, Janssen, Schiff, Zee, & Dubocovich, 2005). Hence, these biopsychosocial and behavioral forces converge to constrain time available for sleep, resulting in very high rates of youth obtaining insufficient sleep (Carskadon, 2002; Carskadon, Mindell, & Drake, 2006; Hansen et al., 2005). Compounding this vicious cycle, most attempts to "catch up" on sleep occur on weekends on a phase-delayed schedule. This is a problem because the circadian system adapts more easily to phase delays; endogenous rhythms are able to reset quickly to later bed and wake times and have more difficulty accommodating phase advances (earlier sleep schedules). Thus, many youth are struggling with the burdens of sleep deprivation and the consequences of repeated circadian shifts (Carskadon, 1990). While the basic biological shift toward eveningness during this phase may be difficult to modify, the psychosocial and behavioral contributors can be targeted in treatment. Moreover, modifying the psychosocial and behavioral contributors may well eliminate key factors that exacerbate the biological shift.

A second reason to develop a transdiagnostic intervention for sleep and circadian problems (TranS-C) is that sleep disturbance can occur as the sole presenting problem, but it is very commonly comorbid across one or more mental disorders. Indeed, many of the DSM symptom lists, across the major disorders, include sleep problems. Even when sleep problems are not specifically listed, they are often a common feature. Moreover, in the context of comorbid mental disorders, it appears that sleep disturbance is "mechanistically transdiagnostic." A mechanistically transdiagnostic process is causally or bidirectionally related to the comorbid mental disorder. This is suggested on the basis of the evidence that inadequate sleep contributes to emotion regulation problems that are core symptoms in mental disorders (Yoo, Gujar, Hu, Jolesz, & Walker, 2007), sleep problems constitute a risk for developing mental health problems (Dolsen, Asarnow, & Harvey, 2014), and there is even evidence that sleep problems contribute to suicide risk (Liu & Buysse, 2006). If sleep problems are common across mental disorders and contribute mechanistically, then to target the sleep problems transdiagnostically, rather than devising a disorder-specific sleep treatment for each mental disorder, should be a powerful approach.

The final reason to develop a transdiagnostic treatment for sleep and circadian problems is that sleep and circadian dysfunction has been identified as a biologically (Harvey et al., 2011) and theoretically (Harvey, 2008) plausible transdiagnostic contributor to mental disorders. More specifically, there is a reciprocal relationship with emotion regulation and its shared/interacting neurobiological substrates in (1) genetics—genes known to be important in the generation and regulation of circadian rhythms have been linked to a range of disorders—and (2) dopaminergic and serotonergic function—there is quite strong evidence for the interplay between these systems and sleep/circadian biology (Harvey et al., 2011).

TOWARD A UNIFYING THEORY OF SLEEP DISTURBANCE IN YOUTH TO GUIDE TREATMENT DEVELOPMENT

Ehrenreich-May and Chu (2013) note that "a good transdiagnostic approach draws from a unifying theoretical model that explains disparate conditions via common mechanisms" (p. 3). Regardless of whether the sleep disturbance is the sole presenting problem or it is combined with one or more mental disorders, the proposed common mechanisms that drive youth sleep problems, across the various overlapping presentations (i.e., insomnia, hypersomnia, delayed sleep phase) are grounded and derived from the "two-process model," which specifies the two biological processes that govern the sleep–wake cycle (Borbely & Wirz-Justice, 1982). As described elsewhere (Harvey, 2016), the first is the circadian process, which arises from the endogenous pacemaker in the suprachiasmatic nuclei (SCN; Reppert & Weaver, 2002). At the molecular level, intrinsically rhythmic cells within the SCN generate rhythmicity via an autoregulatory transcription–translation feedback loop regulating the expression of circadian genes. The process by which the pacemaker is set to a 24-hour period and kept in appropriate phase with seasonally shifting day length is called *entrainment*, which occurs via zeitgebers. The primary zeitgeber is the daily alteration of light and dark (Roennebert & Foster, 1997). The light-entrainable SCN synchronizes networks of subordinate circadian oscillators controlling fluctuations in other brain regions and, in particular, in neural circuitry supporting reward seeking (centered on the ventral striatum) (Venkatraman, Chuah, Huettel, & Chee, 2007) and emotion processing (centered on the amygdala and orbitomedial prefrontal cortex) (Yoo et al., 2007), two highly relevant circuits to youth that continue developing well into the teenage years (Blakemore, Burnett, & Dahl, 2010; Giedd et al., 1999). Hence, TranS-C-Youth incorporates timed light exposure. The SCN is also responsive to nonphotic cues such as arousal/locomotor activity, social cues, feeding, sleep deprivation, and temperature (Mistlberger, Antle, Glass, & Miller, 2000). Hence, TranS-C-Youth takes advantage of powerful nonphotic cues such as mealtimes and exercise.

The second process within the two-process model that governs the sleep–wake cycle is the homeostatic process that regulates the duration and structure of sleep based on prior sleep and wakefulness; sleep pressure increases during wake and dissipates during sleep. TranS-C-Youth includes methods for increasing homeostatic drive to sleep (e.g., reducing after school naps, not sleeping in on weekdays). Together, these basic sleep principles informed the sources for deriving TranS-C-Youth.

A second set of theoretical inputs to the development of TranS-C-Youth come from the theories underlying three existing evidence-based interventions. These were selected and combined because they were deemed to intervene on the variables outlined in the prior section. The first is cognitive-behavioral therapy for insomnia (CBT-I). There is robust evidence for the effectiveness of CBT-I in adults (Morin et al., 2006). The evidence for CBT-I in adolescents is small but promising (e.g., Bootzin & Stevens, 2005; Gradisar et al., 2011; Paine & Gradisar, 2011; Schlarb, Liddle, & Hautzinger, 2010). TranS-C-Youth draws on the CBT-I components that increase homeostatic pressure (stimulus control and sleep restriction) and reduce arousal (cognitive therapy).

We also paid attention to the evidence-based treatments for delayed sleep phase type (DSPT) disorder. The broader spectrum of eveningness, rather than the extreme end represented by DSPT disorder, is very common in teens. So the broader spectrum has been our focus. TranS-C-Youth has been informed by the small treatment literature on DSPT in teens (e.g., Gradisar et al., 2011; Gradisar, Smits, & Bjorvatn, 2014; Okawa, Uchiyama, Ozaki, Shibui, & Ichikawa, 1998; Regestein & Monk, 1995), as well as practice parameters (Sack et al., 2007) that indicate evidence for timed light exposure (with a light box) and planned and regular sleep schedules (chronotherapy) in adults. TranS-C-Youth includes the latter two interventions, with adaptations. First, teens tend not to be motivated to use a light box; hence, TranS-C-Youth incorporates a module to build daily habits of ensuring exposure to natural morning light and evening dim light with youth-selected electronic curfews. Second, traditional chronotherapy involving progressively delaying bedtimes and wake times until reaching the desired alignment can be highly disruptive to family and work schedules, so TranS-C-Youth adopts a planned sleep modification protocol derived from circadian principles involving moving bedtimes earlier by 20–30 minutes per week.

The third input is interpersonal and social rhythms therapy (IPSRT). One aspect of IPSRT is to help clients maintain stability in social rhythms. The evidence base for stabilizing circadian rhythms with IPSRT in bipolar disorder and depression is growing, including in adolescence (Frank et al., 2005; Hlastala, Kotler, McClellan, & McCauley,

2010; Miklowitz et al., 2007). We believe the focus on social rhythms in IPSRT is important because teens tend to have irregular sleep–wake cycles and social and personal schedules. In particular, waking early on weekdays for school, college, or work, then sleeping in on weekends can result in a chronically jet-lagged state to which the human circadian system cannot adjust. Accordingly, TranS-C-Youth includes aspects of IPSRT deigned to stabilize bedtime and wake rhythms, as well as other social rhythms (e.g., mealtimes, socializing, exercise), drawing from the treatment manual developed by Frank and colleagues (2005). This is because the sleep and circadian systems are surprisingly sensitive to nonphotic cues, including physical activity and social interaction. Hence, stabilizing these daily rhythms help stabilize the sleep–wake schedule.

TRANSDIAGNOSTIC SLEEP AND
CIRCADIAN ASSESSMENT AND PROGRESS MONITORING

The assessment strategy briefly described below is recommend to prepare for TranS-C and determine which of the TranS-C optional modules need to be delivered.

As described in various sources elsewhere (e.g., Harvey & Spielman, 2011; Morin et al., 2014; Morin & Espie, 2003), the Clinical Sleep History Interview for TranS-C should cover type of complaint (not enough sleep, trouble falling asleep, difficulty staying asleep, early morning awakening, light or nonrefreshing sleep, inability to sleep without sleeping pills, sleeping too much, sleeping at inconvenient times of the day, or sleep that is unpredictable), presence of specific sleep disorders (insomnia, hypersomnia, circadian rhythm disorders, etc.), frequency of nights affected and night-to-night variability, daytime impairment, and comorbid medical and psychiatric disorders, including use of medications.

As self-report measures, PROMIS-Sleep Disturbance (Buysse et al., 2010; Yu, Buysse, Germain, & Moul, 2011) and PROMIS-Sleep-Related Impairment (Buysse et al., 2010; Yu et al., 2011) are recommended because they are brief, comprehensive, and well-validated measures of nighttime impairment and daytime impairment, respectively. As will become evident, sleep in the night and functioning in the day are *both* important treatment targets in TranS-C. We use the short forms (8 items) of these scales, which are scored 1 = "not at all" to 5 = "very much." These scales are ideal for TranS-C because they are not specific to a particular diagnosis (e.g., insomnia or sleep apnea). Instead, the questions capture the broad range of sleep and circadian problems targeted by TranS-C.

The daily sleep diary is a critically important tool for assessing the sleep problem and monitoring progress across the course of TranS-C. The daily sleep diary is kept for at least 7–14 days prior to the beginning of TranS-C. There are many different sleep diary versions. The consensus sleep diary, developed by Carney and colleagues (2012), is recommended as its development was based on expert agreement and qualitative patient input. It is often helpful to add additional questions to the sleep diary to monitor other treatment targets, such as a rating of daytime energy or nightmare occurrence. Additional sleep diary questions may also be included (e.g., questions pertaining to technology use). We also ask patients to keep the sleep diary throughout the treatment sessions.

As a final note, a current, seriously unmet need in the field is for developmentally adapted sleep and circadian measures for youth. If measures that have been developed and validated for adults are used to assess youth, care should be taken to interpret the results in a way that respects the recommendation that most youth obtain 8.5 to 9.5 hours per night, as opposed to 7–8 hours of sleep per night for adults.

TRANS-C-YOUTH IN PRACTICE

As we have described elsewhere (Harvey, 2016), TranS-C includes four "crosscutting" modules that are introduced in the first session and typically featured in every session thereafter, four "core modules" that apply to the vast majority of clients, and four "optional modules" used less commonly, depending on the presentation. Four to ten 50- to 60-minute sessions are typically sufficient, depending on the complexity of the presentation and the number of modules that need to be delivered.

Crosscutting Modules

The four modules described in this section are introduced in the first session and are typically featured in every session thereafter.

Functional Analysis

We begin the functional analysis by working with the client to choose a *very specific* recent example of a *typical* night of sleep during which the problem was evident. A very specific episode is a situation that occurred on a particular day (e.g., last Monday) and at a particular time (e.g., while trying to get to sleep). Choosing a recent example is a good idea because the client is more likely to remember the details and this will make the process much easier. Examples of some very specific recent episodes follow: "Last Tuesday night I was on an Internet chatroom until 3:00 A.M. and then I couldn't get to sleep" and "On Monday I had a terrible day. I was worried about money and getting a job. I couldn't get to sleep and I woke up hundreds of times across the night."

Based on this recent typical night, we then seek to elicit sleep-related behaviors, thoughts, feelings, and consequences at bedtime (e.g., on an Internet chatroom late into the night), during the night (e.g., television left on), on waking (e.g., sleepiness, lethargy), and during the day (e.g., caffeine use) via Socratic questioning and guided discovery. This process uncovers several modifiable behaviors and thoughts that will be targeted by TranS-C.

We then use this information as the basis for introducing the cognitive-behavioral model—the framework of reciprocal loops whereby thoughts contribute to feelings and behaviors, and feelings and behaviors contribute to thoughts. Then we brainstorm the points (the thoughts, feelings, behaviors) that we can target in treatment. We also try to give a sense of hope that these are all modifiable variables. A fuller description of the case formulation process in the context of sleep problems is available elsewhere (Harvey, 2006).

Although this functional analysis is completed in Session 1, further functional analyses may be completed in subsequent sessions, as needed. For example, in a future session, if we are unable to make sense of why a client had a bad night's sleep, it can be very helpful to consider going through everything that happened, step-by-step. This process typically helps to identify the modifiable cognitive and behavioral factors that fueled the poor night of sleep and helps clarify where skills learned during treatment can be applied within specific episodes.

Goal Setting

At the outset, let's keep in mind that our hope is that youth can obtain around 9 hours of sleep per night across the adolescent years (Carskadon et al., 1980; Wolfson & Carskadon, 1998). This amount of sleep is thought to be important to facilitate the rapid body and brain development that continues well into the early 20s (Casey, Jones, & Somerville, 2011; Giedd, 2004). Youth presenting for treatment for sleep problems are usually sleeping much less than this. So, typically, the clinician keeps this in mind as treatment goals are discussed.

We set goals for the night and goals for the day. Goals must be specific and operationalizable. An example of a goal for the night is "Get into bed by 10:00 P.M. so I will fall asleep by about 10:30 P.M." rather than "I want more sleep," which is too vague. An example of a goal for the day is "Wake up at a more similar time every day, including on the weekend and feel more energetic" rather than "Feel better in the day," which, again, is too vague.

Selecting goals that are acceptable to the client is important, but these goals must be realistic. When the client identifies goals that are not realistic, we provide education about sleep. For example, if a client wishes to fall asleep within 5 minutes, the therapist may need to negotiate a more realistic objective. The therapist can let the client know that the process of falling asleep is more like a dimmer than a light switch: it takes time. In fact, taking *more than* 30 minutes to fall asleep on three or more nights a week is the typical cutoff value to determine whether a person has sleep-onset insomnia. Therapy goals are set in the first session, but they may need to be reevaluated and readjusted periodically as the intervention unfolds. Often the therapist will add questions to the daily diary to enable tracking of the goals that are set.

Motivational Interviewing

Starting from the first treatment session, motivational interviewing (MI) is a core feature interwoven across all sessions. Core values within MI are accepting the client as an individual, avoiding argumentation or confrontation, and avoiding giving lectures or ultimatums (Burke, Arkowitz, & Menchola, 2003; Miller & Rollnick, 2002). MI also involves eliciting and shaping client language in favor of change (i.e., change talk). When a behavior change idea is being discussed, the MI approach is to discuss it in a nonjudgmental, empathic, and collaborative manner. The idea is that an open discussion and additional reinforcement concerning sleep deprivation and its manifold repercussions will help build motivation to change.

MI was chosen as a crosscutting module because it helps build intrinsic motivation. Promoting autonomy is a key developmental task for youth and a core value of MI. It is designed to capitalize on youths' experience and the potential benefits of developing/adapting sleep-friendly habits by asking clients what they think the pros and cons of change are. The latter helps individuals recognize their ambivalence about change and enhances their intrinsic motivation for change.

Within the context of MI, the sleep treatment is provided in a nonprescriptive manner. The therapist first elicits the teen's current knowledge about the importance and health effects of increasing and/or maintaining sleep-friendly behaviors. He or she then offers recommendations in a nonconfrontational manner that support and respect the youth's autonomous decision making. The youth's reactions are then elicited. Together, therapist and youth evaluate the pros and cons of change, and the therapist nonjudgmentally hears and empathizes. In other words, with this approach, the client is not a passive recipient of information; rather, he or she is an active collaborator in the change process.

In MI we recognize that some youth can find that getting into bed is aversive, boring, and a waste of precious hours during which parents and school are not bothering them. We use Socratic questioning to unpack and seek to understand the client's perspective and to raise awareness about the science documenting the adverse consequences of insufficient sleep. We try to find a connection between the interests and motivation of the young person and sleep—this often includes domains such as improving athletic performance, personal attractiveness, and improving grades for college. We also try adding sources of daytime impairment to the sleep diary because sometimes a clear link between sleep and daytime functioning emerges.

Sleep and Circadian Education

The process of teaching a client the basic building blocks that underpin sleep and circadian functioning is important because this forms the rationale for the delivery of the interventions. This module starts in Session 1, unfolds across all subsequent sessions, and includes environmental influences (e.g., light); circadian and social rhythms (following IPSRT); the tendency for the sleep–wake cycle to delay if left unchecked by regular bedtimes; and the importance of sleep for mood regulation and cognitive functioning.

Core Modules

Table 18.2 provides a summary of the core modules.

Behavioral Components

IRREGULAR SLEEP–WAKE TIMES

Drawing from IPSRT (Frank et al., 2005; Frank, Swartz, & Kupfer, 2000) and stimulus control (Bootzin, 1972), a first goal is to work toward regularizing sleep–wake times across the weekdays and weekends and avoid naps after school. In particular, we focus on regularizing bed and wake times from weekday and weekend. Weekday and weekend bed and wake times should definitely be within 2 hours, but less of a discrepancy is better. Sleep disturbance can be reduced by this simple intervention (Kaplan & Harvey, 2013) because it optimizes the functioning of and interplay between the circadian and homeostatic systems (Processes S and C), and ensures that the central biological clock (the SCN) is synchronized with external time and with all the other body clocks. We

TABLE 18.2. Road Map for the TranS-C-Youth Core and Optional Modules

Problems addressed	Treatment module
Difficulty regularizing bedtime–wake times?	Core Module 1, Part a
Difficulty winding-down?	Core Module 1, Part b
Difficulty waking-up?	Core Module 1, Part c
Difficulty functioning across the day?	Core Module 2
Holding unhelpful sleep-related beliefs?	Core Module 3
Maintenance of behavior change	Core Module 4
Poor sleep efficiency?	Optional Module 1
Need to reduce time in bed?	Optional Module 2
Dealing with delayed phase (being a night-owl)?	Optional Module 3
Presence of sleep-related worry/vigilance?	Optional Module 4

make the adjustments *slowly*—typically 20–30 minutes per week. These small adjustments are more achievable than large adjustments. Also, once a teen starts to experience some mastery in making these small adjustment and start to notice positive impacts on his or her functioning, the motivation to engage in the treatment increases.

More broadly, the steps in stimulus control are to work collaboratively with the client to go to bed only when he or she is tired (and to develop pre-bedtime habits to ensure that he or she is tired at an appropriate and desired time of the day); to limit activities in bed to sleep; to get out of bed at the same time every morning; and when sleep-onset does not occur within 15–20 minutes, to get up and go to another room or another place in the bedroom. We may adapt the latter for youth if it seems that it would be difficult for him or her to get up without getting caught up in technology use. For such teens, it may be better to stay in bed and in darkness. A core recommendation of stimulus control is to suggest not napping. The rationale is that this discharges the homeostatic pressure to sleep, which makes it very difficult to get to sleep that night.

The rationale underlying stimulus control is that sleep problems arise, at least in part, as a result of maladaptive conditioning between the environment (bed/bedroom) and sleep incompatible behaviors (e.g., worry/frustration at not being able to sleep). The stimulus control intervention aims to reverse this association by limiting the sleep incompatible behaviors engaged in within the bedroom environment. These techniques also promote consistent sleepiness in the evening. Together, they ensure that both the circadian and homeostatic processes described earlier are aligned and set to promote sleep around the optimal time of the day. We also aim to help our client to regularize his or her daily social rhythms (e.g., timing of meals, exercise, socializing), which help build on and scaffold regular bed and wake times.

DIFFICULTY WINDING DOWN

To support regular bedtimes, we co-create (with our client) a highly individualized "wind down" of 30–60 minutes. Our hope is to establish habits of relaxing and sleep-enhancing activities that are conducted in dim light conditions. This facilitates the circadian phase advance among participants who are evening types, and maintains entrainment (Wyatt, Stepanski, & Kirkby, 2006). Many older youth are evening types, such that they feel active and alert later in the day.

A central issue is the use of interactive electronic media (Internet, cell phones, MP3 players). MI and individualized experiments (Ree & Harvey, 2004) are used to facilitate the client's voluntary choice of an electronic curfew. We suggest doing experiments such as watching just 15 minutes of videos each night versus 24 minutes of *Seinfeld* versus a 1.5-hour movie. For example, one teen found that reading books was a problem—he couldn't put them down after 1–2 hours. For him, watching one episode of *Seinfeld* was better. There are some teens who *will not* give up technology. For them, we try to move in the direction of reducing exposure to light during the wind down, taking a harm reduction approach.

DIFFICULTY WAKING UP

Drawing on IPSRT principles, one of our team members, Dr. Kate Kaplan, developed the RISE-UP routine, which aims to help clients who experience extended *sleep inertia,* which is the transitional state of lowered arousal and impaired performance following sleep. For most people, this period of 5–20 minutes of grogginess, heavy eyes, sore shoulders, and a feeling of wanting to go back to sleep, and so on, resolves relatively quickly. Others may experience a longer period of sleep inertia, up to several hours. Hence, it is very helpful to normalize the unpleasant feelings on waking and point out that these are not good data on which to make judgments about staying in bed and snoozing some more versus getting up. Instead, it is usually better to get up and get moving.

In both cases, an individualized version of the RISE-UP routine can be very helpful. RISE-UP involves the following: Refrain from snoozing, Increase activity, Shower or wash face and hands, Expose yourself to sunlight, listen to Upbeat music, and Phone a friend. But these are starting points. We add or delete parts of RISE-UP based on the teens preferences. The goal of RISE-UP is to use activity scheduling and goal setting to reinforce getting out of bed. We suggest allowing room for creativity. For example, one older teen rigged up a set of string pulleys, so that all the bedroom lights could go on at once with the pull of a string near his bed. This helped motivate him to get out of bed in the morning. Another teen created a wake-up playlist of his favorite upbeat music on his iPod.

Daytime Impairment

Because nighttime and daytime impairment associated with the sleep problem may be functionally independent (Lichstein, Durrence, Riedel, & Bayen, 2001; Neitzert Semler & Harvey, 2005), daytime impairments require specific attention. For example, an unhelpful but commonly held belief is that the only way one can feel less tired in the daytime is to sleep more. We have developed an experiment to help our clients to experience the energy-generating effects of activity (Ree & Harvey, 2004). This seems to be a very helpful part of learning to deal with daytime impairment. We begin this module by reviewing a diary in which sleep and energy during the day have been tracked daily for about a week. In examining the diary together, we point out examples in which there is a discrepancy between the night and the day (i.e., when nighttime sleep was good but energy levels in the day were poor *and* when nighttime sleep was poor but energy levels during the day were good). Often this allows us to introduce the following idea: "Well, that's really interesting. So if sleep isn't the full account of how you feel during the day, then there must be other things that can account for it." Together, we brainstorm possibilities and write them down (e.g., "The job I had to do that day was boring or stressful" or "I had a fight with my partner").

We then devise and complete the generating energy versus conserving energy experiment. We try to devise the experiment collaboratively and target the following beliefs: "Energy is increased only by rest or sleep" and "I don't have much energy, so I need to take care to conserve it." We hope to use the experiment to illustrate that there may be factors other than sleep that influence energy levels. The energy-generating experiment typically looks something like this (but may be adapted/individualized for the client):

- Specific target belief: "The only way I can get my homework done is to nap when I get home."

- A youth's prediction about what might happen in the experiment: "After a nap I am better able to do my home project, and the nap has nothing to do with my nighttime sleep."

The experiment itself can take various forms but one option would be to compare 2 days of the youth doing as he or she usually does (i.e., nap) versus 2 days doing the opposite (and brainstorm exactly what that would be: exercise, sunlight, visit with a friend, etc.).

We devise a way to collect data on the experiment as it unfolds. For example, we often ask teens to text their therapist a rating of how they felt after the nap, on a scale of 1 to 10, or how their homework went, and we carefully examine the sleep diary that night.

The client typically learns that many factors influence his or her energy levels during the day. In particular, we typically conclude that daytime energy levels are elastic and can be stretched quite easily. This is in contrast to the original view that energy levels progressively deplete throughout the day. We are then well positioned to start to develop a list of energy-generating and energy-sapping activities to better manage daytime tiredness.

Unhelpful Beliefs about Sleep

There is robust evidence that, in adults, altering unhelpful beliefs about sleep is important for outcome (e.g., Edinger, Wohlgemuth, Radtke, Marsh, & Quillian, 2001). Unhelpful beliefs are common and include "The TV helps me fall asleep"; "There is no point going to bed earlier because I won't be able to fall asleep"; "Sleep is a waste of time"; and "I can train myself to get less sleep." Guided discovery and individualized experiments test the validity and utility of the beliefs (Harvey, Sharpley, Ree, Stinson, & Clark, 2007; Ree & Harvey, 2004). It is exciting to see that research on unhelpful beliefs about sleep in youth has begun, with the publication of a measure of this construct for children (Blunden,

Gregory, & Crawford, 2013). However, much research is needed to establish the role of unhelpful beliefs about sleep among youth.

Maintenance of Behavior Change

The goal is to consolidate gains and prepare for setbacks using an individualized summary of learning and achievements. In the next to last session of the course of treatment we prepare to create a summary video of the top five tips. This might be in the form of a commercial for other teens or a mock interview with a "journalist" (the therapist). We record the "movie" in the last session as a way to consolidate learning and treatment gains. The movie is just for the teen—no one else will see it unless the teen decides to show it. If the client does not want to make a commercial, he or she might consider drawing a comic strip or writing a song—any activity that will help consolidate learning. Feel free to be creative!

Optional Modules

Table 18.2 provides a summary of the optional modules.

If Average Sleep Efficiency Is Less Than 85% on a 7-Day Sleep Diary

Sleep efficiency is calculated by the following formula: Total Sleep Time/Time in Bed × 100. If sleep efficiency is less than 85% across a 7-day sleep diary, we follow stimulus control (Bootzin, 1972) and sleep restriction (Spielman, Saskin, & Thorpy, 1987) procedures to limit time in bed to the time slept, then gradually go back to an optimal sleep time. As we already mentioned, the goal is to associate the bed with sleep, not with being awake. Also, basic stimulus control instructions (e.g., "Only go to bed when sleepy") are occasionally modified to reduce risk of goal-seeking and/or rewarding behaviors that reduce sleep opportunity. Because these strategies can cause some short-term sleep deprivation, it is important that they be delivered with wisdom. For example, when delivering a sleep restriction, it is very important to not recommend an amount of sleep that would be risky to youth who are riding bikes, driving or operating tools at work, or studying for important exams. This is an optional module because we find that many of our youth clients have acceptable sleep efficiency.

If Average Time in Bed Is Too Long

Spending too much time in bed often contributes to being late for school, missed days of school, and conflict with parents and family members. Given that the recommended nightly sleep for youth is 9.2 hours, we consider this module for youth who are spending 10.5 hours or more in bed to be an amount of time appropriate to the developmental stage of the client. To achieve this, we set goals for the night and goals for each day. In terms of the goals for the night, we slowly reduce time in bed week by week, in 30-minute increments, an amount that is small enough for the circadian system to adapt. We set goals for the day because "having nothing to get up for" seems to be a key contributor to spending too much time in bed. Then one small step toward these goals is set for the coming week, and possible obstacles are identified and discussed.

If Bedtime Is Later Than Preferred

For clients who go to bed too late, we begin with MI and education about the importance of getting sufficient sleep. Then we work collaboratively with our client to progressively adjust his or her bedtime to be earlier by 20–30 minutes per week. The circadian system can tolerate larger shifts, but we adopt 20–30 minutes to ensure that the circadian rhythm adjusts and youth experience mastery. To support the earlier bedtimes, we review the importance of regularity in wake up *and* bedtime, referring back to the client's sleep diary to check regularity/variability. We note that the homeostatic sleep drive helps us to feel sleepy at night and can be discharged by late afternoon or evening naps. We also create a "plan of action" with the teen to achieve this. We write the plan down and provide the teen a copy to help him or her remember. Then we review strategies to enhance success with advancing the bedtime: (1) Ask if the client would like to consider setting him- or herself an electronic curfew and earlier bedtime (e.g., setting a cell phone alarm); (2) ask if he or she would like to secure support from family and friends; (3) ask if he or she would like to use an alarm clock to maintain a regular arising time; (4) brainstorm alternative strategies to daytime napping or caffeine use; and (5) emphasize key points about the circadian rhythm, with a focus on delayed phase. For example, it is very helpful to keep our biology in alignment via light exposure at around the same time each morning. Also, we remind our client that the circadian system is the conductor of an orchestra—keeping bedtime and rise times consistent helps to keep the orchestra "in tune."

If the Client Worries Excessively about Sleep

Given that anxiety is antithetical to sleep (Espie, 2002), we develop a menu of options with our clients who report that they have difficulty sleeping because of worry, rumination, or vigilance. Potential menu items include diary writing, a scheduled "worry period," and training in imagery to gently direct the mind to disengage from worrisome thoughts. When these simple offerings are not helpful, we introduce formal cognitive therapy. The cognitive therapy "bibles" are quite helpful (A. T. Beck, 1979; J. S. Beck, 2005), and their application in the context of sleep problems has also been described (Harvey, 2005a, 2005b; Harvey et al., 2014).

We also introduce the adverse consequences of suppressing thoughts. For example, as soon as a client mentions something along the lines of "I try to suppress my thoughts" or "Then I try to clear my mind," we illustrate the paradoxical effects of though suppression by doing the white bear experiment, which involves asking the client to find a comfortable seating position then close his or her eyes and spend several minutes trying to suppress all thought, particularly thoughts of big, white, fluffy polar bears (or something that we know the client really likes—for example, cars, football teams, cats). We do this thought exercise at the same time as the client does it. After a few minutes, we stop and discuss each of our experiences, then explore this experience by asking, "How was that?" and "What do you conclude about the link between suppressing a thought and experiencing a thought?" We use these responses, and share our own experience, to educate youth about the paradoxical effects of thought suppression. Note that in the spirit of the behavioral experiment approach, wherever possible we set up an experiment to demonstrate a point by "doing" rather than just talking about it—*doing* is much more powerful!

Also, we look out for clients who punish themselves for not being able to control their thoughts (e.g., "I am so stupid for thinking this way" or "There must be something wrong with me"). Unwanted thoughts are normal—we normalize them with the aim of reducing some of the distress associated with them. The message to give is for the client to be gentle and kind to him- or herself. We also consider introducing a self-compassion exercise.

A NOTE ON PARENTS/GUARDIANS/CARERS

During the teen years, parents have less influence over their teen's sleep and often this has become a major form of conflict in the household. Hence, we carefully titrate the role of parents during the sleep intervention, depending on the family dynamics and the developmental stage of the teen. We try to move the responsibility for sleep to the teen. This can shift the dynamic away from parent–child battles, and the teen may feel proud to be trusted with control over such an important domain of his or her life. However, we invite parents to contribute to an emotional sense of safety at bedtime, positive emotions, and good associations at bed- and wake-up time, and to be careful not to create noise and distractions when the teen wishes to go to bed earlier.

In addition, typically, parents are invited into the last 5 minutes of each session, so their child can summarize the major points covered in the session and request the parents' practical and/or emotional support for his or her specific sleep goals in the coming week.

Sometimes we have found that it is better not to bring parents of older youth into the session. Instead we often place phone calls to the caregivers between sessions, with the client's permission, to explain our progress and perhaps facilitate change in any parent behaviors that are causing problems for the teen's sleep (e.g., making noise in the house, criticizing the teen as being lazy) after his or her bedtime.

CONCLUSION

The potential advantages of a transdiagnostic perspective are that it contribute to progress in classification of mental disorders, it provides an approach to think about and treat comorbidity, and it may encourage rapid transfer of advances made in the context of one disorder to other disorders. In many ways, developmental psychopathologists have been leading the way in developing treatments that cut across multiple disorders. This progress is perhaps necessitated by the complexity of the questions that are inherent to studying youth, including age, pubertal development, and context.

Given the evidence for sleep disturbance as a mechanistic transdiagnostic process that is commonly comorbid across mental disorders in youth, the rationale for, and process of deriving, TranS-C has been described—as have the various modules that comprise

TranS-C. Domains for future research have been outlined throughout this chapter. In addition, TranS-C needs to be empirically tested, a process that is currently in progress. One characteristic of TranS-C is that the modules are specified, so as to be useful across the age range, with adaptations for different developmental stages. The focus of this effort is to move toward one protocol that clinicians can learn in order to tackle various sleep problems, across various mental disorders and various age ranges, so as to contribute to reducing the "too many empirically supported treatments problem" (Weisz et al., 2014, p. 68) that impedes the dissemination and uptake of treatments. However, these assumptions await empirical testing. Also, TranS-C comprises several modules. To optimize the efficiency of the treatment and the outcome, it will be helpful if we empirically establish which modules are most powerful for bringing about sleep improvements. There is already a tradition of testing individual behavioral experiments, in one or two sessions (Harvey, Clark, Ehlers, & Rapee, 2000; Tang & Harvey, 2006). More work of this kind would be valuable.

ACKNOWLEDGMENT

This research was supported by Grant No. R01 HD071065 from the National Institute of Mental Health.

REFERENCES

Angold, A., Costello, E. J., & Erkanli, A. (1999). Comorbidity. *Journal of Child Psychology and Psychiatry and Allied Disciplines, 40,* 57–87.

Barlow, D. H., Allen, L. B., & Choate, M. L. (2004). Toward a unified treatment for emotional disorders. *Behavior Therapy, 35,* 205–230.

Beck, A. T. (1967). *Depression: causes and treatment.* Philadelphia: University of Pennsylvania Press.

Beck, A. T. (1979). *Cognitive therapy of depression.* New York: Guilford Press.

Beck, J. S. (2005). *Cognitive therapy for challenging problems: What to do when the basics don't work.* New York: Guilford Press.

Bentall, R. P., Rowse, G., Shryane, N., Kinderman, P., Howard, R., Blackwood, N., et al. (2009). The cognitive and affective structure of paranoid delusions: A transdiagnostic investigation of patients with schizophrenia spectrum disorders and depression. *Archives of General Psychiatry, 66*(3), 236–247.

Bilek, E. L., & Ehrenreich-May, J. (2012). An open trial investigation of a transdiagnostic group treatment for children with anxiety and depressive symptoms. *Behavior Therapy, 43*(4), 887–897.

Blakemore, S. J., Burnett, S., & Dahl, R. E. (2010). The role of puberty in the developing adolescent brain. *Human Brain Mapping, 31,* 926–933.

Blunden, S., Gregory, A., & Crawford, M. (2013). Development of a short version of the Dysfunctional Beliefs about Sleep Questionnaire for use with Children (DBAS-C10). *Journal of Sleep Disorders, 6,* 8–10.

Bootzin, R. R. (1972). Stimulus control treatment for insomnia. *Proceedings of the American Psychological Association, 7,* 395–396.

Bootzin, R. R., & Stevens, S. J. (2005). Adolescents, substance abuse, and the treatment of insomnia and daytime sleepiness. *Clinical Psychology Review, 25,* 629–644.

Borbely, A., & Wirz-Justice, A. (1982). Sleep, sleep deprivation and depression. *Human Neurobiology, 1,* 205–210.

Breslau, N., Roth, T., Rosenthal, L., & Andreski, P. (1996). Sleep disturbance and psychiatric disorders: A longitudinal epidemiological study of young adults. *Biological Psychiatry, 39,* 411–418.

Burke, B. L., Arkowitz, H., & Menchola, M. (2003). The efficacy of motivational interviewing: A meta-analysis of controlled clinical trials. *Journal of Consulting and Clinical Psychology, 71,* 843–861.

Buysse, D. J., Yu, L., Moul, D. E., Germain, A., Stover, A., Dodds, N. E., et al. (2010). Development and validation of patient-reported outcome measures for sleep disturbance and sleep-related impairments. *Sleep, 33,* 781–792.

Carney, C. E., Buysse, D. J., Ancoli-Israel, S., Edinger, J. D., Krystal, A. D., Lichstein, K. L., et al. (2012). The consensus sleep diary: Standardizing prospective sleep self-monitoring. *Sleep, 35,* 287–302.

Carskadon, M. A. (1990). Patterns of sleep and sleepiness in adolescents. *Pediatrician, 17,* 5–12.

Carskadon, M. A. (Ed.). (2002). *Adolescent sleep patterns: Biological, social, and psychological influences.* Cambridge, UK: Cambridge University Press.

Carskadon, M. A., Acebo, C., & Jenni, O. G. (2004). Regulation of adolescent sleep: Implications for behavior. *Annals of the New York Academy of Sciences, 1021,* 276–291.

Carskadon, M. A., Harvey, K., Duke, P., Anders, T. F., Litt, I. F., & Dement, W. C. (1980). Pubertal changes in daytime sleepiness. *Sleep, 2*(4), 453–460.

Carskadon, M. A., Mindell, J. A., & Drake, C. (2006). *Sleep in America Poll.* Washington, DC: National Sleep Foundation.

Casey, B., Jones, R. M., & Somerville, L. H. (2011). Braking and accelerating of the adolescent brain. *Journal of Research on Adolescence, 21*(1), 21–33.

Clarke, G., Harvey, A. G., McGlinchey, E., Hein, K., Gullion, C., Dickerson, J., et al. (2015). Cognitive-behavioral treatment of insomnia and depression in adolescents: A pilot randomized trial. *Behavior Research and Therapy, 69,* 111–118.

Cole, D. A., Truglio, R., & Peeke, L. (1997). Relation between symptoms of anxiety and depression in children: A multitrait–multimethod–multigroup assessment. *Journal of Consulting and Clinical Psychology, 65,* 110–119.

Craske, M. G., Stein, M. B., Sullivan, G., Sherbourne, C., Bystritsky, A., Rose, R. D., et al. (2011). Disorder-specific impact of coordinated anxiety learning and management treatment for anxiety disorders in primary care. *Archives of General Psychiatry, 68*(4), 378–388.

de Graaf, R., Bijl, R. V., Smit, F., Vollebergh, W., & Spijker, J. (2002). Risk factors for 12-month comorbidity of mood, anxiety, and substance use disorders: Findings from the Netherlands Mental Health Survey and Incidence Study. *American Journal of Psychiatry, 159,* 620–629.

Dolsen, M. R., Asarnow, L. D., & Harvey, A. G. (2014). Insomnia as a transdiagnostic process in psychiatric disorders. *Current Psychiatry Reports, 16*(9), 1–7.

Edinger, J. D., Wohlgemuth, W. K., Radtke, R. A., Marsh, G. R., & Quillian, R. E. (2001). Does cognitive-behavioral insomnia therapy alter dysfunctional beliefs about sleep? *Sleep, 24,* 591–599.

Egan, S. J., Wade, T. D., & Shafran, R. (2011). Perfectionism as a transdiagnostic process: A clinical review. *Clinical Psychology Review, 31*(2), 203–212.

Ehrenreich-May, J., & Chu, B. C. (2013). *Transdiagnostic treatments for children and adolescents: Principles and practice.* New York: Guilford Press.

Ellard, K. K., Deckersbach, T., Sylvia, L. G., Nierenberg, A. A., & Barlow, D. H. (2012). Transdiagnostic treatment of bipolar disorder and comorbid anxiety with the unified protocol: A clinical replication series. *Behavior Modification, 36*(4), 482–508.

Espie, C. A. (2002). Insomnia: Conceptual issues in the development, persistence, and treatment of sleep disorder in adults. *Annual Review of Psychology, 53,* 215–243.

Fairburn, C. G., Cooper, Z., Doll, H. A., O'Connor, M. E., Bohn, K., Hawker, D. M., et al. (2009). Transdiagnostic cognitive-behavioral therapy for patients with eating disorders: A two-site trial with 60-week follow-up. *American Journal of Psychiatry, 166*(3), 311–319.

Fairburn, C. G., Cooper, Z., & Shafran, R. (2003). Cognitive behaviour therapy for eating disorders: A "transdiagnostic" theory and treatment. *Behaviour Research and Therapy, 41,* 509–528.

Farchione, T. J., Fairholme, C. P., Ellard, K. K., Boisseau, C. L., Thompson-Hollands, J., Carl, J. R., et al. (2012). Unified protocol for transdiagnostic treatment of emotional disorders: A randomized controlled trial. *Behavior Therapy, 43*(3), 666–678.

Fraire, M. G., & Ollendick, T. H. (2013). Anxiety and oppositional defiant disorder: A transdiagnostic conceptualization. *Clinical Psychology Review, 33*(2), 229–240.

Frank, E. (2005). *Treating bipolar disorder: A clinician's guide to interpersonal and social rhythm therapy.* New York: Guilford Press.

Frank, E., Kupfer, D. J., Thase, M. E., Mallinger, A., Swartz, H., Fagioli, A., et al. (2005). Two year outcomes for interpersonal and social rhythm therapy in individuals with bipolar I disorder. *Archives of General Psychiatry, 62,* 996–1004.

Frank, E., Swartz, H. A., & Kupfer, D. J. (2000). Interpersonal and social rhythm therapy: Managing the chaos of bipolar disorder. *Biological Psychiatry, 48,* 593–604.

Garber, J., & Weersing, V. R. (2010). Comorbidity of anxiety and depression in youth: Implications for treatment and prevention. *Clinical Psychology: Science and Practice, 17,* 293–306.

Giedd, J. N. (2004). Structural magnetic resonance imaging of the adolescent brain. *Annals of the New York Academy of Sciences, 1021,* 77–85.

Giedd, J. N., Blumenthal, J., Jeffries, N. O., Castellanos, F. X., Liu, H., Zijdenbos, A., et al. (1999). Brain development during childhood and adolescence: A longitudinal MRI study [Letter]. *Nature Neuroscience, 2,* 861–863.

Giglio, L. M., Magalhães, P., Andersen, M. L., Walz, J. C., Jakobson, L., & Kapczinski, F. (2010). Circadian preference in bipolar disorder. *Sleep and Breathing, 14,* 153–155.

Gradisar, M., Dohnt, H., Gardner, G., Paine, S., Starkey, K., Menne, A., et al. (2011). A randomized controlled trial of cognitive-behavior therapy plus bright light therapy for adolescent delayed sleep phase disorder. *Sleep, 34*(12), 1671–1680.

Gradisar, M., Smits, M. G., & Bjorvatn, B. (2014). Assessment and treatment of delayed sleep phase disorder in adolescents: Recent innovations and cautions. *Sleep Medicine Clinics, 9*(2), 199–210.

Hansen, M., Janssen, I., Schiff, A., Zee, P. C., & Dubocovich, M. L. (2005). The impact of school daily schedule on adolescent sleep. *Pediatrics, 115,* 1555–1561.

Harvey, A. G. (2005a). A cognitive theory of and therapy for chronic insomnia. *Journal of Cognitive Psychotherapy, 19,* 41–60.

Harvey, A. G. (2005b). Unwanted intrusive thoughts in insomnia. In D. A. Clark (Ed.), *Intrusive thoughts in clinical disorders: Theory, research, and treatment* (pp. 86–118). New York: Guilford Press.

Harvey, A. G. (2006). What about patients who can't sleep?: Case formulation for insomnia. In N. Tarrier (Ed.), *Case formulation in cognitive behaviour therapy: The treatment of challenging and complex clinical cases* (pp. 293–311). New York: Brunner-Routledge.

Harvey, A. G. (2008). Insomnia, psychiatric disorders, and the transdiagnostic perspective. *Current Directions in Psychological Science, 17,* 299–303.

Harvey, A. G. (2009). A transdiagnostic approach to treating sleep disturbance in psychiatric disorders. *Cognitive Behavior Therapy, 38,* 35–42.

Harvey, A. G. (2016). A transdiagnostic intervention for youth sleep and circadian problems. *Cognitive and Behavioral Practice, 23*(3), 341–355.

Harvey, A. G., Bélanger, L., Talbot, L., Eidelman, P., Beaulieu-Bonneau, S., Fortier-Brochu, E., et al. (2014). Comparative efficacy of behavior therapy, cognitive therapy and cognitive behavior therapy for insomnia: A randomized controlled trial. *Journal of Consulting and Clinical Psychology, 82,* 670–683.

Harvey, A. G., Clark, D. M., Ehlers, A., & Rapee, R. M. (2000). Social anxiety and self-impression: Cognitive preparation enhances the beneficial effects of video feedback following a stressful social task. *Behaviour Research and Therapy, 38,* 1183–1192.

Harvey, A. G., & Gumport, N. B. (2015). Evidence-based psychological treatments for mental disorders: Modifiable barriers to access and possible solutions. *Behaviour Research and Therapy, 68,* 1–12.

Harvey, A. G., Murray, G., Chandler, R. A., & Soehner, A. (2011). Sleep disturbance as transdiagnostic: Consideration of neurobiological mechanisms. *Clinical Psychology Review, 31,* 225–235.

Harvey, A. G., Sharpley, A. L., Ree, M. J., Stinson, K., & Clark, D. M. (2007). An open trial of cognitive therapy for chronic insomnia. *Behaviour Research and Therapy, 45,* 2491–2501.

Harvey, A. G., & Spielman, A. (2011). Insomnia: Diagnosis, assessment and outcomes. In M. H. Kryger, T. Roth, & W. C. Dement (Eds.), *Principles and practice of sleep medicine* (5th ed., pp. 838–849). Philadelphia: Elsevier.

Harvey, A. G., Watkins, E., Mansell, W., & Shafran, R. (2004). *Cognitive behavioural processes across psychological disorders: A transdiagnostic approach to research and treatment.* New York: Oxford University Press.

Hlastala, S. A., Kotler, J. S., McClellan, J. M., & McCauley, E. A. (2010). Interpersonal and social rhythm therapy for adolescents with bipolar disorder: Treatment development and results from an open trial. *Depression and Anxiety, 27,* 456–464.

Insel, T., Cuthbert, B., Garvey, M., Heinssen, R., Pine, D. S., Quinn, K., et al. (2010). Research domain criteria (RDoC): Toward a new classification framework for research on mental disorders. *American Journal of Psychiatry, 167*(7), 748–751.

Kaplan, K. A., & Harvey, A. G. (2013). Behavioral treatment of insomnia in bipolar disorder. *American Journal of Psychiatry, 170*(7), 716–720.

Kendall, P. C., & Hedtke, K. A. (2006). *Cognitive-behavioral therapy for anxious children: Therapist manual* (3rd ed.). Ardmore, PA: Workbook.

Kessler, R. C., Chiu, W. T., Demler, O., Merikangas, K. R., & Walters, E. E. (2005). Errors in byline, author affiliations, and acknowledgment in prevalence, severity, and comorbidity of 12-month DSM-IV disorders in the National Comorbidity Survey Replication. *Archives of General Psychiatry, 62*(7), 768.

Kring, A. M., & Sloan, D. M. (2009). *Emotion regulation and psychopathology: A transdiagnostic approach to etiology and treatment.* New York: Guilford Press.

Lee, T. M., Hummer, D. L., Jechura, T. J., & Mahoney, M. M. (2004). Pubertal development of sex differences in circadian function: An animal model. *Annals of the New York Academy of Sciences, 1021,* 262–275.

Lichstein, K. L., Durrence, H. H., Riedel, B. W., & Bayen, U. J. (2001). Primary versus secondary insomnia in older adults: Subjective sleep and daytime functioning. *Psychology and Aging, 16,* 264–271.

Liu, X., & Buysse, D. J. (2006). Sleep and youth suicidal behavior: A neglected field. *Current Opinion in Psychiatry, 19,* 288–293.

Liu, X., Buysse, D. J., Gentzler, A. L., Kiss, E., Mayer, L., Kapornai, K., et al. (2007). Insomnia and hypersomnia associated with depressive phenomenology and comorbidity in childhood depression. *Sleep, 30,* 83–90.

Mansell, W., Harvey, A., Watkins, E., & Shafran, R. (2009). Conceptual foundations of the transdiagnostic approach to CBT. *Journal of Cognitive Psychotherapy, 23*(1), 6–19.

McManus, F., Shafran, R., & Cooper, Z. (2010). What does a transdiagnostic approach have to offer the treatment of anxiety disorders? *British Journal of Clinical Psychology, 49*(4), 491–505.

Miklowitz, D. J., Otto, M. W., Frank, E., Reilly-Harrington, N. A., Wisniewski, S. R., Kogan, J. N., et al. (2007). Psychosocial treatments for bipolar depression: A 1-year randomized trial from the systematic treatment enhancement program. *Archives of General Psychiatry, 64,* 419–426.

Miller, W. R., & Rollnick, S. (2002). *Motivational interviewing: Preparing people to change.* New York: Guilford Press.

Mistlberger, R. E., Antle, M. C., Glass, J. D., & Miller, J. D. (2000). Behavioral and serotonergic regulation of circadian rhythms. *Biological Rhythm Research, 31,* 240–283.

Morin, C. M., Bootzin, R. R., Buysse, D. J., Edinger, J. D., Espie, C. A., & Lichstein, K. L. (2006). Psychological and behavioral treatment of insomnia: An update of recent evidence (1998–2004). *Sleep, 29,* 1396–1406.

Morin, C. M., Drake, C. L., Harvey, A. G., Krystal, A. D., Manber, R., Riemann, D., et al. (2014). Insomnia disorder. *Nature Reviews Disease Primers, 1,* 15026.

Morin, C. M., & Espie, C. A. (2003). *Insomnia: A clinician's guide to assessment and treatment.* New York: Kluwer Academic/Plenum Press.

Neitzert Semler, C., & Harvey, A. G. (2005). Misperception of sleep can adversely affect daytime functioning in insomnia. *Behaviour Research and Therapy, 43,* 843–856.

Nolen-Hoeksema, S., & Watkins, E. R. (2011). A heuristic for developing transdiagnostic models of psychopathology explaining multifinality and divergent trajectories. *Perspectives on Psychological Science, 6*(6), 589–609.

Norton, P. J. (2012). A randomized clinical trial of transdiagnostic cognitve-behavioral treatments for anxiety disorder by comparison to relaxation training. *Behavior Therapy, 43*(3), 506–517.

Okawa, M., Uchiyama, M., Ozaki, S., Shibui, K., & Ichikawa, H. (1998). Circadian rhythm sleep disorders in adolescents: Clinical trials of combined treatments based on chronobiology. *Psychiatry and Clinical Neurosciences, 52,* 483–490.

Paine, S., & Gradisar, M. (2011). A randomised controlled trial of cognitive-behaviour therapy for behavioural insomnia of childhood in school-aged children. *Behaviour Research and Therapy, 49*(6), 379–388.

Pavlov, I. (1928). *Lectures on conditioned reflexes.* New York: New York International.

Ree, M., & Harvey, A. G. (2004). Insomnia. In J. Bennett-Levy, G. Butler, M. Fennell, A. Hackman, M. Mueller, & D. Westbrook (Eds.), *Oxford guide to behavioural experiments in cognitive therapy* (pp. 287–305). Oxford, UK: Oxford University Press.

Regestein, Q. R., & Monk, T. H. (1995). Delayed sleep phase syndrome: A review of its clinical aspects. *American Journal of Psychiatry, 152,* 602–608.

Reppert, S. M., & Weaver, D. R. (2002). Coordination of circadian timing in mammals. *Nature, 418,* 935–941.

Riley, C., Lee, M., Cooper, Z., Fairburn, C. G., & Shafran, R. (2007). A randomised controlled trial of cognitive-behaviour therapy for clinical perfectionism: A preliminary study. *Behaviour Research and Therapy, 45*(9), 2221–2231.

Roennebert, T., & Foster, R. G. (1997). Twilight times: Light and the circadian system. *Photochemistry and Photobiology, 66,* 549–561.

Sack, R. L., Auckley, D., Carskadon, M. A., Wright, K. P. J., Vitiello, M. V., & Zhdanova, I. V. (2007). Circadian rhythm sleep disorders: Part II. Advanced sleep phase disorder, delayed sleep phase disorder, free-running disorder, and irregular sleep-wake rhythm: An American Academy of Sleep Medicine review. *Sleep, 30,* 1484–1501.

Sanislow, C. A., Pine, D. S., Quinn, K. J., Kozak, M. J., Garvey, M. A., Heinssen, R. K., et al. (2010). Developing constructs for psychopathology research: Research domain criteria. *Journal of Abnormal Psychology, 119*(4), 631–639.

Schlarb, A., Liddle, C., & Hautzinger, M. (2010). JuSt—a multimodal program for treatment of insomnia in adolescents: A pilot study. *Nature and Science of Sleep, 3,* 13–20.

Skinner, B. F. (1959). *Cumulative record.* New York: Appleton-Century.

Spielman, A. J., Saskin, P., & Thorpy, M. J. (1987). Treatment of chronic insomnia by restriction of time in bed. *Sleep, 10*, 45–56.

Tang, N. K. Y., & Harvey, A. G. (2006). Altering misperception of sleep in insomnia: Behavioural experiments versus verbal explanation. *Journal of Consulting and Clinical Psychology, 74*, 767–776.

Venkatraman, V., Chuah, Y. M., Huettel, S. A., & Chee, M. W. (2007). Sleep deprivation elevates expectation of gains and attenuates response to losses following risky decisions. *Sleep, 30*, 603–609.

Watkins, E. R., Mullan, E., Wingrove, J., Rimes, K., Steiner, H., Bathurst, N., et al. (2011). Rumination-focused cognitive-behavioural therapy for residual depression: Phase II randomised controlled trial. *British Journal of Psychiatry, 199*(4), 317–322.

Watson, J. B., & Rayner, R. (1920). Conditioned emotional reactions. *Journal of Experimental Psychology, 3*, 1–14.

Weisz, J. R., Chorpita, B. F., Palinkas, L. A., Schoenwald, S. K., Miranda, J., Bearman, S. K., et al. (2012). Testing standard and modular designs for psychotherapy treating depression, anxiety, and conduct problems in youth: A randomized effectiveness trial. *Archives of General Psychiatry, 69*(3), 274–282.

Weisz, J. R., Ng, M. Y., & Bearman, S. K. (2014). Odd couple?: Reenvisioning the relation between science and practice in the dissemination-implementation era. *Clinical Psychological Science, 2*(1), 58–74.

Wolfson, A. R., & Carskadon, M. A. (1998). Sleep schedules and daytime functioning in adolescents. *Child Development, 69*, 875–887.

Wolpe, J. (1958). *Psychotherapy by reciprocal inhibition.* Stanford, CA: Stanford University Press.

Wyatt, J. K., Stepanski, E. J., & Kirkby, J. (2006). Circadian phase in delayed sleep phase syndrome: Predictors and temporal stability across multiple assessments. *Sleep, 29*, 1075–1080.

Yoo, S., Gujar, N., Hu, P., Jolesz, F., & Walker, M. (2007). The human emotional brain without sleep: A prefrontal–amygdala disconnect? *Current Biology, 17*, R877–R878.

Yu, L., Buysse, D. J., Germain, A., & Moul, D. (2011). Development of short forms from the PROMIS Sleep Disturbance and Sleep-Related Impairment item banks. *Behavioral Sleep Medicine, 10*, 6–24.

Author Index

Subject Index

Page numbers that are in *italic* indicate a figure or table